STENTING THE URINARY SYSTEM

STENTING THE URINARY SYSTEM
Second Edition

Edited by

Daniel Yachia MD

Head, Department of Urology, Hillel Yaffe Medical Center
Hadera, Israel
University of Tel Aviv, Sackler Medical School
Tel Aviv, Israel

Peter J. Paterson FRCS

Consultant Urologist, Glasgow Royal Infirmary
Glasgow, UK

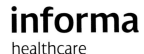

First published in 1998 by Isis Medical Media Ltd. This edition published in 2011 by Informa Healthcare, London, UK.

Simultaneously published in the USA by Informa Healthcare, 52 Vanderbilt Avenue, 7th Floor, New York, NY 10017, USA.

Informa Healthcare is a trading division of Informa UK Ltd. Registered Office: 37–41 Mortimer Street, London W1T 3JH, UK. Registered in England and Wales number 1072954.

A CIP record for this book is available from the British Library.

Library of Congress Cataloging-in-Publication Data available on application

ISBN-13: 9781841843872

Orders may be sent to: Informa Healthcare, Sheepen Place, Colchester, Essex CO3 3LP, UK
Telephone: +44 (0)20 7017 5540
Email: CSDhealthcarebooks@informa.com
Website: http://informahealthcarebooks.com/

For corporate sales please contact: CorporateBooksIHC@informa.com
For foreign rights please contact: RightsIHC@informa.com
For reprint permissions please contact: PermissionsIHC@informa.com

Contents

VII URETERAL STENTS: NON-UROLOGICAL DISEASES

VIII PROSTATIC STENTS IN BENIGN PROSTATIC HYPERPLASIA

IX PROSTATIC STENTS IN PROSTATE CANCER

X STENTS IN URETHRAL STRICTURES

XI STENTS IN DETRUSOR–SPHINCTER DYSSYNERGIA

XII VASCULAR STENTS

XIII THE FUTURE

List of contributors

John E. Abele
Boston Scientific Corporation, One Boston Scientific Place, Natick, MA 01760-1537, USA

Massoud Ahmadzadeh
Oberarzt der Urologischen Klinik, Mathias-Spital, Frankenburg Str. 31, 48431 Rheine, Germany

Marco M. Altaras
Associate Professor and Senior Vice Chairman, Gynaecological Oncology Unit, Department of Obstetrics and Gynaecology, Sapir Medical Centre, Kfar Saba, 44281, Israel; affiliated to Sackler Faculty of Medicine, University of Tel-Aviv, Israel

Yuriy G. Andreev
MIT Ltd, Novaya Str., 20, 143987 Zheleznodorozny, Russia

I. Atilla Aridogan
Assistant Professor, Department of Urology, University of Çukurova, Faculty of Medicine, Balcali, 01330 Adana, Turkey

Gopal H. Badlani
Program Director and Professor of Urology, Long Island Jewish Medical Center, 270-05 76th Ave., New Hyde Park, NY 11040, USA

David M. Bailey
Specialist Registrar in Histopathology, Department of Histopathology, King's College Hospital, Denmark Hill, London, SE5 9RS, UK

George A. Barbalias
Professor and Chairman, Department of Urology, University of Patras, School of Medicine, Patras 26500, Greece

Douglas G. Barnes
Consultant Urologist, Burnley General Hospital, Casterton Avenue, Burnley, Lancs, BB10 2PQ, UK

Gabriel Bartal
Department of Urology, Hillel Yaffe Medical Center, P.O. Box 169, Hadera 38100, Israel

H. P. Beerlage
Urologist, University Hospital Nijmegen, Department of Urology, Geert Grooteplein 10, P.O. Box 9101, 6500 HB Nijmegen, The Netherlands

Darren T. Beiko
Assistant Professor, Department of Urology, Queen's University, Kingston, Ontario, Canada

Itzhak Ben Hasid
Department of Diagnostic and Interventional Radiology, Hillel Yaffe Medical Center, Hadera 38100, Israel

F. A. G. Bloem
Resident in Urology, University Hospital Nijmegen, Geert Grooteplein 10, P.O. Box 9101, 6500 HB Nijmegen, The Netherlands

Christopher M. Booth
Consultant Urologist, Colchester General Hospital, Turner Road, Colchester, Essex, CO4 5JL, UK

Martin Cederbaum
Physics Section, Department of Oncology, Rambam Medical Center, Ha'alia Hashnia 8, Bat Galim, Haifa 31096, Israel

Michael B. Chancellor
Associate Professor, Urologic Surgery, University of Pittsburgh Medical Center, Kaufman Building, Suite 700, 3471 Fifth Avenue, Pittsburgh, PA 15213, USA

Christopher R. Chapple
Consultant Urological Surgeon, Department of Urology, The Royal Hallamshire Hospital, Glossop Road, Sheffield S10 2JF, UK

Aziz A. Chaudry
Staff Urologist, Department of Urology, Colchester General Hospital, Turner Road, Colchester, Essex, CO4 5JL,UK

Simon K. S. Choong
Institute of Urology and Nephrology, 48 Riding House Street, London W1P 7PN, UK

Alberto G. Corica
Department of Microbiology and Molecular Cell Biology, Eastern Virginia Medical School, Norfolk, VA, USA

Alberto P. Corica
Cuyo National University, 5500 Mendoza, Argentina

Federico Corica
Medical University of South Carolina, Charleston, SC, USA

John D. Denstedt
Division of Urology, The University of Western Ontario, 268 Grosvenor Street, London, Ontario N6A 4V2, Canada

Enrique Diaz-Lucas
Associate Professor of Radiology, Chief, Unit of Interventional Radiology, Department of Radiology, San Cecilio University Hospital, Faculty of Medicine, Las Margaritas 37, 18110 Las Babias, Granada, Spain

John W. Duckett Jr (deceased)
Director, Pediatric Urology, Children's Hospital of Philadelphia, Philadelphia PA 19104, USA

David M. Eiley
Fellow in Endourology and Laparoscopic Surgery, Long Island Jewish Medical Center 270-05 76th Ave., New Hyde Park, NY 11040, USA

Adam Eldin
Bedford Hospital South Wing, Kempton Road, Bedford MK42 9DJ, UK

Brian W. Ellis
Consultant Urological Surgeon, Ashford and St Peter's Hospitals, Ashford, Middlesex TW15 3AA, UK

Nachum Erlich
Department of Urology, Hillel Yaffe Medical Center, P.O. Box 169 Hadera 38100, Israel

Gabriel Faragi
Department of Urology, Hillel Yaffe Medical Center, P.O. Box 169, Hadera 38100, Israel

D. Filippas
Department of Urology, School of Medicine, Johannes-Gutenberg University, 55131 Mainz, Germany

Amiram Fishman
Director Gynaecological Oncology Unit, Department of Obstetrics and Gynaecology, Sapir Medical Centre, Kfar Saba, 44281, Israel; affiliated to Sackler Faculty of Medicine, University of Tel-Aviv, Israel

Uwe Friedrich
Professor of Paediatric Surgery, Paediatric Surgical Clinic, Medical Centre Erfurt Nordhauser Strasse 74, D-99089 Erfurt, Germany

S. Gabellon
Medecin associé, Service d'Urologie, CHUV, 1011 Lausanne, Switzerland

Eliahu Gez
Department of Oncology, Rambam Medical Center, Ha'alia Hashnia 8, Bat Galim, Haifa 31096, Israel

Jonathan M. Glass
Specialist Registrar, Department of Urology, Hammersmith Hospital, Du Cane Road, London W12 0H3, UK

Irena Gotman
Senior Research Associate, Faculty of Materials Engineering, Technion, Haifa 32000, Israel

H.-W. Gottfried
University of Ulm, Department of Virology, Prittwitzsstrasse 43, 89070 Ulm, Germany

Andrei Gremitsky
Department of Urology, Hillel Yaffe Medical Center, P.O. Box 169, Hadera 38100, Israel

Rizwan Hamid
Registrar Neuro-Urology, Spinal Injuries Unit, Royal National Orthopaedic Hospital, Stanmore, Middlesex, UK

Henrik Harboe
Engineers and Doctors, Oldenvej 13, Dk-3490, Denmark

David Hassin
Department of Internal Medicine 'C', B. Rappaport Faculty of Medicine, Technion, Haifa, Israel

Syed F. A. Hossainy
Senior Scientist, Johnson & Johnson, Corporate Biomaterial Center, Rt. 22 West, P.O. Box 151, Somerville, NJ 08876-0151, USA

Marcelo Houlne
Cuyo National University, 5500 Mendoza, Argentina

Valeriya Istomin
Department of Internal Medicine 'C', B. Rappaport Faculty of Medicine, Technion, Haifa, Israel

Bernd Jansen
Department of Hygiene and Environmental Hygiene, Johannes-Gutenberg University, 55131 Mainz, Germany

Hrishikesh B. Joshi MD, FRCS
Specialist Registrar in Urology, Department of Urology, Norfolk and Norwich University Hospital, Norwich NR4 7UY, UK

Miriam Kaufstein
Bacteriological Laboratory, Hillel Yaffe Medical Center, Hadera, Israel

Francis Xavier Keeley Jr.
Consultant Urologist, Southmead Hospital, Westbury on Trym, Bristol BS10 5NB, UK

Andrew J. Kirsch
Division of Pediatric Urology, The Children's Hospital of Philadelphia, Philadelphia, PA 19104, USA

Christopher Knight
University Hospital of North Staffordshire (Royal Infirmary) Princes Road, Hartshill, Stoke on Trent ST4 7LN, UK

W. Kohnen
Department of Hygiene and Environmental Medicine, Johannes-Gutenberg University, 55131 Mainz, Germany

V. N. Kuleznev
Head of the Chair of Plastics Processing and Chemistry, Moscow State Academy of Fine Chemical Technology, Vernadskii Ave. 86, Moscow 117571, Russia

Ravi Kulkarni
Consultant Urological Surgeon, Ashford and St Peter's Hospitals, Ashford, Middlesex TW15 3AA, UK

Thayne Larson
13400 E Shea Blud, Scottsdale, Arizona, AZ85259-5404, USA

Dov. M. Lask
Institute of Urology, Rabin Medical Center, Golda Campus, 7 Keren Kayemet Street, Petach Tikva 49372, Israel

H. Leenknegt
Department of Urology, Academic Medical Center, Meibergdreef 9, 1105 AZ Amsterdam, The Netherlands

H. J. Leisinger
Chef du Service d'Urologie, Centre Hospitalier Universitaire Vaudois, 1011 Lausanne, Switzerland

Raymond J. Leveillee
Head of Endourology, University of Miami School of Medicine, P. O. Box 016960 (M814), Miami, Florida 33101, USA

Ronnie Levy
Allium, Inc., Cesarea, Israel

Evangelos N. Liatsikos
Lecturer, Department of Urology, University of Patras, School of Medicine, Patras 26500, Greece

Marcelo L. de Lima
Assistant Professor, Division of Urology, University of Campinas Medical Center, UNICAMP, Sao Paulo, Brazil

Terryl Mack
Circon ACMI, 300 Stillwater Avenue, Stamford, Connecticut 06902-3695, USA

Robert Marcovich
Assistant Professor of Urology, Director, Section of Endourology, University of Texas Health Sciences Center, San Antonio, TX, USA

Zeljko Markovic
Associate Professor of Radiology, Head of Interventional Radiology Department, University Clinical Center–Belgrade, Visegradska 26, Belgrade 11000, Yugoslavia

José L. Martinez-Torres
Associate Professor of Urology, Chief of Section of Urology, Department of Surgery, San Cecilio University Hospital, Faculty of Medicine, Cardenal Parrado 1, 18012 Granda, Spain

Alexey G. Martov
Head of Endourology and New Urotechnology Department, Institute of Urology, 3 Parkovaya, 51, 105425 Moscow, Russia

Johan J. Mattelaer
Head of Department of Urology, St. Maarten Clinic, Burgemeester Vercruysselaan 5, B 8500 Kortrijk, Belgium

Euan J. G. Milroy
Consultant Urologist, Institute of Urology, The Middlesex Hospital, London WIN 1AA, UK

Nelson Rodrigues Netto Jr
Professor and Chairman, University of Campinas Medical Center — UNICAMP, R. Augusta 2347, 30 Andar, 01413-000 Sao Paulo, Brazil

K. J. Ng
Senior Registrar, Department of Urology, St. Thomas's Hospital, London, SE1 7EH, UK

Israel Nissenkorn
Professor and Chairman, Department of Urology, Sapir Medical Center, Meir General Hospital, 44281 Kfar-Saba, Sackler School of Medicine, University of Tel-Aviv, Israel

Jørgen Nordling
Professor of Urology, Department of Urology, Herlev Hospital, University of Copenhagen, DK-2730 Herlev, Denmark

Peter J. Paterson
Consultant Urologist, Glasgow Royal Infirmary, Alexander Parade, Glasgow, G31 2ER, UK

Margaret S. Pearle
Professor of Urology, Department of Urology, The University of Texas Southwestern Medical Center, 5323 Harry Hines Boulevard, Dallas, TX 75390-9110, USA

Sava Perovic
Professor of Pediatric Urology, University Pediatric Clinic, Tirsova 2, Belgrade 11000, Yugoslavia

Anssi A. Pétas
Consultant in Urology, Helsinki University Central Hospital, Haartmaninkatu 4, 00290 Helsinki, Finland

Aleš Petřík
Department of Urology, Region Hospital, B. Němcové 54, 370 87 České Budějorice, Czech Republic

Konrad Planz
Professor of Urology, Director, Department of Urology and Paediatric Urology, Fulda Medical School, Philipps University of Marburg, Pacelliallee 3–5, D-36043 Fulda, Germany

Jin Chye Damian Png
Urological Surgeon, Division of Urology, Department of Surgery, Singapore University Hospital, 5 Lowe Kent Ridge Road, Singapore 119260

Santiago Richter
Senior Vice-Chairman and Lecturer, Department of Urology, Sapir Medical Centre, Kfar Saba 44281, Israel; affiliated to Sackler Faculty of Medicine, University of Tel-Aviv, Israel

David A. Rivas
Suite 112, College Building, 102S Walnut Street, Philadelphia, PA 19107, USA

Jean J. M. C. H. de la Rosette
Director, Prostate and Endourology Center, University Hospital Nijmegen, 426 Department of Urology, Geert Grootplein 10, P.O. Box 9101, 6500 HB Nijmegen, The Netherlands

Alejandro Sagaz
Cuyo National University,

Ruediger W. Schlick
Assistant Medical Director, Department of Urology and Pediatric Urology, Fulda Medical School, Philipps University of Marburg, Pacelliallee 3-5, D-36043 Fulda, Germany

Darshan K. Shah
Department of Urology, Long Island Jewish Medical Center, New Hyde Park, NY 11040, USA

Julian Shah
Consultant Urologist, Spinal Injuries Unit, Royal National Orthopaedic Hospital, Stanmore, Middlesex, UK

Bella Shohat
Department of Internal Medicine 'C', B. Rappaport Faculty of Medicine, Technion, Haifa, Israel

Dimitrios Siablis
Associate Professor, Department of Radiology, University of Patras, School of Medicine, Patras 26500, Greece

Marvin J. Slepian
Director, Interventional Cardiology, University Heart Center, University of Arizona, 1501 North Campbell Avenue, Tucson, Arizona 85724,USA

Arthur D. Smith
Chairman, Department of Urology, Long Island Jewish Medical Center, 270-05, 76th Avenue, New Hyde Park, NY 11040, USA

P. V. Surikov
Plastics Processing and Chemistry Department, Moscow State Academy of Fine Chemical Technology, Vernadskii Ave. 86, Moscow 117571, Russia

Martti T. Talja
Senior Lecturer in Urology, Paijat-Hame Central Hospital, Surgical Department, Urological Unit, Fin-15800 LAHTI, Finland

William Taylor
Clinical Assistant Professor, Department of Surgery, Division of Urology, University of British Columbia, 855 West 12th Avenue, Vancouver V5Z 1M9, Canada

Anthony G. Timoney
Consultant Urological Surgeon, Southmead Hospital, Westbury on Trym, Bristol BS10 5NB, UK

Sun-De Tong
Senior Project Scientist, Baxter Healthcare Corporation, 17511 Armstrong Avenue, P. O. Box 19522, Irvine, CA 92614, USA

Pertti Törmälä
Academy Professor, Head of Department, Institute of Biomaterials, Tampere University of Technology, PO Box 589, FIN-3310, Tampere, Finland

Margarita F. Trapeznikova
Head of Department of Urology, Professor, Corresponding Member of the Russian Academy of Medical Sciences, Moscow Regional Research Clinical Institute, Schepkina Str., 61/2 Moscow, 129110, Russia

Luc Turmel-Rodrigues
Vascular Radiologist, Clinique St. Gatien, 8-Place de la Cathedrale, 37000 Tours, France

Michael Uder
Radiologist, Department of Radiology, University of the Saarland Medical School, D-66421 Homburg/Saar, Germany

Sergey B. Urenkov
Department of Urology, Moscow Regional Research Clinical Institute, Schepkina Str, 61/2, Moscow 29110, Russia

Tero Välimaa
Senior Researcher, Institute of Biomaterials, Tampere University of Technology, PO Box 589, FIN-33101 Tampere, Finland

R. Vetter
Paediatric Surgical Clinic, Medical Centre, Erfurt, Nordhäuser, Strasse 74, D-99089 Erfurt

Hans Wallstén
Wallsten Medical SA, Box 2036, Avenue Riond-Bosson 14, CH-1110 Morges 2, Switzerland

Graham M. Watson
Consultant Urologist, Eastbourne District General Hospital, King's Drive, Eastbourne, East Sussex, BN21 2UD, UK

James D. Watterson
Assistant Professor, Division of Urology, The University of Ottawa, Canada

George D. Webster
Division of Urology, Duke University Medical Center, Box 3146, Durham, NC 27715, USA

Hugh N. Whitfield
Director of Stone Unit and Consultant Urologist, Institute of Urology and Nephrology, 48 Riding House Street, London W1P 7PN, UK

Gordon Williams
Consultant Urologist, Hammersmith Hospital, Du Cane Road, London W12 0H3, UK

M. Wisard
Medecin associé, Service d'Urologie, GHUV, 1011 Lausanne, Switzerland

E. James Wright
Division of Urology, University of Kentucky Medical Center, 800 Rose St., Lexington, KY 40536, USA

Bernd Wullich
Associate Professor of Human Genetics, Urologist, Division and Clinic for Urology and Pediatric Urology, University of the Saarland Medical School, D-66421 Homburg/Saar, Germany

Daniel Yachia
Head, Department of Urology, Hillel Yaffe Medical Center, P.O. Box 169, Hadera 38100, Israel

Alkassim Yakabu
Trust Urologist, Burnley General Hospital, Burnley, Lancs, BB10 2PQ, UK

Sergey S. Zenkov
Roentgenoendourological Department, The First City Clinical Hospital, Leninsky Ave. 10, K12, Moscow, 117049 Russia

Thomas B. H. Zwergel
Professor of Urology, Division and Clinic for Urology and Pediatric Urology, University of the Saarland Medical School, D-66421 Homburg/Saar, Germany

Ulrike E. Zwergel
Associate Professor of Urology, Urologist, Division and Clinic for Urology and Pediatric Urology, University of the Saarland Medical School, D-66421 Homburg/Saar, Germany

Preface to the first edition

As a practising urologist seeing the immense and rapid changes occurring in medicine, and as a person involved in the development of some of the stents used today, I can say that modern surgery is becoming limited only by our imagination. As Jules Verne wrote: "Anything one man can imagine, another one can make real". It was this imagination that brought to mind, almost a century ago, the possibility of using supports for failing conduits in the human body. These supports were developed and have become the stents we use today, creating a novel approach for reaching the same results obtained with open surgical means in a minimally invasive way. During the last few decades we have changed from being urosurgeons to endo-urologists. Max Hosel's vision in 1963 on endo-urology has become a reality to a far greater extent than expected, with the introduction of stents into our armamentarium. Those readers who are following the use of stents in various medical disciplines see that the use of stents resembles a snowball; the more it rolls the bigger it grows and the more we know about stents, the longer the list of indications is becoming.

Since their introduction, urological stents have gained momentum in the armamentarium of urologists, interventional radiologists and vascular surgeons. The names of such developers as Wallsten, Strecker, Palmaz, Schneider, Gianturco, Cragg, and Sigwart, as well as the names of stents such as Double-J, Pigtail, Endostent, IUC, Prostakath, Urolume, UroCoil, ProstaCoil, VascuCoil, Memotherm, Memokath and Ultraflex, have already become a part of our daily medical vocabulary. This list is becoming enlarged by the introduction of new generations of stents that are changing our conventional treatment concepts. Increasingly and rapidly stents are taking the place of various open surgical procedures or are becoming adjuncts to new therapeutic procedures. As a result of these changes, use of the conventional urethral and ureteral catheters is rapidly declining. The Double-J and the Pigtail stents have already sidelined ureteral catheterization for drainage of the upper urinary tract, and urethral stents are taking the place of indwelling catheters. We are at the beginning of an era in medicine where many body passages with disease-induced narrowing are being stented. This approach is developing more rapidly than that of any other treatment modality and is becoming an accepted procedure in many medical disciplines. Urologists have been stenting the urinary tract for more than 20 years. Cardiologists, vascular surgeons and interventional radiologists began to stent the vascular system about 10 years ago. Gastroenterologists, who have been stenting the biliary tract for many years, together with general surgeons, are now stenting the obstructed bowel, and even ophthalmologists are stenting the lacrimal canals.

Because it differs from other systems, the urinary tract is being stented using various stents based on very different concepts. The renal artery is now stented by metallic vascular stents, the ureter is stented with biostable (and of late, biodegradable) polymers, the prostate and the anterior urethra are being stented with various metals, alloys and biostable or biodegradable materials. The increasing use of all these devices has engendered not only new approaches and effective treatments but also some new problems, side effects and complications.

The close cooperation between industry and physicians, and also combined meetings bringing together various medical disciplines, bioengineers and industry, are resulting in cross-fertilization, creating new ideas and improved devices for obtaining better results as well as for preventing problems and complications associated with these new devices, all for the benefit of our patients. Despite my intensive involvement in the development and use of some of these devices for several years, because of the rapid changes in the field, at times I am finding it difficult to keep pace with developments. For the less experienced or uninitiated, this lack of experience is discouraging them from using stents, especially urethral stents, in their practice. I hope that this book will help them in overcoming their reluctance and will persuade them to join urologists using the various stents in their practice.

This book was planned to bring together a multidisciplinary faculty, each of which has made a profound contribution in the field of stents in general and of urological stents in particular. I deeply appreciate the painstaking efforts of all of the contributors who have been so helpful (and quite prompt!) in preparing their manuscripts. They all responded to my invitation to contribute to this book and produced up-to-date and informative chapters. I hope that this book will become the standard working and reference text on urological stents for years to come.

Daniel Yachia

Preface to the second edition

Since the first edition of this book a number of changes have occurred in the field of stents. Some of the developments were up to expectation and some were disappointing. Unfortunately this was, and still is, the great tragedy of science and technology: experience sometimes demolishes elegant hypotheses and expectations by unsatisfactory results. That is why, after a period of great enthusiasm for technologies we should always try to understand their deficiencies to be able to investigate better tools for treating our patients. These new tools may direct us to develop better or new treatments. When stents were first introduced, many medical practitioners thought that they represented a passing fashion. Time showed that they were wrong. Experience proved that stents have an established role in the treatment of many conditions and the indications for their use are constantly increasing. We all know that stents are now being routinely used not only in coronary obstructions but also in aortic aneurisms, carotid, iliac and femoral stenoses, the biliary tree, oesophagus, colon, trachea and bronchi, and the upper urinary tract.

More than 2000 years ago the Greek philosopher Heraclitus said that 'there is nothing more permanent than change'. This is what we are seeing in medicine in general and in the field of stents in particular.

In the area of stents, the search for a perfect stent has been likened to the surfer's pursuit of the perfect wave. The entire stenting concept was developed by researchers investigating a method of holding tissues apart and tubes open, especially the arteries. Current stents are primarily mechanical, static devices doing this mechanical work for treating strictures or preventing restenosis. Since their appearance about two decades ago we have been searching for better stents. This task not only helps to further develop those we have in hand, but also encourages us to invent new ones. Tomorrow's stents will be mechanically and therapeutically active.

If we look to the near future we see that no new metals or alloys are on the horizon for metallic stent making. The outlook seems to be in the use of polymers, alone or combined with the currently used metals or alloys. Intensive work is being done for developing better biodegradable polymers which will replace those in current use. The new generation of biodegradable stents should either degrade by breaking into small pieces, or much better, gradually dissolve. The technology for drug-eluting polymers is developing rapidly. Probably, some future stents will be made of polymers that contain sustained drug-delivery features. Also, new polymers with shape memory characteristics are being developed. These new polymers are similar to metal alloys in that they can be bent and twisted as necessary, and like the metal alloys, at the right temperature, they will bounce back to their original shape. It is likely that they will be used in the manufacture of the next generation of urological stents. There is no doubt that second-generation shape memory polymers will also have biodegradable properties, which will also be used for producing urological stents.

In the field of permanent mesh stents, one of the most disturbing problems is stent occlusion caused by hyperplastic tissue growth, especially when they are used in post-traumatic urethral strictures. Some work should be done to prevent such tissue proliferation by coating the stents with pharmaceutical agents that release in a sustained form. These techniques began to be successfully used in vascular stents and most probably they will also be used in the urinary tract stents.

If we want to use permanent stents in the urinary tract we should develop them according to the needs of this tract and its limitations. Experience in using permanent stents developed for other tubular organs in the urethra showed that they do not always fulfil needs or expectations. All cylindrical stents developed for organs that have a cylindrical lumen, fit the shape and the calibre of the cylindrical tubular organ but they do not always fit the irregular shapes of the urinary tract. These findings were described by Ng and Milroy who recommended new stent shapes for the prostatic urethra; however, no changes have occurred in the shape of the prostatic stents since their work was published in 1994. To overcome this we have to design and develop site-specific permanent stents for the urinary tract, and not adopt, adapt or copy them from other systems.

Stents may cause the development of a reactive proliferative tissue at their end, if they are left indwelling a few months. In vascular use this phenomenon is named the 'candy wrap effect'. This effect may cause partial or complete obliteration of the stent. In urology, we observe this usually at the sphincteric end of the temporary stents. This problem has not been investigated in depth to find a solution.

In this second edition, we have added new chapters to update the knowledge developed since the first edition. We hope that, in this edition, we cover the entire subject of stents used in the urinary system, and we contribute to the science we call 'stentology'. We also decided to add a few chapters on the history of the main urological stents which have influenced us. We hope that these chapters will allow us to understand better the background of the urological stents. The new chapters we added on the use of stents in the renal arteries and pelvic veins show the possibilities of using stents not only in the urinary tract but also in the vascular system related to the urinary tract.

We hope that the readers will appreciate this second edition.

Daniel Yachia
Peter Paterson

Acknowledgements

Our special thanks to Alan Burgess, Senior Publisher, Martin Dunitz Ltd. who joined us in our vision of collecting the available updated and state-of-the-art data on urological stents in this 2nd edition of a book dedicated to this subject. We would like to thank Mark Sanderson, Senior Production Editor and his team for their patience, guidance and excellent cooperation. We are also grateful to Ariela Ehrlich, Head Librarian of the Hillel Yaffe Medical Center for her generous help during all the correspondence with the contributors and editing of all the chapters.

Dedication

To my wife Mengi, for her understanding. I am fortunate to have her.

To all those who taught me, especially to the late Professor Necati Güvenç who introduced me to urology and became my first teacher.

Daniel Yachia

Urological stents: material, mechanical and functional classification

M. J. Slepian and D. Yachia

Introduction

Endoluminal mechanical support utilizing prosthetic implant devices known as stents has emerged as a major therapeutic approach for the therapy of lumen stenosis and obstruction in many clinical fields over the past few years. In cardiology the implantation of metal stents for the treatment of obstructive atherosclerotic coronary artery disease has emerged as a dominant mode of therapy, with stents being utilized in 50% or more of angioplasty procedures. In urology, for many years, non-metallic stents have been utilized for the management of a variety of conditions throughout the urinary tract. More recently, temporary metal stents, as well as balloon-expandable and self-expanding metal stents, similar to those utilized in cardiology, have found increasing clinical use, particularly in the lower urinary tract. As new stents emerge in urology, it is valuable to organize and develop a classification of urological stents based upon design characteristics, materials and mechanical properties and clinical use characteristics.

The purpose of this introductory chapter is to provide, at the outset of this text, an overview of stents currently in use or undergoing development in urology. Similarities and differences in stent design and mode of operation between vascular and urological stents are highlighted. Stents have been categorized according to construction geometry, mode of expansion, material composition, anatomical size of implantation and therapeutic indication. At the end of the text a 'gallery' of photographs of current urological stents is provided for reference: Figures 1.1–1.4 show ureteral stents; Figures 1.5–1.16 are temporary urethral stents; Figures 1.17–1.20 are permanent urethral stents and Figures 1.21 and 1.22 are renal artery stents.

Stent classification

History

Although catheter-based drainage systems have existed in urological practice for centuries, it was not until the development of the Double-J ureteral intracorporeal device that the term 'stent' entered the urological vocabulary. The Double-J stent and its derivatives were upper-tract temporary devices placed to manage ureteral obstruction. Subsequently, temporary intra-urethral stents were devised. Simultaneously, in the vascular field, permanent metal stents were developed that later found application in the lower urinary tract. Also in the vascular field, biodegradable polymers, used either in the form of spiral stents or as lumen-coating systems known as 'polymeric endoluminal paving', were developed, which more recently have found urological applications. An outline of the history of specific stents is provided in Table 1.1.

Stent geometry

Significant differences exist in the overall configuration and surface topography of stents currently in use in urology. The external surface of stents may be either

Table 1.1. *Urological stents: history of development*

Year	Stent (and inventor)
1970	Double-J ureteral stent (Finney)
1980	Partial catheter (Fabian)
1985	Prostakath
	Urospiral
1987	Biodegradable polymer spirals (Slepian)
1988	Polymeric endoluminal paving (Slepian)
1989	IUC* (Nissenkorn)
1990	Urolume (1986 Sigwart, Wallsten vascular stent)
1991	UroCoil (Yachia, Beyar)
1992	Titan (1985 Palmaz vascular design)
1993	ProstaCoil (Yachia, Beyar)
	Biofix (Kemppainen, Törmälä)
1994	Memotherm
	Ultraflex (1992 Strecker self-expanding vascular stent)
1996	IUC* (Barnes)
1997	Trestle (Devonec)

* *IUC = intra-urethral catheter.*

solid or contain apertures. Openwork surfaces may be fashioned out of perforations created in a solid tube or from winding, spiralling or weaving of metal wire or strips. Differing designs afford varying degrees of hoop strength, trans-stent permeability and barrier creation. Stent topography also may influence lumen flow characteristics and late epithelialization. A classification of stents based on geometric considerations is provided in Table 1.2, and photographs of current urological stents are provided in the 'gallery' at the end of this chapter.

Deployment configuration

Deployment of stents utilized in urology varies widely. Several stents in use today have identical configurations both before and after deployment. As such, they are deployed by placement into the desired anatomical location directly without reconfiguration. Other stents possess a low-profile configuration before deployment but, once inserted into the desired anatomical location for deployment, they are then expanded, increasing their cross-sectional area. Expandable stents utilize several differing mechanisms for expansion, including balloon expansion, self-expansion and temperature-dependent expandability. Polymeric endoluminal paving, an alternative to conventional stenting, utilizes a combination of mechanical deformation and heating to deploy solid structural polymers in situ. This technique, as opposed to conventional stenting, results in the creation of custom-contoured conformal endoluminal wall supports. The various stent deployment configurations are summarized in Table 1.3.

Table 1.3. *Urological stents: deployment configuration*

Deployment type	Stents
Fixed-calibre	Ureteral stents; partial catheter; Prostakath; Urospiral; IUCs; Trestle; Biofix A; Polymer coils
Expandable	
Balloon expandable	Titan
Self-expanding	UroCoil, ProstaCoil, Urolume, Ultraflex, Biofix B
Heat-expandable	Memotherm, Memokath
Form in situ	Polymeric endoluminal paving

Material composition

A variety of materials, including metals, alloys, rubbers and polymers, have been used to make stents for urological applications. The majority of early stent devices were constructed from rubbers and polymers; more recently, superelastic memory metals and alloy steels have been employed. These materials afford the potential for low-profile deployment with significant local expansion coupled with excellent crush resistance. The materials currently used in urological stents are listed in Table 1.4.

Implant duration

Urological stents may also be classified on the basis of implant duration. Currently, there are stents that may be implanted as temporary devices to maintain lumen patency and prevent obstruction, for example after ablation of the prostate, in order to maintain the flow of

Table 1.2. *Urological stents: construction geometry*

Construction	Stents
Solid tube	Ureteral stents; Trestle; IUCs; Polymer paving
Slotted tube	Titan; Memotherm; Polymer paving
Spiral or coil	Partial catheter; Urospiral; Prostakath; UroCoil; ProstaCoil; Biofix
Woven mesh	Urolume; Ultraflex

Table 1.4. *Urological stents: material composition*

Material	Stents
Polyurethane	Nissenkorn; Barnes
Silicone	Trestle
Stainless steel	Urospiral; Prostakath
Superalloy	Urolume
Titanium	Titan
Nitinol	UroCoil; ProstaCoil; Memokath; Memotherm; Ultraflex
Biodegradable polymers	Biofix; Polymer paving

urine and prevent obstruction of the urinary tract. Alternatively, stents may be implanted for prolonged periods to facilitate moulding of the urethra during healing, with eventual stent removal. Finally, several stents have been designed as permanent implants to provide long-term wall support. Recently, biodegradable stents have also been introduced, which provide temporary lumen support followed by degradation in situ, obviating the need for procedure-based removal. A classification of stents based on implant duration is given in Table 1.5.

Mode of action

Stents in the urological system are generally employed to maintain lumen patency in the urethra, prostate or ureter, which they accomplish by several mechanisms of action. Early stents were designed to be placed in the ureter to prevent stone-based obstruction (lithiasis). Such stents act as endoluminal devices, freely suspended within the lumen and providing a bridging mechanism between urinary structures to ensure urinary flow in the space between or within the concentric stent and the urinary tract tubular structure. Other stents ensure lumen patency by providing direct wall support. Several of these stents have been fashioned to provide a temporary wall support while the urinary tract structure tissue heals. These devices thus act as endoluminal moulds, facilitating controlled healing and remodelling of the surrounding tissue, and are ultimately removed once the tissue has healed. Other stents have been designed to provide a permanent wall support; they are progressively epithelialized and become incorporated into the urethral wall. A classification of urological stents based on mode of action is shown in Table 1.6.

Anatomical site of implantation

Stents have been used in numerous anatomical locations in the urological system. In the urethra, stents have largely been employed for the management of strictures. Stents have been utilized in the prostate for benign prostatic hypertrophy, as well as for obstruction related to carcinoma. In the ureter, stents have been

Table 1.5. *Urological stents: implant duration*

Permanence	Composition	Stents	Duration (months)
Temporary	Metal	Fabian; Urospiral; Urethrospiral; Prostakath	≤ 12
		UroCoil system; ProstaCoil; Memokath	≤ 36
	Non-degradable polymers	IUC	≤ 6
		Trestle	≤ 3
	Biodegradable polymers	Biofix	≤ 6
		Polymeric endoluminal paving	≤ 12
Permanent		Urolume (Wallstent); Titan; Memotherm; Ultraflex	

Table 1.6. *Urological stents: mode of action*

Wall contact	Action	Stents
No (lumen maintenance)		Ureteral
Yes (lumen support)	Temporary wall support only	Partial catheter; Urospiral; Prostakath; ProstaCoil; Memokath 028; IUCs; Trestle; Biofix; Polymer paving
	Temporary wall support plus lumen moulding and remodelling	UroCoil system; Urethrospiral; Memokath 044; Polymer paving
	Permanent, giving continuous wall reinforcement	Urolume (Wallstent); Titan; Memotherm; Ultraflex

used to maintain lumen patency, primarily in stone disease. Finally, vascular stents have been used for urological purposes in the management of renovascular hypertension. A list of stents based on anatomical site of implantation is given in Table 1.7.

Clinical indications

Since the introduction of stents for use in the urological system, the indications for stenting have grown progressively. Stents were initially used for the management of ureteral obstruction; subsequently the list of clinical indications has expanded to include management of luminal obstruction throughout the urinary tract. Stents have been used where the patency of the lumen has been compromised as a result of benign or malignant strictures, obstructing calculi, infiltrative processes, including malignancies, and also extrinsic compression. Further, stents in the form of temporary lumen-stabilizing and lumen-supporting systems have been used to facilitate lumen healing and wall remodelling after various procedures. Intra-arterial stenting of renal arterial stenoses has also been valuable in the management of renovascular hypertension. A summary of current clinical indications for the use of stents in urology is given in Table 1.8.

Table 1.7. *Urological stents: anatomical site of implantation*

Site	Stents
Penile urethra	UroCoil; Polymer paving
Bulbar urethra	UroCoil S; Memokath 044; Urolume; Ultraflex; Polymer paving
Prostate	Urospiral; Prostakath; ProstaCoil; Memokath 028; IUCs; Trestle; Biofix; Polymer paving; Urolume; Titan; Memotherm; Ultraflex
Bladder neck	Urolume; ProstaCoil
Bladder	Polymer paving
Ureter	Double-J and derivatives; Urolume; Memotherm; UreteroCoil; Polymer paving
Ureteropelvic junction	Intracorporeal endopyelotomy stents
Renal artery	Palmaz; Wallstent; Strecker; Polymer paving

Table 1.8. *Urological stents: clinical indications*

Location	Indications
Anterior urethra	Strictures
External sphincter, membranous urethra	Detrusor–sphincter dyssynergy, traumatic strictures
Posterior urethra	Traumatic strictures, post-prostatectomy stenosis
Prostate	Benign hypertrophy, cancer
Bladder neck	Post-radical prostatectomy anastomotic strictures, post-prostatectomy stenosis
Bladder	Ureterovesical strictures, post-ureteral reimplantation
Intestinal bladder substitute	Uretero-reservoir anastomotic strictures
Orthotopic bladder	Uretero-neobladder anastomotic strictures, urethro-neobladder anastomotic strictures
Ureter	Benign and malignant strictures, calculi obstructions, extra-ureteral compression
Ureteropelvic junction	Post-ureteropelviplasty
Renal artery	Atherosclerotic obstruction, renovascular hypertension

Stents currently used in urology

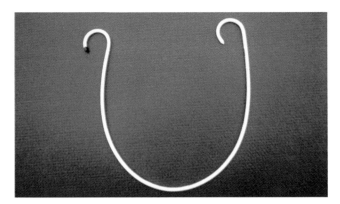

Figure 1.1. *Double-J stent.*

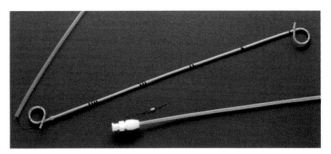

Figure 1.2. *Pigtail stent.*

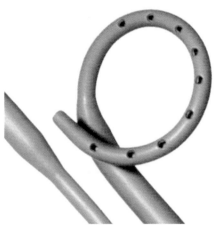

Figure 1.3. *Endopyelotomy stent.*

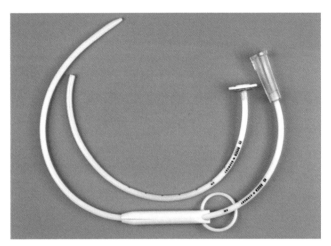

Figure 1.4. *Endostent.*

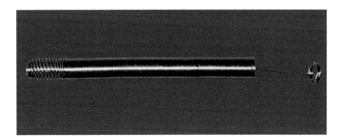

Figure 1.5. *Urospiral.*

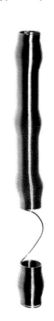

Figure 1.7. *ProstaCoil.*

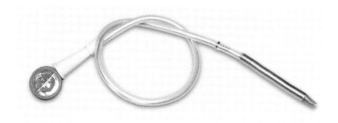

Figure 1.6. *Prostakath.*

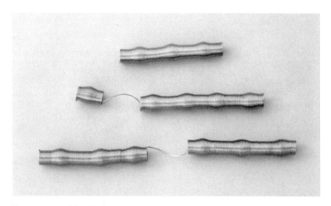

Figure 1.8. *UroCoil-system stents.*

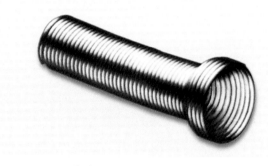

Figure 1.9. *Memokath 028.*

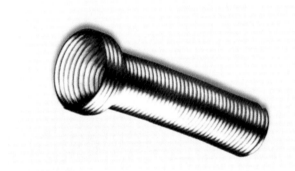

Figure 1.10. *Memokath 044.*

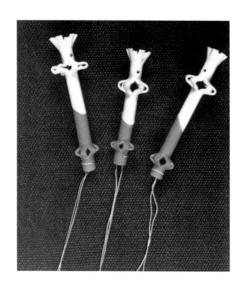

Figure 1.11. *Intra-urethral catheter (IUC): Nissenkorn design.*

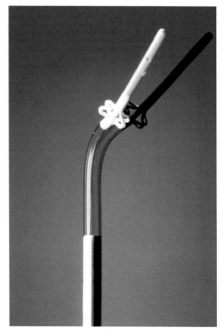

Figure 1.12. *Intra-urethral catheter (IUC): Barnes design.*

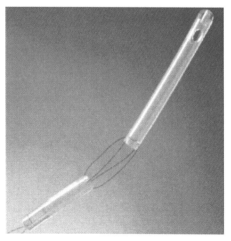

Figure 1.13. *Trestle.*

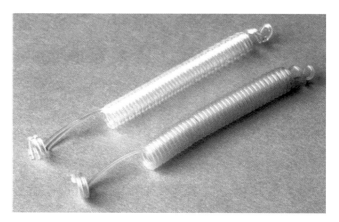

Figure 1.14. *Biofix.*

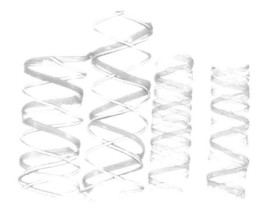

Figure 1.15. *Polymeric spirals.*

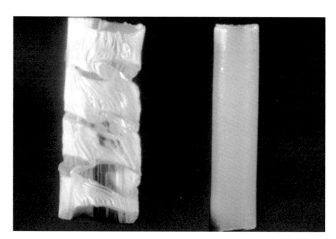

Figure 1.16. *Polymeric endoluminal paving.*

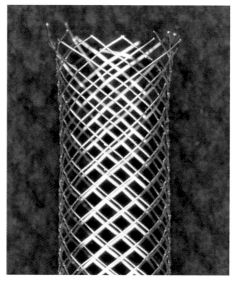

Figure 1.17. *Urolume (Wallstent).*

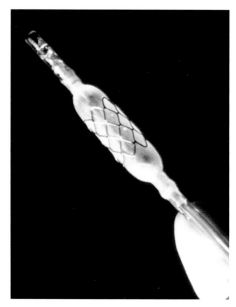

Figure 1.18. *Titan.*

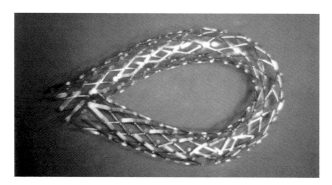

Figure 1.19. *Memotherm.*

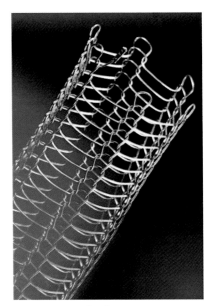

Figure 1.20. *Ultraflex.*

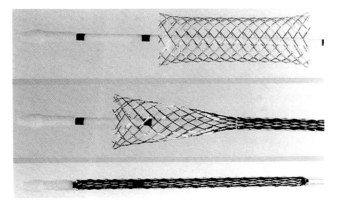

Figure 1.21. *Wallstent-vascular.*

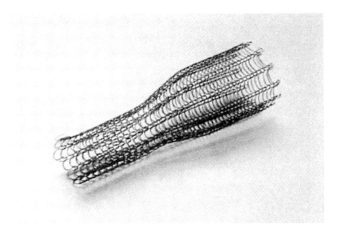

Figure 1.22. *Strecker stent-vascular.*

Evaluating new medical technologies: issues and opportunities

J. E. Abele

Introduction

In its broadest definition, a 'stent' is a device that is intended to keep a biological passageway open. It can vary in shape, length and dimension, as well as in physical and biological properties, and can be designed for permanent or temporary application (in the ureter, urethra or prostate).

A great many varieties of stents are either in commercial use or in development, and more are being conceived every day. They may be fabricated in polymer, metal, biological material, or combinations of these.[1–8]

The challenge for the urological community is to evaluate which type of stent is best suited for a specific application with a specific patient. Unfortunately, there is no comprehensive set of performance criteria, including standardized methods for measurement of these criteria, that can enable the clinician to make meaningful comparisons of one design versus another.

It is the purpose of this chapter to discuss (a) various attributes of stent design that can influence their performance, (b) some of the ways in which those attributes can be measured on the bench or in animals, (c) how these attributes contribute to overall clinical function and, finally (d), the issues and opportunities associated with the evaluation of new technology generally.

Stent design and performance

Unfortunately, there is not a clear understanding of what constitutes the characteristics of an 'ideal stent' for a specific application, or even if an 'ideal stent' for a specific application in a specific patient is ideal for that same application in another patient. The answer to that question will never be known unless the various performance characteristics are understood in a way that allows them to be compared one with another, and unless there are clinical evaluation methods of measurement of the contribution of the various performance characteristics to both short-term and long-term clinical behaviour in the patient.

'Stent function' can be broken down into several components, the first of which is introduction into the body. In this step, the design goal is to minimize trauma to the patient and to simplify manipulation and access for the physician, to reduce the time needed for the procedure and the likelihood of complications. The desirable properties for this step include a low and smooth profile, good flexibility, pushability and trackability (over a guidewire). When stents are introduced trans-cystoscopically, these properties are generally not crucial (as opposed to biliary or arterial stents), but they can be important in tight strictures.

The next step, deployment, controls the accuracy of positioning, as well as the security of its location. A good system design may include such attributes as good visualization, repositioning ability and good anchoring function.

The next component is the function of the stent in situ. Once the stent has been deployed, the only properties that should be 'visible' to the body are those that contribute to maintaining patency. The patient should not be aware of the presence of the stent, and the response to injury (or foreign body) of the local tissue should not lead to any compromise of function or to a complication.

The *physical* properties that affect stent function include tensile strength, compliance, flexibility, elasticity and the uniformity or variation of these properties along its length (Figure 2.1). Each of these properties must be understood in separate 'dimensions' to predict stent behaviour in the patient. Surface characteristics, including roughness and wettability, can also affect the friction between the stent and the tissues. Smoother is not always slipperier. For ureteral stents, at least some of these properties have been described and test methods have been developed in a draft standard for the American Society for Testing and Materials (ASTM).[9]

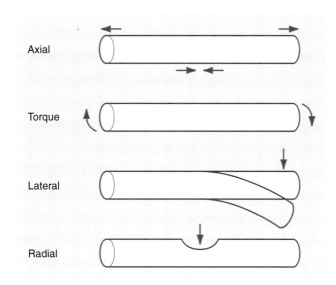

Figure 2.1. *Various compliance elements of a stent.*

- Ureteral perforation or dissection
- Ureteral rupture
- Misplacement
- Migration
- Misfit (too large, too small, too short, too long)
- Spasm
- Encrustation
- Tissue erosion
- Tissue inflammation
- Infection.

It should be apparent that attributes that are beneficial for some functions may be negative to others. The design challenge is to manage these trade-offs and, wherever possible, to try to build innovative elements that achieve 'the best of both worlds'.

Evaluation of stent design and function

The challenge to the medical profession is how to evaluate new stents or other technologies in a cost-effective and timely fashion that protects the public safety but encourages innovation. There is considerable controversy over this topic.[12,13] The United States Food and Drug Administration is quite restrictive, with a comprehensive set of regulations that require extensive testing and analysis, and the evolving European Medical Device regulations are considerably more rigorous than in past years.

Unfortunately, the benefits of greater scientific rigour and accuracy may be more than offset by the liabilities of increased cost and time to develop and assess, as well as the decreased relevance of scientific results that are obsolete by the time they are published. Furthermore, even the most rigorous trials have difficulty in dealing with bias driven by not-so-hidden agendas. Financial conflict-of-interest disclosures may help to contain the inventive physician entrepreneur (positive bias), but not the establishment guru whose professional stature and livelihood may be threatened by a new technology (negative bias). The first step taken by the defender of the status quo is to insist on a long-term randomized trial comparing the new rapidly changing immature technology with the stable mature old one.

There are a number of issues. Technological developments will continue to accelerate. This will occur

The *biological* properties of stents refer to their interactions with tissue and body fluids. Whatever surface is presented to the organ, it should at least be neutral, in terms of not producing an undesirable reaction, and possibly active, such as releasing a drug to suppress bacterial growth or to resist encrustation. Much has been written on this topic.[10,11]

An important component of stent function concerns removal or repair. Some stents are designed to be removed or to degrade and disappear. Permanent stents may migrate, occlude or otherwise malfunction. Understanding and anticipating complications or failures is a good approach to successful product and procedure design, and a good 'stent system' design anticipates failures and/or complications and provides the physician with options to manage these difficulties.

The unique anatomical and biological characteristics of every individual patient require a stent that is appropriately matched for best performance. The 'matching' process strongly influences patient satisfaction and complication rate. Examples of complications with ureteral stents, for example, include the following:

- Obstruction
- Kinking (stent and/or ureter)
- Stent fracture or fragmentation

because more people have improved access to information and experts — through databases, the continually evolving Internet, computer programs and specialized service organizations. The availability of low-cost modelling software, rapid prototyping capabilities and low-cost, desktop analytical tools (mass spectrometers, electron microscopes, gas chromatographs, even particle accelerators) all bring capabilities to small research laboratories that were previously limited to large university, business and government laboratories. As this expanded 'capacity to develop' continues to accelerate the flow of new medical devices, the infrastructure for evaluating new and potentially beneficial technologies will be swamped.

It seems logical to ask why the same innovative spirit that is being applied to accelerating the *development* of new technology cannot be applied to improving and accelerating its *assessment*. Further, since technology and the procedures that it engenders can be assessed only in the context of the people who perform such procedures, how can physicians best be trained to employ this new technology — and how do they stay current?

Finally, who is going to pay for it — the technology *and* the assessment? These are fundamental 'back-to-basics' questions that must be asked in the light of present inefficient and ineffective technology-assessment practices.

In designing studies to evaluate the status of a new procedure, product or technology, it is important to know who the study is for. Different groups have different needs that require different information to address:

1. *Clinical physician researchers*, acting on behalf of their practitioner colleagues, need evidence to evaluate the relative merits and risks of the new technology compared with the present methods of diagnosis and treatment. Although regulatory-driven trials can be helpful, clinicians appreciate broader postapproval trials for a more comprehensive understanding of performance and appropriateness.
2. *Payers* want to know which tests and treatments should be reimbursed and at what level. Reducing or eliminating reimbursement for a procedure restricts its use just as much as lack of approval. Evidence is now being demanded for demonstration of improved

quality of life, together with clinical and economic outcomes. These studies have 'softer' endpoints and are consequently more difficult to conduct and analyse but, with the prominence of the health care cost crisis, there is a growing requirement for this method of determining health care investment priorities. Technology developers must focus increasingly on producing productivity improvements for health care.
3. *Manufacturers* and related parties have several objectives regarding clinical studies. One is to determine whether the technology warrants continued investment or needs to be modified, redirected or dropped. They wish to know not only how well the procedure worked, but what did *not* work, why, and what might be done to make it better. These are more than just 'feasibility studies': they involve a continuing review of the risk–benefit analysis to determine the size of the commercial opportunity, the cost of failure and the likelihood of both. A second objective for manufacturers is to achieve favourable publicity from a well-conducted study.
4. Finally, the *regulatory agencies*, in their role as guardians and protectors of public health, want to know the clinical benefits, but with a much greater emphasis on understanding and reducing the risks.

These different audiences, and the different types of information desired, demonstrate the difference between safety (what is its potential to cause harm?), efficacy (will it produce the intended result?), effectiveness (can many people use it?) and efficiency (is it cost effective?). Regulatory approval is based on the first two factors, clinical acceptance is influenced by the third and reimbursement is determined by the fourth.

The earliest types of trials, sometimes called feasibility trials or design studies, are performed only after safety issues have been worked out on the bench and in animals. They are performed for the benefit of the developer or manufacturer. These trials tend to involve significant change or iteration from case to case and tend to be performed on patients for whom there are no acceptable alternatives. They help to determine critical performance issues as well as procedures, protocols and physician criteria for subsequent trials.

Differences between clinical trials of drugs and of devices

In recent years it has become fashionable to apply the lessons of pharmaceutical trials to the device field. The distinctions between drugs and devices are significant, however. Understanding these differences is essential to the development of an effective evaluation system.

Factor: influence of physician technique on result (drug, low; device, high)

When a device is used in a procedure, it may be handled by a number of people as well as by a physician. Its successful function is heavily influenced by the knowledge and experience of that team. Although drug efficacy is influenced by dosage and timing, these are more easily documented than the many subtleties of technique involved with device use. Trauma produced by a clumsy introduction, for example, can easily mask the positive effect of the device's function. Frequently, physicians will push a therapeutic device to failure when they recognize that the risk of device failure is less than the risk of not achieving the intended outcome, such as bursting a balloon in an angioplasty procedure.

Factor: rate of technical change (drug, low; device, high)

New devices can be bench-tested more easily than drugs, and performance attributes can be characterized more completely. The effect of a change is more readily understood and its behaviour in vivo better modelled and predicted. A single device, such as a guidewire, can lead to many hundreds or thousands of variations. Advances tend to be more rapid with devices because the functional requirements are better understood and the physician can *see* what is happening. Product life-cycles are measured in months for devices and in years for drugs. In addition to rapid changes in device technology, there are continuing improvements in patient selection capabilities, follow-up and analysis capabilities and general methodologies for assessment.

Factor: ability to evaluate performance attributes in vitro (drug, low; device, high)

As mentioned above, device performance is easier than drug performance to describe as well as to model. The effect of small changes is easier to isolate and tests are more readily developed that can challenge performance to extremes in order to predict and control failure modes.

Factor: ability to visualize performance during and after use (drug, low; device, high)

As imaging technology continues to improve, it is increasingly possible to see not only the device and the anatomy but also the physiological (and, in some cases, metabolic) responses to its use. This enables the physician literally to titrate the application of the device to the optimal patient response. Complications are more readily observed, understood and managed, and, since the intended effect of devices tends to be more physical than biological, the longer-term effects can frequently be observed using the same imaging techniques.

Factor: effect of accessories and environment on performance (drug, low; device, high)

Having a complete armamentarium for a device intervention is essential for maintaining procedural success rates. Good imaging equipment, a wide variety of sizes and shapes and a collection of accessories for access, monitoring, measuring and documentation help to determine the quality of the procedure and the quality of the data.

Factor: developer (drug, large with many resources; device, small with limited resources)

The average drug company is larger than the average device company. 50% of device companies employ fewer than 30 people. The critical mass necessary for drug development is many times that for the average device. As a result, the average drug company has more resources and experience in the design and management of trials for its drugs than a device manufacturer has for its devices. Because there is more money invested in drug assessment, and more physicians and technical personnel are involved and knowledgeable, device studies are sometimes inappropriately conducted using the drug model for their design.

Factor: (a) technology influencing (drug, chemical; device, physical); (b) mechanism of action (drug, biological; device, materials)

The implications of these differences have been discussed earlier — the ease of seeing the effect of its use is greater with a device than a drug. Although the use of a mechanical device can have a biological effect, its impact tends to be local and more predictable than that of a drug administered systemically.

Shortcomings of current assessment methods

It should be clear that present assessment methods are not very effective for dealing with fast-moving technologies. The time required to evaluate and approve a new device may be longer than the useful life-cycle of the device. In addition to being insensitive to the iterative nature of device and procedure development, such methods also do not effectively capture continuing improvements in patient selection capability, follow-up capability, user skills, accessory improvements and advances in imaging, sensing and other facilitating technologies.

To deal with these idiosyncrasies of device technology assessment, an effective system needs to be dynamic, not static. Too many developers maintain that it is 'too early for a trial' because, to them, that implies a controlled clinical trial in which changes are not allowed. As a result, they fail to capture valuable information. An alternative is the registry type of trial, which allows incremental changes but requires that they be documented. Some trials of this type are being conducted today.

Conclusions

It is the hope of some health care futurists that, over time, it will become possible to track on-line, in real time, every physician, every laboratory, every procedure and every device, as well as every patient, in a cost-effective manner.[14]

Admittedly, this is a tall order. On the surface, the technological, economic and legal hurdles appear to be insurmountable. Nevertheless, continuing advances in communication technologies are redefining the environment. Improved imaging capabilities, together with better ways of sending images and data at low cost, make it possible for a multicentre research team to collaborate on-line. New cases can be added daily for real-time review and analysis by all parties. Virtual forums already exist on the Internet, making it possible for participants to discuss complications and to receive advice. Over 100,000 physicians are plugged into the Internet through Physicians On Line. Equipping patients or family with measuring instruments and/or a video conference system for the home is being viewed by some as a more cost-effective and patient-friendly follow-up technique than periodic hospital visits.

There is great potential for capturing device experience information along with inventory, laboratory and physician performance data seamlessly in conjunction with patient case data. With point-of-care data-entry techniques (e.g. 'palm-top' computers, devices embedded with data chips) data management should look more like a rapid courier service than the slow, cumbersome process that exists today.

The future technology assessment model must serve many constituencies: it must provide (a) *developers* with the information necessary to guide and finalize device design, (b) *manufacturers* with a timely and cost-effective device approval process, (c) *physicians* with the information on effectiveness (sometimes with regard to non-approved uses) that is necessary for optimum treatment of their patients, (d) *payers* with the information on patient outcome and cost effectiveness that is necessary to make reimbursement decisions, (e) *regulatory agencies* with the information regarding safety and efficacy that is necessary to satisfy their statutory obligations, and (f) *patients* with timely access to beneficial new technologies. The key to the model will be the phasing of the information: device approval cannot be the final phase.

The challenges to making changes of this sort are immense, but the benefits are even greater. The system needs to be changed; it can, and must, be changed.

References

1. Saltzman B. Ureteral stents. Indications, variations, and complications. Urol Clin North Am 1988; 15(3): 481–491
2. Mardis H K et al. Comparative evaluation of materials used for internal ureteral stents. J Endourol 1993; 7(2): 105–115
3. Lugmayr H F, Pauer W. Wallstents for the treatment of extrinsic malignant ureteral obstruction: midterm results. Radiology 1996; 198(1): 105–108
4. Phan C N, Stoller M L. Helically ridged ureteric stent facilitates the passage of stone fragments in an experimental porcine model. Br J Urol 1993; 72(1): 17–19
5. Saporta L, Beyar M, Yachia D. New temporary coil stent (Urocoil) for treatment of recurrent urethral strictures. J Endourol 1993; 7(1): 57–59
6. Dobben R L, Wright K C, Dolenz K et al. Prostatic urethra dilatation with Gianturco self-expanding metallic stent: a feasibility study in cadaver specimens and dogs. AJR 1991; 156(4): 757–761

7. Gottfried H W et al. Thermosensitive stent (Memotherm) for the treatment of benign prostatic hyperplasia. Arch Esp Urol 1994; 14(9): 933–943

8. Chiou R K et al. Long-term outcome of prostatic stent treatment for benign prostatic hyperplasia. Urology 1996; 48(4): 589–593

9. American Society of Testing and Materials Subcommittee F.04.70.01. Standard test specifications for ureteral stents — Draft, Chicago, Ill.; 10 May 1995

10. Talja M et al. Biodegradable self-reinforced polyglycolic acid spiral stent in prevention of postoperative urinary retention after visual laser ablation of the prostate—laser prostatectomy. J Urol 1995; 154(6): 2089–2092

11. Kemppainen E et al. A bioresorbable urethral stent. An experimental study. Urol Res 1993; 21(3): 235–238

12. Health Industry Manufacturers Association. Report on public policy reform and the U.S. health care technology industry. Washington DC; 5 May 1995

13. Brook R H et al. Health system reform and quality. JAMA 1996; 476–480

14. Fortin D. On-line/Internet/real-time: future realities for outcomes management. Summit Medical 1st Annual Outcomes Conference, 22 October 1996. Unpublished.

History of stents

History of ureteral and urethral stenting: 1870–1990

J. J. Mattelaer

History of ureteral stenting

The Hindu Ayurveda of Sucrutu describes two organs that make urine and convey it into a waterbag in the lower part of the abdomen to be expelled later.[1,2]

In the fourth century BC, Hippocrates surmised that the kidney had the faculty of extracting and separating moisture from the blood; this moisture descends into the bladder.[1,2]

Detailed description of the anatomy and function of the ureter, however, was left to Claudius Galen, who demonstrated, by controlled experiments, the function of the kidneys and the flow of urine down the ureters into the bladder.[3,4]

Other classical descriptions of the ureter were provided by Andreas Vesalius in 1541 and Leonardo da Vinci in 1680. Both described and illustrated the ureters as starting at the pelvis of the kidney and ending in the bladder.[1,5]

Morgagni is credited with the description of an autopsy where he found that a stricture of the ureter had produced ipsilateral hydro-ureter and hydronephrosis.[6]

The first ureteral stents were utilized during open surgery to facilitate upper tract drainage or to align the ureter. The first reported case was described by Gustav Simon, in the 19th century; he placed a tube in the ureter while performing an open cystostomy. It was necessary to wait for the development of the cystoscope by Max Nitze in 1876 and the refinement of this instrument by Joseph Leitner in 1879 before doctors were able to see the ureteric orifices and to introduce a catheter endoscopically into the ureter.

Catheterization of the female ureter to obtain separated urine from both kidneys was attempted at an early stage and with a fair degree of success. A water cystoscope for catheterization of the ureter, designed by Alexander Brenner of Vienna, appeared in Leiter's catalogue of 1887. This unit-built, direct-vision, single catheter bore some resemblance to the modern instrument. Brenner was able to catheterize the female but not the male ureter. James Brown of Johns Hopkins University, using the Brenner instrument, accomplished male catheterization, apparently for the first time in 1893.[8]

Around 1895, Boisseau du Rocher introduced his megaloscope.[9] This was the first double-catheterizing instrument and was similar to that of Brenner, except that it had two tubes inside the sheath (Fig. 3.1). Following these modifications of the cystoscope, many others were developed.

Nitze, in the early 1890s, used a catheterizing cystoscope. The distal part of the beak was movable and carried the lightsource; the stationary section had a hole for emergence of the catheter.[10] Casper's cystoscope, developed in 1895,[11] had an offset telescope with two prisms, so that the eyepiece was a short distance below the catheterizing groove. The catheter passed through the groove in the top of the shaft (Fig. 3.2).

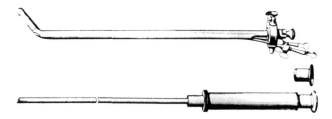

Figure 3.1. *Boisseau du Rocher's megaloscope is especially interesting, because the inventor intended this as a double-catheterizing instrument.*

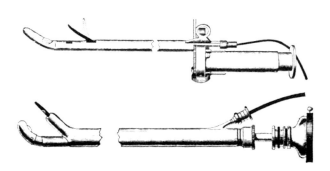

Figure 3.2. *Nitze's (above) and Casper's (below) catheterizing cystoscopes. The development of these instruments was a major advance in urological diagnosis.*

In 1897, Joachim Alberran y Dominguez, born in Cuba but working in Paris, invented the elevator, which is still used in most modern cystoscopes to control the movement of the ureteral catheter[12] (Fig. 3.3).

The ureteral catheter, which was introduced endoscopically or by open surgery and was exteriorized through the urethra or the bladder, has remained the unchanged standard device.

Initially, ureteral catheters used for stenting were constructed of fabric coated with varnish; subsequently, they were constructed of plastic, which made them rigid and easier to place. The ureteral catheters were connected to external drainage devices. These early ureteral catheters caused significant irritation to the bladder mucosa and, since the catheters were partly external, infection of the urinary tract was common. This infection caused rapid formation of encrustations, often limiting ureteral stenting to a few days because of patient discomfort and poor drainage. When silicone rubber tubing became available, some urologists used straight lengths of tubing in the ureter for internal stenting. Although drainage was improved for a time, the straight stents impinged on the bladder, causing discomfort. Unfortunately, the straight stent was frequently expelled into the bladder because of ureteral peristalsis. In 1952, Tulloch published an article reporting the successful restoration of the continuity of both ureters and ureterovaginal fistula by means of polythene tubing[13] (Fig. 3.4). This long period of hiatus, when little work was directed toward refining ureteral stents, ended in 1967, when a report by Zimskind and associates[14] touched off an explosion in research into

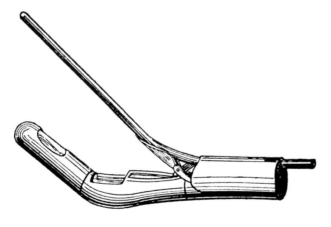

Figure 3.3. *In 1897, Albarran demonstrated his cystoscope fitted with a moveable lever to guide the catheter, and the problem of ureteric catheterization was solved.*

the development of ureteral stents. In that report the authors described the use of a long-term indwelling silicone stent introduced cystoscopically as a method of treatment in patients with carcinomatous obstruction of the ureter, ureterovaginal fistula and ureteral stricture. Those stents easily migrated, as they had no distal or proximal features to hold them in place. Nevertheless, when they were not expelled and had enough side-holes, excellent drainage continued for many months.

In 1967, another step was taken when Gibbons devised silicone ureteral stents moulded with pointed barbs, which greatly reduced the frequency of expulsion.[15] Often he was able to bypass lower ureteral obstruction, usually caused by pelvic malignancy (Fig. 3.5). This stent was available in calibres of 7 and 9 Fr, and lengths of 15 and 23 cm. After dilatation of the obstructed ureter by ureteral catheters, the Gibbon stent was introduced into the ureter over a ureteral catheter-guide, using a 24 Fr cystoscope sheath (Fig. 3.6a). However, the barbs significantly increased the outer diameter relative to the inner diameter and so made proper placement difficult and decreased the urinary flow rate. In addition the distal flange was not capable of preventing antegrade stent migration (Fig. 3.6b).

There was an evident need for a design that would prevent upward or downward migration without an increase in the diameter. The proximal and distal ends of a silicone tube were coiled in the shape of a 'J'. Such tips were malleable and could be straightened and strengthened by an internal guidewire that was utilized for stent passage. Once the wire was removed, the 'J' structure would prevent stent migration.

In 1978, Hepperlen and colleagues[16] developed a single-pigtail configuration that could be straightened with a wire stylet and passed in to the kidney (Fig. 3.7). Effective placement was achieved and downward migration was greatly reduced. However, there was no means to prevent migration above the bladder. Until that time, stents were primarily designed to be passed endoscopically in a retrograde fashion and not during an open operation.

In 1978, Finney[17] described the Double-J stent, which since has been adapted for passage cystoscopically or percutanously (Fig. 3.8). They saw the need for a stent incorporating specific characteristics: it should be of a uniform diameter; it had to pass easily through an endoscope into the ureter; it should not migrate upwards

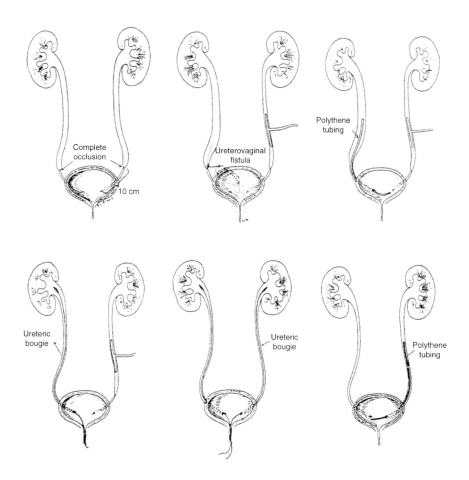

Figure 3.4. *Various stages of restoration of the continuity of the ureters by means of polythene tubing . (From ref. 13 with permission).*

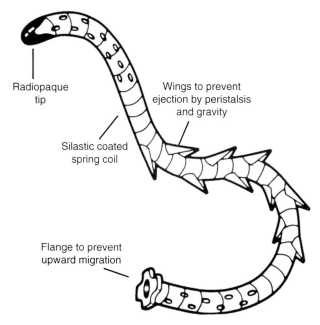

Figure 3.5. *Radiopaque ureteral Gibbons stent designed to resist downward expulsion and upward migration.*

into the kidney or downwards into the bladder; it should produce minimal trauma to the endothelial surfaces, and be radiopaque; last but not least, it should utilize the best material available, to prevent encrustation.

In 1978 the stent was named the 'Double-J' and Surgitek (Racine, WI, USA, acquired in August 1995 by Circon Corporation) took this simple design and began hand-producing ureteral stents with the distal and proximal 'J's moulded in.

The 'Double-J' was developed before the evolution of external shock-wave lithotripsy (ESWL); in those days, ureteral and renal stones were removed by open surgery. Without an indwelling stent, urine frequently drained from the incision for days or weeks. The 'Double-J' greatly reduced leakage, allowing patients to be discharged much earlier.

Initially, the 'Double-J' stent was primarily used to bypass obstruction caused by such factors as malignancy, stones or pregnancy. In the case of malignancy, a

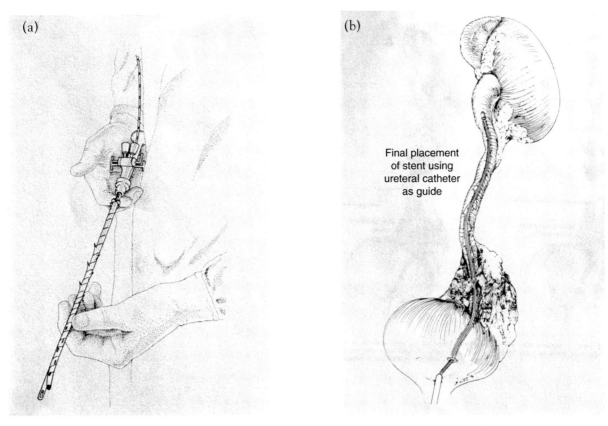

Figure 3.6. *(a) Gibbons stent and ureteral catheter guide are ready to be introduced into a 24 Fr cystoscope sheath. (b) The Gibbons stent is advanced up into the ureter in a retrograde manner until the distal flange is in contact with the ureteral orifice.*

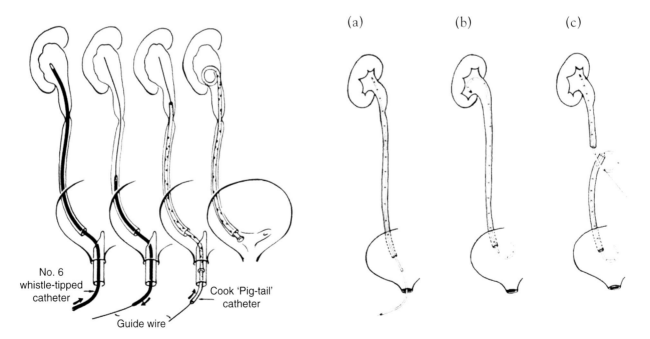

Figure 3.7. *Single-pigtail, self-retained internal ureteral stent developed by Hepperlen et al.*

Figure 3.8. *Double-J ureteral catheter stent by Finney:[17] (a) endoscopic passage with stylet and push catheter; (b) stent positioned in renal pelvis and bladder; (c) open surgical passage using stylet only.*

nephrostomy was not required, and the patient could be kept on permanent indwelling ureteral stenting with occasional stent changes. ESWL also led to other stent designs, such as the Uro Pass® Obstruction ureteral stent, and new placement techniques. In addition, the 'Single-J' stent was designed to promote drainage following ureteral diversion into a bowel segment. Over the course of time, special stents were developed to help treat various specific types of obstruction, including ureteral and renal stones, cancer and surgical anastomosis.

The original 'Double-J' was constructed of silicone rubber, which is an excellent material but not perfect. In the event of an infection, a mucous coating can form on its surface and encrustation can become attached to this coating. New materials appeared to reduce this risk. (Fig. 3.9). Today the 'Double-J' is widely used and is considered to be the 'Gold standard' of stents.

This chapter does not cover the topic of alloplastic ureteric replacements, and the reader is referred to the excellent article and overviews in references 18 and 19. Surgical replacement of the ureter by a bladder flap described by van Hook at the end of the 19th century[20]

and popularized by Boari in 1894,[21] is also beyond the scope of this chapter.

History of urethral stenting

Temporary urethral stents

The 'prehistory' of stenting the urethra is the history of bladder catheterization. Emptying the painful, overfilled bladder has been one of the problems of mankind since ancient times. Catheterization was reported to have been accomplished with reeds, straw and rolled palm leaves. The Chinese used leaves of *Allium* (*Allium* is the generic name of the onion family, and the long thin leaves are hollow).[22] Over the ages, mankind developed urethral catheters made of silver, gold, iron, paper, wood or leather. The introduction of catheters made of elastic gum or rubber was an important step forward,[22] but this rubber could not be formed and shaped as desired until 1839, when Goodyear invented vulcanization. Although these catheters were used only to empty the bladder, some of them had to remain in place; one of the developments needed, therefore, was a catheter that could be retained in place through its own configuration.

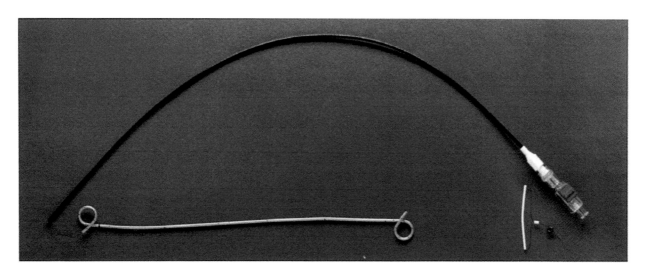

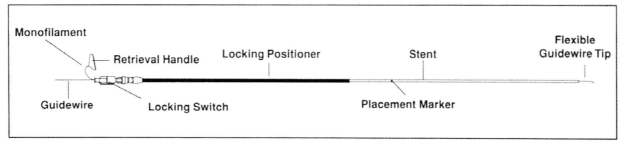

Figure 3.9. *Speed Lok™ ureteral stent set with Hydroplus™ Coating Sets (Microvasive).*

After some attempts by Reyland in 1841, and subsequently by Lebreton, Desnos, Holt and Dowse,[22] Foley of St Paul, Minnesota, USA, commissioned the manufacturer Bard to construct a longitudinally grooved catheter, to which he attached an inflating tube and a balloon by means of a fine silk thread and waterproof cement. Later, the Anode Company, with the help of Foley, produced a practical balloon catheter, now known as the 'Foley catheter'. This was described in 1937 as 'a self-retaining bag catheter for use as an indwelling catheter for constant drainage of the bladder'.[22]

It was necessary to wait until 1980, when Fabian[23] first used and tested the intraprostatic partial catheter termed the 'Urological Spiral' and manufactured by Uromed. This intraprostatic 'partial catheter' (urological spiral) represents a completely new concept. The material is stainless steel and it enables a patient to discard his indwelling catheter. The spring-shaped spiral inserted in the prostatic urethra keeps the enlarged prostate lobes compressing the urethra so far apart that spontaneous voiding is again possible (Fig. 3.10).

Implanting such devices into the urinary tract is likely to lead to encrustation and recurrent infection. To reduce the incidence of these complications, modifications of the original stainless steel spiral have taken place and several new stents have been introduced. Harrison and De Souza[24] described a modified spiral developed under the name of Prostakath by the Engineers

and Doctors Corporation, Kvistgaard, Denmark. This is a gold-plated, spring-shaped spiral with an outside diameter of 21 Fr. It is available in five lengths, ranging from 45 to 85 mm. The gold plating is said to reduce encrustation and bacterial growth (Fig. 3.11). These stents are

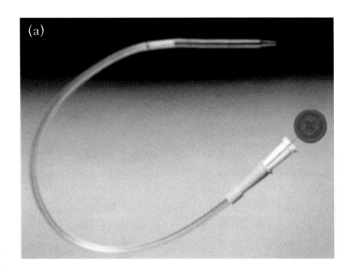

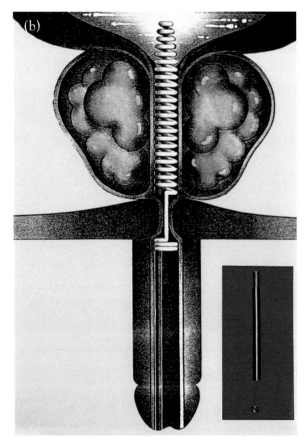

Figure 3.11. *(a) The Prostakath™ gold-plated intra-urethral stent can be introduced under ultrasonic control, like a normal urethral catheter; (b) the Urospiral: flexible stainless steel endoprostatic 'partial catheter'.*

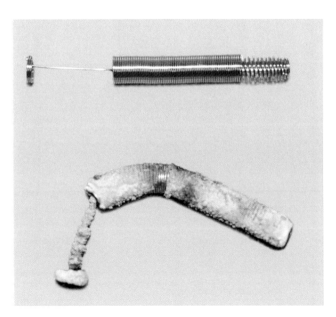

Figure 3.10. *Fabian's spring-shaped spiral before insertion (above) and covered with encrustations after removal (below).*

referred to as temporary stents, in that they are not incorporated into the urinary tract and can be removed with relative ease. They have been used in the treatment of both prostatic obstruction and urethral stricture.

In 1989, Nissenkorn introduced the 'self-retaining intra-urethral catheter' (IUC), a double-Malecot 16 Fr catheter in polyurethane[25] (Fig. 3.12). More recently, temporarily implanted self-expanding spirals of Nitinol (nickel-titanium alloy), the UroCoil and ProstaCoil (InStent USA) have been used in cases of urethral stricture and prostatic obstruction.[26,27]

Permanently implanted urethral stents

The finding that stents manufactured from a woven mesh of superalloy, titanium or nickel–titanium would become covered with normal epithelium when the stent was held against the wall of the urinary tract by the radial force of the device, led to the introduction in 1987 of so-called permanently implanted stents. These have been used to treat prostatic obstruction, urethral stricture and neurological voiding disorders. These stents are still undergoing modification and, as a result, the reported follow-up period is often short. Whereas temporary prostatic stents are becoming more permanent, with the follow-up of some patients, permanently implanted prostatic stents appear to be becoming more temporary.[28]

In 1988, Milroy et al.[29] reported the use of the original Urolume™ (American Medical Systems, Minnetonka, MN, USA) permanently implanted stents for the treatment of bulbar strictures that had recurred after previous treatments. In 1989, Williams et al.[30] used the same Urolume™ stent in patients with prostatic obstruction, and in 1990 Shaw et al.[31] used this stent in patients with neurological voiding disorders as a result of spinal injury. Later, Angiomed developed a stent from woven Nitinol — the Memotherm™.

An original stent manufactured by ASI (California, USA) and known as the ASI Prostate Dilatation System (PDS) was a pure titanium mesh stent (Fig. 3.13). This

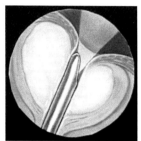

1. Measure urethra
Using a graduated sheath, measure the prostatic urethra from a point 2 mm distal to the bladder neck to the apex.

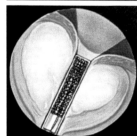

2. Position stent
Place a scope lens through the inner sheath. Position the distal tip of the stent 2 mm from the bladder neck.

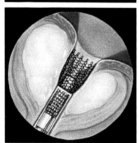

3. Deploy stent
Using the finger ring, gently retract the outer sheath. The stent will self-expand to its full diameter. If necessary, the trailing suture can be used to adjust stent position.

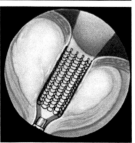

4. Confirm position
Confirm that the stent is in desired position. Remove trailing suture and the delivery system.

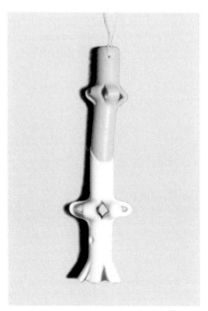

Figure 3.12. *'Self-retaining' intra-urethral catheter of Nissenkorn in polyurethane.*

Figure 3.13. *Manufacturer's instructions for introduction of a permanently implanted urethral stent of woven mesh.*

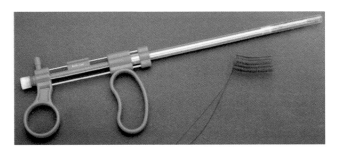

Figure 3.14. *Ultraflex: exclusive woven stent design and advanced Elastalloy™ construction (Microvasive).*

was subsequently modified to the Titan™ intraprostatic stent. Recently, Microvasive have developed the Ultraflex stent, which is an exclusive woven stent design made of Elastalloy™ (nickel–titanium alloy) (Fig. 3.14). Details of urethral stents are covered in subsequent chapters of this volume.

References

1. Lewis B. History of urology. Vol. 1. Baltimore: Williams and Wilkins, 1933
2. Welcome H S. The evolution of urine analysis : lecture memoranda. London: Burroughs and Wellcome, 1911
3. Smith H W. Highlights in the history of renal physiology. Bull Georgetown Univ Med Cent 1959; 13: 4.
4. Hovnanian A P. Ureteral replacements. Surg Gynecol Obstet 1972; 135: 801–810
5. Vesalius A. De humani corporis fabrica. Basel, 1543.
6. Long E R. A history of pathology. Baltimore: Williams and Wilkins, 1928
7. Saltzman B. Ureteral stents, indications, variations, and complications. Urol Clin North Am 1988; 15: 481–491
8. Brown J. Catheterisation of the male ureter. Bull Johns Hopkins Hosp 1993; 4: 73
9. Boisseau du Rocher. De la mégaloscopie. Ann Mal Org Genito-Urin 1890; 8: 65–93
10. Nitze M. Uber kystoskopische Diagnostik chirurgischer Nierenerkrankungen mit besonderer Berücksichtigung des Harnleiterkatheterismus. Berl Klin Wochenschr 1895; 32: 350–353
11. Casper L. Der Katheterismus des Ureteren. Dtsch Med Wochenschr 1895; 21: 104–106
12. Albarran J. Technique du Cathétérisme Cystoscopique des Uretères. Rev Gynecol Chir Abd 1897; 1: 457
13. Tulloch W B. Restoration of the continuity of the ureter by means of polythene tubing. Br J Urol 1952; 24: 42–45
14. Zimskind P D, Fetter T R, Wilkerson J L. Clinical use of long-term indwelling silicone rubber ureteral splints injected cystoscopically. J Urol 1967; 97: 840–844
15. Gibbons R P, Mason J T, Correa R J. Experience with indwelling silicone rubber ureteral catheters. J Urol 1974; 111: 594
16. Hepperlen T K, Mardis H K. Pigtail stent, termed means of lessening ureteral surgery. Trends Clin Urol 1978; 1: 405
17. Finney R P. Experience with new 'double J' ureteral catheter stent. J Urol 1978; 120: 678–681
18. Wagenknecht L V, Furlow W L, Auvert J. Genitourinary reconstruction with prostheses. Stuttgart: Thieme, 1981.
19. Cormio L, Ruutu M. Alloplastic ureteric replacements and ureteric stents: history, surgical procedures, indications and results. In: Buzelin J M (ed) Implanted and Injected Materials in Urology. Oxford: Isis Medical Media, 1995
20. Reed R H. A review of ureteral surgery. Columbus Med J 1895; 15: 492
21. Boari A. Contributo sperimentale alla plastica delle uretere. Atti Accad Sci Med Nat Ferrara 1894; 14: 444
22. Mattelaer J J. Catheters and sounds: the history of bladder catheterisation. In: Mattelaer J (ed) Kortryk De Historia Urologiae Europaeae, Vol 3. 1996: 201–223
23. Fabian K M. Der Intraprostatische "Partielle Katheter". Urologe A 1980; 19: 236–238
24. Harrison N W, De Souza J V. Prostatic stenting for outflow obstruction. Br J Urol 1990; 65: 192–196
25. Nissenkorn I. Experience with a new self-retaining intra-urethral catheter in patients with urinary retention: a preliminary report. J Urol 1989; 142: 92–94
26. Yachia D, Beyar M. New treatment modality for penile urethral strictures. Using a self-expanding and self-retaining coil stent: UroCoil. Follow-up of 16 months after removal of the stent. Eur Urol 1993; 24: 500–504
27. Yachia D, Beyar M, Aridogan I A. A new, large caliber, self-expanding and self-retaining temporary intraprostatic stent (ProstaCoil) in the treatment of prostatic obstruction. Br J Urol 1994; 74: 47–49
28. Williams G. Urethral stents: history, surgical procedure, indication and results for treating BPH, urethral stricture and neurological voiding dysfunction. In: Buzelin J M (ed) Implanted and injected materials in urology. Oxford: Isis Medical Media, 1995: 74–90
29. Milroy E J G, Cooper J E, Wallsten H et al. A new treatment for urethral strictures. Lancet 1988; 1: 1424–1427
30. Williams G, Jager R, McLoughlin J et al. Prostatic stents: a new treatment for prostatic outflow obstruction in patients unfit for surgery. Br Med J 1989; 298: 1429–1430
31. Shaw J P R, Milroy E J G, Timoney A G, Mitchell N. Permanent external sphincter stents in spinal injured patients. Br J Urol 1990; 66: 297–302

4

The Double-J®: then and now
T. Mack

Introduction

Dr Roy P. Finney developed the Double-J® closed-tip ureteral stent in 1978. Its availability increased the use of indwelling stents for placement during both open surgery and endoscopic procedures. The Double-J has been widely used, and its innovative design was the basis for stents as we know them today. This chapter is adapted from an interview with Dr Finney (Uro Trends© 1996; 1(2)) in which the history and development of the Double-J and its role in minimally invasive therapy were discussed.

History

Before the mid-1970s, ureteral stenting was accomplished by inserting ureteral catheters through the flank or bladder during open surgery or cystoscopy. This was generally considered to be an effective method for bypassing ureteral obstructions or ureterovesical fistulas. However, cystoscopic insertion required the use of a long standard ureteral catheter, a part of which remained outside the patient and extended distally beyond the urethra. This technique limited patient mobility, caused significant irritation to the bladder mucosa, and increased the risk of intrarenal infection.[1] Infection caused rapid formation of encrustations, resulting in patient discomfort and poor drainage that often limited the duration of ureteral stenting to a few days.

Initially, ureteral catheters were relatively simple devices made of a variety of materials. In 1839, vulcanization — which imparted the properties of firmness, flexibility and durability to crude rubber — led to the development of the rubber catheter. By the late 1800s, the prototype of the modern gum elastic-type catheter had been developed in France. In the early 1930s, catheters constructed of gum elastic incorporating varnish-coated woven nylon were in widespread production. Subsequent catheters were made of polyethylene or polyvinyl, resulting in a more rigid device that was easier to place. Stents of silicone elastomer, a substance with a consistency similar to that of latex rubber, had the added advantages of improved elasticity for ease of placement and maintenance of proper position, and increased resistance to encrustation by urinary deposits. Silicone became the standard against which other materials were measured for tissue compatibility, and was preferred for urinary drainage tubes and other self-retaining catheters.[2]

In 1967 Zimskind and colleagues[3] reported using open-ended silicone tubing as an indwelling stent on patients with ureteral obstruction. A straight length of silicone tubing was connected to a 4 Fr whistle-tip catheter and endoscopically inserted into the renal pelvis. The tubing was held in position with grasping forceps while the catheter was removed. Advantages for patients treated with this method were no external catheters (thus less risk of retrograde infection) and good drainage for several months.[1]

Although drainage was improved, the straight stents impinged on the sensitive bladder wall and caused discomfort. Ureteral peristalsis also frequently caused straight stents to be expelled into the bladder. Occasionally the straight stent migrated proximally where it could not be removed cystoscopically and an open surgical procedure was required to remove it.

Stent design evolution

Several design modifications were developed to prevent migration. In 1970, Marmar[4] modified the straight silicone stent by closing the proximal end to facilitate its placement. The stent was introduced onto the proximal tip of a guidewire. The stent and wire were then passed through the working port of a cystoscope as a unit. The combined stent and guidewire were stiffer than a stent alone, allowing the catheter to be placed through more severely obstructed ureters.[1]

By 1973, Orikasa and co-workers[5] had modified Marmar's insertion technique. A ureteral catheter and guidewire (as described above) were inserted into the renal pelvis using a hard polymer tube to act as a 'pusher'. The stent was held in position by the pusher while the guidewire was removed (Figure 4.1). However, once indwelling stents had been placed, maintaining their correct position remained problematic.[1]

The Gibbons stent (1974)[6] (Figure 4.2) was the first stent that successfully prevented downward migration and explusion. This stent had multiple barbs along its silicone shaft and a distal flange. The Gibbons was effective and provided adequate drainage, but the barbs along the stent shaft increased the nominal 7 Fr diameter to 11 Fr, making passage of the stent through tight obstructed areas more difficult. In addition, the barbs caused some stents to migrate upward towards the kidney.

In 1978, Hepperlen and Mardis[7] (Figure 4.3) developed a unique stent incorporating a single pigtail, or coil, with a distal flange at the proximal end of the stent that could be straightened with a wire stylet and passed to the renal pelvis. Ease of placement was enhanced and downward migration was greatly reduced. However, there was no means of preventing retrograde migration.

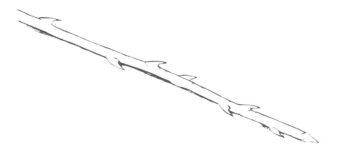

Figure 4.2. *Gibbons.*

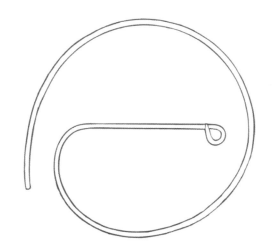

Figure 4.3. *Single pigtail.*

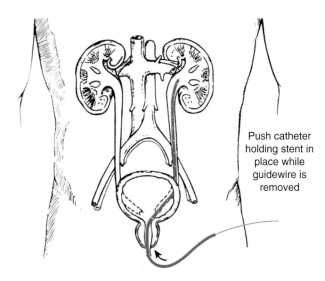

Push catheter holding stent in place while guidewire is removed

Figure 4.1. *Closed-tip stent.*

Double-J design

Until 1978, stents were designed primarily to be passed endoscopically in a retrograde fashion, not placed during open surgical procedures. A stent incorporating specific characteristics to overcome existing limitations was needed. The ideal stent had to be of uniform diameter, pass easily through an endoscope into the ureteral orifice and ureter, and pass in either direction during an open operation. It had to have a means to prevent migration upward into the kidney or downward into the bladder. Additionally, it had to produce minimal trauma to the endothelial surfaces, and it had to be radiopaque for fluoroscopic visualization. Finally, it had to be made of a material that reduced or prevented encrustation.[8]

To solve the problem of migration, a stent design using a very fine strand of silicone tubing to bow both the distal and proximal ends to form J-shaped hooks was chosen. This design prevented upward or downward migration. (A pigtail configuration was not used, as it was possible for a knot to form within the renal pelvis, requiring open surgery for stent removal.) The 'Js' formed in opposite directions, allowing the proximal J to hook into a lower calyx, or the renal pelvis, while the distal J curved into the central bladder cavity. This design prevented the distal tip of the stent from impinging directly into the bladder mucosa, especially in the highly innervated, sensitive trigone area, thus minimizing patient discomfort and inflammation. The double-J stent was of uniform diameter, tapered, with both ends closed (Figure 4.4).[8]

The stent was initially available in calibres of 7 and 8.5 Fr, and lengths of 16, 26, and 28 cm. These lengths were measured along the straight segment of the stent, from the onset of one curl to the other (Figure 4.5). This enabled the length of the ureter to be estimated radiographically and the proper size stent selected. Drainage holes were located at 1 cm increments and standard markings used at each 5 cm increment on the main shaft. The stent had a printed medial line along the side opposite the proximal J to allow easy determination of the direction in which the J would form when the stylet was removed during endoscopic or open surgical passage.[8] In 1978, the stent was named the Double-J.® Surgitek* (Racine, WI, USA) took this simple design and began hand-producing ureteral stents with the distal and proximal Js moulded in.

*Surgitek was acquired by Circon Corporation in August 1995.

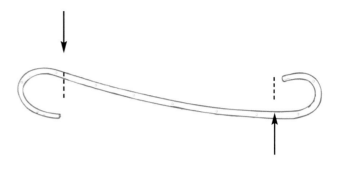

Figure 4.5. *Measure stent from base of curl to base of curl.*

Placement and removal techniques

To insert the Double-J, a guidewire can be passed through a distal side-hole, up to the proximal (closed) end to straighten the stent for cystoscopic placement. The distal tip can also be cut as an alternative for insertion of the wire (Figure 4.6), or both ends can be removed to use the over-the-wire technique (Figure 4.7). The stent is held in place by hand or with a haemostat. Once the stent is placed, the guidewire is withdrawn, allowing the Js to form in the kidney and then the bladder. During an open procedure each closed end is placed by inserting the guidewire through a side-hole at the middle of the stent (Figures 4.8, 4.9). The stent is removed endoscopically using rigid or flexible forceps to grasp the distal coiled end in the bladder, withdrawing it simultaneously with the cystoscope.[1]

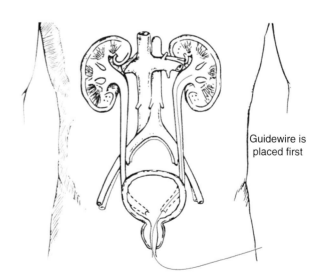

Guidewire is placed first

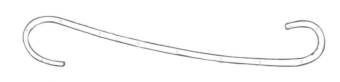

Figure 4.4. *Double-J®.*

Figure 4.6. *Open-tip stent.*

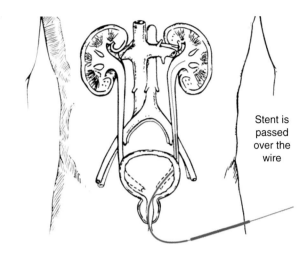

Figure 4.7. *Open-tip stent.*

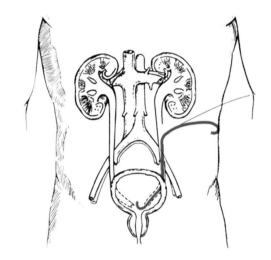

Figure 4.8. *Open surgical technique.*

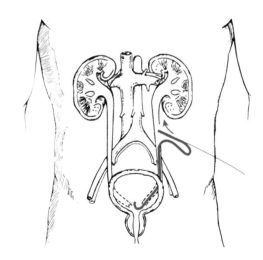

Figure 4.9. *Open surgical technique.*

Evaluation and results

The initial evaluation[8] of the Double-J stent in 1978 included 51 patients with varied diagnoses. This new design provided excellent drainage with no migration or loss of function. The Double-J was used to bypass obstruction and maintain urinary drainage in 12 patients: it was placed endoscopically in eight and through an open route in four. Less common procedures led to the use of the Double-J in the remaining 39 patients, including the following:

- *Extended pyelolithotomy (Gil–Vernet) and pyeloplasty without a nephrostomy tube.* Recovery was achieved with no leakage of urine postoperatively, and with stent removal cystoscopically with topical anaesthesia.
- *Nephrolithotomy.* The Double-J was used in conjunction with a temporary nephrostomy tube in situations where heavy bleeding was anticipated. An antegrade pyelogram through the nephrostomy tube was performed to verify patency of the stent. Following removal of the nephrostomy tube, any residual urine leakage generally ceased. Stent removal took place 3–4 weeks postoperatively, as warranted by the patient's recovery.
- *Ureteroneocystostomy.* Rare pathologies, such as total obstruction or a solitary kidney, demanded immediate drainage through a stent. Complicated procedures, involving tapering of the ureter, were also enhanced by the use of the Double-J for a period of 3–4 weeks.
- *Urinary diversion.* Stents were placed in one or both ureters and exited through a stoma with a collection bag placed over the stents. The results were positive, with no detectable urine leakage despite prior radiation therapy. Good drainage was maintained after the stents were removed, 10 days to 4 weeks postoperatively, as dictated by renal function, prior irradiation, infection and type of anastomosis used. Because of the risk of infection with a stent that was not indwelling, patients received antibiotic cover following stent removal.

The advantages of an endoscopically placed indwelling ureteral stent for long-term drainage have been well documented. The unique design features of the Double-J eliminated the flaws inherent in previous stent designs. For the first time, indwelling stents could be placed for prolonged periods without the inevitable development of sepsis, encrustation or migration. The stent could be inserted and removed easily with minimal patient discomfort. Patient comfort was so great with the Double-J that some patients failed to remember to return to have the stent removed. This necessitated implementation of a log to track patients to ensure that they were not lost to follow-up.[8]

The Double-J preceded the external shock-wave lithotripsy (ESWL) revolution. Prior to ESWL, ureteral and renal stones were commonly removed through open surgical procedures. Without the availability of an indwelling stent, urine would drain from the incision for days or weeks, inhibiting healing and increasing the likelihood of infection. The Double-J markedly reduced leakage, allowing patients to be discharged from the hospital much sooner. As the Double-J became widely available, the indications for its use multiplied extensively.

Impact of the Double-J on clinical management

The Double-J has been in use for 20 years. Initially, the primary application was to bypass obstruction caused by pregnancy, malignancy, stones and other pathologies within the urinary tract. In the case of malignancy, a nephrostomy was not required, and the patient could be easily managed with long term indwelling ureteral stents with occasional replacement. Use of an indwelling stent provided the benefit of ureteral dilatation, facilitating spontaneous passage of stones following temporary stent drainage.

The advent of ESWL markedly increased the demand for indwelling stents. Generally, fragmentation of larger stones produces a greater stone burden to be expelled through the ureter. *Steinstrasse*, the accumulation of fragments in the ureter, may create a difficult obstruction, requiring longer to resolve. Placement of a stent following ESWL treatment aids in preventing the formation of *steinstrasse* and facilitates the passage of stone fragments.

Over time, unique stent designs and refined biocompatible materials have been introduced,

promoting more efficient drainage, ease of placement and retrieval, enhanced patient comfort and reduced morbidity. However, the Double-J stent remains a popular design today.

State of the art

Over the years, attempts have been made to improve on the design of the basic Double-J, but until recently have met with limited success. The efficacy of the Double-J's basic design has been excellent; however, the silicone rubber, although an excellent material, leaves room for improvement. Silicone is soft and non-irritating, enhancing patient comfort, especially for long-term use. However, silicone has a higher coefficient of friction than other available materials, increasing the difficulty of initial passage. In addition, silicone is less resistant to encrustation if bacteriuria is present.

Alternative materials, such as thermoplastic elastomers — which include polyurethane and other similar compounds — have been available for several years. These materials allow for varying degrees of stiffness and, when fashioned into a more rigid stent, passage over a guidewire is facilitated. Furthermore, stents made from elastomers such as polyurethane have thinner walls than silicone stents, resulting in larger lumens with the same outer diameter and, therefore, a higher capacity for urine drainage. However, other properties associated with thermoplastic elastomers prevent these materials from exhibiting the same resistance to encrustation as silicone. This characteristic, when coupled with the degree of stiffness, can cause more irritation when stents are left indwelling for long periods.

Recent innovations in materials and design continue to advance the state of the art for ureteral stents. New materials and hydrophilic coatings on the external and/or internal stent surface serve to increase long-term lubricity, which is highly desirable. A slick, smooth stent greatly reduces surface friction, allowing for easier passage over the guidewire and facilitating proper placement.

Other design enhancements include (a) composite stents (dual durometer), which provide a firm proximal curl for retention in the renal pelvis and a soft distal curl in the bladder for ease of placement and increased patient comfort; (b) new thermosensitive materials, which are stiff initially to allow for rapid and easy placement and which soften at body temperature to ensure patient comfort; and (c) stents with new curl designs and multilength configurations that offer the advantages of better retention and decreased proximal migration.

Even with all these advances, the original concept of the ureteral stent has changed very little since its inception — and the Double-J stent has maintained its widespread appeal over the years. In a relatively short time the Double-J has been the impetus for numerous refinements in procedural techniques and has made a significant impact on the management of stone disease and other endourological disorders.

References

1. Bagley D H, Huffman J L, Lyon E S. Ureteral catheterization, retrograde ureteropyelography, and self-retaining ureteral stents. In: Bagley D H et al. (eds) Urologic endoscopy — a Manual and Atlas. Boston, MA: Little, Brown, 1985: 163–184

2. Lytton B. Catheters and sounds. In: Landes R R, Bush R B, Zorgniotti A W (eds) Perspectives in urology — the official American Urological Association (AUA) history of urology, vol 1. Nutley, NJ: AUA and Hoffman LaRoche, 1976: 117–134

3. Zimskind P D, Fetter T R, Wilkerson J L. Clinical use of long-term indwelling silicone rubber ureteral splints inserted cystoscopically. J Urol 1967; 97: 840

4. Marmar J L. The management of ureteral obstruction with silicone rubber splint catheters. J Urol 1970; 104: 386

5. Orikasa S, Tsuji I, Siba T, Ohashi N. A new technique for transurethral insertion of a silicone rubber tube into an obstructed ureter. J Urol 1973; 110: 184

6. Gibbons R P, Mason J T, Correa R J Jr. Experience with indwelling silicone rubber ureteral catheters. J Urol 1974; 104: 386

7. Hepperlen T K, Mardis H K. 'Pigtail stent' termed means of lessening ureteral surgery. Clin Trends Urol 1976; 405: 1

8. Finney R. Experience with new Double-J ureteral catheter stents. J Urol 1978; 119: 678

5

History of the Wallstent

Hans Wallstén with the collaboration of:
Christopher Knight, Adam Eldin and Euan Milroy

Introduction

The Wallstent is now well known in urology for the treatment of recurrent urethral strictures and prostate obstruction and is being marketed as the Urolume™. Few urologists realize, however, that this important device was first proposed for the management of vascular obstructions particularly in the coronary blood vessels, also for obstructed peripheral vascular disease and the treatment of aneurysm. It has also been widely used in other areas of the body for the relief of obstruction. We felt that urologists and others would be interested to learn how these useful modern devices were invented, designed and developed, and in the case of the Wallstent, more than 20 years ago.

The original concept

If one reviews the literature of the late 1970s and early 1980s concerning the haemocompatibility of vascular prostheses it would have appeared that transluminally implanted prostheses had a poor chance of success. It was known that vascular grafts made from woven polyester or microporous PTFE (polytetrafluorethylene) could only be used in large diameters in the arterial system, but that graft prostheses of 5 mm in diameter or less were not satisfactory for coronary artery replacement. Neither biomaterial could be considered as a suitable candidate for venous system replacement. Many materials have also been evaluated for their haemocompatibility in artificial heart valves but it was found that although some biomaterials might be superior to others, the nature of the blood flow could completely overwhelm the physiochemical properties of the basic material.

It is very unlikely, therefore, that researchers familiar with all the problems of biomaterials research at that time would have invested time, let alone large sums of money, in the search for an intraluminal prosthesis primarily destined for the cardiovascular system. There is a saying that 'a little knowledge is a dangerous thing',

but I think that in my case the opposite was true, namely, that 'a little ignorance can be helpful'. Quite simply, because I was ignorant of the possibilities of failure, I was encouraged to try something that was 'not obvious to someone skilled in the art'.

Although being a Swedish industrialist, inventions have played a large part in my life, specifically in the paper industry where I have invented and developed a number of innovative coating technologies. Because of my continuing interest in this area, in 1974 the Swedish multinational Bonnier Group and I co-founded a company 'Inventing SA' in Lausanne, Switzerland, with the purpose of industrializing my own paper-coating inventions and of pioneering research and development in new ideas from any other manufacturing sector.

In 1980, therefore, while working with Inventing SA, I was approached by a fellow Swede, the celebrated cardiac surgeon Professor Åke Senning, who was then at the University Hospital in Zürich. In the light of his previous work with one of his former clinical assistants, Dr Andreas Grüntzig, the pioneer of Percutaneous Transluminal Coronary Angioplasty (PTCA), Professor Senning began to appreciate the benefits of engineering and entrepreneurial support. He therefore invited me to collaborate with him in the development of a new concept.

Professor Senning and Dr Dirk Maas had been experimenting with the implantation of large diameter spiral endoprostheses in the aorta and vena cava. Their initial results, even though they were in relatively large vessels, were certainly encouraging, but they were beset by fundamental engineering problems. The spirals they wished to implant were quite short and of large diameter but made from fine stainless steel wire. Due to this the spirals lacked geometric stability and had a tendency to tilt. They therefore needed a more stable spiral design and, of course, a catheter or introducer that would permit accurate placement of the device.

The collaboration began and led to the development of the 'double helix' spiral, where the geometric stability was increased by using spirals in the form of steel strips and these were rendered even more stable by the use of steel bridging elements between pairs of spirals (Fig. 5.1). The introducing device we developed for this new 'double helix' was a steerable articulated arm comprised of over 600 individual elements. This work was originally presented at the annual meeting of European Society for Artificial Organs in 1982,[1] and also is well described in later publications.[2,3]

Animal models had clearly shown that the improved geometrical stability led to a radical improvement. However, the whole concept of intravascular stenting and its wider clinical potential, particularly for treatment of restenosis by using the percutanous technique (developed by another Swede, Dr Seldinger), proved fascinating and led me to make two major decisions. The first of these was to totally rethink our engineering approach to stenting and to propose a much superior geometrical design and more practical method of catheter-based introduction. I wanted a high expansion rate combined with stability and flexibility. In particular, I wished to retain the 'self-expanding' property, or diametric flexibility of the spiral concept and still have a stented vessel that had a similar 'elasticity' to the native vessel.

It became clear that we should use another approach, namely, to combine the spirals into clockwise and counter-clockwise pairs that would support each other but still offer great flexibility of the prosthesis with respect to both length and diameter. Such a stent would also be self-expanding for an improved compliance with blood vessels. This then was the basic thinking behind the 'braid' prosthesis approach and its coated and uncoated variants outlined in a number of patents (Fig. 5.2).

But the braided stent also needed a new approach for the delivery catheter. As a result of innumerable experiments with my wife's rubber kitchen gloves, I found that it was possible to peel back an inverted elastic and flexible tube from the stent in its compressed state without creating frictional forces on the stent itself, like peeling a banana. This became the concept for the flexible rolling membrane stent catheter. These then were the basic ideas of the cardiovascular form of the 'Wallstent', which was featured in many publications relating to both animal models and clinical applications.

It was clear that these ideas now needed a group of people to take them from the lab and drawing board,

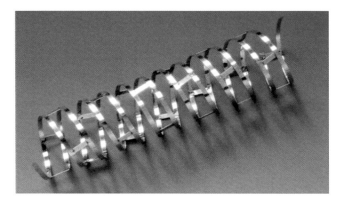

Figure 5.1. *The double helix spiral stent with bridging elements.*

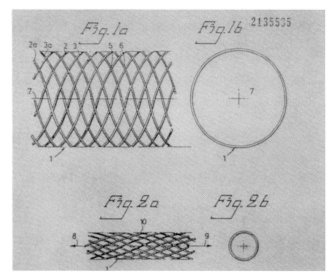

Figure 5.2. *In the first patent of the Wallstent: self-expansion properties from the constrained to the expanded state.*

through development, and on to the factory and clinic. Consequently, the second major decision in 1982 was the creation of the company Medinvent SA in Lausanne, Switzerland and the recruitment of major European specialists. This multinational team of some fifteen people was considerably influential in the future success that the company was to enjoy.

Relatively quickly we became aware that spiral or braided stents have a unique feature. Analysis after they had been implanted in animal blood vessels for some weeks showed that the metal surface had been overgrown with endothelium. That cells would grow on a metal surface was, of course, a surprise but it appeared that the cells could form tissue bridges over the metal wire, at least for relatively short distances. It was known that pseudo-endothelium could proliferate over the first few millimetres of a vascular graft but would not progress much further, and that they often appeared deformed and non-functional, while those on our stents appeared perfectly normal and functional.

In reviewing past literature we discovered the work of Dotter (1969), who had implanted small 'memory' metal spirals as a form of vascular graft in the small arteries of dogs.[5] In general, vascular grafts in the popliteal arteries of dogs do not remain patent, and yet here was proof of patency at 18 months or more. It was clear, therefore, that the mechanism of endothelialization in stents was totally different to that encountered with conventional prosthetic grafts, and that the endothelium so created was not just covering the wire surface but that the cells themselves appeared to have normal endothelial function. It was the healthy status of these cells that presented the prospect of long-term antithrombogenesis.

This led us to appreciate that since we needed a radial force to hold the stent in position against the vessel wall, this force must not be so strong as to damage the intima, media or adventitia which are so vital in nourishing the endothelium. Here again, it was very clear that the 'braid' approach to stenting had distinct advantages over the spiral approach in terms of the lower normal pressures engendered.

Much of our early engineering work was therefore aimed at finding the most suitable alloy or metal with high 'spring' properties since this is fundamental to gaining the greatest possible expansion ratio of the braid from its constrained form on the catheter to its fully opened form. We selected a very well-documented stainless steel that had been widely used in medical implants for many years. Consequently, much experimentation was devoted to finding the best and safest combination of these characteristics and also for the development of production equipment for the braiding of the stents in different configurations and sizes and the corresponding implantation devices (Figs 5.3, 5.4).

Of equal importance was our awareness that between the time of implantation of the vascular stent and the completion of the endothelialization process some weeks later, the naked surface of the stent offered some risk of thrombosis. Although anticoagulation was possible, we were also very active in investigating modifications of the material surfaces of the stent. Heparin bonding to the surface was evaluated and also the use of a novel plasma-deposited synthetic carbon coating which was shown to inhibit platelet deposition in baboons.

In addition to research and development, we began European clinical trials with selected volunteers with clinical symptoms of coronary, iliac, femoral, popliteal, renal and venous defects. From my notes of that period, I saw that before we instigated commercial sales of our devices, we had implanted over 1000 prostheses in animals or humans. The panels of leading clinicians who performed these trials and their institutions, all freely gave their time and resources in support of advancing this revolutionary technology. It was a period of unparalleled excitement, partnership and cooperation and it was a privilege to share this experience with the medical community.

Despite the evident enthusiasm in the cardiovascular sector, highlighted by the successful first 50 coronary

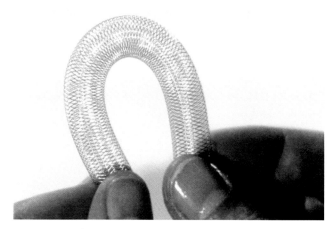

Figure 5.3. *The spring properties of the material in the Wallstent provide a high axial flexibility in constriction and expansion, in contrast to balloon-expanded stents.*

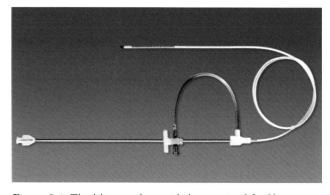

Figure 5.4. *The delivery catheter with the constricted flexible stent at the distal tip. Based on the rolling membrane principle, it is very flexible and allows percutanous implantation over a guidewire.*

stent implantations in the world performed in the university hospitals of Toulouse and Lausanne, our thinking at Medinvent had quite quickly appreciated that our expandable stents also held great promise in the non-vascular channels of the human body. We could foresee possible applications in the urethra, ureter, oesophagus, lungs, fallopian tubes, bile duct, pancreatic duct, etc. Just as easily, we could foresee that we would be confronted by major fundamental questions: would the stents still endothelialize; was this important; would the ductal fluids erode or attack the material of the prosthesis or render it brittle? And, of course, another important question: would we need a new set of introducing catheters or devices specific to each application? These considerations led us to take the decision to establish, within the company, a team specifically dedicated to the non-vascular applications of our technology.

Early urological experiments

The urinary tract seemed an ideal organ system because of the tubular nature of ureters and urethra. They are both lined by modified epithelial structures and quite frequently experience a variety of stenotic lesions often requiring difficult and complex surgery.

During 1984 and 1985, we carried out a number of implants of the Wallstent at the Royal College of Surgeons of England experimental station at Downe House, Kent, UK. Originally the home of Charles Darwin, this building with its associated laboratories, was his bequest to the College. This site was chosen because John Cooper, the College's veterinary officer, and the urologist Euan Milroy, had earlier developed techniques for cystourethroscopy in dogs and other mammals for veterinary and experimental diagnostic and treatment purposes.

A Wallstent, measuring 10 mm in length and 4.5 mm in fully expanded diameter, was inserted into the normal urethras of four anaesthetized, male, crossbred dogs using the standard rolling membrane delivery catheter developed for endovascular use. The stents were implanted so that they lay in the bulbar portion of the urethra, just beyond (proximal to) the os penis. The position of the stents was checked endoscopically and radiologically and were seen to open fully in the correct position. After insertion, the stents did not seem to cause any problems for the dogs and no subsequent

urinary tract infection or difficulties were noted. The dogs were sacrificed 2, 4, 6, and 12 months after insertion and the excised fixed urethra was opened to allow scanning electron microscopy of the surface of the device. The stent was then removed and tissue subsequently submitted for histological examination of deeper tissues.

These animal studies confirmed the earlier cardiovascular work that the stent covered with urothelium. At 6 months, partial covering of the stent was seen and this was virtually complete at 12 months. On light microscopy, no abnormalities were seen in the deeper tissues of the urethra, other than minor inflammatory changes in the first few months after implantation.[6]

Early clinical studies

The frequent occurrence of complex urethral strictures and the limited availability of the surgical skills necessary to repair them seemed to us an ideal opportunity to use the Wallstent to maintain the lumen of a strictured urethra, in the same way that it had been used to keep open coronary and peripheral vessels obstructed by atheroma.

We had already shown in our animal models that the Wallstent was tolerated within the dog urethra and, more importantly, confirmed that as in the cardiovascular system, the stent was covered with what appeared to be normal urothelium. In 1987, we were therefore encouraged to implant the stent into eight male patients, aged between 33 and 78 years with recurrent strictures. These strictures had all failed multiple previous attempts at treatment, including urethrotomy and urethroplasty, and in each case the only alternative was further urethroplasty surgery. Other than this, the patients were unselected in so far as aetiology and duration of stricture history were concerned. All the patients gave their fully informed consent for the use of this new device. In seven of these first patients the recurrent stricture was situated in the bulbar urethra. We were anxious to avoid the membranous urethra because of the risk of damaging urethral sphincter function, and the penile urethra because of possible difficulties in erection during sexual activity. The eighth patient had a Wallstent inserted into the membranous urethra in order to relieve obstructed ejaculation because of a membranous urethral stricture following an earlier total cystectomy and urinary diversion.

In 1988, these cases were reported in the first publication of clinical results on the Wallstent in urology.[6] Excellent results were reported of a minimal follow-up of 6 months, the first two patients treated having a 12 month follow-up.[6] These stents were all mounted on a delivery catheter covered by a rolling membrane compressing the stent to a small diameter similar to that used in cardiovascular cases and the subsequent dog urethral experiments. Implantation was carried out with the delivery catheter alongside a standard cystoscope. There were obvious practical difficulties with this technique, although the stent could easily be observed as it was released in position in the urethra covering the previously dilated urethral stricture.

The success of these first patients demonstrated that the technique of implantation was simple and safe. Up to one year, the material of the stent caused no problems in the male urethra. Using cystoscopy and urethrograms, the stent was seen to be well-covered by epithelium at between 6 and 9 months after implantation. These seemed to be excellent results from the point of view of stricture treatment (Fig. 5.5 a,b). Further clinical experience in the treatment of urethral strictures was rapidly gained with this device, thus confirming its value in this condition.[7,8]

Development of a new (current) delivery system

Although the clinical results of the Wallstent in urethral strictures were good it rapidly became apparent that while the catheter-mounted rolling membrane delivery system was ideally suited for endovascular use it was far from ideal in the lower urinary tract. It was pointed out by Euan Milroy that urologists would prefer to use a device mounted on equipment that was compatible with their existing cystoscopic equipment. We agreed that this was of even more importance when we considered the possibilities of using the Wallstent not only for urethral strictures but also for the more common problem of prostate obstruction, particularly in the unfit patient.

In conjunction with our clinical collaborators we then developed a Wallstent delivery system especially designed for the lower urinary tract. This used an identical Wallstent which was mounted in a compressed and elongated form between two tubular sheaths down the centre of which passed a standard 0 or 30 urology telescope. The device was fitted with finger grips very similar to those on a resectoscope, which allowed the outer metal sheath to be retracted once the whole device had been slid up the urethra into position. The stent then expanded under direct vision. The location could be checked far more readily with this device than with the earlier catheter-mounted system. In addition, with the help of safety catches preventing final release of the stent, it could be repositioned if necessary to

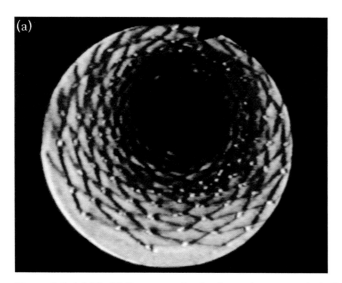
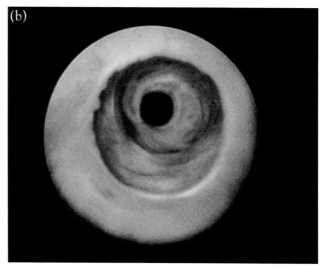

Figure 5.5. *(a) The Wallstent immediately after implantation in the bulbar urethra. (b) The Wallstent at 12 months follow up.*

ensure perfect deployment. Following early clinical trials of the device, resulting in some modification and improvements to the prototype, we achieved a delivery system almost identical to that in current use (Fig 5.6).

Further clinical studies

Following the first clinical reports of the use of the Wallstent for the treatment of urethral strictures from Euan Milroy at the Middlesex Hospital, London, further large scale studies were carried out in both Europe and North America.[9,10] These results confirmed that the Wallstent was very successful in the treatment of urethral strictures with up to two years follow-up, although more difficulties were found in strictures following complete urethral rupture and failed urethroplasty procedures.

The best results were obtained with strictures measuring 1–2 cm in length lying within the bulbar part of the urethra. However, interestingly, some experience was gained in using the Wallstent for treating strictures in the sphincter-active membranous urethra in carefully selected patients, in combination with an artificial urinary sphincter.[11] The device was also used in patients with obstructed urethral sphincters after high spinal injuries and failure of sphincterotomy.[12]

Following these encouraging results, it was decided to use the Wallstent as a treatment for prostate obstruction in the elderly unfit patient. This followed earlier reports of a variety of metal and plastic stents, which when used in the prostatic urethra, had risks of

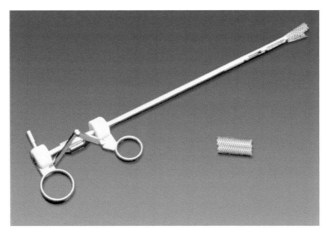

Figure 5.6. *The delivery system for urology application under direct vision (developed in 1987), is almost identical to that in present use. (Reproduced with permission from Journal of Urology.)*

stent displacement, infection and encrustation. Because we had already demonstrated epithelial covering of the Wallstent in urethral strictures we anticipated that this stent would be more satisfactory as a permanent cure for prostatic obstruction in those patients unfit for surgery. As the stent would be covered by epithelium, this should avoid the risk of displacement, infection and encrustation. Early results from Williams et al. and Milroy and Chapple were encouraging, although difficulties were noted in positioning the stent accurately within the prostatic urethra.[13,14] It was vital to ensure that no part of the stent protruded into the bladder lumen as it would then fail to be covered by epithelium and would cause encrustation.

A large European study of patients who were fit for surgery but who were offered the Wallstent for treatment of their prostate obstruction also showed excellent results, and a large North American study also reported encouraging results.[15,16] A report from Schneider et al. demonstrated how useful the Wallstent could be as a rapid outpatient treatment for prostate obstruction in relieving waiting list pressure on busy hospitals in Britain.[17]

Other clinical applications

While work continued on the use of the Wallstent for urethral strictures, with good 5 year long-term results reported from Milroy and Allen,[18] and in benign and even malignant prostate obstruction, Pauer and Lugmayr in Austria had started using the Wallstent mounted on its original catheter delivery system for treating ureteric strictures that were difficult to manage or which recurred after balloon dilatation.[19] Excellent results were obtained, although some problems with the development of hyperplastic tissue within the lumen of the stent were experienced.[12] This hyperplasia is a normal reaction to the stent implanted into the urinary tract. In cases of urethral stricture or prostate obstruction, presumably because of the relatively large diameter of the stent, this hyperplasia is rarely of any significance and settles in the majority of patients within the first 6 months. However, in the narrow bore of the ureteric stricture the hyperplasia did on occasion cause repeated obstruction, although this could easily be circumvented by means of a temporary ureteric catheter through the stent.

Excellent results were also found when the Wallstent was used transhepatically and endoscopically, mounted on the rolling membrane catheter for the treatment of biliary strictures. It is also used for the treatment of tracheal and bronchial strictures.

Subsequent history

As the enormous potential of the Wallstent began to emerge, it became rapidly clear that the number of clinical indications, the scale of clinical trials and the very large number of geographical markets would stretch the resources of our small company (Table 5.1). We, and indeed our medical colleagues, were particularly reluctant to delay the introduction of this remarkable technology to the wide range of medical disciplines that could benefit from it.

In view of the strict regulatory requirements for the introduction of one, let alone innumerable products onto the US market via the Food and Drug Administration, it can be appreciated that we had pressing need for partners in this area. As a result, Medinvent SA became a joint venture company in association with the large American medical group, Pfizer, in 1988. This gave Medinvent access to a very substantial sales and marketing organization with many years of regulatory affairs experience. In 1989 Pfizer acquired the remainder of Medinvent.

Currently, the urology applications of the Wallstent, under the name Urolume™, are owned by American Medical Systems and the other Wallstent applications, under the trademark Wallstent™, are owned by Boston Scientific Corporation.

Conclusions

The Wallstent, originally developed to meet the challenge of recurrent atheromatous obstruction of coronary and other blood vessels, has proved remarkably successful in its use in the urinary tract and elsewhere. The structure of the stent with its woven open meshwork of fine biocompatible wire and its self-expanding properties ensures that a radial force is maintained to hold open the lumen of whatever tube is being stented, while allowing covering of the wire by normal epithelium. Once this has occurred, the stent is excluded from contact with the contained body fluid and in this regard has many advantages over the numerous other metallic stents used in these areas.

The basic structure and design of the stent and delivery system would be difficult to improve. However, there remains many interesting possible developments in stent coating to reduce the risk of intrastent hyperplasia and possible recurrent fibrotic stenosis, and to treat surrounding malignant tissue, particularly in the prostate and biliary tract to prevent the tumour from growing within the lumen of the stent. Although the initial considerable enthusiasm for the Wallstent may have diminished it remains a popular, simple, safe, effective and very useful means of relieving obstruction in many areas of the body.

Table 5.1. *Wallstent™ clinical implantation: 1989*

Application	Patients	Centres
Vascular		
Coronary	300	6
Peripheral		
iliac arteries	120	
superficial femoral artery	100	
other peripheral vessels	70	
Total peripheral	290	10
Total vascular	**590**	**16**
Non-vascular		
Biliary	250	
Urethral strictures	90	
Prostate obstruction	85	
DESD	60	
Trachea and bronchi	30	
Oesophagus	30	
Pancreatic duct	40	
Total non-vascular	**585**	**34**
Grand total	**1175**	**50**

References

1. Maas D, Kropf L, Egloff L, Demierre D, Turina M, Senning A. Transluminal Implantation of Intravascular 'Double Helix' spiral prostheses; technical and biological considerations. ESAO Proc 1982; 9: 252–256
2. Maas D, Demierre D, Deaton D, Largiarder F, Senning A. Transluminal implantation of self-adjusting expandable prostheses: Principles, techniques and results. Progress in Artificial Organs 1983
3. Radiological follow-up of transluminally inserted vascular endoprostheses: An experimental study using expanding spirals. Radiology 1984; 152(3): 659–663
4. US Patent no 4655771 11 April 1983. Swedish Patent 8202739 30 April 1982

5. Dotter C T. Transluminally placed coilspring endarterial tube grafts; long-term patency in the canine popliteal artery. Invest Radiol 1969; 4: 329–332

6. Milroy E J G, Cooper J E, Wallsten H, Chapple C R, Eldin A, Seddon A M, Powles P M. A new treatment for urethral strictures. Lancet 1988; 1: 1424–1427

7. Milroy E J G, Chapple C R, Eldin A, Wallsten H. A new stent for the treatment of urethral strictures. Br J Urol 1989; 63: 392–396

8. Milroy E J G, Chapple C R, Eldin A, Wallsten H. A new treatment for urethral strictures; a permanently implanted urethral stent. J Urol 1989; 141: 1120–1122

9. Ashken M H, Coulange C, Milroy E J G, Sarramon J P. European experience with the urethral Wallstent for urethral strictures. Eur Urol 1991; 19: 181–185

10. Badlani G H, Press S M, Defalco A. Urolume endourethral prosthesis for the treatment of urethral stricture disease. Urology 1995; 45: 846–856

11. Milroy E J G. Treatment of sphincter strictures using permanent Urolume stents. J Urol 1993; 150: 1729–1733

12. Shaw P J R, Milroy E J G, Timoney A G, Eldin A, Mitchell N. Permanent external striated sphincter stents in patients with spinal injuries. Br J Urol 1990; 66: 297–302

13. McLoughlin J, Jager R, Abel P D, Williams G. The use of prostatic stents in patients with urinary retention who are unfit for surgery. Br J Urol 1990; 66: 66–70

14. Milroy E, Chapple C R. The Urolume stent in the management of benign prostatic hyperplasia. J Urol 1993; 150: 1630–1635

15. Guazzoni G, Montorsi F, Coulange C, Milroy E, Pansodoro V, Rubben H, Sarramon J P, Williams G. A modified prostatic Urolume Wallstent for healthy patients with symptomatic benign prostatic hyperplasia; a European multicentre study. Urology 199; 44: 364–370

16. Oesterling J E, Kaplan S A, Epstein H B, Defalco A J, Reddy P K, Chancellor M B. The North American experience with the Urolume endoprosthesis as a treatment for benign prostatic hyperplasia; long term results. Urology 1994; 44: 353–362

17. Schneider H J, De Souza J U, Palmer J H. The Urolume as a means of treating urinary outflow obstruction and its impact on waiting lists. Br J Urol 1994; 73: 181–184

18. Milroy E J G, Allen A. Long term results of Urolume urethral stents for recurrent urethral strictures. J Urol 1996; 155: 904–907

19. Pauer W, Lugmayr H. Metallic Wallstents as a new therapy for extrinsic ureteral obstruction. J Urol 1992; 148: 281–284

6

From Prostakath® to Memokath® stents

Henrik Harboe and Jørgen Nordling

Introduction

Prostakath® was one of the first metallic prostate stents. It was introduced in 1987 and used mainly for relief of prostatic obstruction in men with severe concomitant diseases preventing safe anaesthesia and surgery.

Several articles were published between 1988 and 1996 including some from Herlev University Hospital in Copenhagen, Denmark.[1–30] The general experience was summarized in 1992 and concluded that the Prostakath® was a useful alternative to an indwelling catheter.[24]

Ideal prostatic stent definition

The experience with Prostakath® constituted the background for the definition of an ideal prostatic stent (Table 6.1). The definition was later published as follows:

The ideal prostatic stent should be easy to insert and position under topical urethral anaesthesia. Cystoscopy through the stent should be possible. The stent should not extend outside the prostatic urethra. It should not give any local reaction or give rise to encrustations. Finally it should be easy to remove if necessary.[31]

During the Third International Consultation on Benign Prostatic Hyperplasia, 1995,[32] three further criteria were added:

1. Stents should be malleable to conform to the shape of the prostatic urethra.

2. Stents should not migrate.
3. Stents should be inexpensive.

Design and development of Memokath®

The definition of the ideal prostatic stent was used as a guideline for development of the Memokath® 028 prostatic stent. Subsequent research led to the construction of a nickel-titanium (NiTi) wire coil stent (Fig. 6.1). This stent was introduced in 1992. The first stent was 22 Ch with the distal segment expanding to 34 Ch. Two years later a slightly larger stent was made available; 24 Ch with segment expanding to 44 Ch.

The distal segment of the stent expands in response to flushing the stent with water at approximately 50°–55°C. This response is termed 'thermally induced shape memory' and is unique to the NiTi alloy used for Memokath®. The expanded distal segment anchors the stent in the desired position in the prostatic urethra.

The NiTi stent also has a lower temperature thermal response at approximately 10°C where the alloy becomes 'supersoft' and thus facilitates removal of the stent, which easily uncoils and comes out as a twisted wire. NiTi is attractive as an implant material because it is highly biocompatible and can be constructed to have excellent corrosion resistance.

Table 6.1. *The ideal prostatic stent*

- Easy to insert
- Easy to remove if required
- Free lumen large enough to alleviate the obstruction and allow cystoscopy
- No sphincter involvement
- No creation of tissue reaction or infection
- No encrustation even after long indwelling time

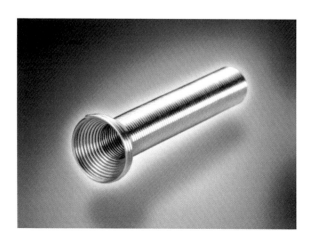

Figure 6.1. *Memokath® stent with bell-shaped expansion and tightly coiled design.*

The Memokath® stent was further constructed with insertion systems to enable direct vision control of stent insertion, positioning and deployment. As a unique feature, Memokath® can be inserted with a flexible cystoscope. The coil design allows normal function of the active tip of the cystoscope (Fig. 6.2) and consequently permits a truly minimally invasive procedure.

The release of the stent from the insertion system is an integral function of the expansion of the distal segment (Fig. 6.3).

Clinical experience of Memokath®

Many articles have been published reporting consistently positive outcome after prostatic stenting with Memokath®.[33–45] Treatment results are good and complications are acceptable. Chapter 44 describes clinical experience in more detail.

Conclusion and future prospects

The Memokath® 028 prostatic stent fulfils most of the criteria for the ideal prostatic stent:

1. it is easy to insert and position under local anaesthesia;
2. it is possible (with caution) to pass a flexible cystoscope through the stent;
3. the stent does not extend outside the prostatic urethra;
4. local discomfort is rare;
5. encrustations occur but are infrequent;
6. stent removal, if necessary, is easy;
7. the stent is malleable and the migration rate is low.

The cost of Memokath® 028 prostatic stent treatment equals that of one year of treatment with an indwelling Foley catheter – and is far more acceptable for the patient.

References

1. Mandresi A. Prostakath®. Un' endoprotesi uretrale prostatica per la risoluzione della patalogia ostruttiva da causa prostatica. Riv Med Prat 1989; 288: 32–34
2. Shalkow P E, Jiménez V D. Alternative en el tratimento temporal de la retención urinaria por crecimiento prostático. Rev Mex Urol 1989; 49(5): 127–130
3. Nielsen K K, Kromann-Andersen B, Nordling J. Relationship between detrusor pressure and urinary flow rate in males with an intraurethral prostatic spiral. Br J Urol 1989; 64: 275–279
4. Nordling J, Holm H H, Klarskov P et al. The intraprostatic spiral: a new device for insertion with the patient under local anesthesia and with ultrasonic guidance with 3 months of follow-up. J Urol 1989; 142: 756–758
5. Nielsen K K, Klarskov O P, Nordling J et al. Prostataspiral. En ny behandling af urinretention hos mænd. Kliniske Erfaringer med 6 Måneders Observationstid. Ugeskr Læger 1989; 151(44): 2888–2889
6. Baert L. De Prostaatspiraal. Alternatief voor een verliljfcatheter bij patienten met prostaatadenoom. Tijdschr Geneeskd 1989; 45: 309–311
7. Yachia D, Lask D, Rabinson S. Self-retaining intraurethral stent: an alternative to long-term indwelling catheters or surgery in the treatment of prostatism. AJR 1990; 154: 111–113

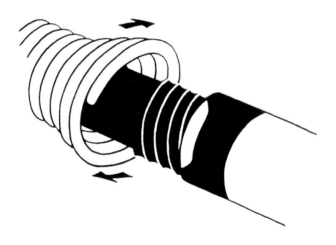

Figure 6.2. *The Memokath® stent flexes easily with the active movement of the tip of the flexible cystoscope.*

Figure 6.3. *Expansion of the Memokath® stent also releases the stent from the insertion sheath.*

8. Nielsen K K, Nordling J, Holm H H et al. Prostataspiral – en nz behandling af urinretention hos mænd: kliniske erfaringer med 6 Måneders Observationstid (Article of the Month). Nord Med 1990; 105(2): 50–51, 60

9. Harrison N W, De Souza J V. Prostatic stenting for outflow obstruction. Br J Urol 1990; 65: 192–196

10. Billiet I, Amattelaer J, Van Brien P. The use of transrectal longitudinal sonography in the placement of a prostatic coil. Eur Urol 1990; 17: 76–78

11. Nielsen K K, Klarskov P, Nordling J et al. The intraprostatic spiral. New treatment for urinary retention. Br J Urol 1990; 65: 500–503

12. Chevallier D, Quientens H, Amiel J et al. La spirale intraprostatique dans le traitment de l'hypertrophie bénigne de la prostate. J Urol (Paris) 1990; 96(4): 203–206

13. Ovesen H, Poulsen A L, Nordling J. Differentiation between neurogenic and prostatic obstruction using the intraprostatic spiral. A case report. Scand J Urol Nephrol 1990; 24: 179–180

14. Chen J, Matzkin H, Braf Z. Intraprostatic urethral catheter in benign prostatic hyperplasis: six-month follow-up study. J Endourol 1990; 4(2): 199–207

15. Yachia D. Spontaneous breakage of self-retaining intraprostatic stent. J Urol 1990; 144: 997–998

16. Sandermann J, Bearmani M, Mikkelsen I. Infravesical obstruktion kan avhjälpes med prostataspiral. Läkertidningen 1990; 87(47): 3967–3970

17. Magnusson A, Lönnemark M, Ahlström H, Brekkan E. Forändrad teknik förbättrer behandlingen med prostataspiral. Läkertidningen 1991; 68(16): 1485

18. Holmes S A V, Miller P D, Crocker P R, Kirby R S. Encrustation of intraprostatic stents – a comparative study. Br J Urol 1992; 69: 383–387

19. Poulsen A L, Ovesen H, Nielsen K K et al. Intraprostatic spiral during waiting time for transurethral prostatectomy. Urol Int 1991; 146: 172–175

20. Chiu A W, Lin A T L, Lee Y-H et al. Stone incrustration: a relevant complication of the intraprostatic spiral. Eur Urol 1991; 19: 304–307

21. Ovesen H, Poulsen A L, Nielsen K K et al. Intraprostatic spiral: alternative to permanent indwelling catheter in men with senile dementia. J Endourol 1991; 5: 329–332

22. Rosenkilde P, Pedersen J F, Meyhoff H-H. Late complications of Prostakath® treatment for benign prostatic hyperplasia. Br J Urol 1991; 68: 387–389

23. Yasumoto R, Yoshihara H, Kishimoto T, Maekawa M. Clinical study of a metallic prostatic stent. Acta Urol Jpn 1991; 37: 1467–1470

24. Nordling J, Ovesen H, Poulsen A L. The intraprostatic spiral: clinical results in 150 consecutive patients. J Urol 1992; 147: 645–647

25. Krogh J. Long term complications of the intraprostatic spiral. Case report. Scand J Urol Nephrol 1992; 26: 191–192

26. Thomas P J, Britton J P, Harrison N W. The Prostakath stent; four years experience. Br J Urol 1993; 71: 430–432

27. Ala-Opas M, Talja M, Tiitinen J et al. Prostakath® in urinary outflow obstruction. Ann Chir Gynaecol 1993; 82: 14–18

28. Nordling J, Ovesen H, Poulsen A L et al. Den intraprostatiske spiral: langtidsresultater hos 150 konsekutive patienter. Ugeskr Læger 1993; 155: 4064–4066

29. Nielsen K K, Kromann-Andersen B, Poulsen A L et al. Subjective and objective evaluation of patients with prostatism and infravesical obstruction treated with both intraprostatic spiral and transurethral prostatectomy. Neurourol Urodyn 1994; 13: 13–19

30. Braf Z, Chen J, Sofer M, Matzkin H. Intraprostatic metal stents (Prostakath® and Urospiral®): more than 6 years clinical experience with 110 patients. J Endourol 1996; 10: 555–558

31. Nordling J, Harboe H, Othel-Jacobsen E. A thermoexpandable stent for treatment of prostatic obstruction. Oral presentation. SIU (International Society of Urology), 22nd Congress, 3–7 November 1991, Seville, Spain

32. Crockett A T, Aso Y, Denis L et al. Recommendations of the International Consensus Committee concerning: 4. Treatment recommendations for benign prostatic hyperplasia (BPH): Proceedings of the 3rd International Consultation on Benign Prostatic Hyperplasia, Monaco, 26–28 June 1995: 625–640

33. Poulsen A L, Schou J, Ovesen H, Nordling J. MEMOKATH®: A second generation of intraprostatic spirals. Br J Urol 1993; 72: 331–334

34. Soni B M, Vaidyanathan M S, Krishnan K R. Use of MEMOKATH®, a second generation urethral stent for relief of urinary retention in male spinal cord injured patients. Paraplegia 1994; 32: 480–488

35. Kuriki O, Ohshima S, Matsuura O, Ono Y, Kato N, Yamada S, Kinukawa T, Hattori R. A thermosensitive stent for the treatment of benign prostatic hyperplasia. Jpn J Endourol ESWL 1995; 2: 192–194

36. Booth C M, Chaudry A A, Lyth D R. Alternative prostate treatments: Stent or catheter for the frail. J Manag Care 1997; 1: 24–26

37. Derry F, Fellows G, Frankel H. Methicillin-resistant Staphylococcus aureus cleared using a spiral thermoexpandable urethral stent. Br J Urol 1997; 80: 683–684

38. Shah N C, Foley S J, Edhem I, Shah J P R. Use of MEMOKATH®; Temporary urethral stent in treatment of detrusor-sphincter dyssynergia. J Endourol 1997; 11: 485–488

39. Chaudry A A, Booth C M. Clinical and cost comparison of long-term catheterisation and MEMOKATH®; prostatic stenting. In: Yahia D (ed) Stenting the urinary system. Oxford: ISIS Medical Media 1998: 297–300

40. Eichenauer R H, Koll B, Schüller J. Der thermolabile Stent als Therapiemöglichkeit obstruktiver Prostataerkrankungen. Med Bild 1998; 5(5): 23–28

41. Itoh H, Shinomiya T, Matsumoto Y, Arai T, Katoh M, Okada K. Clinical experience of intraurethral catheter made of shape-memory alloy (MEMOKATH®). Jpn J Urol Surg 1999; 12(4): 511–517

42. Mahnken A H. Einwachsens eines MEMOKATH® 028 Prostatastent —Ein Fallbericht. Akt Urol 1999; 30: 492–494

43. Hara H, Ishii N, Deguchi M, Kawakami T, Nakajima K, Kurita M, Miura K, Ishii N, Harada M, Matsumoto H, Nozawa E, Suzuki R, Harada T, Morokuma F, Sato S. Clinical experience of intraurethral stent made of shape memory alloy (MEMOKATH®) for refractory urethral strictures. Jpn J Urol Surg 2000; 13(11): 1431–1437

44. Shigeta M, Nakamoto T, Nakahara M, Usui T. Efficacy of intraurethral catheter made of shape-memory alloy for complete posterior urethral rupture complicated with pelvic bone fracture. Jpn J Urol Surg 2000; 13(7): 929–932

45. Perry M J A, Roodhouse A J, Gidlow A B, Spicer T G, Ellis B W. Thermo-expandable intraprostatic stents in bladder outlet obstruction: an 8-year study. BJU Int 2002; 90(3): 216–223

History of the UroCoil and ProstaCoil stents
Daniel Yachia

7

Introduction

Insertion of a urethral catheter is the simplest form of urinary diversion. Despite the well-known complications associated with long-term catheterization, it is still widely used in chronic or acute obstructions of the lower urinary tract. Since the introduction of urethral stents, having the indwelling catheter removed and regaining the ability to urinate spontaneously through the stent, proved to ease the medical and psychological burden of the patient.

In urology, the use of prostatic stents instead of indwelling catheters was introduced in 1980 by Fabian in Germany.[1] Fabian developed a fixed calibre (21 Fr) stainless steel coil to be inserted into the prostatic urethra, instead of an indwelling catheter for the management of severe prostatic obstruction. He named this device a 'Partial Catheter' or 'Urologic Spiral'. Initially, the Fabian stent was used for patients who were poor operative risks or who refused surgery because of fear of impotence. Subsequently, this stent, and the other new intraurethral stents introduced for urological use, gained increasing acceptance in daily urological practice, especially in Europe.[2–6] Later, self-expanding temporary stents were developed. Either the fixed calibre or the self-expanding temporary stents were intraluminal devices left temporarily in the prostatic urethra to hold the urethral lumen open. They remained in the urethral lumen, without becoming incorporated into the urethral wall. Then, they were either removed or replaced with a new one.

In parallel to the temporary urethral stents, a second group of stents based on a different concept were introduced for opening prostatic obstructions.[7,8] These were either balloon expandable or self-expanding permanent stents, which were initially developed as vascular stents and later adapted for urological use. The permanent stents were intended to be covered ultimately by the urethral epithelium and to remain permanently in the body. The use of the balloon expandable prostatic stents was limited and they disappeared from the urologist's armamentarium.

In urology, the era of permanent stenting started with the introduction of the self-expanding Wallstent developed by Hans Wallstén. This stent became a widely popular one in many medical disciplines as well as in urology and its original design or its many modifications are still widely used. The design of this stent was based on the well-known 'Chinese finger trap' in which one can insert a finger which is trapped when the finger is retracted. For many years this wire-braiding principle was used industrially in the manufacture of coaxial cables and some catheter braids, but until it was redesigned by Wallstén it was not used as a stent. In Chapter 5 the development and history of the Wallstent is described by its inventor.

Based on these concepts, some of these stents were developed further for the treatment of urethral stricture disease. Since then, the use of various stents in benign and malignant prostatic obstructions and recurrent urethral strictures has resulted in high success rates (up to 80%) in overcoming obstructions along the urethra.

In this chapter I will describe the history of the development of the first self-expanding temporary stent.

History

My experience with prostatic stents began during the late 1980s with the use of the Prostakath. This stent was a modification of the device developed by Fabian, which originally was made of medical-grade stainless steel to be inserted endoscopically (Urologische Spirale, Uromed, Kassel, Germany). Although the design of the Prostakath was based on the Fabian stent, its insertion mechanism was redesigned by a team of Danish physicians and engineers. An introducing catheter temporarily locked to the stent was added to allow easier insertion under sonographic guidance, and the stainless steel wire was plated with 24-carat gold to reduce contact allergy and incrustation (Prostakath, Engineers & Doctors A/S, Copenhagen, Denmark).[5] Although it was an excellent alternative to an indwelling catheter, it had the major problem of distal and proximal, partial

(42%) or complete (12%) migration.[9] In our initial experience with this device on 26 patients, six were incontinent immediately after the procedure. In six patients, the device had to be repositioned to restore continence. Urinary retention developed in two others on the day of insertion and in an additional patient, a day after insertion. In two patients the stent was removed because of severe frequency and urgency, which did not respond to treatment.[9]

The possibility of using a temporary stent as a mould in the treatment of recurrent urethral stricture disease occurred to me on using the first-generation intraprostatic stent (Prostakath) in 1986 in prostatic obstructions, and being impressed by its performance. The idea was of developing a long-term but easily removable intraurethral mould-stent to allow better healing of the urethral incision obtained by optical urethrotomy. The Prostakath was unsuitable for use in urethral strictures because of its small calibre (21 Fr) and its very high migration rates. The idea of developing a new stent to insert into the bulbar or penile urethra after optical urethrotomy was discussed with the team which developed the Prostakath stent. Despite several attempts to reach a new design for this indication, its effectiveness could not be backed by clinical experience because the new stent always migrated. The failed search for a better stent gave birth to a new concept for a large calibre stent to be introduced in reduced profile and to self-expand when deployed, for use in urethral strictures.[10] The first generation of this self-expanding stent was made of stainless steel by InStent (Minneapolis, MN, USA) (Fig. 7.1). Its expanded calibre was 26/34 Fr and it could be reduced in calibre to 22 Fr by winding it on to a 20 Fr catheter. Differing from the 21 Fr fixed calibre stents, which had a smooth surface, this new stent was designed to self expand to a larger calibre and change its shape to a wavy outline after deployment in order to reduce migration. It was named the 'UroCoil'. This stent had a single-segment design anchored by its large 'shoulders'. The first UroCoil stent was bench-tested in 1989. The initial results of the use of this removable temporary stent in 18 patients were published in 1991.[10] This first-generation design could anchor much better than the 21 Fr smooth stents in the penile urethra, which has a natural calibre of up to 28–30 Fr. Initially, the single segment UroCoil was designed for use along the entire urethra. However, because of the differences in calibre along the urethra, the UroCoil was later found suitable to be used only in post-bulbar and pendulous urethral strictures. However, when used in the bulbar urethra it still migrated downstream because of the very large calibre of the bulbar urethra (which can reach up to 45 Fr). In order to prevent this migration and be able to use the UroCoil in bulbomembranous strictures, the stent was redesigned in order to anchor it in place. This new design was designated as the 'UroCoil-S' (Fig. 7.2). This design allowed the long segment of the UroCoil-S to stent the bulbar or membranous urethra, while its short prostatic segment, attached to the main body by a single helical trans-sphincteric wire passing along the external sphincter, to anchor the entire device in place. Because of the natural angulation between the bulbar and prostatic segments of the urethra, a straight connecting wire, such as that in the original Fabian stent or in its various modifications, would not allow the two segments of the stent to conform themselves to this

Figure 7.1. *The first-generation, stainless steel UroCoil stent.*

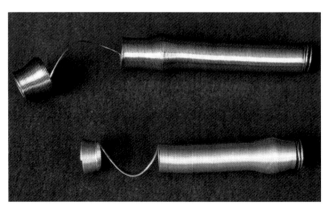

Figure 7.2. *Two first-generation UroCoil-S prototype stents (stainless steel and gold-plated stainless steel).*

angulation, because of the relative stiffness of the connecting wire. The helical connecting wire was designed to allow more flexibility to the device and prevent constant pressure of its bulbar segment on the posterior wall of the bulbar urethra, thus preventing decubitus or even perforation. A second advantage of the helical trans-sphincteric wire was to allow passage of rigid and flexible instruments up to 17 Fr through its lumen (Fig. 7.3). This was not possible with the first generation of the prostatic stents. Shortly afterwards, and based on the same principle, the 'ProstaCoil' design was developed as a by-product of the UroCoil-S stent, for use in the prostatic urethra (Fig. 7.4, top). The ProstaCoil had exactly the same design as the UroCoil-S but was mounted on the delivery catheter upside down: the long tubular part to 'tutor' the prostatic urethra (prostatic segment) was mounted distally and the short anchoring part (bulbar segment) was mounted proximally. The short bulbar segment was for anchoring the stent and to prevent its migration toward the bladder. These two segments again were connected by a helical trans-sphincteric wire. The ProstaCoil also was mounted on a delivery catheter, constricted to 22 Fr (Fig. 7.4, bottom). The ProstaCoil was used in benign and malignant prostatic obstructions.[11] The necessity of stenting a patient who had an obstructing prostate and a concomitant long bulbar stricture gave rise to the third configuration – the 'UroCoil-Twins' (Fig. 7.5). This configuration was designed to stent combined stenoses below and above the external sphincter. In this configuration, the prostatic and bulbar segments were almost equal in length and they were attached to each other, again by a single trans-sphincteric helical wire.

The introduction of UroCoil stents as a different approach in the treatment of urethral stricture disease opened a new era. The novel concept involved the placement of an internal mechanical 'tutor' in the dilated or incised stenotic urethra, leaving it in place long enough to act as a mould to prevent scar contraction and until stabilization of the scarring process around it, and then to be removed.

The initial experience with first-generation UroCoils also demonstrated their deficiencies. Because of the elastic limitations of stainless steel, which caused deformation of the stent after a certain point, the insertion calibre of the first-generation UroCoils and the ProstaCoil could not be reduced further. Design

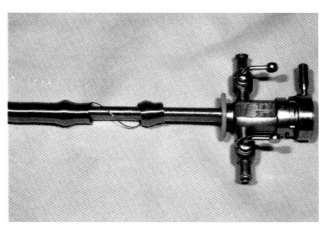

Figure 7.3. *A 17 Fr cystoscope passing through the entire length of a UroCoil/ProstaCoil stent.*

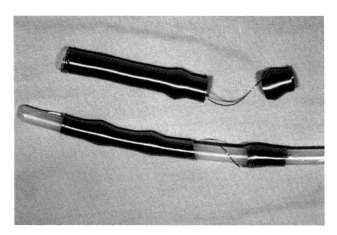

Figure 7.4. *The prototype of the stainless steel ProstaCoil stent.*

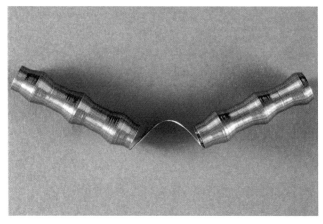

Figure 7.5. *Stainless steel UroCoil-Twins.*

modifications were carried out and also in the material these stents were made of: the stainless steel wire was replaced with a nickel-titanium alloy (Nitinol) wire. The Nitinol wire was preferred because of its super-elastic properties, allowing reducing the insertion calibre of the stent to 17 Fr without becoming deformed after its deployment. The stent, by self-expansion, became wavy with an alternating calibre of 24/30 Fr – 24 Fr at its narrow part and 30 Fr at its 'shoulders' after deployment. Although Nitinol allowed further reduction (even to 12 Fr) without causing deformation, this made the insertion length of the stent too long and very difficult to accurately position.

The urethral segments of all the UroCoil-System stents were available in lengths of 40–80 mm, in 10 mm increments, and the prostatic segment of the ProstaCoil stent was also similarly available in lengths of 40–80 mm. The length marked on the package of all the UroCoil/ ProstaCoil stents was the length of the urethral or prostatic segment of the released device. Before release, the length of the constricted stent was about 40% longer than its final released form (Fig. 7.6).

Differing from the 'Partial Catheter', which was inserted under endoscopic control, and the Prostakath, which was inserted under abdominal or transrectal sonographic control, the UroCoil and the ProstaCoil stents were inserted under fluoroscopy. To accurately measure the length of the occluded part of the urethra a fluoroscopic measuring catheter ruler was developed. This

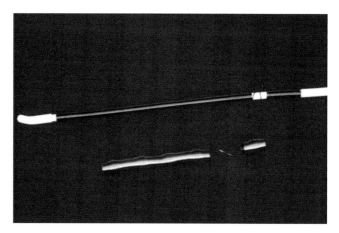

Figure 7.6. *Mounted and released Nitinol ProstaCoil stents.*

catheter ruler had radiopaque dots embedded at each 1 cm along its length (Fig. 7.7 a,b). Trials for endoscopic delivery of the UroCoil and ProstaCoil using a delivery mechanism to deploy the stents under vision was not successful and the idea was abandoned (Fig. 7.8).

By using one, or a combination of two or more of the three second-generation UroCoil stents, the entire urethra, from the bladder neck to the urethral meatus, could be covered in cases of recurrent strictures. This possibility was not – and still is not – provided by any other stent.

(a)

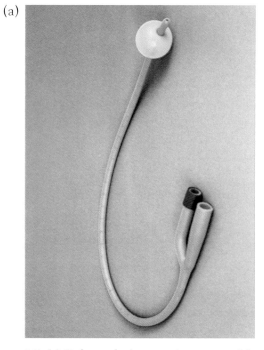

(b)

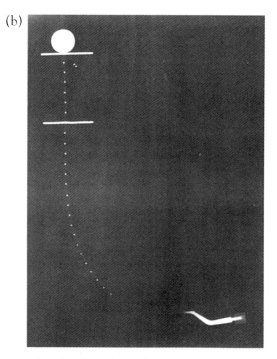

Figure 7.7. *(a) Catheter ruler for measuring segments of the urethra. (b) Radiopaque dots along the catheter ruler (the balloon is filled with contrast). The straight lines are radiopaque markers put on the skin to mark the bladder neck (top) and the external sphincter (bottom).*

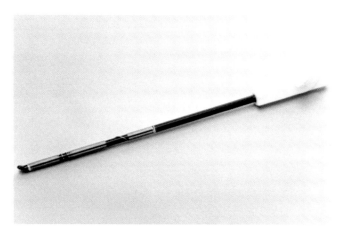

Figure 7.8. *Prototype of an endoscopic delivery mechanism for the UroCoil and ProstaCoil stents which was not clinically successful.*

The introduction of these first self-expanding temporary urological stents opened a new era in temporary stenting of other systems as well. Based on the same calibre-reducing technological principle of the UroCoil and ProstaCoil, new, non-urological stents were developed to be used in various parts of the body, such as the EndoCoil for the common bile duct, or the EsophaCoil for the oesophagus. Again, based on the same calibre-reducing technological principle the VascuCoil and the CardioCoil were developed for the peripheral vascular system and the coronary arteries.

References

1. Fabian K W. Der intraprostatische 'Partial Katheter' (urologische Spirale). Urologe A 1980; 19: 236–238
2. Fabricius P G, Matz M, Zepnick H. Die Endourethralspirale: eine alternative zum Dauerkatheter. Z Arztl Fortbild (Jena) 1983; 77: 482–485
3. Reuter H J, Oettinger M. Las primeras experiencias con la espiral de acero en lugar del cateter permanente. Arch Esp Urol 1986; 39 (suppl): 65–68
4. Nordling J, Holm H H, Klarskov P et al. The intraprostatic spiral: a new device for insertion with the patient under local anesthesia and with ultrasonic guidance with 3 months followup. J Urol 1989; 142: 756–758
5. Yachia D, Lask D, Rabinson S. Self retaining intraurethral stent: an alternative to long term indwelling catheters or surgery in the treatment of prostatism. AJR 1990; 154: 111–113
6. Nissenkorn S, Richter S. A new self-retaining intraurethral device. An alternative to an indwelling catheter in patients with urinary retention due to intravesical obstruction. Br J Urol 1990; 65: 197–200
7. Milroy E J G, Cooper J E, Wallstén H et al. A new treatment for urethral strictures. Lancet 1988; 1: 1424–1427
8. Williams G, White R. Experience with the Memotherm permanently implanted prostatic stent. Br J Urol 1995; 76: 337–340
9. Yachia D, Aridogan I A. Comparison between first generation (fixed calibre) and second generation (self-expanding, large calibre) temporary prostatic stents. Urol Int 1996; 57: 165–169
10. Yachia D, Beyar M. Temporarily implanted urethral coil stent for the treatment of recurrent urethral strictures: a preliminary report. J Urol 1991; 146: 1001–1004
11. Yachia D, Beyar M. Preservation of sexual function by insertion of 'ProstaCoil' instead of indwelling catheter in surgically unfit BPH patients. In: Proceedings of the Second International Congress in Therapy in Andrology, Bologna: Monduzi Editore, 1991: 399–402

History and status of bioabsorbable and biodegradable materials in urology

M. Talja

8

Introduction

The use of medical implants has a long history. Mention of the use of implant materials can be found in the medical writings of the early Hindu, Egyptian and Greek civilizations. Organ or tissue transplantation (autologous) from the same body is now a well-tried procedure, but donor site morbidity is a problem of concern. The use of non-living materials for implants has therefore become a logical and promising alternative in modern surgical practice.

Modern synthetic materials for applications in biological environments (biomaterials) may be classified as metals, polymers, ceramics and composites. Polymeric materials and their composites have been used in medical and surgical applications for 40 years. Typical indications for polymeric biomaterials are tissue replacement, tissue augmentation, tissue support, or delivery of therapeutic substances such as antibiotics or hormones.

On the basis of their behaviour in living tissue, polymeric biomaterials can be divided into three categories — biostable, biodegradable (absorbable or resorbable) and partially biodegradable. Typical biostable polymers (such as polyethylene and polypropylene) are widely used in permanent prostheses and sutures. However, in many cases the tissues need only the temporary presence of a biomaterial. In such cases, bioabsorbable polymeric materials (such as polyglycolide and polylactide) are more suitable than the biostable materials. The bioabsorbable polymeric or composite surgical materials retain their tissue-supporting properties for specific periods (from a few days to a year) and they are gradually degraded biologically into tissue-compatible components that are absorbed by living tissues and replaced by healing tissue. In general, the choice of the bioabsorbable material depends on the surgical target, the physical forces in that area and the speed of the healing process. The material and the device itself should retain their strength during the critical days of healing and the tissue response to the material should be minimal. The main benefit of the use of bioabsorbable

materials is, however, that there is no need for a second operation for their removal. The inflammatory reaction induced by cellular phagocytosis of degradation debris is minimal and varies according to the material and site of implantation.[1,2]

Bioabsorbable polymers in surgery

The first significant indication for bioabsorbable polymers was their use, since the 1960s as surgical suture materials. Kulkarni and co-workers reported the manufacture of bioabsorbable poly (lactic acid) (PLA) sutures in 1966.[3] In 1967, Schmitt and Polistina[4] developed the manufacture of poly (glycolic acid) (PGA) sutures, which led in 1970 to the first commercial synthetic bioabsorbable suture (Dexon®). Subsequently, there was intensive development of medical devices made of bioabsorbable polymers. As a result, a variety of different types of fixation implants in orthopaedics and maxillofacial surgery became available (Biofix®).[5] Biodegradable materials are regarded as highly biocompatible, with few side effects.[2,6,7]

Bioabsorbable materials in urology

Since 1980, different types of temporary and permanent stent have been introduced into urological practice to prevent obstruction of the prostatic urethra.[8–11] Stents are also used to prevent restenosis of the urethra.[12,15] Such stents previously were made of biostable polymers and metals.

The development of biodegradable devices for urological use started in the late 1980s in Finland as a result of encouraging experimental and clinical experience, mainly in the field of orthopaedics, with bioabsorbable implants. Nowadays a variety of biodegradable devices are available for experimental and clinical studies in urology.

The configuration of the first biodegradable urological device, selected from numerous models, was a helical spiral. The benefit of this device was that the mass of polymer material was relatively small in relation to the size of the device. The spiral configuration also conferred flexibility. The first spiral stents were relatively rigid and had a fixed calibre (non-expanding); the rigidity was achieved with use of supporting microspirals.[1] With progress in production technology, the benefits of material elasticity were discovered. The new generation of spiral stents gradually achieved their properties of self-expansion and controlled degradation.

Currently, the bioabsorbable materials used for urological spiral stents are PLA and PGA; these belong to the group of poly-alpha hydroxy acids which are derived from polyesters.

To achieve the precise mechanical properties specified, urological spiral stents (Biofix®, Bioscience Ltd, Tampere, Finland) are manufactured from PGA and PLA wires by extrusion and die-drawing.[7] After this self-reinforcing procedures (SR), filamentous (long polymer chains) material and matrix material have the same chemical composition. When the molecular microstructure is orientated parallel to the mechanical force, the modulus of elasticity and toughness of absorbable polymers increase significantly.[7] Mechanical properties depend also on the basic molecule and the length of the polymer chain. In addition, the configuration and thickness of the material are important factors in the degradation process.

Experimental and clinical experience in urology

Bacterial adherence

The ability of uropathogens to adhere to the urothelium or to the surface of urinary tract prosthetic devices is a well-known key event in the pathogenesis of urinary tract infection (UTI) and prolonged infection of the device. PGA and PLA have no antibacterial properties.[14] To investigate a possible method of preventing bacterial adhesion to the bioabsorbable materials, samples of SR-PGA and SR-PLA were immersed for one minute in tobramycin, ceftriaxone and ciprofloxacin solutions before incubation with two common uropathogenic bacteria (Enterococcus faecalis and Escherichia coli). Immersion in ciprofloxacin solution (200 mg in 100 ml saline) prevented the adherence of both bacteria; immersion in ceftriaxone solution prevented only the adherence of the E. coli and

immersion in tobramycin solution had no effect on either of the bacteria. After immersion in ciprofloxacin, the stent segments retained significant antibacterial activity even after 1 day's incubation in saline.[14] It is of great importance to confer more potent antibacterial properties on bioabsorbable polymer devices.

Anterior urethra

The anterior urethra was the first anatomical location for the use of bioabsorbable spiral stents in urology. After Milroy and co-workers[12] published their results in 1988 regarding the use of metallic urethral spiral stents to maintain patency of the strictured part of the urethra,[12] a programme to develop a bioabsorbable urethral stent was started. PLA was chosen as the material because of its degradation properties and prolonged (1 year) degradation time. The helical spiral was chosen as the configuration of the device and it was supported by three microspirals. The spirals were made of self-reinforcing poly-L-lactic acid (SR-PLLA; molecular weight 660, 000 Da) coated with PDLA (D configuration of PLA, molecular weight 100, 000 Da). Stainless steel helical spirals were used as controls in experimental studies with male rabbits. The study showed that the SR-PLLA spirals were totally covered by urethral epithelium after 6 months, at which time the mechanical strength of the spiral had already started to decrease. After 12 months the spirals were mostly degraded macroscopically. With the stainless steel devices, tissue penetration was less than that with the bioabsorbable spirals. Marked encrustation was also observed on the metallic stents. Microscopic analysis revealed extreme biocompatibility of the bioabsorbable stents, as well as their superior tissue penetration.[1]

Clinical results

Anterior urethra

The preliminary clinical results of a multicentre study in Finland with the expandable SR-PLLA double-helix spiral stent have been encouraging. A total of 16 patients with recurrent bulbous urethral stricture were included in the study. After internal urethrotomy, an SR-PLLA spiral stent with self-expansion properties was inserted into the stricture site. There was no need for external fixation of the stent because the outer diameter of the stent increases by 70% from the initial 8 mm

(24 Fr); this expansion is rapid, occurring mostly during the first 30 minutes. Urine was drained through a suprapubic catheter during day 1 and patients were allowed to void normally from postoperative day 2.[15] During the 6-month follow-up period, in two patients a recurrent stricture developed between the stent and the membranous urethra. In one case an epithelial overgrowth obstructed the device. Only in one case was stent migration observed.[15]

Bioabsorbable SR-PGA spiral stents have also been used as a tutor during free skin graft urethroplasty in cases of bulbar urethral stricture. The preputial free skin graft was mounted over the spiral stent. After internal urethrotomy, the graft was positioned endoscopically and sutured percutaneously to the site of the stricture. Suprapubic urinary diversion was used for 10 days. The preliminary results have been successful in all five patients with recurrent bulbar urethral strictures who underwent this procedure.[16]

Posterior urethra

In the management of bladder outlet obstruction caused by benign prostatic hypertrophy, many minimally invasive new methods have been introduced during the last decade. These methods are based on the effect of thermal energy on the prostate gland.

Such treatment induces transient tissue oedema, which leads to temporary exacerbation of the obstructive symptoms. In such procedures a biodegradable stent would be ideal to prevent the oedematous prostatic lobes from occluding the urethra, and thus to allow spontaneous voiding.

Biodegradable SR-PGA stents have been used with good results after visual laser ablation of the prostate (VLAP) to prevent postoperative retention.[17,18] The configuration of the spiral stent used is reminiscent of the shape of the Fabian spiral stent:[8] it has an outer diameter of 8 mm (24 Fr) and a prostatic portion 45 mm in length; the neck of the spiral located at the external sphincter is 20 mm long. At body temperature the outer diameter of the spiral stent increases by more than 60% because of the tendency of the spiral to straighten. The spiral was inserted by pushing it with the tip of the cytoscope into the prostatic urethra over a ureteral catheter as a guidewire. The neck of the stent was located in the membranous urethra under endoscopic guidance. The patients were allowed to void immediately.

In the early pilot study, the SR-PGA spiral stent was used after VLAP therapy in 22 patients to prevent postoperative retention. All patients urinated on postoperative day 1 or 2. Four cases of late retentions were noted: two were caused by too short a spiral and two by premature degradation of the prostatic part of stent. Some patients were aware of the early degradation of the stent because their obstruction intensified, as degradation occurred before the oedema induced by VLAP had totally resolved. Only a few patients detected soft fragments of the stent in the urine during voiding. The change in the peak urinary flow rate was from 8.1 (range 2.8–12.9) ml/s to 14.1 (5.3–30.9) ml/s ($p<0.002$) at 6 months. The change in symptom score (DAN PSS1) was from 16.2 to 3.0 ($p<0.01$). Only three patients developed UTI; no late complications were noted.

To date, experience with the SR-PGA spiral stent after VLAP therapy has involved more than 150 patients, and has shown its efficacy in preventing postoperative retention after VLAP. Because, in some patients, the degradation period of this spiral was too short, a material with a longer degradation period has been developed, to construct the SR-PLA 96 spiral stent. Experience with this stent in the same indication has also been encouraging. The total degradation period of the SR-PLA 96 stent was more than 6 months, but the spiral lost its mechanical strength after 3 months. However, this degradation period was too long and many patients suffered from irritative symptoms, caused by the softened device becoming bent in the prostatic fossa (see chapter 50).

SR-PGA spiral stents have also been used in combination with high-energy transurethral microwave thermotherapy (TUMT) to prevent postoperative urinary retention. Dalhstrand and co-workers have reported encouraging results.[19] Instead of requiring an indwelling catheter after TUMT for 14.1 ± 3 days in patients with a large prostatic volume (75.1 ± 21 cm^3), all patients fitted with a prostatic SR-PGA spiral stent were able to urinate immediately after therapy. The peak flow of these patients had increased from 6.1 ± 2.8 to 13.9 ± 3 ml/s when measured after 3 months. In the catheterized group, the peak flow rate was similar (13.3 ± 2.1 ml/s).

To prevent urinary retention, prostatic spiral stents could also be used in combination with other treatment modalities, such as transurethral needle ablation (TUNA), high-intensity focused ultrasound (HIFU), interstitial laser coagulation (ILC) of the prostate and cryotherapy. Other indications for the spiral stent might be temporary management of urinary retention in patients awaiting surgery, or in the early phase resolution of bladder outlet obstruction in patients waiting for medical therapy to take effect, or in cases of recurrent bladder neck stricture.

Upper urinary tract

There are many indications for stenting of the ureters, and bioabsorbable or biodegradable materials can also be used in the production of ureteral stents. In most cases only part of the ureter requires stenting. Results of preliminary animal experiments with such ureteral stents have been encouraging. In dogs, after transverse ureterotomy and insertion of a stent, the ureteral patency and healing process have been found to be comparable to that with conventional polyurethane stents. However, in two of 16 ureters stented with the SR-PLA 96, hydronephrosis and hydro-ureter were noted; in one of these cases the stent dislocated distally. The stents used in this experiment were not self-expanding;[20] stent migration may be prevented by using rapidly expanding stents.

The main indications for biodegradable stents in the ureter will be for postoperative stenting of the upper ureter after ureteropelvic junction incision and local ureteral trauma or defects. The degradation speed of the stents can be adjusted during the manufacturing process, so that the lower end of the stent will degrade more rapidly than the upper end; ureteral occlusion by stent fragments can thus be prevented.

Conclusions

The use of biodegradable and bioabsorbable devices is a new departure in urology. The spiral stent model has proved its efficacy in early experiments. However, further experimental and controlled clinical studies are needed to explore all the indications for the use of such devices in urology. An intensive study to pinpoint the best possible materials, models, coating materials and additives for bioabsorbable urological stents is on going. The use of biomaterials will probably also lead to new treatment methods in the future.

References

1. Kemppainen E, Talja M, Riihelä M et al. A bioresorbable urethral stent; an experimental study. Urol Res 1993; 21: 235–238

2. Bergsma J E, Rozema F R, Bos R R M et al. Biocompatibility and degradation mechanisms of predegraded and non-degraded poly(lactide) implants; an animal study. Mater Med 1995; 6: 715–724

3. Kulkarni R K, Pani K C, Neuman C, Leonard F. Polylactic acid for surgical implants. Arch Surg 1966; 93: 839

4. Schmitt E E, Polistina R A. Surgical sutures, US Pat 3,297,033, 1967

5. Vainionpää S, Rokkanen P, Törmälä P. Surgical applications of biodegradable polymers in human tissues. Prog Polym Sci 1989; 14: 679–716

6. Majola A, Vainionpää S, Vihtonen K et al. Absorption, biocompatibility and fixation properties of polylactic acid in bone tissue; an experimental study in rats. Clin Orthop 1991; 268: 260–269

7. Tormala P. Biodegradable self-reinforced composite materials; manufacturing structure and mechanical properties. Clin Mater 1992; 10: 29–34

8. Fabian K M. Der intraprostatische 'partielle Katheter' (urologische Spirale). Urologe A 1980; 19: 236

9. Nordling J, Holm H H, Klarskov P et al. The Intraprostatic Spiral: a new device for insertion with the patient under local anesthesia and with ultrasonic guidance with 3 months follow-up. J Urol 1989; 142: 756–758

10. Yachia D, Beyar M, Aridogan I A. A new, large caliber, self-expanding and self-retaining temporary intraprostatic stent (ProstaCoil) in the treatment of prostatic obstruction. Br J Urol 1994; 74: 47–49

11. Nissenkorn I, Richter S. A new self-retaining intraurethral device. Br J Urol 1990; 65: 197–200

12. Milroy E, Cooper J, Wallsten H et al. A new treatment for urethral strictures. Lancet 1988; 1: 1424

13. Yachia D, Beyar M. Temporarily implanted urethral Coil stent for the treatment of recurrent urethral stricture: a preliminary report. J Urol 1991; 146: 1001–1004

14. Cormio L, La Forgia P, Siitonen A et al. Immersion in antibiotic solution prevents bacterial adhesion onto biodegradable prostatic stents. Br J Urol 1997; 79: 409–413

15. Isotalo T, Tammela T, Talja M et al. Bioabsorbable SR-PLLA urethral stent in the treatment of recurrent urethral stricture. Endourol 11: Suppl 1; abstr BS2–8, 1997

16. Oosterlink V. Endoscopic urethroplasty with a free skin graft around resorbable polyglycolic acid urethral stent. XIIth Congress of the European Association of Urology, 1–4 September 1996, Paris. Eur Urol 1996; 30 (suppl 2): abstr 668

17. Talja M, Tammela T, Petas A et al. Biodegradable self-reinforced polyglycolic acid spiral stent in prevention of postoperative urinary retention after visual laser ablation of the prostate — laser prostatectomy. J Urol 1995; 154: 2089–2092

18. Pétas A, Talja M, Tammela T et al. A randomized study to compare biodegradable self-reinforced polyglycolic acid spiral stent to suprapubic and indwelling catheters after visual laser ablation of the prostate. J Urol 1997; 157: 173–176

19. Dahlstrand C, Grundtman S, Pettersson S. High energy TUMT and the use of resorbable stent for large benign prostatic hyperplasia. XIIth Congress of the Association of Urology, September 1-4, 1996, Paris. Eur Urol 1996; 30 (suppl 2): abstr 975

20. Lumiaho J, Heino A, Tunninen V et al. Kidney function after a ureteric lesion treated with a bioresorbable polylactide stent. Proc First ISUS Symposium: Jerusalem, October 1996 (abstr 012.3)

Radiation protection of patients and personnel during urological stenting

G. Bartal and I. Ben-Hasid

9

Introduction

The expanding use of image-guided urological procedures that require the use of fluoroscopy is associated with extensive radiation exposure of patients and personnel. Advances in radiological equipment have led to the incorporation of more powerful X-ray sources into the standard fluoroscopy systems. Basic training in interventional image-guided urological interventions barely includes some of the fundamentals of radiation protection. Radiation protection must be implemented in the daily practise of each image-guided physician (interventional radiologist, radiographer and endourologist). The image-guided surgeon must master all modern imaging modalities in order to choose the most effective and least hazardous one. Endourological procedures that comprise use of fluoroscopy require the same radiation protection practice as other interventional radiology procedures. The purpose of this chapter is to present a comprehensive and pragmatic approach to radiation protection for the practising image-guided endourologist.

Any medical exposure should be justified by weighing the benefits against the radiation detriment. Dose limits are not applied to medical exposures, yet any such exposure must be clinically justified and utilized only for the benefit of the patient, while the personnel are subject to strict dose constraints.[1-3]

X-rays initiate ionization of atoms and molecules in biological tissues through the deposition of energy. Ionization can initiate series of events that may lead to a biological effect.

Absorbed dose. Energy with potential biological effects deposited per unit mass. Absorbed dose is measured in units of gray (Gy) or milligray (mGy). An outdated unit of RAD is equivalent to 0.01 Gy.

Entrance skin dose (ESD). A measure of radiation dose absorbed at the skin entrance.

Organ dose (OD). Radiation absorbed by a particular organ in the exposed field. Various organs have different radiosensitivity that can be characteristic for any tissue and depends on the rate and intensity of biosynthesis and ferment activity.[4-7] Bone marrow has the highest radiosensitivity followed by lymphoid tissue, gonads, gastric epithelium, etc.

An *intensity* (*I*) of the X-ray beam decays while passing through space as the inverse square of the distance (*D*) from the X-ray tube: $I_2/I_1 = D_1^2/D_2^2$.

Doubling of the distance from the X-ray source is followed by a decrease in radiation intensity to one quarter, and so on.

During urological interventions, the gonads and most of the bone marrow (about 60%) are in the unattenuated primary radiation beam. The kidneys, pancreas, stomach and liver are situated in the attenuated secondary radiation zone.[8] As a result, fluoroscopically guided urological procedures carry a potentially high radiation dose to the patient and consequently to the staff.

Collimation. Adjustment of the irradiated field to the field of view (FOV) necessary for the procedure. Proper collimation reduces scattered radiation and improves image quality.

Two important technical variables have a great impact on patient dose-saving. Source (X-ray tube) to skin distance should be as far as possible, while patient to image intensifier distance must be kept at a minimum. Mobile C-arm fluoroscopy units that are used in operating rooms have a fixed X-ray tube to image intensifier distance. In such situations the X-ray tube should be positioned as far as possible from the patient and always situated under the operating table. Image magnification is always at the expense of a higher radiation dose and its use should be restricted.

The endourologist must be skilled in the use of endoscopic as well as fluoroscopic equipment and be able to integrate these methods intelligently. The goal is to reach the necessary minimum amount of radiation based on the ALARA (As Low As Reasonably Achievable) principle. Techniques that reduce patient dose also reduce scattered radiation, and provide an additional benefit of reducing exposure to the operator and the other staff members.

Any interventional procedure requires detailed preparation of the equipment and method. When sophisticated new devices are introduced, little if any attention is paid to the radiation protection during deployment. We routinely use a detailed flow-chart for each procedure, which is based on patient dose saving, without interfering with optimal procedural performance. The procedural flow-chart shows the order in which the entire procedure is routinely performed with special attention to the contrast media injection time, including only essential and the shortest necessary fluoroscopy time. Special attention is paid to the collimation of the exposed field. We managed to reduce the use of fluoroscopy to only five out of the nine routinely used components.

The endourologist usually performs interventional procedures in the operating room using a mobile fluoroscopy system that does not incorporate any radiation protection devices. Proper use of lead apron, lead collar, protective gloves and protective glasses, as well as the routine use of personal dosimeter and ring dosimeter are vital for the practising physician (Fig. 9.1). The working environment of the endourologist usually comprises a sitting position between the legs of the patient or standing alongside the patient in percutaneous procedures, very close to the irradiated area, adding another variable that contributes considerably to his/her radiation exposure (Fig. 9.2 a,b). Minimal and only necessary use of fluoroscopy using optimal collimation significantly reduces the exposure to the patient and the physician. Accurate monitoring and recording of patient exposure in each procedure is advocated.

Female personnel

Special consideration should be given to the female members of staff (the operator, assistant, nurse or radiographer). There might be a possibility of pregnancy in any one of the female staff members. During the

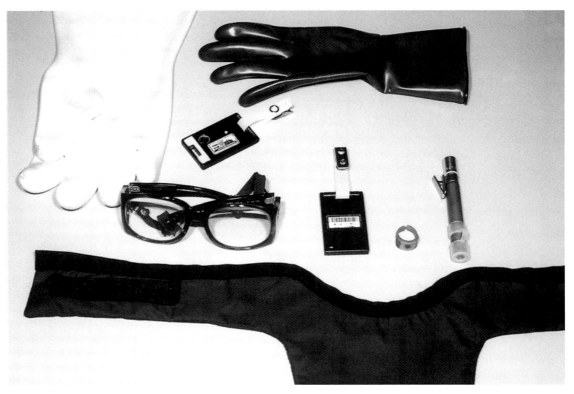

Figure 9.1. *Protective equipment for endourological procedures (in addition to the standard lead apron). Heavy and soft protective lead gloves, lead collar, protective glasses with lead lenses, dosimetric badges, dosimetric ring, personal dosimetric meter.*

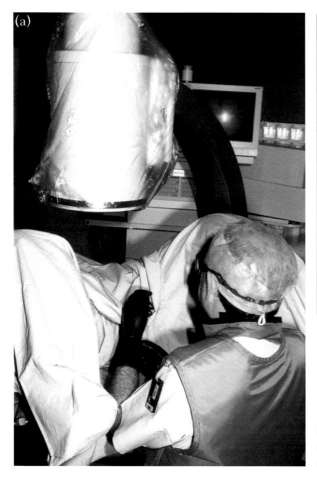

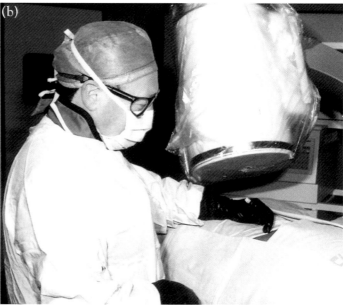

Figure 9.2. *Position of the urologist in endourological procedures. (a) Sitting at the end of the table with hands between patient's legs. (b) Standing alongside the table, with the tube at cranial-caudal angle.*

first trimester of pregnancy, female personnel are recommended not to be present during use of radiation. They should be outside the room while fluoroscopy is going on. If they must be in the room at this time, special precautions must be taken for the fetus' safety, such as, use of protective screens in addition to the lead aprons.

Any woman considered for urological imaging and/or endourological procedure that requires use of radiation, which may affect the uterus, should be asked if she is or might be pregnant, and be regarded as such unless the answer is a definite "no"[9].

Female patients

When a patient is regarded as pregnant, special care should be taken to determine whether the procedure is necessary or not. During the first trimester of pregnancy, use of fluoroscopy should be avoided, unless absolutely necessary. In the following trimesters, special measures should be taken to minimize possible exposure of the fetus.

The referring physician must enquire and make a written request that clarifies the necessity of the procedure despite pregnancy. All information shall be documented in writing in, the patient's record, including a description of the measures taken to protect the fetus, fluoroscopy time and if possible the amount of patient exposure.

Staff exposure must be closely monitored using special badges (TLD–S) in most instances. The operator requires at least two badges; chest, worn underneath the lead apron, and neck badge that should be worn outside the apron at the upper chest level. Ring badges are useful for image-guided procedures when the hands of the operator are close to or in the area of irradiation. Protective gloves are useful only for scattered radiation and not for the unattenuated beam. One must remember that the radiation protection gloves may provide a false feeling of security. It is strongly recommended to never expose the hands to the primary unattenuated beam. A practical tip is to cut off tips of the protective gloves for keeping the fingertips free, in order to preserve the skills of the endourologist, and use sterile gloves over the protective ones.

A bleeping personal dosimeter may be useful for trainees and for the evaluation of new fluoroscopy equipment or any new interventional procedure. Radiation protection must be an integral part of any procedural planning as well as the training of staff. Similar techniques of dose saving may be applied to any endourological procedure such as the following described method.[10–13]

Modified dose-saving method[14]

Prostatic urethral stent insertion under fluoroscopy (ProstaCoil)

We prepared an examination manifest, which showed the order of patient manipulation, time of contrast media administration, and quantity and time of X-ray execution. A study of the technological card performance process shows that there is no need for fluoroscopy accompaniment during any phase of the examination. Only five out of nine general elements required fluoroscopy.

The following are elements that are associated with higher radiation in fluoroscopy:

- external sphincter identification and marking
- measurement of the prostatic urethra
- ProstaCoil insertion and placement.

Following the standardization of the fluoroscopy time programme, we succeeded to save patient dose by 53.8%. Fluoroscopy time-recording is conducted routinely (fluoroscopy time must be displayed on the X-ray machines). Last image hold (LIH) must be used routinely in order to understand the images and to plan further procedural phases, using fluoroscopy only when obligatory. The use of new and modern technology with incorporated LIH provides a 0.3 minute (18 s) decrease in fluoroscopy time during the urethral length measurement phase, which represents about 5% of the procedural fluoroscopy time.

During invasive urological procedures performed both by radiologist and urologist, the main role is that of the urologist. The radiologist has a secondary role. The radiologist must create optimal fluoroscopy conditions for the urologist and document the procedure. In some institutions, the radiographer is a person in charge of the equipment and a surgeon performs the fluoroscopy. This division of roles provides the urologist with the option of observing obtained images (LIH) as much as possible, and using fluoroscopy only when necessary. Due to the increase in fluoroscopy time, the patient and the personnel are also exposed to a greater amount of radiation. Therefore, urological procedures, which use ionizing radiation, belong to the group of procedures with higher level patient exposure.

A solution for decreasing the problem of patient radiation would be to standardize the entire cycle of the urological procedure. We recommend a comprehensive approach to standardize invasive procedures:

1. Study of invasive and non-invasive examination protocols performed under fluoroscopy control.
2. Accurate recording of fluoroscopy time and patient exposure for each phase of the procedure.
3. Method standardization.

Fluoroscopically guided endourological procedures carry considerable and, in some instances, high patient doses. Critical analysis of the examination protocols based on the dose saving regulations provides good quality diagnostic images with reduced patient dose. For example: changing posterior/anterior (PA) projection to oblique (about 30°) can reduce patient dose by 20% (Fig. 9.3 a,b,c).

Conclusions: practical recommendations[15–18]

1. ALARA principle must be maintained.
2. Predefined method should be followed step-by-step using fluoroscopic guidance only during required phases of examination. Precise knowledge of procedural method and expected results (what we want to see and can acquire).
3. Reduce fluoroscopy time using intermittent fluoroscopy and last-image hold.
4. Use only dose-saving projections.
5. Collimate and use an optimal and only necessary field of view.
6. Proper use of protective apron, lead collar, protective glasses and personal dosimeters (badges) for the personnel. Always keep in mind that the front of the wrap-around apron has a double lead equivalent compared to its back (i.e. 0.5 mm/0.25 mm).

X-Ray field size in PA projection (mSv)

(a)

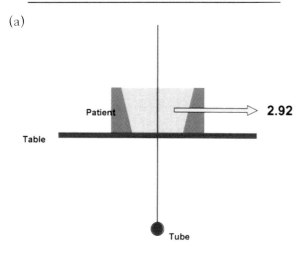

X-Ray field size in PA projection (30⁰ table tilt)

(b)

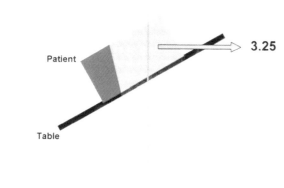

X-Ray field size in oblique projection (30⁰ RPO)

(c)

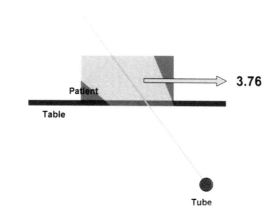

Figure 9.3. *Changing posterior/anterior (PA) projection of the tube to oblique (about 30°) can reduce patient dose by 20%. (a) X-ray field size in PA projection. (b) X-ray field size in PA projection (30° table tilt). (c) X-ray field size in oblique projection (30° right posterior oblique).*

Therefore, the staff members should never turn their backs towards the radiation source (the tube and/or examination table).

7. Precise location and movement of all persons present in the room during the procedure.

References

1. National Radiological Protection Board. Patient dose reduction in diagnostic radiology. Report by the Royal College of Radiologists and NRPB: Documents of the NRPB. Vol. 1, No. 3. London: HMSO, 1990

2. Radiological protection for medical exposure to Ionizing Radiation. Safety Guide. Safety standard series No. RS-G-1.5. Vienna: International Atomic Energy Agency (IAEA), 2002

3. Avoidance of radiation injuries from medical interventional procedures Annals of the ICRP (International Commission on Radiological Protection) Vol. 30, Issue 2, Publication 85. Vienna: ICRP, 2000

4. Feinedegen L E, Loken M K, Booz J, Muhlensiepen H, Sondhaus C A, Bond V P. Cellular mechanisms of production and repair induced by radiation exposure and their consequences for cell system responses. Stem Cells 1995; 13 (Suppl 1): 7–20

5. Sandborg, M. Radiology UK 1996. Applications of Monte Carlo methods in diagnostic imaging. Department of Radiation Physics, Faculty of Health Sciences, Linkoping University, Sweden

6. O'Donnell C, Gallacher D, Wilkinson M L, Ede R J, Batchelor S. Radiology UK 1996. Radiation protection: Radiation protection in endoscopic retrograde cholangiopancreatography (ERCP) procedures for staff and patients. Medical Physics Directorate and Department of Gastroenterology, Guy's and St. Thomas' Hospital Trust, London, UK

7. Cohen B E. Cancer risk from low-level radiation. Review. AJR 2002; 179: 1137–1143

8. Bartal G, Ben-Hasid I. The effect of pulse fluoroscopy in patient radiation exposure in vascular interventional radiology. Annual CIKSE Meeting 1998, Venice, Italy.

9. Sharp C, Shrimpton J A, Bury R F. Diagnostic Medical Exposures: Advice in exposure to ionizing radiation during pregnancy. National Radiology Protection Board, 1998

10. Quinn A D, Sabharwal T, Taylor C, Sikdar T. Physics: Radiation Protection: Radiation protection awareness in non-radiologists. X-ray Department, Charing Cross Hospital, Hammersmith, UK

11. Njeh C F, Goldstone K E. Physics: Radiation Protection. Significance of shielding and location of personnel around couch to the radiation dose in interventional cardiology. East England Regional Radiation Protection Service, Addenbrooke's Hospital, Cambridge, UK

12. Beaconsfield T, Safar-Aly H K, Shorvon P J. Physics: Radiation protection. Radiation and fluoroscopy: are you getting an eyeful? Department of Radiology, Central Middlesex Trust Hospital, Acton Lane, London, UK

13. Bailey E, Cole P R, Crawford P, Moores B M. infoRAD™. Simulation learning in radiation protection (SLIRP). Research and Development Department, Integrated Radiological Services Ltd, Liverpool and Physics and Astronomy Department, University of Central Lancashire, UK

14. Bartal G, Ben-Hasid I, Yachia D. Method of stenting bladder outlet obstruction using low-dose radiation. 1st International Symposium on Urological Stents Jerusalem, Israel, October 1996

15. Gray J E, Ragozzino M W, Van Lysel M S, Burke T M. Normalized organ doses for various diagnostic radiology procedures. AJR 1981; 137: 463–470

16. Vano E, Arranz L, Sastre J M, et al. Dosimetric and radiation protection considerations based on some cases of patient skin injuries in interventional cardiology. Br J Urol 1998; 71: 510–516

17. Koenig T R, Wolff D, Mettler F A, Wagner L K. Skin injuries from fluoroscopically guided procedures. AJR (2001); 177(1,2): 3–20

18. Vano E, Gonzalez L, Beneytez F, Moreno F. Lens injuries induced by occupational exposure in non-optimized interventional radiology laboratories. Br J Urol 1998; 71: 728–733

Stent materials

Characteristics of materials used in implants: metals
I. Gotman

Introduction

Metals are by far the oldest materials used in surgical procedures. The earliest records of the use of metallic implants in surgery go back to the 16th century, with most cases representing the application of a noble metal to repair a localized structural defect. For example, Ambroise Paré described, in 1546, the use of gold plates for the repair of traumatic defects in the skull and of gold wire for the repair of abdominal hernias, and Petronius, in 1565, suggested the use of gold plates for the repair of cleft palates. In 1666, Fabricius described the use of gold, bronze and iron wires in surgical procedures. More than a hundred years later, in 1775, the first fixation of a bone fracture with an iron wire was performed. It was also during this period that the first animal experiments were conducted to determine tissue tolerance to implant materials. In 1829, Levert tested silver, gold, lead and platinum wires in dogs and concluded that platinum was the least irritating metal. It is very difficult, however, to interpret the results of any implant operation performed in those early days when tissue reaction to an implant could not be distinguished from inflammation due to infection. This became possible in the 1880s, with Lister's introduction of antiseptic surgical techniques that sharply reduced the incidence of infection. The following years saw a rapid development in implant surgery accompanied by the introduction of newly developed metals and alloys into clinical practice. In the 1950s, materials other than metals started to find their way into implant surgery. At present, a wide range of materials are used in medical applications including metals, ceramics and polymers.

Generally speaking, the performance of any biomedical material is controlled by two characteristics — biofunctionality and biocompatibility.[1] Biofunctionality defines the ability of the device to perform the required function, while biocompatibility determines the compatibility of the material with the body. For metallic biomaterials that are typically used in orthopaedic implants and prosthetic heart valves, the functional requirements are high mechanical properties — yield strength, ductility, fatigue strength and fracture toughness. These requirements are usually not as stringent as those found in many advanced engineering applications where hundreds of metals and alloys are used successfully. At the same time, the number of metals and alloys currently being used in surgical applications is extremely limited. It is clear that the reason for this resides not so much within the considerations of biofunctionality as within the considerations of biocompatibility. Phenomena covered by the term biocompatibility relate to the interactions between an implant and a physiological environment — an environment that is both extremely hostile and yet sensitive to, and unforgiving of, irritating foreign species. The result of such interaction is material degradation or, in the context of metals, corrosion. Unlike most engineering applications, the importance of corrosion in surgery lies not so much in the effect that it has on structural integrity of the implant as in the release of corrosion products into the surrounding tissue. Since the adverse effect of corrosion products on the patient can lead to rejection of the implant, the history of implant metal development has been largely one of seeking the most corrosion-resistant materials. At the beginning of the century, a large number of metals and alloys — such as aluminium, copper, zinc, iron and carbon steels, silver, nickel and magnesium — were tested for implantation, and all were found to be too reactive in the body and, therefore, unsuitable for implant use. Today, in the early 21st century, commonly used metallic biomaterials belong to one of the three good corrosion-resistant alloy systems, and these are iron–chromium–nickel alloys (austenitic stainless steels), cobalt–chromium-based alloys, and titanium and its alloys. Other metals that find miscellaneous uses in surgery include tantalum and some precious-metal alloys for electrodes.

Stainless steel

The most widely used stainless steel in medical applications is type 316L austenitic stainless steel. This is an alloy primarily of iron, chromium and nickel with the composition shown in Table 10.1. At room temperature, iron exists in a crystal structure termed ferrite, and it transforms to a high-temperature phase called austenite when heated above 910°C. Nickel is added to the alloy to stabilize the austenitic phase down to room temperature; hence the name 'austenitic' stainless steel. The most important alloying constituent in stainless steel is chromium, which should have a concentration of at least 12% for the steel to develop a passive chromium oxide film necessary for corrosion resistance. Minimal carbon content is highly desirable,

as carbon precipitation in the form of chromium carbides, in the temperature range 450–900°C, can severely impair corrosion resistance.

Cobalt–chromium-based alloys

The compositions of two representative Co–Cr-based surgical alloys are shown in Table 10.2. These alloys owe their excellent corrosion resistance to the high content of chromium (approx. 30 %). The carbon-containing cast Co–Cr alloy is characterized by the presence of block carbides in its microstructure that contribute to the material's superior wear resistance. Therefore, cast Co–Cr alloy is the metal of choice for the articulating surfaces of joint replacements. The MP35N alloy was developed for the manufacture of highly stressed

Table 10.1. *Chemical composition of surgical 316L stainless steel*

Element	Percentage composition (w/w)	
	ASTM F55 (1982)	ASTM F138 (1986)
C (carbon)	0.03 (max.)	0.03 (max.)
Mn (manganese)	2.00 (max.)	2.00 (max.)
P (phosphorus)	0.03 (max.)	0.025 (max.)
S (sulphur)	0.03 (max.)	0.010 (max.)
Si (silicon)	0.75 (max.)	0.75 (max.)
Cr (chromium)	17.00–20.00	17.00–19.00
Ni (nickel)	12.00–14.00	13.00–15.50
Mo (molybdenum)	2.00–4.00	2.00–3.00
N_2 (nitrogen)	0.10 (max.)	—
Cu (copper)	0.50 (max.)	—
Fe (iron)	Balance	Balance

Table 10.2. *Chemical composition of Co–Cr surgical alloys*

Element	Percentage composition (w/w)	
	Cast Co–Cr–Mo [ASTM F85 (1982)]	Wrought MP 35N [ASTM F562 (1984)]
Cr (chromium)	27.0–30.0	19.0–21.0
Mo (molybdenum)	5.0–7.0	9.0–10.5
Ni (nickel)	1.0 (max.)	33.0–37.0
Fe (iron)	0.75 (max.)	1.0 (max.)
C (carbon)	0.35 (max.)	0.025 (max.)
Si (silicon)	1.0 (max.)	0.15 (max.)
Mn (manganese)	1.0 (max.)	0.15 (max.)
P (phosphorus)	—	0.015 (max.)
S (sulphur)	—	0.010 (max.)
Ti (titanium)	—	1.0 (max.)
Co (cobalt)	Balance	Balance

anchorage stems of total hip prostheses. The high strength of this alloy is the result of a cold work-induced phase transformation from alpha-Co to epsilon-Co followed by the precipitation of intermetallic phases.

Titanium and its alloys

Titanium and titanium alloys are relatively new materials compared with stainless steels and cobalt-based alloys. Unalloyed titanium exists in two different structural modifications — as alpha phase at room temperature and as beta phase above 883°C. The addition of alloying elements stabilizes either the alpha or beta phase, and titanium alloys are classified as alpha, beta or alpha-beta alloys on the basis of the phases present at room temperature. An alpha-beta Ti-6 Al-4 V alloy (Table 10.3) is most commonly used in medical applications. Three other alpha-beta alloys used to a lesser extent are Ti-3 Al-2.5 V, Ti-5 Al-2.5 Fe, and Ti-6 Al-7 Nb. The development of low-modulus beta-titanium alloys with high strength, such as Ti–Nb–Ta, Ti–Nb–Ta–Zr, Ti–Mo–Ta–Zr and Ti–Mo–Nb–Zr, is also attracting greater attention.[2] The main drawback of titanium and its alloys is their inadequate wear resistance.

Table 10.3. *Chemical composition of Ti-6 Al-4 V surgical alloy [ASTM F136 (1984)]*

Element	Percentage composition (w/w)
N_2 (nitrogen)	0.05 (max.)
C (carbon)	0.08 (max.)
H_2 (hydrogen)	0.012 (max.)
Fe (iron)	0.25 (max.)
O_2 (oxygen)	0.13 (max.)
Al (aluminium)	5.50–6.50
V (vanadium)	3.50–4.50
Ti (titanium)	Balance

Fundamentals of implant metal corrosion

With the exception of a few noble metals, metallic materials never occur in their elemental form and are usually found in nature in combination with non-metallic elements in ores. Pure metals produced by reduction from ores are thermodynamically unstable, and will tend to lower their free energy by reacting with the environment to form a compound. This spontaneous chemical reaction of a metal with a liquid or a gas is known as corrosion.

Surgical implants are expected to function in the body fluids consisting of an aqueous solution of various anions, cations and biological macromolecules. The severe corrosivity of the bioenvironment is largely determined by the presence of chloride ions (0.11 N, interstitial fluid). In addition, biological macromolecules, and specifically the proteins in extracellular fluids, are able to influence corrosion considerably. It has long been established that the process of metal corrosion in an aqueous medium of the sort provided by the body fluids is electrochemical in nature. When a metal surface is exposed to an aqueous solution, it becomes the site for two types of chemical reaction. There is an oxidation, or anodic reaction that produces electrons:

$$Me \rightarrow Me^{n+} + ne^{-} \qquad (1)$$

and a reduction, or cathodic reaction that consumes the electrons produced by the anodic reaction. The reduction of dissolved oxygen and the reduction of hydrogen ions with the release of gaseous hydrogen are the two principal cathodic reactions:

$$O_2 \text{ (diss)} + 4e^{-} + H_2O \rightarrow 4OH^{-} \qquad (2)$$

$$2H^{+} + 2e^{-} \rightarrow H_2(g) \qquad (3)$$

Since the body fluids are characterized by nearly neutral pH values, reaction (2) is typically the one most relevant to implant corrosion. However, reaction (3) must be considered in confined areas where pH can reach acidic values because of the restricted oxygen supply or the large concentrations of H^{+} ions that cannot readily move out.

The immediate consequence of the anodic oxidation process is metal loss, or corrosion. The flow of electrons produced by the anodic reaction to the cathode constitutes the corrosion current, the value of which is determined by the rate of corrosion. In order for electrons to flow between the anodes and the cathodes there must exist a driving force. This driving force is the difference in potential between the anodic and cathodic sites. The difference exists because each oxidation or reduction reaction has associated with it a potential determined by the tendency for the reaction to take place spontaneously. The potential is the measure of this tendency.

A metal in contact with a solution containing its metal ions at unit activity establishes a fixed potential difference with respect to every other metal in the same condition. The list of these potentials comprises the standard electrochemical series given in Table 10.4. This electrochemical series is arranged with the most noble metals, such as gold or platinum, at the top and increasingly electronegative or base metals as one proceeds down the list. The greater the negative potential of a metal, the greater its reactivity and the lower its corrosion resistance in pure water.

While the standard electrochemical series in Table 10.4 is frequently very useful as a guide to corrosion behaviour, its main drawback is that it does not take into consideration factors other than equilibrium thermodynamics. In reality, the potentials obtained will differ considerably if the metal surface is bare or if it is passivated, i.e. covered by a thin, adherent, continuous protective oxide film. A slightly better indication of corrosion behaviour of metals and alloys can be obtained by measuring their electrode potentials when immersed in specific solutions, for example in saline solutions (Table 10.5). The most notable difference between the series in Tables 10.4 and 10.5 is that in saline solutions titanium moves well up the list,

reflecting the highly insoluble nature of the TiO_2 passivation layer that forms spontaneously in air.

As can be seen from Eqns (1)–(3), the reactions involved in metal corrosion are governed by the transfer of electrons and/or by the concentration of hydrogen or hydroxyl ions. Therefore, the two main variables that control electrochemical corrosion are the electrode potential of the metal and the pH of the solution. The relationship between the corrosion behaviour and the dual parameters of electrode potential and pH are displayed graphically by Pourbaix diagrams. A simplified version of the diagram for titanium is given in Figure 10.1. Such diagrams are much more useful for predicting the behaviour of a metal in a specific environment than are simple standard electrode potentials. Using the Pourbaix diagrams it can be determined, on a thermodynamic basis, whether a metal surface is in a region where no corrosion is possible (*immunity*), in a region where corrosion is expected (*corrosion*), or in a region where the tendency for corrosion still exists but where a corrosion product film forms that may confer protection against corrosion (*passivation*). Whether the film is protective (passive) or not is a kinetic consideration and not a thermodynamic one and cannot be deduced from the Pourbaix diagram. Lines A and B

Table 10.4. *The electrochemical series of metals**

NOBLE END	
Gold	+ 1.45
Platinum	+ 1.20
Silver	+ 0.80
Copper	+ 0.34
Hydrogen	0.00
Molybdenum	− 0.20
Nickel	− 0.25
Cobalt	− 0.28
Iron	− 0.44
Chromium	− 0.73
Titanium	− 1.63
Aluminium	− 1.66
Magnesium	− 2.37
Lithium	− 3.05
ACTIVE END	

*Normal electrode potentials measured in volts at 25°C.

Table 10.5. *The galvanic series in saline solutions*

NOBLE END
Platinum
Gold
Silver
Titanium
316 Stainless steel (passive)
304 Stainless steel (passive)
410 Stainless steel (passive)
Nickel (passive)
Copper
Nickel (active)
Tin
Lead
316 Stainless steel (active)
304 Stainless steel (active)
410 Stainless steel (active)
Wrought iron
Aluminium
Zinc
Magnesium
ACTIVE END

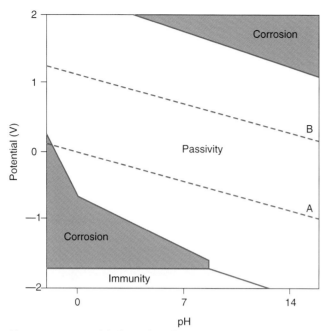

Figure 10.1. *Simplified Pourbaix diagram for titanium showing the gaseous evolution lines A and B.*

represent, respectively, Eqns (2) and (3): above A the conditions are sufficiently oxidizing for oxygen to be released, and below B water is reduced and hydrogen is evolved. Thus all stable aqueous solutions lie between lines A and B.

As indicated above, the suppression of corrosion by the continued presence of a stable oxide on the surface constitutes the phenomenon known as passivity, and those metals and alloys that rely on such a film for their resistance to corrosion are referred to as passive materials. All the metallic materials used in surgery fall into this category: stainless steels and cobalt–chromium alloys are protected by a chromium oxide layer, Cr_2O_3, whereas titanium and its alloys are protected by a titanium oxide/rutile layer, TiO_2. The important point about their passivity and corrosion resistance is the nature of the conditions that will cause breakdown of the oxide film and produce corrosion. The tendency of passive alloys to undergo loss of passivity after prolonged exposure to body fluids can be predicted by suitable electrochemical measurements.

When placed in an aqueous saline solution, an implant metal tends to dissolve until the reversible potential of the anodic reaction (Eqn 1) — the potential where the metal is in equilibrium with its ions — has been reached. The amount lost at this stage

would generally be insignificant. This equilibrium, however, is upset by the cathodic reaction removing the excess electrons from the metal. As a result, a current flows between the anodic and the cathodic areas, and the potentials of both are changed. The anode and cathode are said to be polarized, and the potential difference between them is reduced, as shown schematically in Figure 10.2. When the potential difference is reduced to zero, an open circuit or rest potential is reached, which is also called corrosion potential, E_{corr}, because it is a potential at which corrosion is occurring. The corrosion current density, i_{corr}, is directly proportional to the corrosion rate.

When the rest potential of a metal or alloy immersed in a simulated physiological solution, such as Hanks' or Ringer's solution, is plotted as a function of time, three types of behaviour are observed depending on the character of the metal (Fig. 10.3). The potential that drops rapidly and remains low (curve a) indicates that there is a complete film breakdown after immersion and general corrosion is taking place. A curve rising to a high level and remaining there over a long period of time (curve b) is indicative of a passive metal or alloy. In the early stages, any imperfections in the air-formed film are made good by reactions with the solution and the film may thicken slightly. Thereafter, the situation stabilizes with slight chemical dissolution of the outer film surface and very slow diffusion of metal through the oxide, but no gross corrosion. In between is curve c which refers to a material in which there is initial film thickening but some film breakdown thereafter. This

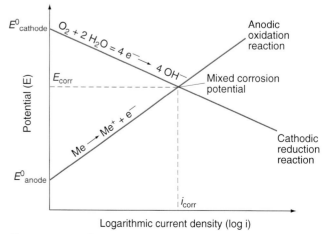

Figure 10.2. *Schematic representation of polarization of anodic and cathodic reactions.*

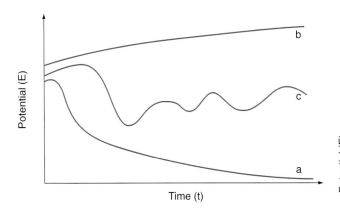

Figure 10.3. *Isolated electrode potentials as a function of time for (a) metal that exhibits film breakdown after immersion, (b) metal with intact film, and (c) metal that exhibits film breakdown after initial thickening.*

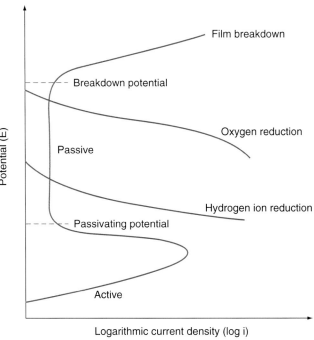

Figure 10.4. *Typical anodic polarization curve of a passive metal showing oxygen and hydrogen ion reduction reversible potentials.*

represents the condition of localized corrosion known as pitting, in which small areas on the metal surface are rapidly attacked while the remainder of the surface remains passive and unaffected.

Of the metals relevant to surgical applications, titanium and its alloys, cobalt–chromium alloys and tantalum exhibit a truly passive behaviour described by curve b. Unlike this, the potential–time curve for the most corrosion-resistant 316 stainless steel is of a fluctuating nature, indicating a strong propensity toward film breakdown.

In establishing the corrosion resistance of implant metals, the relation between the rest potential and the potential at which breakdown of passivity occurs is most important. The breakdown potential is determined from an anodic polarization curve which, for a system exhibiting passivity, looks like that shown in Figure 10.4. With an increase in potential, the current initially increases, but when the potential reaches the value of the passivating potential, E_{pp}, the critical current density is observed. This is the onset of passivity, and, even though the potential is increased to higher values, the current density, i_p (corrosion rate) remains low. When the potential reaches the value of E_b, film breakdown occurs and pitting ensues.

In Table 10.6, the values of the rest potential after 480 h in de-aerated 0.17 M saline and the breakdown potential in the same solution are given for several surgical metals.[3] It can be seen that with stainless steel the two potentials are about the same, so that the alloy

Table 10.6. *Resting and breakdown potentials of major surgical metals and alloys*

Material	Resting potential (V) after 480 h*	Breakdown potential (V)*
304 Stainless steel	0.20	0.20
316 Stainless steel	0.3–0.5	0.4–0.48
Cast cobalt–chromium alloy	0.5	0.87
Titanium	0.37	9.0
Typical titanium alloy	0.23	25.0
Tantalum	0.36	24.0

*In de-aerated 0.17 M sodium chloride.

is unlikely to resist pitting in the body. Many other stainless steels and nickel fall into this category. With the cobalt–chromium alloy, the rest potential is below the breakdown potential so that film breakdown is unlikely but possible under exceptional conditions.

With titanium, the difference between the two potentials is so great that breakdown is impossible under conditions in the body. A further point here is that, in media containing oxygen and water, breakdown at high potential is avoided if the breakdown potential is more positive than the oxygen reduction reversible potential, as shown in Figure 10.4. Similarly, activity at low potential (as in crevices) is avoided if the passivating potential is more negative than the water (hydrogen ion) reduction reversible potential. Titanium and its alloys — and probably some alloys based on zirconium, niobium and tantalum — appear to be the only materials in this category. For the cobalt–chromium alloy, the breakdown potential and the oxygen reduction reversible potential are very close, so that film breakdown is extremely unlikely but not impossible.

Corrosion in clinical practice

It can be understood from the above discussion that titanium and its alloys should never corrode in body fluids, that cobalt–chromium-based alloys should become the subject of corrosive attack only very rarely and under exceptional circumstances, and that 316L stainless steel is quite susceptible to film breakdown and local corrosion. These conclusions are confirmed by clinical observations of corrosion in vivo. Indeed, corrosion is never a clinical problem with titanium alloy implants, and the cases of corrosive attack on cobalt–chromium medical devices are extremely rare. At the same time, corrosion occurs to a significant extent in stainless steel implants, the major mechanisms being intergranular corrosion, crevice corrosion, pitting, fretting corrosion, and galvanic corrosion.

It could be instructive to consider the spontaneous breakage of a gold-plated stainless steel urological coil reported by Yachia[4] (Fig. 10.5), apparently caused by coupling steel with gold which gave rise to galvanic corrosion. Figure 10.6 shows a schematic of a gold-plated stainless steel wire. As long as the coating is intact, it will effectively protect the steel substrate from contact with

the body fluids. The corrosion of such a device will be minimal, owing to the very high corrosion resistance of gold. However, if there is a small scratch or another defect in the gold coating, the situation will change drastically. Now, both stainless steel and gold are exposed to the body fluid, and a galvanic couple will be formed. As can be seen from the galvanic series (Table 10.5), stainless steel is a much less noble metal than gold, and it will become the anode, i.e. the corroding electrode of the galvanic couple. The magnitude of the corrosion current depends on the reactions at the cathode (gold), and it will be the stronger the larger the cathodic area. Since the anodic area, i.e. the area of exposed steel, is very small, the current density will be very high. In this case, the rate of corrosion may be several orders of magnitude greater than it would be in the same steel without the gold plating, and it will soon lead to the breakage of the

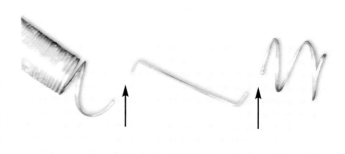

Figure 10.5. *Removed parts of a broken gold-plated stainless steel coil. Spontaneous breakage points (arrows).*

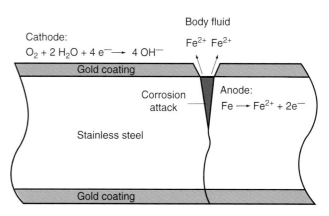

Figure 10.6. *Schematic of a gold-plated steel wire illustrating the formation of a galvanic couple.*

thin wire. Thus, coating stainless steel with a more noble metal may result in enhanced corrosion, and from this point of view, the use of gold-plated urological coils should be re-evaluated.

In spite of numerous reports of stainless steel implant corrosion in the body environment, it is only in rare cases that corrosion attack leads to failure of the device. At the same time, corrosion products are found in the tissues, and signs of corrosion attack are often observed on implants that had to be removed only because the patient complained of associated pain. The growing recognition of the adverse long-term effect of corrosion debris and dissolved metal ions on the patient's health has led to the decision not to use stainless steels as permanent implants. At present, the use of 316L stainless steel is limited to temporary devices with service life not exceeding 12 months.

Even in the absence of frank corrosion, as it is the case for Co–Cr-based and Ti alloys, elevated concentrations of metal ions are detected in tissues around the implant, as well as in serum, urine and remote tissue locations. This is the result of the slow passive dissolution of ions from the protective layer that takes place even in the most corrosion-resistant passivated metals. In the case of Ti, passive ion dissolution often results in the characteristic tissue discolouration around the implant. No negative clinical implications of such discolouration have been reported, and Ti is generally considered as a very toxicologically benign metal. Nevertheless, the presence of V and Al in the most commonly used Ti-6Al-4V alloy arouses some concern, and much effort is currently being directed towards the development of V- and Al-free Ti alloys.

Local tissue response to metal implants is closely related to the amount and toxicity of the corrosion products. Thus, minimal fibrosis is typically observed around Ti alloys, whereas fibrous layers up to 2 mm thick are encountered with Co–Cr and, especially, steel implants. The presence of a fibrous layer results in the lack of firm union between the implant and the surrounding tissue, and it is obviously detrimental when rigid fixation of the implant is sought. However, in the cases where ease of removal is desired, as, for example, with temporary urological stents, a certain degree of fibrosis may even be beneficial. Clearly, of the three widely used surgical alloys generally accepted as good biomaterials, stainless steel is the least biocompatible.

Both cobalt–chromium and titanium alloys offer a clear advantage in corrosion resistance and general biocompatibility; however, none of these materials can be considered 'ideal' or permanent.

A separate issue of biocompatibility is thromboresistance, or blood compatibility. Blood compatibility is an important requirement of vascular implants, and thrombogenicity is a major complication of intravascular stenting during the postinsertion period.[5] In the case of metals, thrombogenicity is related to the electrode potential, and the higher the electronegativity of a metal, the more antithrombogenic it is. This creates a controversy in the choice of a metal which is both thromboresistant and tissue compatible, since the higher the electronegativity of a metal, the less corrosion resistant it is and, thereby, the less tissue compatible. Among surgical metals, cobalt–chromium and titanium alloys display relatively good thromboresistant properties. The nature of the metal surface is crucial to blood compatibility: non-uniformly oxidized surfaces, or dirty or contaminated surfaces, are most likely to cause thrombus formation around the implant.

Metal alloys as stenting materials

In order to discuss the parameters of biofunctionality of a material for a stent, it is necessary to describe the functions that are required of such a device. An ideal stent should be self-anchoring, it should be easily inserted and must allow a reasonable flow through its lumen.[6] Depending on the design, different material characteristics may be required in order for the stent to meet the devised objectives. For the sake of distinctness, the discussion here is focused on the functional requirements of a self-expanding urological coil (Fig. 10.7). This coil comes wound on an introducing catheter in its reduced calibre and expands by itself when released. The major requirement of a material for

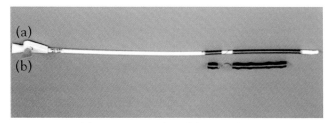

Figure 10.7. (a) Stent mounted on delivery catheter is reduced in calibre; (b) released stent has wavy shape after full expansion.

Table 10.7. *Selected properties of surgical metals and alloys*

Metal/alloy		Density ρ (g/cm^3)	Young's modulus E (GPa)	Yield stress σ_y (MPa)	Tensile strength σ_{UTS} (MPa)
316L stainless steel:	annealed			170	480
	30% cold work	7.9	200	840	910
	80% cold work			1100	1350
Co–Cr–Mo alloys		8.3–9.2	210–240	300–1500	800–1800
CP Titanium		4.5	110	280	345
Ti-6Al-4V		4.5	110	900–1000	1050–1100
Ti-6Al-7Nb		4.7	100	900	1050
Ti-5Al-2.5Fe		4.5	110	780	860
Ti-13Nb-13Zr		5.6	80	900	1030
55 Nitinol		6.45	70	103–138	860
60 Nitinol		6.71	113	900–1000	945–1060
Hard-drawn Nitinol wire		—	33	close to σ_{UTS}	1585–1725

such a stent is high resilience, i.e. the ability to return to the original shape after having been deformed. Resilience is directly proportional to the maximum amount of elastic strain that the material can endure before starting to deform plastically: $\varepsilon_{el}^{max} = \sigma_y/E$, where σ_y is the yield stress, and E is the modulus of elasticity, or Young's modulus. Therefore, a material will have high resilience when it has a high yield stress coupled with a low modulus of elasticity. The material typically used for such stents is 316 stainless steel, and it would be instructive to compare the major surgical metals with this steel in terms of σ_y and E (Table 10.7). For Co–Cr–Mo alloys, both characteristics are slightly higher than those of the stainless steel, with the values of maximum elastic strain being close for both materials (0.55 and 0.62% for the stainless steel and Co–Cr–Mo alloys, respectively). This means that, from the point of view of resilience, Co–Cr–Mo offers no advantage over stainless steel. Taking into account that the forming and shaping of most Co–Cr alloys by mechanical means is extremely difficult, it does not seem likely that Co–Cr will become a feasible material for urological stents in the near future.

Unlike Co–Cr–Mo alloys, the modulus of elasticity of the typical Ti alloy, Ti-6Al-4V, is almost twofold lower than that of the stainless steel. At the same time, the values of yield stress of Ti-6Al-4V and the stainless steel are comparable. With the maximum elastic strain approaching 1%, Ti-6Al-4V is noticeably more resilient than the stainless steel, which makes it an attractive

material for stenting applications. This is even more true for the novel beta-Ti alloys, such as Ti-13Zr-13Nb, which have an even lower modulus of elasticity without compromising the yield stress. An additional advantage of Ti alloys is their low density which can allow the fabrication of lightweight urological stents.

Shape memory alloy: Nitinol

In addition to the major surgical metals discussed, another group of alloys is gaining increasing popularity in many biomedical applications, including urological stenting. These are titanium–nickel Nitinol alloys based on the equiatomic intermetallic compound NiTi and containing 54–60% (w/w) Ni. A typical composition of a Nitinol wire is given in Table 10.8. Owing to the high titanium content, Nitinol alloys exhibit good biocompatibility and corrosion resistance in vivo.

Nitinol alloys belong to a very special group of the so-called shape memory alloys — materials that can

Table 10.8. *Typical composition of a Nitinol alloy wire*

Element	Percentage composition (w/w)
Ni (nickel)	54.1
Co (cobalt)	0.64
Cr (chromium)	0.76
Mn (manganese)	0.64
Fe (iron)	0.66
Ti (titanium)	Balance

'remember' their original shape after having been plastically deformed. The shape memory effect is illustrated in Figure 10.8. A coil spring is fabricated at a high temperature, cooled to a lower temperature and deformed. If the spring is now heated above a certain temperature, it will recover its original shape. The shape memory effect in Nitinol is related to the crystallographically reversible martensitic transformation — a diffusionless structural change where the resulting structure is obtained by a coordinated movement of large blocks of atoms. The martensitic transformation is induced by changes in temperature, and it is characterized by its transition temperatures M_s, M_f, A_s and A_f (Fig. 10.9). M_s and M_f refer, respectively, to the start and finish of the formation and growth of

the low-temperature phase martensite on cooling, and As and A_f refer to the start and finish of the formation and growth of the high-temperature phase *austenite* on heating. As can be seen in Figure 10.10, the transformation temperature strongly depends on the alloy composition: an increase in Ni content above the stoichiometric composition results in a decrease in M_s. The same effect can be achieved by adding cobalt as a substitute for Ni.[7] The martensite transformation in Nitinol brings about an abrupt change in Young's modulus and yield stress. This gives the rare possibility of tailoring the properties of Nitinol to a specific application by slightly changing the alloy composition.

The rationale for using Nitinol in stenting applications is threefold. First, the shape memory effect can be utilized in the design. Here, the great advantage is that the device can be implanted in an optimal shape for surgery, after which the desired functional shape is obtained in situ simply by the action of the body heat.

Another working principle that can be involved in the design is termed *pseudoelasticity*, or *superelasticity*. Pseudoelasticity is defined as the ability of the material to recover an apparently plastic strain upon unloading.

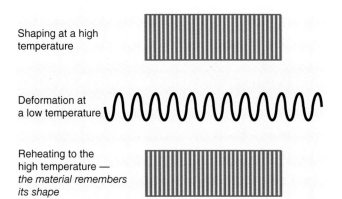

Figure 10.8. *Schematic illustration of the shape memory effect.*

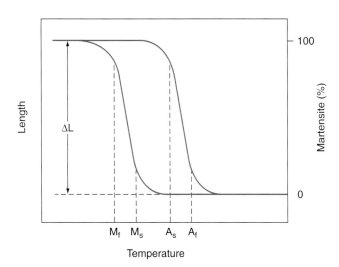

Figure 10.9. *Typical transformation versus temperature curve for a shape-memory specimen under constant load as it is cooled and heated. M_s, martensite start; M_f, martensite finish; A_s, austenite start; A_f, austenite finish.*

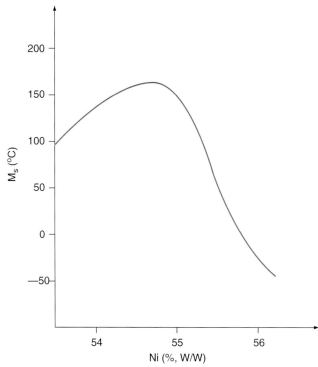

Figure 10.10. M_s *temperature of Nitinol as a function of Ni content.*

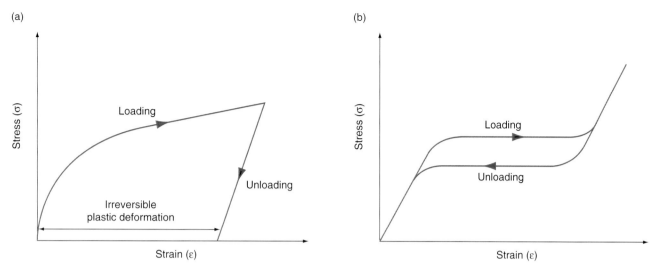

Figure 10.11. *Schematic stress–strain curves for (a) regular metal and (b) pseudoelastic material.*

The amount of this reversible deformation is much greater than the classical, elastic strain. In Figure 10.11(a), a typical stress–strain curve of a non-pseudoelastic metal is shown. As previously discussed, the loading of such a metal results in a small amount of elastic strain that usually does not exceed 1%. On further loading, irreversible plastic deformation starts to occur, so that when the load is released the metal does not return to its original dimensions. This behaviour is typical of all metals, including stainless steel and Ti alloys.

Consider now the pseudoelasticity effect that is also closely related to the martensitic transformation. A typical pseudoelasticity loop of Nitinol in the austenitic state (at $T > A_f$) is shown in Figure 10.11(b). It can be seen that linear elastic deformation of the austenitic phase is followed by non-linear strain based on the formation of stress-induced martensite plates. On unloading, this strain recovers by the reverse transformation from martensite to austenite, since stress-induced martensite is completely unstable in the absence of stress at temperatures above A_f. In this case, shape recovery occurs not upon the application of heat but upon a reduction of stress. Pseudoelasticity causes the material to be extremely elastic (approx. 8–10% reversible strain), making Nitinol very attractive for stenting applications.

An additional important property of Nitinol that can be utilized in stents is its relatively low modulus of elasticity in the martensitic condition (approx. 30 GPa), which is about three times lower than that of the typical Ti alloy and about six times lower than that of the stainless steel. When drawn into a high-strength wire (Table 10.7), such a Nitinol alloy exhibits an outstanding elasticity ($\varepsilon_{el}^{max} > 4.5\%$) and is much more resilient than both stainless steel and Ti alloys.

As shown, Nitinol alloys have a number of truly remarkable properties, making them feasible materials for stenting applications.

References

1. Williams D F. Biofunctionality and biocompatibility. In: Cahn R W, Haasen P, Kramer E J (eds) Materials science and technology. Vol 14: Williams D F (ed) Medical and dental materials. Weinheim, Germany: VCH, 1991: 1–27

2. Niinomi M. Recent developments in Japanese titanium research and development. Journal of Metals 1996; 48: 55–57

3. Hoar T P, Mears D C. Corrosion-resistant alloys in chloride solutions: materials for surgical implants. Proc R Soc Lon Ser A 1966; 294: 486–510

4. Yachia D. Spontaneous breakage of self-retaining intraprostatic stent. J Urol 1990; 144: 997–998

5. Taylor A. Metals. In: Sigwart U (ed) Endoluminal stenting. London: Saunders, 1996: 29–33

6. Saporta L, Beyar M, Yachia D. New temporary coil stent (Urocoil) for treatment of recurrent urethral strictures. J Endourol 1993; 7: 57–59

7. Porter D A, Easterling K E. Phase transformations in metals and alloys. London: Chapman and Hall, 1992; 431–437

Further reading

Bardos D I. Titanium and zirconium alloys in orthopedic applications. In: Wise DL et al. (eds) Encyclopedic handbook of biomaterials and bioengineering, Part B. New York: Marcel Dekker, 1995; 1: 541–548

Castleman L S, Motzkin S M. Biocompatibility of Nitinol. In: Williams DF (ed) Biocompatibility of clinical implant materials. Boca Raton: CRC Press, 1981; 2: 129–154

Hodgson D E, Wu M H, Biermann R J. Shape memory alloys. In: Metals handbook, 10th ed. ASM International, 1990; 2: 897–902

Kohn D H, Ducheyne P. Materials for bone and joint replacement. In: Cahn R W, Haasen P, Kramer EJ Materials science and technology. Vol. 14: Williams DF (ed) Medical and dental materials. Weinheim, Germany: VCH, 1991: 29–109

Kousbroek R. Shape memory alloys. In: Ducheyne P, Hastings GW (eds) Metal and ceramic biomaterials. Boca Raton: CRC Press, 1984, 2: 64–90

Kruger J. Fundamental aspects of the corrosion of metallic implants. In: Syrett B C, Acharya A (eds) Corrosion and degradation of implant materials. Philadelphia: ASTM, 1979: 107–127

Lycett R W, Hughes A N. Corrosion. In: Ducheyne P, Hastings GW (eds) Metal and ceramic biomaterials. Boca Raton: CRC Press, 1984, 2: 91–141

Mears D C. Metals in medicine and surgery. Int Met Rev 1977; 22: 119–155

Otsuka K, Shimizu K. Pseudoelasticity and shape memory effects in alloys. Int Met Rev 1986; 31: 93–114

Park J B. Metallic biomaterials. In: Bronzino J D (ed) The biomedical engineering handbook. Boca Raton: CRC Press, 1995; 537–551

Pillar R M. Manufacturing processes of metals: the processing and properties of metal implants. In: Ducheyne P, Hastings G W (eds) Metal and ceramic biomaterials. Boca Raton: CRC Press, 1984; 1: 80–105

Semlitsch M. Mechanical properties of selected implant metals used for artificial hip joints. In: Ducheyne P, Hastings G W (eds) Metal and ceramic biomaterials. Boca Raton: CRC Press, 1984; 2: 1–21

Shetty R H, Ottersberg W H. Metals in orthopedic surgery. In Wise D L et al. (eds) Encyclopedic handbook of biomaterials and bioengineering, Part B. New York: Marcel Dekker, 1995; 1: 509–540

Sutow E J, Pollack S R. The biocompatibility of certain stainless steels. In: Williams D F (ed) Biocompatibility of clinical implant materials. Boca Raton: CRC Press, 1981; 2: 45–98

Williams D F. Corrosion of implant materials. Annu Rev Mater Sci 1976; 6: 237–266

Williams D F, Roaf R. Implants in surgery. London: Saunders, 1973

Williams D F. The properties and clinical uses of cobalt-based alloys. In: Williams D F (ed) Biocompatibility of clinical implant materials. Boca Raton: CRC Press, 1981; 2: 99-127

Williams D F. Titanium and titanium alloys. In: Williams D F (ed) Biocompatibility of clinical implant materials. Boca Raton: CRC Press, 1981; 2: 9–44

11

Characteristics of materials used in implants: polymers
M. J. Slepian and S. F. A. Hossainy

Introduction

Catheters and stents, fabricated from a variety of materials, have been utilized throughout the history of urology.[1] In the modern era, numerous endourological devices have been constructed from polymeric materials.[2] The term 'polymeric materials' generally refers to the class of materials composed of polymers, i.e. macromolecules made up of simple repeating units known as monomers. Both natural and synthetic polymers, including organic and partially inorganic polymers, have been employed in fashioning endourological implant devices. The advantages of polymeric materials for this purpose are that they are readily available, easily configurable and have generally acceptable biocompatibility, which affords device comfort to the patient. Despite the above, with increasing clinical experience of polymeric endourological implants over the years, significant limitations in the biocompatibility of specific materials have emerged.[2,3]

The aim of this chapter is to review the polymeric materials used in endourological implant devices. Rubbers, elastomers and plastics, which are traditionally considered non- or minimally-degradable materials will be discussed. Discussion of biodegradable polymers is excluded since it is the focus of a separate chapter. However, the following questions will be addressed here:

- Which polymers have been used in endourological implant devices?
- What are the basic and urologic-specific material properties of these polymers?
- How may these materials be improved for endourological applications?

Which polymers have been used in endourological implant devices?

Over the past few decades a variety of polymeric materials have been used to fashion catheters and stents

for endourological applications. As an introduction to the field of polymeric materials a glossary of terms and definitions is provided in Table 11.1.

Initially, natural polymers such as latex rubber were used for constructing endourological implants. In the past, latex was readily available as an initial polymeric material and afforded advantages in terms of ease of formability, device flexibility and patient acceptibility. While latex is still utilized for specific applications today, over the past few decades, with declining availability and recognized biocompatibility limitations, greater use of synthetic polymers or 'plastics' has occurred.

The polymers, both natural and synthetic, used in endourological implant devices are listed in Table 11.2 and their basic chemistry and general properties are described below.

Polyethylene (PE)

Polyethylenes are polyolefin polymers with numerous medical and non-medical uses (Figure 11.1). PE is typically produced via free radical polymerization of ethylene and selected alpha-olefins using a transition metal catalyst system and may be produced via high and low pressure processes. PEs typically have molecular weights ranging from 10 000 to >50 000 and are thermoplastic resins which exist in several families: ultra-low density (ULDPE), low-density (LDPE), linear-low density (LLDPE) and high-density (HDPE). They are generally tough, light-weight materials which are flexible and readily thermoformable and possess excellent resistance to aqueous solutions and good resistance to various solvents and chemicals. In addition to simple polyolefins such as PE, proprietary olefinic block co-polymers, such as Percuflex™, have been developed for endourological applications.[4]

Polytetrafluoroethylene (PTFE)

Polytetrafluoroethylene is a completely fluorinated polymer synthesized via the free radical-initiated polymerization of the gaseous monomer

Table 11.1. *Glossary of polymer terms*

Polymer	Material composed of macromolecules formed by covalent linkage of one or more repeating units, i.e. monomeric units
Co-polymer	Polymeric material formed by linkage of repeating segments of one or more types (blocks) of polymer
Polymer blend	Polymeric material formed by non-covalent physical mixing of two or more polymers
Natural polymer	Polymer produced by a living organism
Synthetic polymer	A man-made polymer
Organic polymer	Polymer with monomeric subunits which are carbon based, e.g. polyethylene
Partially inorganic polymer	Polymer with a non-carbon backbone. Monomers may contain organic pendant groups, e.g. polydimethylsiloxane
Inorganic polymer	Polymer with monomeric units that are non-carbon based, e.g. polydichlorophosphazene
Elastomer	Polymers possessing segmental mobility of the polymer backbone, low resistance to stress and resilience. Elastomers may be either synthetic or natural polymers although the term is generally identified with synthetic polymers
Rubber	Natural elastomers
Thermoplastic	Non-crosslinked polymers that readily melt and flow with heating and may be fabricated via extrusion or moulding
Thermoset	Typically cross-linked polymers which do not melt with heating and may be further cured with heating

Table 11.2. *Polymers used in endourological implant devices*

- Polyethylene (PE)
- Polytetrafluoroethylene (PTFE)
- Polyurethane (PU)
- Polyvinyl chloride (PVC)
- Styrenic thermoplastic elastomer (STE)
- Silicone
- Latex rubber

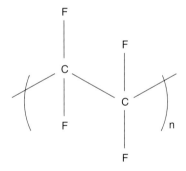

Figure 11.2. *Polytetrafluoroethylene (PTFE).*

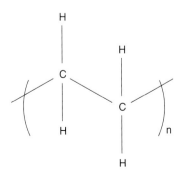

Figure 11.1. *Polyethylene (PE).*

tetrafluoroethylene (Figure 11.2). PTFE is a crystalline polymer that is particularly known for its excellent chemical resistance. It has superb thermal stability (melting point = 620°C) and a useful temperature range of 500°C. The high melt viscosity of this material requires processing techniques more akin to those used for metals and ceramics than those for conventional thermoplastics. One form of PTFE, whose trade name is widely recognized, is Teflon™. PTFE has numerous medical and non-medical uses and has unique surface properties, with both a low critical surface tension and friction coefficient. As a result of these surface properties, PTFE creates an excellent anti-stick or release surface.

Polyurethane (PU)

Polyurethanes, also referred to as urethanes, are a broad group of materials formed by condensation polymerization of polyisocyanates, polyols and chain extenders (Figure 11.3). The wide variety of monomeric components available has resulted in numerous urethanes suitable for a wide range of end-uses. Depending upon the degree of functionality in the starting isocyanate and polyol, urethanes may exist as either thermoplastics or thermosets. In addition, elastomeric polyurethanes have been synthesized. PUs may exist as foams, millable gums, adhesives, coatings or sealants.

Polyvinyl chloride (PVC)

Polyvinyl chloride is produced via free radical polymerization of gaseous vinyl chloride (Figure 11.4). It exists in both flexible and rigid forms and is used widely as a commercial material due to its imminent blendability, the addition of small amounts of

plasticizing additives dramatically altering the material properties of the resin. PVC resins are widely used in the fabrication of pipes, sidings, moulding and windows.

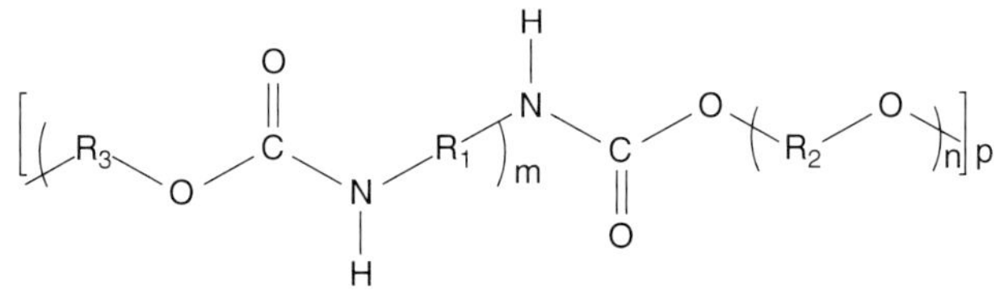

Styrenic thermoplastic elastomer (STE)

Styrenic thermoplastic elastomer is the generic name for a broad class of polymeric materials with the generic formula $(S–E)_nX$, where S represents a polystyrene end segment, E represents an elastomer mid-segment (e.g. polyisoprene, ethylene-butylene, or ethylene-propylene), and X represents a junction point. A representative polymer of this class, C-Flex™, is shown in Figure 11.5. Styrenic block copolymers are typically processed via conventional thermoplastic techniques such as extrusion and moulding. STEs exhibit excellent strength (similar to vulcanized rubber), hydrolytic stability, heat stability, are generally non-toxic and have been employed as adhesives, sealants and coatings and in the fabrication of moulded products, such as baby bottle nipples and shoe soles.

Silicone

Silicone is the generic name which describes polysiloxanes. As a family of synthetic polymers, silicones are typically partially organic, possessing an inorganic Si–O backbone with attached organic side groups (Figure 11.6). They may exist as fluids, gels, elastomers or solids. In general, silicones exhibit low surface tension, high lubricity, extreme hydrophobicity and excellent physiological, chemical and electrical inertness. Silicone fluids are typically employed as lubricants, elastomers as sealants, and solid resins for a wide variety of household and personal care products.

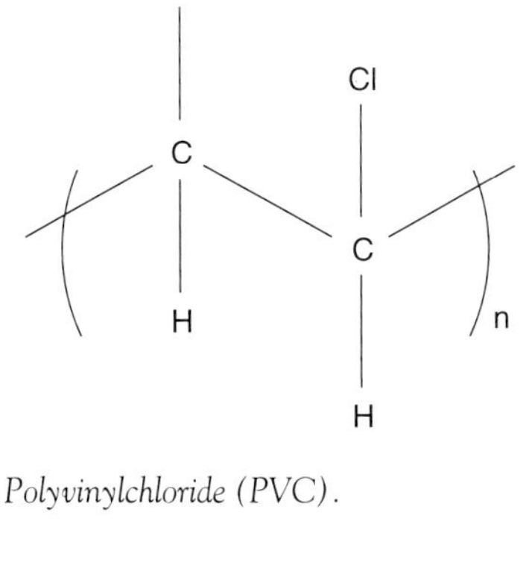

Figure 11.3. Polyurethane (PU). R1 is a hard block e.g. MDI, TDI; R2 is a chain extender e.g. butane diol or other diols, diamines, etc; R3 is the soft segment repeat unit e.g. CH_2-, CH_2-CH_2-.

Figure 11.4. Polyvinylchloride (PVC).

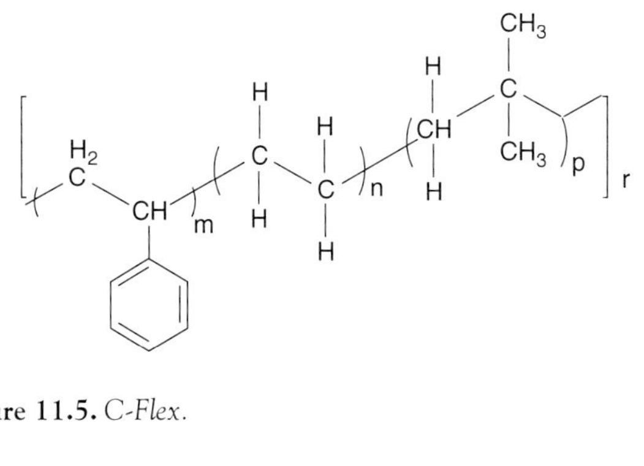

Figure 11.5. C-Flex.

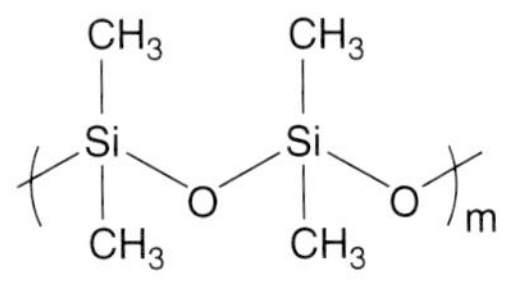

Figure 11.6. *Polydimethylsiloxane (PDMS).*

Latex rubber

Latex rubber is the generic name for the broad class of natural polyisoprenes produced by numerous plants, including the 'rubber tree' *Hevea brasiliensis* (Figure 11.7).[5] It is synthesized by the enzymatic polymerization of isopentenylpyrophosphate. As a material latex rubber is a natural elastomer. Natural rubber typically refers to cis-1,4-polyisopropene and its molecular weight is extremely high, averaging about 1 million. The material properties of rubber may be modified, by the formation of sulphur cross-links in the process of vulcanization, creating a harder, stronger and less tacky material.

The materials described above have been used in a wide variety of urological drainage catheters as well as stents. An outline of specific devices and the materials from which they are fabricated is provided in Table 11.3.

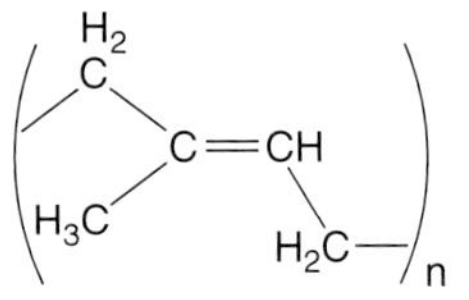

Figure 11.7. *Polyisoprene (natural rubber).*

Table 11.3. *Polymeric endourological implant devices*

Stent	Material
Pigtail	Polyethylene
Hawkins accordion	PTFE
Cope loop	C-Flex
Castenada malecot	Percuflex
Amplatz malecot	C-Flex
Stamey suprapubic malecot	Polyethylene
Argyle	Polyvinyl chloride
Council	Latex or other rubber
Foley balloon	Latex, polyurethane, silastic
Polyurethane Double-J	Polyurethane
Silastic Double-J	Silastic
Smith universal	Silastic
Intraurethral catheter (IUC):	
Nissenkorn design	Polyurethane
Barnes design	Polyurethane
Trestle	Polyurethane

What are the basic and urologic-specific material properties of polymers used in endourological applications?

Polyethylene (PE)

Polyethylenes are thermoplastics that are readily configurable via thermoforming processes including, extrusion, injection moulding and blow moulding. In general, they possess excellent chemical resistance and are employed commercially to manufacture films, bottles and containers. The general material properties of PEs vary with the density of the PE; LDPE is highly flexible (flexural modulus 36 000–53 000 psi) with tensile strengths of 2–3000 psi whereas HDPEs are stiffer (flexural modulus 120 000–225 000 psi), harder materials with tensile strengths as high as 6500 psi. PE exhibits limited water absorption (<0.1% in 24 hours).

Polyethylenes have been used in a variety of drainage catheters and stents. In the 1950s Tulloch reported on the use of indwelling polyethylene tubing to restore continuity and endoluminal patency of obstructed ureters.[6] More recently PE has been used in the fabrication of a variety of temporary drainage catheters as well as in the Stamey suprapubic malecot catheter.[3]

While PEs are user-friendly, they have limitations as endourological materials. For example, they are easily fouled by overflowing biological fluids leading to ready protein deposition. In the urinary tract fouled PE surfaces are well set-up for crystalloid adherence and encrustation leading to an increased likelihood of infection. PE implants have also been found to lose flexibility, becoming brittle and fracture with time.[7,8]

More recently complex polyolefins have been developed for endourological use. Percuflex™ is a proprietary thermoplastic olefinic block co-polymer developed by Boston Scientific Corporation.[4] The superior coil and tensile strength of this material allow it to be extruded while maintaining a superior ID/OD ratio. This guarantees good sidehole efficacy for drainage and debris passage.[4] In vitro studies, using a modified Robbins device which allows continuous urinary flow, have demonstrated intermediate levels of hydroxyapatite deposition, with PE scoring between polyurethane and hydrogel-coated PU.[9] In vivo studies of ureteral stents fabricated from this material have demonstrated lumenal patency for periods beyond 6 months.[10]

Polytetrafluoroethylene (PTFE)

Polytetrafluoroethylene is a hard, tough thermoplastic. It is a unique polymer in that it possesses excellent chemical resistance, largely due to C–F bonds. The general mechanical properties of PTFE are similar to medium density PE, with moderate flexibility (flexural modulus 60 000 psi) and low tensile strength (3000 psi).[11] It exhibits minimal water absorption (<0.05% in 24 hours).

Despite its excellent chemical resistance, PTFE has limited utility as a primary material for endourological applications, partly due to the fact that PTFE catheters are generally stiff. As a coating it also has moderate utility. In an early study using an in vitro human urine system, Srinivasan demonstrated that 7/13 PTFE-coated catheters exhibited encrustation compared with 3/20 PVC or silicone catheters.[12] More recently bacterial adherence to PTFE was examined and reduced, though variable, adherence was observed compared to rubber and silicone catheters.[13] However, PTFE has been employed in 5 and 6 Fr external drainage catheters with good long-term patency.[14]

Polyurethane (PU)

Polyurethanes are a broad class of materials existing as either elastomers (elastic modulus 10^6–10^7 dynes/cm), plastics (elastic modulus 10^8–10^9 dynes/cm) or fibres (elastic modulus 10^{10}–10^{11} dynes/cm). Thermoplastic PUs are moderately flexible (flexural modulus 10 000–100 000 psi) with low to moderate tensile strength (1500–11 000 psi). Thermoset PUs have similar flexibility with higher tensile strength (10 000–15 000 psi).

Unfortunately, PUs are readily fouled in the urinary tract. Protein and crystal deposition, bacterial adherence and biofilm formation have all been reported for urethanes. PU ureteral stents were also shown to cause epithelial ulceration and erosion, partially due to high surface roughness.[15] Surface roughness also plays a role in bacterial attachment, biofilm formation and encrustation.[16] In the upper urinary tract, urethane stent patency has been compromised by fibrin deposition, inflammatory debris generation and clot formation at the level of the renal pelvis. PU stents are generally contraindicated in external shock wave lithotripsy (ESWL) patients, if in use for longer than 6 months, due to observed secondary stone formation, encrustation, infection and urothelial ulceration.[4]

In addition, urethanes have limited durability compared with other polymers. PU implants have been demonstrated to lose flexibility and modulus with time and the material demonstrates slow in vivo biodegradation. Degradation products may also be cytotoxic, particularly if the hard-block segment of the polymer is made of aromatic species, i.e. diphenylmethane diisocyanate monomer (MDI) or toluene diisocyanate monomer (TDI). As a result, urethane catheters and stents are best employed as short-term implants.

Polyvinyl chloride (PVC)

Polyvinyl chloride is a thermoplastic material whose properties vary depending upon the nature of the admixed plasticizer and stabilizer. In the pure 'unplasticized' form, PVC is generally moderately flexible (10 000–16 000 psi) with a high tensile strength (6000–7500 psi). Flexible PVCs are generally plasticized, exhibiting a high degree of flexibility with a low tensile strength (800–3000 psi).

Use of PVC in endourological catheters and stents has been limited, although overall the urinary biocompatibility of PVC is fair. In an in vitro study of surface biofouling and encrustation using a urolithic simulator, significant deposition was observed on PVC tubing compared with silicon elastomer, Teflon™ and ethylenacrylic acid copolymer.[17] Insertion of the Argyle trilumen balloon catheter has been difficult due to the high coefficient of friction associated with PVC.[3]

Styrenic thermoplastic elastomer

Styrenic rubber block co-polymers combine thermoplastic and elastomeric properties in a single material. STEs consisting of poly(ethylene-butylene) are generally tough rubbery materials which are flexible (flexural modulus 1000–4000 psi) and have low tensile strength (1500–2500 psi).

C-Flex is a block co-polymer of styrene–ethylene–butylene and is one of the most suitable materials for endourological catheters and stents.[4] C-Flex catheters show good flow rates and coil retention strength. The in vivo patency of C-Flex internal double-J ureteral stents studied in 35 patients during an average of 5 months follow-up showed an 80% patency rate.[18] Bacterial colonization of C-Flex stents compared to silicone and urethane stents was studied in a prospective study of 266 patients over a 3-month period. Rates of colonization of

55.5% for C-Flex versus 62.6% for silicone and 100% for urethane were found.[19] Interestingly, in another study, hydrogel coating of C-Flex stents was not observed to improve urinary biocompatibility; increased encrustation was observed compared with uncoated C-Flex devices.[20] C-Flex also exhibits superior tissue compatibility in the ureter. In a study comparing silicone, C-Flex and polyurethane stents for local ureteral tissue reaction in the dog, C-Flex caused less reaction overall.[15]

Silicone

Silicone thermoset resins are rubbery materials. Silicones are generally flexible (flexural modulus 200–2000 psi) with a low tensile strength (350–1000 psi). In addition to pure polysiloxane, a silicone-based polymer, Silitek, has found applicability as a material for endourological application.[2]

Silicones show superior urinary biocompatibility and are generally resistant to encrustation. In a study examining encrustation of materials in vitro, silicone demonstrated superior compatibility with limited encrustation.[12] Similarly, in an in vivo study in patients with chronic indwelling catheters, silicones were demonstrated to be preferable catheter materials since limited encrustation was observed.[21] Recently the urinary biocompatibility of silicone was compared to polyurethane using a modified Robbins device which allows continuous urinary flow in vitro.[22] Despite similar levels of hydroxyapatite deposition, scanning electron microscopy, atomic absorption spectroscopy and energy dispersive X-ray analysis all demonstrated that silicone was less prone to encrustation than polyurethanes.

Despite superior urinary biocompatibility, silicones have significant limitations as catheter and stent materials. The low tensile strength of silicones has limited the ID and sidehole aperature of catheters leading to low-flow drainage rates[4] and low modulus and stiffness contribute to weak coil strength and a greater propensity for stent migration. A high surface friction coefficient contributes to greater difficulty during stent insertion and may also limit egress of calculi debris following ESWL.

Latex rubber

Natural latex rubber is a flexible material. It has been used for many years in the fabrication of upper tract stents and lower tract catheter devices, e.g. Foley catheters. Encrustation of latex versus PTFE and silicone catheters was examined using a stagnant human urine immersion protocol in vitro.[12] Latex was found to have inferior urinary biocompatibility, manifesting the highest degree of encrustation.

How might these polymers be improved for endourological application?

Ideal biomaterials for endourological stent application are those which provide adequate endoluminal support while resisting biofouling, encrustation, infection, urothelial damage and excessive neoepithelial overgrowth, all of which lead to lumen compromise. Several approaches may be envisioned to improve the in vivo biocompatibility of polymeric materials for use in the urinary tract. Modifications, in the form of coatings or surface grafting, may be made to existing polymers, thus altering the surface free energy, charge or coefficient of friction. Alteration of surface properties may also reduce protein fouling, bacterial adhesion and crystal deposition. Slippery surfaces may also facilitate stone and fragment passage following ESWL.

Using this approach desirable materials such as C-Flex may be enhanced further through grafting of hydrophilic polymers to its surface. Examples of potential graft polymers include polyacrylic acid, polyacrylamide, polyvinyl pyrollidone, polyvinyl alcohol, heparin or heparin-like sulfonated dextrans or hyaluronic acid. Grafting can be achieved by radiation of polymer solutions with grafting onto the underlying substrate. Care must be exerted in this process to limit homopolymerization versus graft co-polymerization. An alternative approach may be photolytic grafting, achieved by adsorbing photosensitizers onto the substrate surface and irradiating the polymer solution. Thioxanthene or benzophenone may be used as photosensitizers. Azide activated polymer molecules may also be grafted. This may be achieved by abstracting H- from the substrate surface. Chemical coupling is also possible on available surface functional groups such as CHO, NCO, OH, COOH, epoxy or NH$_2$. For example, NH is available on PU surfaces. These surfaces may be reacted with an NCO-terminated hydrophilic polymer of choice via allophanate or biuret linkages.

Hydrogel materials may be grafted to structural polymeric surfaces to enhance surface properties and reduce fouling. Non-ionic, hydrogel polymer systems that do not have metal ion chelation potential are the best candidates for this type of surface modification for urological applications. Polyethylene glycol (PEG), a hydrogel demonstrated in the vascular system to be non-fouling,[23] is unfortunately not a good choice in urinary application due to its high Ca^{2+} chelation potential. Its crown ether-like structure tends to selectively chelate Ca^{2+} resulting in calcification. Polysaccharide-based hydrogels also may pose potential problems since they may host uropathogens.

Engrafted hydrogels also may serve as a means for local drug incorporation and delivery. Incorporated bacteriocidal or antimicrobial agents may serve to reduce biofilm formation. Further, hydrophobic drug delivery particles or capsules may be suspended in the surface hydrogel to sustain the delivery of ionic hydrophilic bacteriocidal drugs. Agents such as ethylene hydroxydiphosphonate (EHDP), a very potent anti-calcifying agent, and its derivatives may also be incorporated into hydrogels to prevent initial crystal formation. Unfortunately, these agents are extremely water soluble. However, efficacy may be enhanced further if they are physically bound directly to the implant polymer surface.

In addition to surface grafting to existing polymers, new polymers, co-polymers and polymer blends, which take advantage of the desirable properties of one class of material to synergistically enhance another material, may also be developed. An interesting possibility will be the development of new materials based on pyrolytic carbon. Pyrolytic carbon is unique as a cardiovascular material in that it is relatively free of calcification. Carbonizing of different substrates may be achieved via chemical vapour deposition, electrode discharge, and sputtering at the subsurface level of implant. New polymer or polymer blends which have pendant groups

of EHDP also may be developed as potential urocompatible materials. All of the above approaches potentially may be used to reduce implant fouling, encrustation, infection and obstruction and enhance the long-term clinical efficacy of endourological implants.

Conclusions

Numerous natural and synthetic elastomers and plastics have been utilized as materials for endourological catheters and stents. Styrenic thermoplastic elastomers e.g. C-Flex, polysiloxanes and olefinic block co-polymers, e.g. Percuflex, are generally the most desirable non-degradable polymers available for endourological applications to date. Despite the limitations of existing materials, advances in polymer chemistry and surface science have opened new pathways for potential improvement of existing materials and the creation of new ones. It is becoming increasingly clear that through advances in surface grafting and new material formulation, the next generation of endourological materials on the horizon will emerge with superior long-term implant characteristics.

References

1. Lange P H. Diagnostic and therapeutic urologic instrumentation. In: Campbell's Urology. Walsh P C, Gittes R F Perlmutter A D, Stamey T A (eds.) Philadelphia: W. B. Saunders Co., 1986, pp. 510–540.
2. Mardis H K, Kroeger R M. Ureteral stents: materials. Urol Clin N Am 1988; 15: 471–479.
3. Brazzini A, Castaneda-Zuniga W R, Coleman C C et al. Urostent designs. Semin Intervent Radiol 1987; 4: 26–35.
4. Mardis H K, Kroeger R M, Morton J J, Donovan J M. Comparative evaluation of materials used for internal ureteral stents. J Endourol 1993; 7(2): 105–15.
5. Rodriguez F. Principles of Polymer Systems. New York: Hemisphere Publishing Co., 1989, p. 109.
6. Tulloch W S. Restoration of the continuity of the ureter by means of polyethylene tubing. Br J Urol 1951; 24: 42.
7. Hepperlen T W, Mardis H K, Malshock E. Spontaneous breakage of polyethylene double pigtail ureteral stents (abstr). Proceedings of the American Urological Association, 1982, p. 198.
8. Papo J, Waizbard E, Merimsky E. Sponatneous breakage of a double pigtail stent and bladder stone formation. J Urologie 1986; 92(9): 617–19.
9. Tunney M M, Keane P F, Gorman S P. Assessment of urinary tract biomaterial encrustation using a modified Robbins device continuous flow model. J Biomed Materials Res 1997; 38(2): 87–93.
10. Rackson M E, Mitty H A, Losef S V. Biocompatibility of a co-polymer ureteral stent: maintenance of patency beyond 6 months. Am J Radiol 1989; 153: 783.
11. Fifoot R E. Fluoroplastics. Mod Plastics 1989; 65: 24–28.

12. Srinivasan V, Clark S S. Encrustation of catheter materials in vitro. J Urol 1972; 108: 473.

13. Roberts J A, Kaack M B, Fussell E N. Adherence to urethral catheters by bacteria causing nosocomial infections. Urology 1993; 41: 338–342.

14. Hawkins I F. Single-step placement of a self-retaining catheter. Semin Intervent Radiol 1984; 1: 60–62.

15. Marx M, Bettmann M A, Bridge S et al. The effects of various indwelling ureteral catheter materials on the normal canine ureter. J Urol 1988; 139: 180–185.

16. Axelsson H, Schoenebeck J, Winblad B. Surface structure of unused and used catheters. Scand J Urol Nephrol 1977; 11: 283–287.

17. Weissbach L, Lunow R, Gebhardt M, Bastian H P.[Scanning electron microscopy of different materials after urine contact in vitro]. Rasteelektronenmikroskopische Untersuchungen vershiedener Natur- und Kunststoffe nach Urineinwirkung in vitro. Urologe-Ausgabe A 1979; 18: 175–179.

18. Cardella J F, Castaneda-Zuniga W R, Hunter D W et al. Urine-compatible polymer for long-term ureteral stenting. Radiol 1986; 161: 313–18.

19. Farsi H M, Mosli H A, Al-Zemaity M F et al. Bacteriuria and colonization of double pigtail ureteral stents: long-term experience with 237 patients. J Endourol 1995; 9(6): 469–472.

20. Desgrandchamps F, Moulinier F, Daudon M et al. An in vitro comparison of urease induced encrustation of JJ stents in human urine. Br J Urol 1997; 79: 24–27.

21. Kunin C K, Chin Q F, Chamber S. Formation of encrustations on indwelling urinary catheters in the elderly: a comparison of different types of catheter materials in 'blockers' and 'non-blockers'. J Urol 1987; 138: 899–902.

22. Tunney M M, Keane P F, Jones D S, Gorman S P. Comparative assessment of ureteral stent biomaterial encrustation. Biomaterials 1996; 17: 1541–1546.

23. Slepian M J, Hubbell J A. Polymeric endoluminal gel paving: hydrogel systems for local barrier creation and site-specific drug delivery. Adv Drug Delivery Rev 1997; 24: 11–30.

12

Bioabsorbable materials in urology

T. Välimaa and P. Törmälä

Introduction

Most living tissues are macromolecular composites (combinations of different macromolecules and possibly other components). For that reason, synthetic polymeric composites are an attractive group of materials for the development of new, tailor-made biomaterials for replacement, support, augmentation or fixation of living tissues.[1]

In several surgical operations the healing tissue needs only a temporary support or guide. In such cases, bioabsorbable polymers are better alternatives than biostable materials. In general, the demand for the bioabsorbable material depends on the surgical target, the forces in that area and the speed of the healing process. The implant construction and material should retain their strength during the critical days of healing and the tissue reaction to the material should be minimal.

The bioabsorbable materials polylactide (PLA, polylactic acid) and polyglycolide (PGA, polyglycolic acid) are both poly-alpha-hydroxy acids and have been widely investigated with regard to their medical use. There have been numerous published reports of their good biocompatibility. The starting monomers and the degradation products are normal metabolic products, such as lactic acid and glycolic acid. The first medical applications were bioabsorbable sutures, such as Dexon, in the 1970s. Subsequently, several other sutures have been developed, with different degradation times and mechanical properties. Recently, bioabsorbable implants have been developed for different applications, such as maxillofacial surgery, orthopaedics, urology and gastoenterology.

In the processing of bioabsorbable polymer implants, special attention must be focused on the hydrolytic stability of these polymers. The degradation rate of the material in processing and storage depends on the moisture content and the temperature; processing, sterilization and storage of these materials should therefore take place in a dry atmosphere and at as low a temperature as possible.

The terminology attached to the degradation of bioabsorbable materials has been numerous. The meaning of biodegradable, bioabsorbable, absorbable, degradable and resorbable has varied, according to the writer. In this chapter the term bioabsorbable means degradation of the material in vivo to carbon dioxide, water and energy; biodegradation means the morphological and chemical degradation of the polymer in vivo to shorter chains and the term degradation represents the general breakdown of the polymer and molecular chains into shorter chains.

Degradation of the polymer is the sum of many factors, and the degradation of PLA and PGA is accelerated by the following:

- The residual monomers and oligomers in the polymer;[2,3]
- The alkalinity of the medium;[4-6]
- Reduction of crystallinity, and orientation;[2,7-9]
- Certain enzymes, e.g. pronase, proteinase-K and bromelaine;[10,11]
- The implantation site, where numerous muscular movements and stresses put a strain on the implant.[12]

Both lactide and glycolide monomer are extremely soluble in water, and PGA as well as PLA degrade mainly by hydrolysis.[2,13,14] In the tissues hydrolysis takes place first in the interstitial space, until the material has degraded to small particles which are phagocytosed by macrophages and giant cells when the particle size is about 10–80 μm. Inside the cells the degradation continues by hydrolysis in the lysosomes.[15,16]

Both PLA and PGA degrade by hydrolysis first into short molecular chains (oligomers), which in turn break down into basic acids: poly-L-lactic acid (PLLA) degrades into L-lactic acid, poly-D-lactic acid (PDLA) into D-lactic acid and PGA into glycolic acid.[17,18]

Lactic acid degrades by lactate dehydrogenase to pyruvate (Fig. 12.11). The pyruvate decarboxylates to acetyl-CoA or is converted by pyruvate carboxylase to oxaloacetate and shifts to the citric acid cycle in the mitochondria. The final degradation products are energy, water and carbon dioxide.[19,20]

The chemical degradation PGA has more intermediate stages than that of PLLA (Fig. 12.1). After these stages it breaks down into pyruvate which degrades in the same way as that from PLA.

Bioabsorbable implants

General criteria

A bioabsorbable surgical implant should fulfil certain criteria from the point of view of material and mechanical properties. The material should be:

- Non-mutagenic
- Non-antigenic
- Non-carcinogenic
- Non-toxic
- Non-teratogenic.

Additionally, the material should have the following properties:

- Good biocompatibility and haemocompatibility
- Sufficient strength
- Appropriate rigidity
- Degradation products that are water-soluble and, preferably, normal metabolic products
- Ease of sterilization and properties that are not unduly altered by the sterilization process.

The speed of degradation and the concentration of degradation products in the tissues surrounding the implant should be within acceptable limits. The material should not have allergenic properties and should lose its strength at the same rate as the tissue regeneration, ideally at the rate depicted in Figure 12.2, which matches the increase in strength of collagen. In such cases the forces affecting the implant in the tissues will be transferred gradually to the healing tissue. An ideal bioabsorbable implant should also be absorbed as soon as possible after the implant has lost its strength and the tissue has healed.

Implantation site

The place of implantation has a major effect on the degradation of absorbable polymers. In vivo these materials degrade in the order shown in Figure 12.3.

The strength retention time and the operational time of the bioabsorbable implant varies according to the material selected, the molar mass of the raw material, the degree of polymerization, the process parameters and the sterilization method. For example, a polymer with low molar mass or degree of polymerization loses its strength very rapidly in vivo.

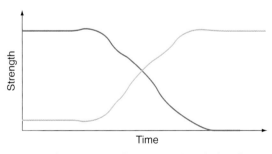

Figure 12.2. *Change in strength over time of an ideal implant material (————) compared with that of collagen (————) (according to refs. 21 and 22).*

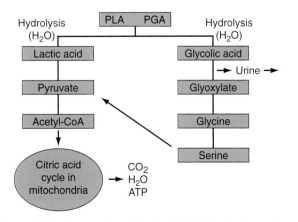

Figure 12.1. *Degradation of PLA and PGA in vivo (according to ref. 19).*

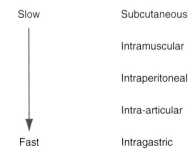

Figure 12.3. *Order of degradation of bioabsorbable polymers in vivo (according to ref. 12).*

The strength of bioabsorbable polymers such as PGA and PLA can be completely lost in a week, or strength can be retained for more than a year, even under exacting conditions. By changing these parameters, the operational time of the implant can be varied to suit the healing time of the relevant tissue.

Materials

As previously stated, PLA and PGA are poly-alpha-hydroxy acids which belong to the group of polyesters. The structural formulae of these materials are depicted in Figure 12.4. Polylactide is polymerized from a lactic acid dimer and polyglycolide is polymerized from a glycolic acid dimer (Table 12.1); they are usually produced in semi-crystalline form. The raw materials and degradation products of these polymers are normal metabolic products.[23,24]

Polylactides

Lactic acid (2-hydroxypropanoic acid; $CH_3CHOHCOOH$) is widely distributed in nature, the trivial name arising from its occurrence in sour milk. It possesses an asymmetrically substituted carbon atom and can exist in two enantiomeric forms — L(+)-lactic acid and D(−)-lactic acid (Fig. 12.5). In the Fischer projection, with the carbon chain vertical and the carboxyl group at the top, the D enantiomer has the hydroxyl group on the right-hand side.[25–27] From these two isomers, copolymers with molecular chains consisting of repeating units of both of these monomers can by polymerized. The degradation rate and amorphous sections of this type of random copolymer increase when the proportion of D-lactide increases from 0 to 50% (w/w).[28]

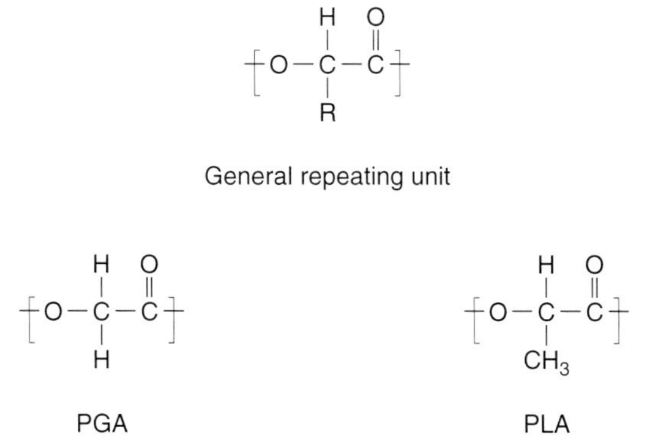

Figure 12.4. *Structural formulae of poly-alpha-hydroxy acids.*

Table 12.1. *Alpha-hydroxy acids, their corresponding dimers and their melting points. (From ref. 24 with permission.)*

Hydroxy acid	Dimer	Melting point (°C)
L-Lactic acid	L-Lactide	97–98
D-Lactic acid	D-Lactide	97–98
Racemic lactic acid	D,L-Lactide (meso lactide)	43–46
	D,D-L,L-Lactide (racemic)	123–125
Glycolic acid	Glycolide	83–86

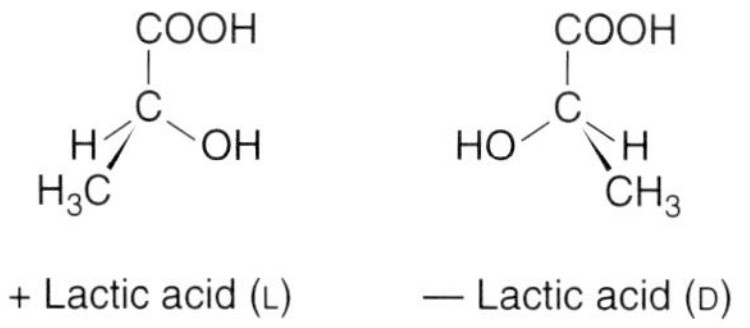

Figure 12.5. *Enantiomers of lactic acid.*

Polylactide is a semicrystalline, bioabsorbable thermoplastic and is obtainable from renewable resources. The starting monomeric compound L-lactic acid can be produced in high yields by many fermentation and chemical treatments of cheap biomass materials such as molasses or potato starch. Once polymerized, the L-lactic acid polymer eventually returns to the same L-lactic acid form after being gradually hydrolysed in the moist environment.[29] Polylactic implants have been used successfully in orthopaedic operations for almost a decade (Biofix®, Bioscience Ltd, Finland).[9,30,31]

Polyglycolide

Glycolic acid (hydroxyethanoic acid; $HOCH_2COOH$) is an important intermediate in some metabolic pathways, and also occurs in cane-sugar juice and unripe grapes. Glycolic acid has no chiral centre in the molecule and therefore does not form enantiomers.[25,32]

Polyglycolide is the simplest aliphatic polyester. It was the first commercially successful synthetic bioabsorbable polymer to be used as a biomedical material. It is usually produced in semi-crystalline form. PGA is of great interest as an implant material because of its good mechanical and absorption properties; in addition, its degradation products are normal metabolic products, like those of polylactides. The oldest and best-known application of PGA is the bioabsorbable Dexon suture (Davis & Geck Ltd).[33]

Development and studies of bioabsorbable spiral stents

Mechanical properties of materials studied

In Figure 12.6 the mechanical strength properties of certain bioabsorbable polymers are presented. The draw ratio is the ratio between the cross-sectional areas of unorientated and of self-reinforced (SR) monofilament. The mechanical strength can be increased considerably by self-reinforcement.[8,9]

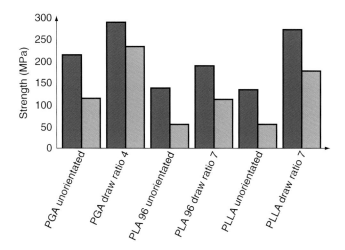

Figure 12.6. *Mechanical strength of bioabsorbable polymers (■ bending strength; ▨ shear strength).*

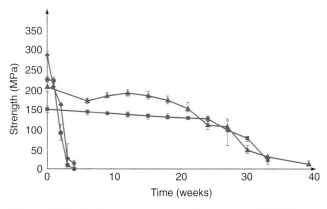

Figure 12.7. *Bending and shear strength retention of SR-PGA and SR-PLA 96 in vitro (37°C, pH 6.1): vertical bars represent ranges;* ● *PGA shear strength draw ratio (dr) 3.8;* ■ *PLA 96 shear strength dr 6.8;* ◆ *PGA bending strength dr 3.8;* ▲ *PLA 96 bending strength dr 6.8.*

Figure 12.7 depicts typical strength-retention curves of SR-PGA and SR-PLA 96 in vitro. SR-PGA typically loses its strength within 3 weeks, whereas the strength retention of SR-PLA 96 and of other polylactides is much longer. The specific batch of SR-PLA 96 shown in Figure 12.7 lost its strength in 34 weeks.

Degradation of SR-PLA 96 and SR-PGA

The degradation of poly-alpha-hydroxy materials can be divided in two main stages. In the first stage the degradation begins in amorphous regions of the material. The molecular chains between crystalline and amorphous areas break down, leading to loss of strength of the material. In the second stage the crystalline areas start to degrade; this can be quite a long process, depending on the degree of crystallinity of the polymer. The degradation behaviour of these polymers can be altered by copolymerization, radiation, thermal treatment or orientation of the material.[34,35]

Figures 12.8–12.11 depict the morphology of degradation of SR-PLA 96. Scanning electron-microscopic images were taken from the end of a SR-PLA 96 wire (diameter 1.15 mm, draw ratio 7) before and after hydrolysis at +37°C in buffer solution pH 6.1. The magnification is 200 X in all images. Figure 12.8 shows the monofilament after processing and gamma sterilization. The wire in Figure 12.9 has been undergoing hydrolysis for 3 weeks and degradation has started in the amorphous areas; the gaps between crystallized areas have started to increase and microfibril bundles have started to separate.

Figures 12.10 and 12.11 show the wires after hydrolysis for 18 and 21 weeks, respectively. The gaps are increasing in size and the microfibrils are starting to break apart. The amorphous areas are dissolving and the microfibrils are breaking down into smaller fragments. At this stage the mechanical strength of the material has started to decrease.

Figures 12.12 and 12.13 depict the morphological degradation of SR-PGA, which separates into microfibrils more rapidly than SR-PLA and breaks down after 4 weeks into small blocks with little, if any, mechanical strength. The blocks change to fine powder as degradation proceeds.

The SEM images show the differences between the degradation of SR-PGA and SR-PLA. The degradation of SR-PGA is so rapid that the polymer degrades first to

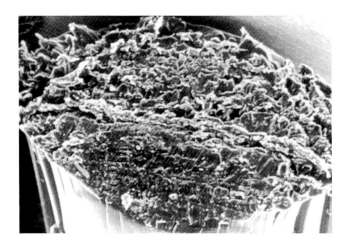

Figure 12.8. *SR-PLA 96 wire (diameter 1.15 mm) after gamma sterilization.*

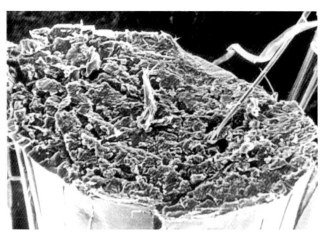

Figure 12.9. *SR-PLA 96 wire (diameter 1.15 mm) after 3 weeks' hydrolysis in vitro.*

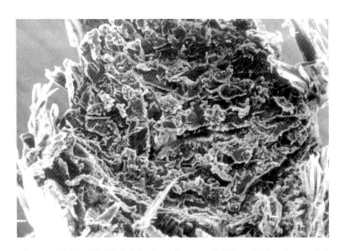

Figure 12.10. *SR-PLA 96 wire (diameter 1.15 mm) after 18 weeks' hydrolysis in vitro.*

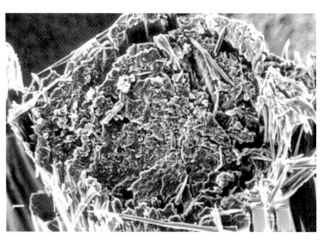

Figure 12.11. *SR-PLA 96 wire (diameter 1.15 mm) after 21 weeks' hydrolysis in vitro.*

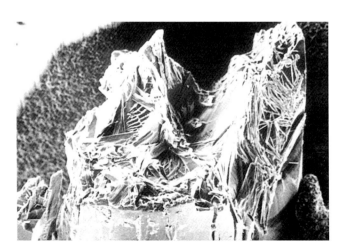

Figure 12.12. *SR-PGA wire (diameter 1.15 mm) after 2 weeks' hydrolysis in vitro.*

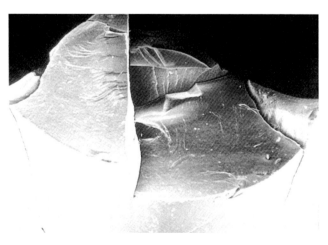

Figure 12.13. *SR-PGA wire (diameter 1.15 mm) after 4 weeks' hydrolysis in vitro.*

blocks and then to a fine powder. The inner fibrous structure of SR-PLA lasts longer than that of SR-PGA, owing to the slower degradation process of the former. Macroscopically the basic degradation process of the two is quite similar: first, the amorphous areas dissolve from the material, followed by degradation of the crystalline areas.

Effects of sterilization of PLLA

Every implant must be sterilized before implantation. Because the mechanical and degradation properties of the implant can be affected by the sterilization method, implants for different indications can be developed from the same material by variation of the sterilization method. Choosing the right sterilization method for PGA and PLA is problematic because heat and moisture cause degradation of both materials.[7,8,36] The authors have studied the effect of sterilization method on the initial strength and strength retention in vitro of SR-PLLA wires.

As Figure 12.14 shows, the sterilization method has a significant effect on the properties of SR-PLLA wires. In accelerated hydrolysis at +70°C the plasma-sterilized SR-PLLA wires retained a great deal of their strength for 8 days, whereas those sterilized by gamma irradiation retained much of their strength for 4 days. The degradation of PLA can be slowed down considerably by plasma sterlization, but gamma irradiation destroys the connecting molecular chains (chain scission) and/or makes crosslinks between them.[37,38] Polymer chain scission causes a sharp fall in molecular weight and also speeds up degradation.[10]

Expansion properties

When the implant is installed in situ it is critical that it remains in place. Bioabsorbable materials are viscoelastic, which means that, with certain processing methods, the stent can be made self-expanding at body temperature.

Figure 12.15 shows the expansion curves of different SR-PLLA stents at body temperature. The stent can be stabilized so that it does not expand at all at body temperature, or the expansion rate can be so slow that the stent will expand by only 20–30% over 2 weeks.

The SR-PLLA stent can also be manufactured for rapid expansion (Fig. 12.16), even by as much as 50% in 30 minutes. The expansion rate depends on draw ratio (dr). Figure 12.16 shows the expansion pressure of the rapidly expanding SR-PLLA stent; pressure increases rapidly and after approximately 40 minutes has attained 65 mmHg.

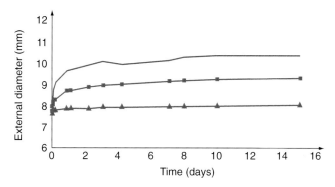

Figure 12.15. *Expansion of SR-PLLA stents (▲ PLLA H; ■ PLLA NH; —— PLLA L) in vitro at 37°C.*

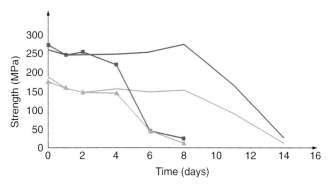

Figure 12.14. *Effect of sterilization method on the retention of the strength of PLLA in vitro (70°C, pH 6.1):* —— *bending strength after plasma sterilization;* ■ *bending strength after gamma irradiation;* —— *shear strength after plasma sterilization;* ▲ *shear strength after gamma irradiation.*

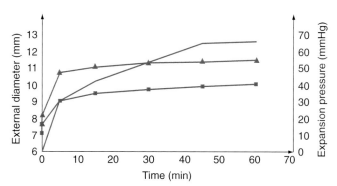

Figure 12.16. *Expansion pressure of a rapidly expanding SR-PLLA stent in vitro at 37°C:* ■ *fast expanding PLLA double helix;* ▲ *fast expanding PLLA double helix WWA dr 10;* —— *expansion pressure, unsterilized.*

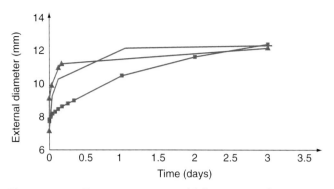

Figure 12.17. *Expansion properties of different materials in vitro at 37°C:* ■ *PGA;* ▲ *PLLA;* —— *PLA 96.*

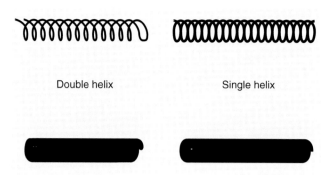

Figure 12.19. *Double- and single-helical spirals of different angles of pitch.*

In Figure 12.17 the expansion properties of stents manufactured from different materials are compared. The SR-PGA stent has the slowest rate of expansion. The SR-PLLA stent can expand more rapidly than the SR-PLA 96 stent, owing to the higher specific rigidity of the former. The rates of expansion of the SR-PLLA and SR-PLA 96 stents are greatest during the first few hours, but subsequently slows down and stops, at a stent diameter that depends on the initial diameter of the spiral, the draw ratio of the wire, the diameter of the wire and the processing conditions.

In Figure 12.18 the smaller spiral is a fast-expanding SR-PLLA urethral stent at its initial size; the larger spiral is the same type of SR-PLLA stent, which has been in the patients urethra for 2 weeks. The stent has clearly expanded in the urethra and the spaces between the rounds of the spiral have widened.

Structure-property relationships of spiral stents

The helical structure of the spiral stent has a significant effect on its properties. Figure 12.19 depicts different types of helical spirals; the helix can be either single or double and the pitch of the spiral can be varied. These alterations can bring about considerable variation in the rigidity and expansion properties of the stent. When the pitch angle increases, the number of rounds in the spiral decreases and the wire is straighter than a spiral with a smaller angle of pitch.[39] This means that the spiral with the greater pitch angle is more rigid (Fig. 12.20). The rigidity of the spiral can also be increased by changing the construction to a double helix. Figure 12.20 shows the elongation force needed to elongate single-helical and double-helical spirals. The force needed to elongate the double-helical spiral is twice that of a single-helical spiral of the same pitch angle, because in a double-helical spiral there are two wires to bear the load.

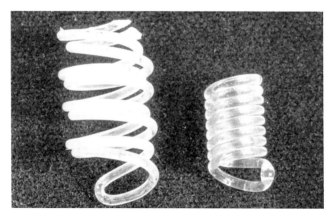

Figure 12.18. *SR-PLLA urethral stent showing initial size, and expanded dimensions after 2 weeks in situ.*

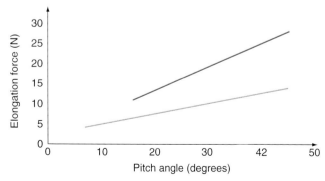

Figure 12.20. *Mathematically estimated force (elongation constant) needed to elongate a helical SR-PLLA spiral, diameter 7 mm, constructed from wire of diameter 1 mm:* —— *single helix;* —— *double helix.*

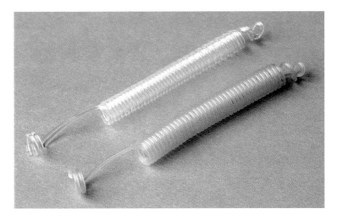

Figure 12.21. *Biofix® SR-PLLA (upper) and SR-PGA (lower) Prostatic Stents (Bioscience Ltd, Finland).*

Figure 12.21 shows two different prostatic stents, the darker one being a single-helical polyglycolide stent and the paler one being a double-helical polylactide stent. By changing the pitch angle of the spiral, the diameter of the wire and the construction of the spiral it is possible to change the rigidity or flexibility, installation expansion and fixation properties of the stent.

Conclusions

There are many possible uses of bioabsorbable materials in surgical operations, and new applications are continuously being devised. In addition, development of these materials is leading to an increased choice and the possibility of tailoring their properties for a specific application. The properties of bioabsorbable stents can be varied by different processing methods and by changes in the structure of the implant. The stents can be made to expand in situ and the expansion time can be varied; furthermore, properties, such as mechanical strength and retention of strength can be varied by different processing methods.

References

1. Törmälä P, Rokkanen P (eds). Self-reinforced Bioabsorbable Polymeric Composites in Surgery. Helsinki, Helsinki University, Department of Orthopaedics, 1995
2. Jamshidi K. Synthesis and properties of polylactides. Thesis, Kyoto University, 1984
3. Bos R R. Poly(L-lactide) osteosynthesis — development of bioresorbable bone plates and screws. Thesis, Rijksuniversiteit Groningen, 1989
4. Reed A, Gilding D. Biodegradable polymers for use in surgery — poly (glycolic)/poly (lactic acid) homo- and copolymers: 2. In vitro degradation. Polymer 1981; 22: 494–498
5. Chu C A comparison of the effect of pH on the biodegradation of two synthetic absorbable sutures. Ann Surg 1982; 1: 55–59
6. Chu C C, Moncrief G. An in vitro evaluation of the stability of mechanical properties of surgical suture materials in various pH conditions. Ann Surg 1983; August: 223–228
7. Li S, Garreau H, Vert M. Structure–property relationships in the case of the degradation of massive poly(-hydroxy acids) in aqueous media. Part 3: influence of the morphology of poly(L-lactic acid). J Mater Sci: Mater Med 1990; 1: 198–206
8. Törmälä P. Biodegradable self-reinforced composite materials: manufacturing structure and mechanical properties. Clin Mater 1992; 10: 29–34
9. Pohjonen T, Törmälä P, Mikkola J et al. Studies on mechanical properties of totally biodegradable polymeric rods for fixation of bone fractures. In: Pantjes A, Cortney J, Feijen J (eds) Proceedings 6th International Conference, Polymers in Medicine and Surgery, Leeuwenhorst Congress Centre, Holland, Leeuwenhorst: The Plastics and Rubber Institute, April 1989; 34/1–34/6
10. Chu C C, Williams D F. The effect of gamma irradiation on the enzymatic degradation of polyglycolic acid absorbable sutures. J Biomed Mater Res 1983; 17: 1029–1040
11. Williams D. Enzymatic hydrolysis of polylactic acid. Eng Med 1981; 10(1): 5–7
12. Scherer M, Früh H-J, Ascherl R et al. Kinetics of resorption of different suture materials depending on the implantation site and the species. In: Planck H, Dauner M, Renardy M (eds) Degradation Phenomena on Polymeric Biomaterials, Proceedings of the 4th International ITV Conference on Biomaterials, Denkendorf, 3–5 September 1991. Berlin: Springer-Verlag, 1992: 133–150
13. Nakamura T, Hitomi S, Watanabe S et al. Bioabsorption of polylactides with different molecular properties. J Biomed Mater Res 1989; 23: 1115–1130
14. Li S, Garreau H, Vert M. Structure–property relationships in the case of the degradation of massive aliphatic poly-(-hydroxy acids) in aqueous media. Part 1: Poly(DL-lactic acid). J Mater Sci: Mater Med 1990; 1: 123–130
15. Bos R R. Poly(L-lactide) osteosynthesis — development of bioresorbable bone plates and screws. Thesis, Rijksuniversiteit Groningen, 1989
16. Majola A. Biodegradation, biocompatibility, strength retention and fixation properties of polylactic acid rods and screws in bone tissue. Thesis, Helsinki University, 1992
17. Sinclair R, Preston J. Degradable thermoplastics from lactides. Int. Pat. WO 90/01521. Appl. 4 August, 1989. Acc. 22 February 1990
18. McNeill I, Leiper H. Degradation studies of some polyesters and polycarbonates—2. Polylactide: degradation under isothermal conditions, thermal degradation mechanism and photolysis of polymer. Polym Degrad Stabil 1985; 11: 309–326
19. Miettinen H. Fracture of the growing femoral shaft. Thesis, Kuopio University, 1992
20. Mayes P. The citric acid cycle: the catabolism of acetyl-CoA. In: Harper's Biochemistry. Connecticut; Appleton and Lange, 1988; 149–157
21. Manninen M. Self-reinforced polyglycolide and poly-L-lactide devices in fixation of osteotomies of weight-bearing bones. Thesis, Helsinki University, 1993
22. Manninen M, Pohjonen T. Intramedullary nailing of the cortical bone osteotomies in rabbits with self-reinforced poly-L-lactide rods manufactured by the fibrillation method. Biomaterials 1993; 4: 305–312

23. Eenink M. Synthesis of biodegradable polymers and development of biodegradable hollow fibres for the controlled relase of drugs. Thesis, Universiteit Twente, 1987
24. Nieuwenhuis J. Synthesis of polylactides, polyglycolides and their copolymers. Clin Mater 1992; 10: 59–67
25. Taylor G. Organic chemistry for students of biology and medicine, 3rd edn. Harlow: Longman Scientific and Technical, 1987: 211–215
26. Daniels A, Chang M, Andriano K. Mechanical properties of biodegradable polymers and composites proposed for internal fixation of bone. J Appl Biomater 1990; 1: 57–78
27. Mälkönen P. Orgaaninen kemia. Helsinki: Otava, 1989: 159–162
28. Kulkarni R, Moore E, Hegyeli A, Leonard F. Biodegradable poly(lactic acid) polymers. J Biomed Mater Res 1971; 5: 169–181
29. Sinclair R, Preston J. Degradable thermoplastics from lactides. Int. Pat. WO 90/01521. Appl. 4 August, 1989. Acc. 22 February 1990.
30. Rokkanen P. Absorbable materials in orthopaedic surgery. Ann Med 1991; 23: 109–115
31. Vainionpää S, Rokkanen P, Törmälä P. Surgical applications of biodegradable polymers in human tissues. Prog Polym Sci 1989; 14: 679–716
32. Streitwieser A, Heathcock C, Kosower E. Introduction to organic chemistry, 4th edn. New York: Macmillan, 1992: 871–878
33. Zederfelt B H, Hunt T K. Wound closure: materials and techniques. New Jersey: Davis & Geck Medical Device Division, 1990: 8–53
34. Chu C. Hydrolytic degradation of polyglycolic acid: tensile strength and crystallinity study. J Appl Polym Sci 1981; 26: 1727–1734
35. Chu C C, Williams D F. The effect of gamma irradiation on the enzymatic degradation of polyglycolic acid absorbable sutures. J Biomed Mater Res 1983; 17: 1029–1040
36. Rozema R. Resorbable poly(L-lactide) bone plates and screws, tests and applications. Thesis, Rijksuniversiteit Groningen, 1991
37. Christel P, Chabot F, Leray J et al. Biodegradable composites for internal fixation. In: Biomaterials 1980. Chichester: John Wiley and Sons Ltd, 1982: 271–280
38. Gupta M, Deshmukh V. Radiation effects on poly(lactic acid). Polymer 1983; 24: 827–830
39. Popov E. Mechanics of materials, 2nd edn. New Jersey: Prentice-Hall, 1976: 221–224

Evaluation of stents

IV

13

Methods of testing the biocompatibility of implantable medical devices
M. Talja

Introduction

The number of implantable medical devices is increasing; their safety is, therefore, a prerequisite for the use of such devices. In the mid-1980s there was international cooperation to start preparing guidelines for the biological evaluation of medical devices because of discrepancies between the various national standards and pharmacopoeial requirements for tissue safety testing. The standardization work was organized by cooperation between ISO (International Organization for Standardization) and CEN (European Committee for Standardization). Both organizations are federations of national standards bodies (member bodies). The work of preparing standards was carried out through technical committees. Each national member body interested in a subject for which the technical committee had been established had the right to be represented on that committee. Acceptance as an International Standard required approval by a least 75% of the member bodies casting a vote.

As a result of the harmonized work between ISO and CEN, it was hoped that parity could be achieved between international standards. However, the legal validity of the standardization differs: for CEN members the standards have to be followed as requirements for biocompatibility but for other countries, as members of ISO, the standards are only guidelines for manufacturers and notifying bodies, on how the biological safety of devices should be evaluated.

Biological evaluation of medical devices

Currently, the biological safety evaluation of medical devices is guided by the revised versions of the documents ISO 10993 and CEN 30993 (ISO/DIS 10993-Part 1:1995),[1] which were harmonized from numerous international and national standards and guidelines. The selection and evaluation of any new material or device intended for use in humans requires a structured programme of assessment. In the design process, an informed decision weighing the advantages/disadvantages of the various materials and test procedure choices should be made. To ensure that the final product will perform as intended and be safe for human use, the programme should include a biological evaluation.

The protection of humans is the goal of the standardization. In the biological evaluation of the devices, the number and exposure of animals should also be minimized; analysis of new materials should therefore start with cell culture tests. If the material does not pass those tests, it should be abandoned without any further evaluation.

Part 1 of the ISO 10993 Standard describes:

(a) The fundamental principles governing the biological evaluation of medical devices;
(b) The definition of categories of devices based on the nature and duration of contact with the body, and
(c) The selection of appropriate tests.

The mechanical and structural guides for medical devices are given in other standards or guidelines.

The definition of a medical device is given in ISO 10993. A medical device is an instrument, apparatus, appliance, material or other article, including software, whether used alone or in combination with other devices, which is intended to be used for the purpose of:

(a) Diagnosis, prevention, monitoring, treatment or alleviation of disease, injury or handicap,
(b) Investigation, replacement or modification of the anatomy or of a physiological process, or
(c) Control of conception.

As materials for medical devices or for their components, any synthetic or natural polymer, metal, alloy, ceramic, or other non-living substance can be used.

General principles for testing

The ISO 10993 standard serves as a framework for planning and carrying out safety analysis. The biological evaluation should be planned, carried out and documented by knowledgeable and experienced individuals capable of making informed decisions based on the advantages and disadvantages of the various materials and test procedures. When materials are selected for use in devices, their chemical, toxicological, physical, electrical, morphological and mechanical properties have to be considered.

When a biocompatibility testing protocol is planned as part of the overall biological evaluation the following aspects of the device should be considered: materials of manufacture; intended additives; process contaminants and residues; leachable substances; degradation products and other components. The interactions of the different components in the final product and the properties and characteristics of the final products should also be evaluated.

The potential device may carry a risk and the occurrence and nature of such side effects should be included in the evaluation programme. Short-term effects to be considered are acute toxicity; irritation of the skin, eyes and mucosal surfaces; sensitization; haemolysis, and thrombogenicity. Long-term or specific toxic effects to be considered are subchronic or chronic toxic effect; sensitization; genotoxicity; carcinogenicity, and effects on reproduction, including teratogenicity (Tables 13.1 and 13.2). All potential hazards should be considered for every material and final product. It is, however, not necessary or practical to test for all potential hazards.

Whenever possible, in vitro screening of the device should take place before in vivo tests are planned or conducted. The device should be re-evaluated, if there are changes in the materials, formulations, processing, packaging, sterilization or storage, or in the intended use of the device. Any adverse effects that may come to light subsequently in humans and that are induced by devices should be considered for biological re-evaluation. For the assessment of such side effects, information about the material and/or device must be amassed from various sources and should be available.

Categorization of medical devices

The medical devices are divided into categories, according to type of body contact and duration of the contact. Certain devices may fall into more than one category, in which case testing appropriate to each category should be considered separately. Tests for biological evaluation for each category are presented in Tables 13.1 and 13.2.

There are two categories of urological devices — surface-contacting devices and implant devices. Indwelling urinary and ureteral catheters, as well as non-implantable urological devices, fall into the surface-contacting device category. Such devices as implantable incontinence and impotence prostheses, long-term tissue-invasive urethral and ureteral stents, and drug supply devices, are all included in the implant devices category.

Test methods and selection of evaluation tests

The only current multiple-purpose test methods for evaluation of medical devices are listed in Tables 13.1 and 13.2. ISO 10993 gives only the guidelines for toxicity testing; the details of testing procedures are presented in national standards and guidelines.

The tests recommended are listed in annexes of standard (ISO/DIS 10993-1, 1995). Table 13.1 identifies the initial evaluation tests that should be considered for each device and duration category; Table 13.2 identifies the supplementary evaluation tests that should be considered for each device and duration category.

In selecting the test procedure, the nature, degree, duration, frequency and conditions of exposure should be taken into account. The evaluation should be based also on the existing information derived from the literature, clinical experience and non-clinical tests. If extracts of the device are used for biological testing, the solvent and conditions of extraction used should be appropriate to the nature and use of the final product. Positive and negative controls should be used wherever they are appropriate. The results of biocompatibility testing cannot ensure freedom from potential biological hazards. Any possible unexpected clinical adverse reactions or events should be analysed in order to ensure the safety of medical devices.

Table 13.1. *Initial evaluation tests for consideration**

Device categories			Biological effect							
Body contact	Contact duration A-limited (≤24 h) B-prolonged (>24 h to 30 days) C-permanent (>30 days)		Cytotoxicity	Sensitization	Irritation or intracutaneous reactivity	Systemic toxicity (acute)	Sub-chronic toxicity (sub-acute toxicity)	Geno-toxicity	Implantation	Haemo-compat-ibility
Surface devices	Skin	A	X	X	X					
		B	X	X	X					
		C	X	X	X					
Surface devices	Mucosal membranes	A	X	X	X					
		B	X	X	X					
		C	X	X	X		X	X		
Surface devices	Breached or compromised surfaces	A	X	X	X					
		B	X	X	X					
		C	X	X	X		X	X		
External communicating devices	Bloodstream, indirect	A	X	X	X	X				X
		B	X	X	X	X				X
		C	X	X		X	X	X		X
External communicating devices	Tissue/bone /dentine communicating	A	X	X	X					
		B	X	X				X	X	
		C	X	X				X	X	
External communicating devices	Circulating blood	A	X	X	X	X				X
		B	X	X	X	X		X		X
		C	X	X	X	X	X	X		X
Implant devices	Tissue/bone	A	X	X	X					
		B	X	X				X	X	
		C	X	X				X	X	
Implant devices	Blood	A	X	X	X	X			X	X
		B	X	X	X	X		X	X	X
		C	X	X	X	X	X	X	X	X

*This table is a framework for the development of an assessment programme and is not a checklist.[1]

Table 13.2. *Supplementary evaluation tests for consideration**

Device categories			Biological tests			
Body contact		Contact duration A-limited (≤24 h) B-prolonged (>24 h to 30 days) C-permanent (>30 days)	Chronic toxicity	Carcinogenicity	Reproductive/ developmental	Biodegradation
Surface devices	Skin	A				
		B				
		C				
Surface devices	Mucosal membranes	A				
		B				
		C				
Surface devices	Breached or compromised surfaces	A				
		B				
		C				
External communicating devices	Bloodstream, indirect	A				
		B				
		C	X	X		
External communicating devices	Tissue/bone/ dentine communicating	A				
		B				
		C		X		
External communicating devices	Circulating blood	A				
		B				
		C	X	X		
Implant devices	Tissue/bone	A				
		B				
		C	X	X		
Implant devices	Blood	A				
		B				
		C	X	X		

*The table is a framework for the development of an assessment programme and is not a checklist.[1]

Conclusions

Biocompatibility evaluation of new medical devices with no history nowadays is based on International Standard ISO 10993, which gives guidelines for selection of tests used for biological safety analysis of materials for use in the manufacturing process and in the final product. On the other hand, changes may be made in the design or materials of established devices and in their indications; the evaluation may therefore include both a study of the relevant experience and actual testing. According to the ISO standard, such an evaluation should be conducted by knowledgeable and experienced individuals, and may result in the conclusion that no further testing is needed if the material has a demonstrable history of use in a specified role that is equivalent to that of the device under design.

Reference

1.   Biological evaluation of medical devices — Part 1: Evaluation and testing. Draft International Standard ISO/DIS 10993-1, 1995.

14

Elasticity of radiopaque ureteral stents
P. V. Surikov, V. N. Kuleznev and S. S. Zenkov

Introduction

The successful clinical use of radiopaque ureteral stents reflects their elasticity, which depends on both the nature of the polymer material and the construction of the catheter. During insertion, ureteral stents become greatly deformed and it is essential that they subsequently regain their original shape. Ureteral stents must be flexible enough to avoid complications in situ,[1] but they must be rigid enough to drain urine and also must have a shape 'memory',[2] to guarantee retention. The purpose of the investigation described in this chapter was to quantify the recovery of shape of the polymer tube after its deformation.

Materials and methods

To investigate the process of elastic recovery of shape of the catheter tube, a method analogous to that for a strip specimen[3] was chosen and test apparatus was designed (Fig. 14.1) to measuring the kinetics of alteration of the angle of bend of the previously deformed specimen (bent at an angle of 90 degrees). The device enabled measurements to be made automatically at intervals of $0.2 \times 10^{0} - 1.0 \times 10^{4}$ and more seconds, thus including practically the entire relaxation process of the elastic component of full deformation. The device was connected to a personal computer program that calculated the alteration in the tube's angle of bend during the experiment; the program was also capable of calculating the experimental results by mathematical statistical methods.

The tubes tested comprised a low-density polyethylene matrix filled with radiopaque material. Their external diameter was 2.0–3.0 mm and their inner diameter 1.0–2.0 mm, which is the calibre commonly used for ureteral stenting. The polymer tube was fixed in the deformed position in the experimental unit for 1–20 minutes and was then released by the operator.

Results

The process of elastic recovery of the bent polymer tube was found to be in close accordance with the Kolraush formula:

$$e = \exp\left(-(t/T_{R})^{k}\right),$$

where e = relative bend deformation (from 1 to 0),
         t = time of experiment,
         T_{R} and k = parameters of this model.

The investigation showed that parameter T_{R} depended on the tube construction (either its inner or outer diameters), the chemical nature of the polymer material, filler contents and period of retention of the deformation. The parameter k was constant and was determined only by the chemical nature of the polymer (Fig. 14.2). The external and internal diameters and the thickness of the catheter wall are the basic construction parameters of the tubes. The analysis of Kolraush constants for tubes of various types and dimensions made from low-density polyethylene showed that, in the range of tube dimensions investigated, the value of k was constant whereas, as previously stated, the value of T_{R} depended on the construction of the tube, the main construction factor being the thickness of the polymer tube wall (Fig. 14.3). An increase in wall thickness

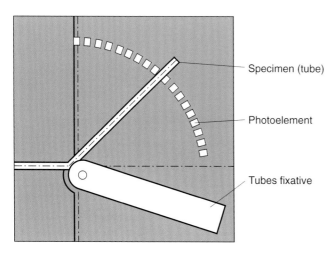

Figure 14.1. *Apparatus for testing the elasticity of ureteral stents.*

Specimen (tube)

Photoelement

Tubes fixative

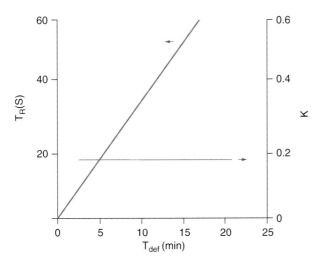

Figure 14.2. *Effect of period of deformation, t_{def} (min) on parameters $T_R(s)$ and k.*

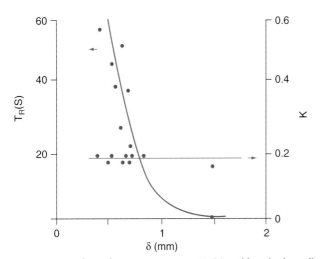

Figure 14.3. *Relation between parameters $T_R(s)$ and k and tube wall thickness δ (mm).*

leads to a reduction in T_R, related to the complex deformation of the tube during bending.

The investigations showed a good correlation between the elasticity of the tube and the relaxation properties of the polymer materials (Table 14.1).

Addition of a radiopaque filler to the polymer composition resulted in a decrease in the tube's elasticity. This effect could be compensated by sterilization with gamma radiation.

It was expected that increasing the temperature would accelerate all relaxation processes; this was confirmed, in that an increase in temperature caused a decrease in both parameters T_R and k.

In accordance with the temperature dependence of the elastic properties of the material, an increase in temperature leads to a decrease of the modulus of elasticity, which in turn brings about increasing flexibility of the radiopaque catheters. Alterations in the mechanical properties despite the small temperature increase were significant and must be taken into account when catheters are being designed. The parameter T_R for a number of polyolefine tubes has a value of between 2 and 30 seconds, these values are compatible with use of such tubes in urological practice.

The mechanical stability of the polymer tubes during bending was also studied. During bending, the cross-section of a tube becomes oval. The tube loses its stability when the lumen of the tube is obliterated; the catheter then loses its properties and cannot be used. When reducing the critical radius of bending, which is characteristic of thin-walled tubes of different materials (such as metal or plastic) during the process of buckling, the tube loses its stability, according to the following equation:[4]

$$r_{cr} = 2R^2/\delta$$

where r_{cr} = critical radius;
          R = tube radius;
          δ = wall thickness.

The experimental and calculated values of the critical radius of bending, for tubes made from polyethylene are shown in Figure 14.4. Good correlation was noted between the experimental and theoretically calculated results.

Thus the 'minimum wall thickness' of a catheter is defined by its mechanical stability during bending. Maximum wall thickness of the tube is limited by the necessity for patency of the internal lumen, stiffness of

Table 14.1. *Elastic properties of tubes of various materials[9]*

Material	Kolraush equation parameters	
	$T_R(S)$	k
Low-density polyethylene	4.5	0.18
Radiopaque polyethylene	12.8	0.18
High-density polyethylene	17.7	0.22
Polypropylene	28.2	0.15

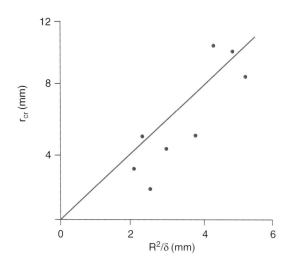

Figure 14.4. *Relation between critical radius r_{cr} (mm), tube radius R (mm) and wall thickness δ (mm).*

the catheter and the medical requirements. Most catheter tubes have an inner diameter of 1 mm or more and an outer diameter of 3 mm or less. These principles are applied in practice for the manufacture of 'pigtail' stents.

Conclusions

The results of this study have shed light on the mechanical properties of polymer tubes used for medical purposes, and may be relevant to the design of new types of radiopaque polymer stents.

References

1. Lennon G M, Thornhill J A, Sweeney P A et al. 'Firm' versus 'Soft' double pigtail ureteric stents: a randomized blind comparative trial. Eur Urol 1995; 28: 1–5
2. Hofman R, Hartung R. Ureteral stents — material and new forms. World J Urol 1989; 7: 154–157
3. Charrier J M, Gent A M. Recovery (spring-back) of polyethylene from imposed bend. Polym Eng Sci 1985; 25: 48–53
4. Thompson J M T, Hunt G W (eds). Collapse. The buckling of structures in theory and practice. Cambridge: Cambridge University Press, 1983

Infections and encrustations on stents

V

Surface modification of polymeric and metal stents coming into contact with blood or urine
S. D. Tong

Introduction

The dramatic increase in demand and use of surgical prostheses in the last decade has been followed recently by questions concerning their overall safety. Urological practice includes a number of devices, both temporary and permanent indwelling, coming into contact with blood or urine, that are made of a wide range of different materials; these include silicone, polyurethane and, most recently, metals. These materials have been selected largely on the basis of their chemical inertness though recent evidence suggests that this may not always correlate with biological inactivity. Bioincompatibility, infection, encrustation and thrombogenicity are the most common causes of urological stent-associated failure. The purpose of this chapter is to discuss viable approaches to the alleviation of the problems identified for stent surfaces.

Common materials and their limitations

Polyethylene was the first synthetic polymer used for the construction of a urological prosthesis,[1] followed by Teflon.[2] In the form of tubes for use as ureteric replacements, these prostheses failed because of a combination of anastomotic leakage, infection and encrustation. Silicone, though susceptible to the same problems when exposed to urine, has subsequently been regarded as the most biocompatible material available and has been used for the construction of urethral catheters[3] and double-pigtail stents. However, there is currently no material that can effectively completely resist infection and encrustation on prolonged exposure to urine.[4] With regard to metallic blood-contacting stents, thrombogenicity and hyperplastic intimal growth have been shown to be significant limiting features in the management of patients undergoing small-vessel stent placement.[5]

Infection

Bacterial adhesion with subsequent infection is a phenomenon common to all prosthetic materials. Once established, the infection is difficult to eradicate, usually necessitating removal of the device. In the presence of a foreign body, normal host defences are impaired, opsonization is inadequate, and polymorphonuclear leucocytes degranulate on contact with the foreign material. Bacteria are thus enabled to grow in the form of a biofilm adherent to the surface of the foreign material. Once attached to the surface, the organisms produce a glycocalyx matrix that protects them from host defence mechanisms and antimicrobial therapy.[6] Several factors are thought to influence bacterial adhesion to devices: these include bacterial surface features,[7] biomaterial surface characteristics[8] and the presenting clinical condition.[9] All prosthetic devices appear to be susceptible to this form of infection,[10] and numerous attempts are being made to develop materials with antimicrobial properties.

Encrustation

The formation of encrustations and stones on foreign materials placed in the bladder was first recognized and documented in 1790 by Austin. Hellstrom[11] established the distinction between sterile metabolic and infective stones and, in 1950, Vermeulen et al.[12] showed that encrustations on various foreign bodies in the bladder were composed of struvite. The association between this struvite and urinary infection with organisms that split urea was subsequently confirmed and the stoichiometry elucidated.[13] Urealysis forms ammonium and hydroxyl ions, which raise the pH of the urine and hence alter the solubility product of the urine with respect to struvite, which is precipitated. This type of encrustation forms readily on urethral catheters, leading to the persistent risk of ascending infection. The severity of encrustation depends on the type of material used, the length of time in contact with the urine and the solute content of the urine. Attempts to prevent the formation of encrustations by eradication of the infection or by alteration of the urinary mineral composition or pH have been largely unsuccessful.[14,15] It has been observed that encrustations also occur on internal stents in sterile urine and appear more likely to affect stents exposed to the urine of known stone-formers.[16,17] The exact mechanism of this kind of encrustation is not understood completely.

Thrombosis

Vascular stents used in blood vessels are in direct contact with blood, until they become covered by endothelium. Blood compatibility is a critical requirement for intravascular devices, since contact of blood with a foreign surface will commonly result in deposition and activation of plasma proteins, platelets, and other cellular elements that lead to thrombus formation. It is generally believed that plasma protein adsorption is the first event to occur following blood–surface contact and that subsequent phenomena are to a large extent determined by interactions of the blood with the adsorbed protein layer.[18] Device thrombogenicity involves surface potential, surface texture and surface free energy. For decades, there has been intensive research in the area of blood-compatible materials.[19]

Tissue response

Urological stents are in close contact with the urothelium during the intubation period. Various biocompatibility parameters for urinary catheters were recognized by clinicians during the 1980s, following reports of severe urethral strictures in patients receiving indwelling latex catheters. A series of investigations revealed that toxic substances added to the catheters during the manufacturing process can leak from the device in situ and cause severe urethritis and scarring, leading to the development of urethral strictures.[20–22] Urethral ischaemia, a condition of reduced blood circulation, was found to play a major role in the development of catheter-induced urethral strictures, owing to the reduced clearance of toxic substances leaking from the catheters.[23,24] The urothelial reaction is dependent on the specific chemical formulation of the stent material.[25,26] In vitro cytotoxicity tests have suggested that latex and rubber catheters induce a greater local reaction than silicone-coated catheters, as indicated by polymorphonuclear neutrophil infiltration and complement activation.

Intimal hyperplasia gradually occurs over endoluminal metallic stents that are deployed in the vascular system. After placement, the endothelium begins to cover the stents in the first 2–7 days, with complete endothelization typically occurring by week 3 in animal models. To date, a specific treatment for intimal hyperplasia and restenosis has not been identified because restenosis is a multifactorial process. The specific stimuli and effectors of intimal hyperplasia have yet to be identified completely. A long list of pharmacological agents have been evaluated in trials,[5] in an attempt to prevent restenosis. (Table 15.1)

Advantages of treating the surface of urological stents

Surface treatment of urological stents offers the unique opportunity of improving current stent designs by selectively altering the surface characteristics. It is hoped that such alteration will decrease infection, encrustation, thrombosis and tissue response, and will allow site-specific delivery of pharmacological or biological agents for incorporation into the epithelial or endothelial wall (Table 15.2).

Surface treatment with antimicrobial properties

Urological prostheses can be broadly categorized into two categories — totally implantable devices and transcutaneous devices (i.e. those with an exit site). Totally implantable devices such as ureteral stents are less prone to becoming infected than are urinary

Table 15.1. *Pharmacological agents evaluated in trials to prevent restenosis*

Antiplatelet	Antithrombin	Antiproliferative
Aspirin	Meparin	Heparin
Persantine	Hirudin	Low-molecular-weight heparin
IIb/IIIa receptor AB	Hirulog	Trapadil
Omega-3 FA		Enoxaprin
Ketanserin		Cilazapril
Salutroban		Fosinopril
GR32191		Lovastatin
Ciprostene		Angiopeptin
Ticlopidine		Nifedipine
		Procardia
		Verapamil
		Interleukin blocker

Table 15.2. *Stent properties altered by surface treatment*

Metallic or polymeric surface no longer exposed
Surface potential neutralized
Surface texture customized
Surface free energy lowered
Surface tension optimized
Antimicrobial/Antiplatelet/antithrombotic/antimitotic agents administered
Toxic substance leakage prevented

catheters. Bacterial adhesion and biofilm formation on indwelling ureteric stents was first described by Reid and co-workers.[27] In their study, the incidence of urinary infection in patients with indwelling silicone Double-J stents was 27%, and as many as 90% of the stents were found to be colonized by adherent uropathogens. In the case of devices with exit sites, such as the urinary catheter, similar to central venous lines or continuous ambulatory peritoneal dialysis catheters, the exit site represents a source of continuous recolonization and infection. The ability of uropathogens to adhere to the urothelium or to the surface of prosthetic devices is multifactorial: electrostatic and hydrophobic interaction, bacterial components (fimbriae, glycocalyx), the suspending fluid and the material itself all have a role. Thus antimicrobial modifications of the material are of the following types:[28]

1. Fixation of antibiotics or antiseptics in the polymer structure or its surface for controlled release.
2. Coating of the surface of devices with heavy metals, such as silver.
3. Modification of the polymer surface to create functional groups with intrinsic antimicrobial activity.
4. Fixation of anti-adhesive agents to device surfaces.

Antibiotics have been incorporated into the catheter surface to prevent catheter-related infections. TDMAC (tridodecyl methylammonium chloride) or benzalkonium chloride are positively charged surfactants, that form strong ionic bonds with anionic antibiotics.[29,30] A TDMAC–cefazolin-treated intravascular catheter (Bio-Guard AB coating, Cook Critical Care, Bloomington, IN, USA, with cefazolin bonded to the surface before insertion) was reported to reduce the infection rate in a

prospective, randomized controlled clinical trial.[31] Ciprofloxacin was absorbed onto urinary catheters and found to be effective for the prevention and early treatment of urinary tract infection.[32] Aminoglycoside sustained release from urethral catheters was reported to be clinically efficacious.[33] The use of catheters coated with antibiotics is generally believed to be effective over the short term, but is, unfortunately, likely to increase a patient's drug resistance.

Central venous catheters have been impregnated with antiseptics such as silver sulfadiazine and chlorhexidine to render them resistant to infection.[34] Similar approaches could very well be used for urological stents, assuming that they do not irritate the urothelium. Ion-beam-assisted deposition of silver, which is applicable to both polymeric or metallic materials, has been reported to possess antimicrobial properties.[35,36] Electric fields and iontophoresis have been demonstrated to have a lethal effect on bacteria and yeasts.[37,38] The application of these technologies to urological stents has yet to come.

Quaternary ammonium polymers, used as polyurethane coatings, are reported to exhibit a high degree of biocidal activity and haemocompatibility.[39–41] Their mode of lethal action is postulated to involve contact of the pendant quaternary ammonium group with the cell membrane of the microorganism in the absence of diffusion of any toxic substance. Initially, the pendant group is adsorbed onto the negatively charged cell surface by electrostatic interaction; the long lipophilic chain then diffuses through the cell wall. This leads to a weakening of the cytoplasmic membrane, causing a loss of cytoplasmic constituents and the death of the cell. The antimicrobial activity may be permanent because the biocidal group is not consumed during the course of interaction with microorganisms. This could be a useful approach for treating urological stents, but application of this technology to urological devices has yet to be developed.

Jansen reported a 1–3 log reduction of Gram-negative and Gram-positive organisms in adherence to hydrogel-coated polyurethane stents in perfusion experiments.[42] This same phenomenon was shown to occur in ophthalmology patients with hydrogel-coated contact lenses. The hydrophobic/hydrophilic nature of a stent surface certainly has an impact on the initial adhesion of a microorganism: the adherence of cell and protein is far less on a hydrogel-coated surface than on a hydrophobic surface. Hydrogel coating is very lubricious and therefore should be applied only to the luminal surface of the urological stent, to avoid stent migration. It is believed that the bacterial adhesion problem is mitigated but not totally eradicated on a hydrogel-coated surface.[43]

Surface treatment with anti-encrustation compounds

Bacterial infection is known to be an important factor in the development of encrustation on urinary catheters. Surface treatment with antimicrobial compounds will lessen the infection-related encrustation. Ramsay and co-workers[44] demonstrated that the physicochemical properties of stent material also play a role in encrustation. They showed that the barium or bismuth used to make the stent radiopaque leached from the polymer and was incorporated into the encrustation material. This study suggests that dissolution of material does occur. Holmes has demonstrated that the incorporation of fluorine-containing components confers significant resistance to the formation of encrustation.[45] His study showed that stent surfaces with fluorinated groups (-CF3 groups), which are known to reduce the surface energy of the bulk polymer, are most resistant to encrustation. This is evidence that changing the surface chemistry, and hence the surface energy, would influence the encrustation process.

Surface treatment with thromboresistance compounds

Several approaches can be taken to reduce thrombosis. Whereas a number of 'passive' coatings, including hydrogels and polyurethane, were found be ineffective against thrombus formation,[46] an 'active' coating that interacts with the circulating blood appeared to be required in order to make a significant impact on thrombogenicity. It has been shown that heparin-like molecules with anticoagulant activity are synthesized on the luminal surface of endothelial cells. The endothelium plays an important part in the inactivation of thrombin and possibly also of other coagulation factors. As a result, heparin has been one of the most extensively investigated substances for adsorption or

binding to biomaterial surfaces. Heparin-coated surfaces have been evaluated in various types of devices where thromboresistance might be of particular clinical value, such as arteriovenous shunts, catheters, arterial filters, oxygenators, cardiopulmonary bypass circuits and vascular endoprostheses.[47,48] The principal anticoagulant mechanism of heparin is mediated by its interaction with antithrombin III. The heparin–antithrombin complex accelerates the inactivation of thrombin and other coagulation factors. The active site of heparin has been shown to contain a specific carbohydrate sequence. When the heparin molecule is modified in the process of surface coating, it is essential that the active sequence responsible for anticoagulation should remain unaltered. Many techniques have been used to immobilize heparin onto various synthetic surfaces.[49] A large number of materials involved in cardiopulmonary bypass circuits have been immobilized with heparin by two commercially available techniques — the Carmeda bioactive surface (Carmeda, Stockholm, Sweden) and the Duraflo heparin coating (Baxter Healthcare Corporation, Irvine, CA).[50] Recently, a Carmeda heparin-coated Palmaz–Schatz Stent was implanted in human coronary arteries and was reported not to cause acute or subacute stent thrombosis in patients under a new antiplatelet drug regimen.[51]

Other than surface-immobilized heparin, phospholipid polymer-coating materials have been reported to exert thromboresistant properties through their reduced protein adsorption and strong affinity toward phospholipids in blood.[52,53] The application of these thromboresistant surface treatments to endoluminal stent or polymeric surfaces is under investigation.

Surface treatment with antimitotic compounds

Hyperplastic growth and fibrotic proliferation have caused restenosis in urological stents. Pharmaceutical agents that inhibit intimal and fibrotic proliferation can be coated on the stent surface and released for localized delivery at high concentrations. Hydrocortisone, colchicine, methotrexate, forskolin, angiopeptin, and nitric oxide-releasing polymers are all potential candidates. Beta-emitting isotopes have also been incorporated into stent material, to deliver localized irradiation to inhibit intimal growth.

Future advances

The future of coated urological stents is promising. The development of new tools for site-specific therapy may have unexpected consequences. Nevertheless, the opportunity to custom-tailor stent surfaces opens an exciting chapter in the advancement of urology.

References

1. Tulloch W S. Restoration of continuity of the ureter by means of polyethylene tubing. Br J Urol 1952; 24: 42–45
2. Ulm A H, Kraus L. Total unilateral teflon ureteral substitutes in the dog. J Urol 1960; 83: 575–582
3. Cox A J, Hukins D W L, Sutton T M. Comparison of in vitro encrustation on silicone and hydrogel coated latex catheters. Br J Urol 1988; 61: 156–161
4. Holmes D A V, Cheng C, Whitfield H N. The development of synthetic materials that resist encrustation on exposure to urine. Br J Urol 1992; 69: 651–655
5. Bailey S R. Coating of endovascular stents. In: Topol E J (ed) Textbook of interventional cardiology. Philadelphia: Saunders, 1994; 2: 754–756
6. Costerton J W, Cheng K J, Geesey G G et al. Bacterial biofilms in nature and disease. Annu Rev Microbiol 1987; 41: 435–464
7. Jones D S, Gorman S P, McCafferty D F et al. A comparative study of the effects of three non-antibiotic antimicrobial agents on the surgace hydrophobicity of certain microorganisms. J Appl Bacteriol 1991; 71: 218–227
8. Gorman S P, Mawhinney W M, Adair C G, Issouckis M. Confocal scanning laser microscopy of CAPD catheter surface microrugosity in relation to recurrent peritonitis. J Med Microbiol 1993; 38: 411–417
9. Mawhinney W M, Adair C G, Gorman S P. Factors influencing the adherence of microbial pathogens to CAPD catheters. Pharmacotherapy 1992; 12: 253
10. Ramsay J W A, Garnham A J, Mulhall A B et al. Biofilms, bacteria and bladder catheters, a clinical study. Br J Urol 1989; 64: 395–398
11. Hellstrom J. The significance of staphylococci in the development of renal and ureteral stones. Br J Urol 1938; 10: 348–350
12. Vermeulen C W, Grove W J, Goetz R et al. Experimental urolithiasis. Development of calculi upon foreign bodies surgically introduced into the bladders of rats. J Urol 1950; 64: 541–548
13. Griffith D P, Musher D M, Itin C. Urease. The primary cause of infection-induced urinary stones. Invest Urol 1976; 13: 346–350
14. Hedelin H, Eddeland A, Larsson L et al. The composition of catheter encrustations, including the effects of allopurinol treatment. Br J Urol 1984; 56: 250–254
15. Griffith D P, Khonsari F, Skurnick J H et al. A randomized trial of acetohydroxamic acid for the treatment and prevention of infection-induced urinary stones in spinal cord injury patients. J Urol 1988; 140: 318–324
16. Finney R P. Double-J and diversion stents. Urol Clin North Am 1982; 9: 89–94
17. Schulz K A, Wettlauffer J N, Oldani G. Encrustation and stone formation: complication of indwelling urethral stent. Urology 1985; 25: 616–619
18. Scott C F. Mechanism of the participation of the contact system in the Vroman effect. Review and summary. In: Bamfort C H, Cooper S L, Tsuruta T (eds) The Vroman effect. Utrecht: Bookcraft, 1992: 75–83
19. Brash J L. Role of plasma protein adsorption in the response of blood to foreign surfaces. In: Sharma C P, Szycher M (eds) Blood compatible materials and devices, perspectives towards the 21st century. Lancaster, Pennsylvania: Tecnomic, 1991: 3–24
20. Ruutu M, Alfthan O, Talja M, Anderson L C. Cytotoxicity of latex urinary catheters. Br J Urol 1985; 57: 82
21. Talja M, Anderson L C, Ruutu M, Alfthan O. Toxicity testing of urinary catheters. Br J Urol 1985; 57: 579
22. Talja M, Ruutu M, Anderson L C, Alfthan O. Urinary catheter structure and testing methods in relation to tissue toxicity. Br J Urol 1986; 58: 443
23. Abdel-Hakim A, Hassouna M, Teijera J, Elhilali R. Role of urethral ischemia in the development of urethral strictures after cardiovascular surgery: a preliminary report. J Urol 1984; 131: 1077
24. Talja M, Vortamem J, Andersson L C. Toxic catheters and diminished urethral blood circulation in the introduction of urethral strictures. Eur Urol 1986; 12: 340
25. Cormio L, Talja M, Koivusalo A et al. Biocompatibility of various indwelling double-J stents. J Urol 1995; 153: 494–496
26. Thijssen A M, Millward S F, Mai K T. Ureteral response to the placement of metallic stents: an animal model. J Urol 1994; 151: 268–270
27. Reid G, Denstedt J D, Kang Y S, Lam D, Nause C. Microbial adhesion and biofilm formation on ureteral stents in vitro and in vivo. J Urol 1992; 148: 1592–1594
28. Jansen B. Bacterial adhesion to medical polymers — use of radiation techniques for the prevention of materials-associated infection. Clin Mater 1991; 6: 65–74
29. Trooskin S Z, Donetz A P, Harvey R A, Greco R S. Prevention of catheter sepsis by antibiotic bonding. Surgery 1985; 97: 547–551
30. Henry R, Harvey R A, Greco R S. Antibiotic bonding to vascular prostheses. J Thorac Cardiovasc Surg 1981; 82: 272–277
31. Kamal G D, Pfaller M A, Rempe L E, Jebson P J R. Reduced intravascular catheter infection by antibiotic bonding. JAMA 1991; 265(18): 2364–2368
32. Reid G, Tieszer C, Foerch R et al. Adsorption of Ciprofloxacin to urinary catheters and effect on subsequent bacterial adhesion and survival. Colloids Surf B: Biointerfaces 1993; 1: 9–16
33. Sakamoto I, Umemurs Y, Nakano H, Nihira H. Efficacy of an antibiotic coated indwelling catheter: a preliminary report. J Biomed Mater Res 1985; 19: 1031–1041
34. Greenfeld J I, Sampath L, Popilskis S J et al. Decreased bacterial adherence and biofilm formation on chlorhexidine and silver sulfadiasine impregnated central venous catheters implanted in swine. Crit Care Med 1995; 23: 894–900
35. Collinge G A, Doll G, Seligson D, Easley K J. Pin tract infections: silver vs. uncoated pins. Orthopedics 1994; 17(5): 445–448
36. McLean R J C, Hussain A A, Sayer M et al. Antibacterial activity of multilayer silver–copper surface films on catheter material. Can J Microbiol 1993; 39: 895–899
37. Davis C P, Anderson M D, Hoskins S, Warren M M. Electrode and bacterial survival with iontophoresis in synthetic urine. J Urol 1992; 147: 1310–1313
38. Pareilleuz A, Sicard N. Lethal effects of electric current on Escherichia coli. Appl Microbiol 1970; 19: 421–424
39. Hazziza-Laskar J, Nurdin N, Helary G, Sauvet G. Biocidal polymers active by contact. I: Synthesis of polybutadiene with pendant quaternary ammonium groups. J Appl Polymer Sci 1993; 50: 651–662
40. Hazziza-Laskar J, Nurdin N, Helary G, Sauvet G. Biocidal polymers active by contact. II: Biological evaluation of polyurethane coating with pendant quaternary ammonium salts. J Appl Polymer Sci 1993; 50: 663–678

41. Hazziza-Laskar J, Nurdin N, Helary G, Sauvet G. Biocidal polymers active by contact. III: Aging of biocidal polyurethane coatings in water. J Appl Polymer Sci 1993; 50: 671–678

42. Jansen B, Goodman L, Ruiten D. Bacterial adherence to hydrophilic polymer-coated polyurethane stents. Gastrointest Endosc 1993; 39: 670–673

43. Khoury A E, Olson M, Villari F. Determination of the coefficient of kinetic friction of urinary catheter materials. J Urol 1991; 145: 610–612

44. Ramsay J W A, Crocker R P, Ball A J et al. Urothelial reaction to ureteric intubation. A clinical study. Br J Urol 1987; 60: 504–505

45. Holmes S A V, Cheng C, Whitfield H N. The development of synthetic polymers that resist encrustation on exposure to urine. Br J Urol 1992; 69: 651–655

46. Lunn A C. Heparin stent coatings. In: Sigwart U (ed) Endoluminal stenting. London: W. B. Saunders Company Ltd, 1996; 80–83

47. von Segesser L K, Turina M. Cardiopulmonary bypass without systemic heparinization. J Thorac Cardiovasc Surg 1989; 98: 386–396

48. Hsu L C. Principles of heparin-coating techniques. Perfusion 1991; 6: 209–219

49. Emanuelsson H, van der Giessen W J, Serruys P W. Benestent II: Back to the future. J Intervent Cardiol 1994; 7(6): 587–592

50. Hsu L C. Principles of heparin-coating techniques. Perfusion 1991; 6: 209–219

51. Serruys P W, Emanuelsson H, van der Giessen W J. Heparin-coated Palmaz–Schatz stents in human coronary arteries. Circulation 1996; 93: 412–422

52. Ishihara K, Ziats N P, Tierney B P et al. Protein adsorption from human plasma is reduced on phospholipid polymers. J Biomed Mater Res 1991; 25: 1397–1407

53. Ishihara K, Oshida H, Endo Y et al. Hemocompatibility of human whole blood on polymers with a phospholipid polar group and its mechanism. J Biomed Mater Res 1992; 26: 1543–1552

Encrustation and microbial adhesion on stents: current understanding of biofilms

J. D. Watterson, D. T. Beiko and J. D. Denstedt

16

Introduction

A biomaterial is defined as any substance, natural or synthetic, used in the treatment of a patient, which at some stage interfaces with tissue.[1] The use of biomaterials within the urinary tract dates back to ancient Egypt where lead and papyrus catheters were used for urinary drainage.[2] In contemporary urological practice, the most routine materials implanted in the urinary tract, urethral catheters and ureteral stents, continue to be constructed from synthetic polymeric compounds. Many millions of devices are used each year, with North American data showing that, for urethral catheters and urinary stents alone, this represents over 100 million per annum.[3]

During the last decade there has been significant advances in the understanding of the association between urinary infection, biofilm formation on biomaterials and encrustation. Despite such advances, biomaterial-related infection and encrustation within the urinary tract are the major limitations in the long-term use of these devices. For urethral catheters, the risk of catheter-associated infection increases by 5–8% per day,[4] and over 90% of patients undergoing long-term catheterization will develop bacteriuria within 4 weeks, despite closed drainage systems.[5] Fifty per cent of patients with long-term indwelling catheters will experience encrustation and catheter blockage.[6] Stent colonization is frequent with rates ranging from 28% to 90%.[7,8] Established device-related infection and encrustation cannot be resolved employing traditional antimicrobial therapy and often require device removal for infection resolution. Furthermore, the use of systemic antimicrobial therapy in these difficult clinical situations may induce the selection of resistant organisms, due to the unique metabolic and physical characteristics of biofilms.

In this chapter, an overview of the existing understanding of biofilm, biomaterial-related infection and encrustation will be presented. Analytical techniques for the evaluation of biomaterials and novel approaches to combat these problems will be reviewed.

Biofilm and device-related infection/encrustation

Encrustation deposition can occur in both infected and sterile systems. However, many of the processes in both systems are intimately related and frequently coexist. Creation of conditioning film on a prosthetic device surface represents the initial stage of device-associated infection and encrustation. A conditioning film is produced by the deposition of host urinary components on the surface of the biomaterial within minutes of placement.[9] The conditioning film is comprised of proteins, electrolytes, and other organic molecules. Protein adsorption following materials–tissue contact is generally nonspecific, with multiple binding sites on the proteins interacting with sites on the material surface. Factors influencing the binding of proteins include Van der Waal's forces, electrostatic and polarity forces between the molecules and the surface, solvent-dependent interactions, hydrogen bonding, hydrophobic interactions, hydration forces and steric forces.[10] The conditioning film alters the surface of the biomaterial and may block or provide receptor sites for subsequent bacterial adhesion.[11]

Development of a biofilm is the next step towards device-related infection and encrustation. Following the formation of the organic conditioning film on the device surface, urease-producing and other bacteria adhere to the conditioning film and develop within a matrix of bacterial exopolysaccharide (EPS). The production of EPS and the formation of a glycocalyx chemically bind this living and constantly changing layer to the polymer surface, which is known as a 'biofilm'.[12] Attached cells up-regulate the genes responsible for the production of enzymes concerned with the synthesis of EPS and evidence now exists that demonstrates the ability of bacteria to transfer genetic information within biofilms.[13] The structure of biofilm is very complex. Many biofilms are defined by three components: a linking film attached to the surface of tissues or materials; a base film containing compact organisms; and a surface film from which planktonic organisms may spread to other sites.[14] The resultant biofilm protects bacteria against antibiotics, antibodies, and urease inhibitors, as well as host defenses.[15]

The development of biomaterial-related encrustation is dependent on the microbiological flora present in the urinary tract. In an infected system, urease-positive bacteria are the main cause of these encrustations. Through the hydrolysis of urea by the action of the enzyme urease, the urinary pH is increased resulting in the precipitation and stabilization of calcium and magnesium within the biofilm matrix, forming magnesium ammonium phosphate ($NH_4MgPO_4 \cdot 2H_2O$) and calcium hydroxyapatite ($Ca_{10}[PO_4]_6 \cdot H_2O$) crystals. In the past few years it has been demonstrated that *Proteus mirabilis* plays a dominating role in encrustation processes.[16] In several studies this species has been detected in nearly all obstructing material of urethral catheters.[17,18] The enzyme urease from *P. mirabilis* hydrolyses urea 6 to 10 times faster than the urease enzymes from other species.[19] Furthermore, *P. mirabilis* has the ability to differentiate into swarming cells that allow the bacteria to migrate significantly faster over biomaterial surfaces,[20] and is accompanied by 30-fold increases in the production of urease.[21]

In a sterile setting, the mechanistic processes responsible for encrustation development have not been fully elucidated but may be dependent on both urinary constituents and the properties of the biomaterial. Sterile encrustations are often composed of calcium oxalate.[22] The precipitation and formation of these crystals may be accelerated kinetically by the presence of rough surfaces, catheter holes and edges. Metabolic disorders such as hypercalciuria, certain physiological states such as pregnancy, and even the intestinal microbial flora may contribute to further accelerated encrustation of devices within a sterile urinary environment.[22] A recent paper by Verkoelen and Schepers challenges that there be a link between the production of proteins in response to renal tissue injury and the subsequent development of nephrolithiasis.[23] The possibility exists that cellular injury in response to the presence of urinary tract biomaterials may be

an important determinant in the promotion and progression of encrustation as many of these up-regulated proteins are also known for their role in wound healing. Further investigation into this novel theory is required. Finally, regardless of system, the interactions involved in the deposition of encrustation onto biomaterials are numerous and appear to be influenced by the following: the chemical composition of the polymer, the physical properties of its surface, the presence of graft polymer coating, conferring on the biomaterial a hydrophilic/hydrophobic nature, contact time with urine, the urine solute content, metabolic disorders, and even the intestinal microbial composition.[24]

Techniques of analysis

Biomaterials research continues to search for the ideal material. The comparison of available and novel biomaterials requires an understanding of the physical and chemical properties of the biomaterials, in addition to evaluating the biomaterial and its response to each unique environment. Before new biomaterials can be tested in an in vivo human setting they must be rigorously tested in vitro and/or in animal models. The evaluation of materials used in the fabrication of urinary tract biomaterials should initially assess tensile strength, flexibility, coefficient of friction, radiopacity, biodurability, biocompatibility, and unit cost.[25] The American Society for Testing and Materials develops standards and tests protocols evaluating various materials, including polymeric biomaterials.[26] The physicochemical assessments must be correlated with the most current methods of biocompatibility testing, encrustation and bacteriological studies, and advanced microscopic and surface analytical techniques.

Biocompatibility is defined as 'the utopian state where a biomaterial presents an interface with a physiologic environment without the material adversely affecting that environment or the environment adversely affecting the material'.[1] At present, all biomaterials have some form of reactive effect on tissue. The most common biocompatibility testing procedures used today include animal models,[27,28] and cell culture techniques.[29] Novel techniques using urinary tract-specific cell lines, such as human urothelial cells (HUC) or human bladder smooth muscle,[30,31] and the use of genetically engineered animals,[32] may provide a bridge between in vitro testing and the final application in the human body.

Standard microbiological testing has evolved to provide more objective data concerning biomaterial-related infection. It is well recognized that the predictive value of urinary cultures in assessing microbial colonization of urinary tract biomaterials is poor. Several studies have shown a 28–44% concordance rate between urine and stent cultures.[33,34] Reid et al. have proposed that sonication prior to culture and plating should be used in microbiological protocols in order to retrieve most of the bacteria adherent to the biomaterial.[8] Failing to do so results in isolation of a portion of bacteria, therefore yielding a falsely low incidence of bacterial colonization. In addition to routine microbiological cultures to evaluate and quantify adherent bacteria, researchers are beginning to evaluate the nature of the interaction between bacteria and biomaterial. As bacterial adherence and spreading are regarded as important steps in the pathogenesis of stent infection and occlusion, several groups have specifically evaluated the ability of Proteus mirabilis to translocate across the surface of various biomaterial surfaces. Stickler and Hughes developed a simple, in vitro model to evaluate this pathogenic ability and found that migration of P. mirabilis was significantly more rapid across hydrogel-coated latex catheters than over all-silicone or silicone-coated latex catheters. Watterson et al. followed up this initial study with an evaluation of ureteral stents confirming silicone's relative resistance to Proteus translocation compared to other polymers.[35] Since the resultant binding, differentiation into swarmers, and migration of P. mirabilis across the surface of a urinary tract device promotes biomaterial-related infection and encrustation, further characterization of a device's ability to retard the migration of Proteus may provide new insights into biomaterial development.

The evaluation of encrusting deposits onto biomaterials has also been subject to recent urological investigation. The susceptibility of a biomaterial to encrustation can also be tested by in vitro or in vivo methods. The variability of in vivo models in terms of fluid intake, diet, urinary components, and infection has made comparison of biomaterials difficult. In vitro testing provides a means of determining the tendency of materials to encrust and the results are not influenced by patient diet or metabolic differences between individuals.[36] Choong et al. have recently developed an in vitro encrustation model using human urine that specifically addresses the inadequacies of previous in vitro models.[37] This validated encrustation model has allowed for the rapid and economical screening of a large number of new and existing polymers intended for urological use. Using their model they have noted several findings. First, the majority of polyurethane alloplastic materials encrust significantly more than silicone, the current gold standard biomaterial. Second, phosphorylcholine (PC), a chemical group found in the membrane of living cells that has been incorporated into eye-care and cardiovascular products, was found to encrust as much as silicone. Third, coating with hyaluronic acid resulted in less encrustation than silicone. Last, hydrogel-coated ureteral stents accumulated significantly more encrustation than the same stents without a coating.

Evaluation of encrustation on the various stents and catheters relies on advanced microscopic and surface analytical techniques, such as X-ray photoelectron spectroscopy (XPS), atomic force microscopy (AFM), scanning electron microscopy (SEM), and energy-dispersive X-ray analysis (EDX), and surface-enhanced laser desorption and ionization (SELDI).[38] XPS can distinguish fine chemical features on large to minute surfaces and involves the irradiation of a freeze-dried specimen by an X-ray beam that induces the ejection of electrons. The kinetic energy of the emitted electrons is analysed, their binding energy determined, and each recorded peak is characteristic of an element (N, C, O, etc.). This achieves a direct elemental analysis of the surface. While the presence of elemental nitrogen, oxygen and sodium characterizes conditioning film formation, the finding of magnesium, phosphorus, and calcium implies the presence of encrustation crystals.[9] Another valuable technique is SEM. The combination of SEM with EDX allows visual selection of a material section, followed by chemical elemental analysis.[39] EDX is based on atomic excitation within the specimen by an electron beam and assessment of the X-ray spectrum that emanates once these atoms return to a lower energy status. Objective quantification of encrustation can be accomplished using calcium atomic absorption spectroscopy (AAS).[37] Atomic absorption spectrometry is based on an atom's ability to absorb and emit energy at a specific wavelength due to its electronic transitions. Since each element has its own absorbance and emission 'signature', atomic absorption spectrometry can be used to quantitatively determine a specific element in a complex sample matrix. Finally, SELDI combines mass spectrometry (MS) analysis with enzymatic and/or chemical modification of target proteins allowing for direct, facile mass spectrometric detection of both major and minor proteins in heterogeneous samples.[40] Arrays of spots containing chemical (ionic, hydrophobic, hydrophilic, etc.) or biochemical (antibody, receptor, DNA, etc.) surfaces are designed to capture proteins of interest. The spots are exposed to pulsed nitrogen laser energy, resulting in the ionization of proteins and subsequent measurement of the mass of each protein species based on its velocity through an ion chamber. This technology has recently been the focus of interest in a study by Cadieux and colleagues evaluating urinary proteins in patients with urolithiasis.[41] These surface science methodologies provide a means to measure changes in the physical and chemical compositions of biomaterials ultimately allowing insights into conditioning film, bacterial biofilm formations and encrustation deposition.

Therapeutic approaches

Efforts to prevent encrustation and device-related infection have largely met with limited and often contradictory results. A variety of methods are currently used in the management of catheter encrustation and infection.[12] Prophylactic catheter and stent replacement before the time of expected encrustation appearance, alteration of the size or type of device, and increasing fluid intake are standard recommendations. Despite these general measures, the search continues for biomaterials or coatings that are more resistant to encrustation and infection. Current strategies involve alteration of the bulk material, coating with inhibitors, biocides, or anti-infectives or manipulation of the urinary environment.

Bulk materials

Silicone has been used extensively in the manufacture of urinary tract biomaterials and is widely considered to be the gold standard for tissue compatibility due to its

non-toxic, inert nature.[42] Existing evidence supports its relative resistance to encrustation, allowing for possible extended device retention compared to other currently used materials.[37] Alteration of the chemical composition of the bulk material has found support in the literature. Studies have indicated that materials with surface energies between 20 and 30 dynes/cm^2 exhibited increased resistance to bacterial, mineral, fungal and thrombus growth.[43] Fluorinated,[44] and carbon-rich[45] devices result in the lowering of device surface energy that has translated into less dense encrustations when tested in vitro and in vivo, respectively. Lastly, the use of bioabsorbable materials designed to disappear before encrustation deposition continues to be the focus of research of many groups and will be discussed elsewhere in the text.[46–50]

Coatings

Hydrogels are common materials used for coating urinary tract biomaterials. Hydrogels are composed of hydrophilic polymers that swell on contact with water and retain a large fraction of this water within their polyanionic structure. The surface water of a hydrogel material reduces its coefficient of friction, which contributes to biocompatibility by reducing frictional irritation and cell adhesion at the biomaterial–urothelial interface.[51] This low interfacial tension may explain observations of hydrogels resisting protein and crystalloid deposition on their surfaces.[1] Contradictory evidence, however, exists in the literature and recent testing by Choong et al. using a validated model has demonstrated significantly more encrustation on hydrogel-coated ureteral stents than uncoated stents.[37]

Coating with inhibitors of encrustation and other various biomolecules represents a relatively novel approach to reducing device-related encrustation. Borrowing from cardiovascular research, investigators have begun evaluating heparin-like compounds for their encrustation-resistance potential. In one recent study, heparin-coated polyurethane ureteral stents were compared with uncoated polyurethane stents. Heparin-coated stents did not show any biofilm formation or encrustation after 6 weeks, and effectively inhibited the encrustation process that was observed on the uncoated stents.[52] This study complements previous findings from a rabbit bladder implantation model published by Zupkas et al. that found when silicone rings were coated with pentosanpolysulfate (PPS), a semi-synthetic polysaccharide chemically similar to heparin, an eightfold reduction of encrustation was observed.[53] Further in vitro studies in rats have shown PPS to inhibit calcium oxalate crystallization,[54] and that PPS is an active inhibitory of calcium oxalate crystal growth and agglomeration.[55]

The production of materials with surface properties that prevent adherence of bacterial cells is another strategy to reduce encrustation. Compounds based on 2-methacryloloxyethylphosphorylcholine copolymerized with long-chain alkyl methacrylates have been produced which have structural and surface properties similar to those of the outer membranes of erythrocytes. These PC coatings have been applied onto catheter base materials where they produce polar surfaces that are extremely hydrophilic. In a clinical study by Stickler et al., the performance of PC-coated ureteral stents was investigated. Scanning electron microscopy and bacteriological analysis on 44 PC-coated stents that had been implanted in patients for 12-week periods and 28 control stents suggested that the PC-coated devices were less vulnerable to encrustation and colonization by bacterial biofilm than normal stents.

A novel approach to reducing biomaterial-related urinary tract encrustation involves coating biomaterials with oxalate-degrading enzymes derived from *Oxalobacter formigenes*. It had been previously demonstrated that this anaerobic bacterium is capable of degrading oxalate through its production of several enzymes, including oxalyl coenzyme A decarboxylase (OXC) and formyl coenzyme A transferase (FRC).[56,57] Watterson et al. successfully demonstrated incubation-based coating of OXC and FRC onto silicone disks. Furthermore, in an in vivo rabbit bladder implantation model, they demonstrated a reduction in the amount of encrustation on the enzyme-coated disks versus control disks after a 30 day implantation period.[58]

Systemic antimicrobial therapeutic agents are of little or no value in preventing or eradicating uropathogen colonization of biomaterial surfaces. Microorganisms deep within the biofilm are characterized by a slow and variable growth rate, and as growth rate is a primary modulator of antibiotic action, may account for the resistance to antimicrobial therapy. However, the incorporation of antimicrobial agents or biocides into the polymers or as coatings remains a common focus of investigative research. Silver, various antibiotic coatings, antibiotic-containing liposomal hydrogels and antimicrobial composite polymer have been investigated with varying results.[59–63] Silver-coated biomaterials continue to spark controversy. Silver exerts its biocidal effect by interacting with surface proteins on the bacterium and, possibly, with other macromolecules within the microbe.[64] Heralded as an effective non-resistance inducing strategy to prevent device-related infections, many researchers have claimed strong antimicrobial activity resulting in the launch of several products on the market. However, randomized clinical trials showing statistically significant antimicrobial efficacy of silver coated medical devices are rare. The largest randomized controlled clinical trial with 1300 patients failed to demonstrate significant differences in infection rates between silver-coated and non-coated catheters. Despite advances in vitro and in short-term use of antimicrobials and biocides, the ability to provide protection for device surfaces represents a continuing challenge. Regardless of agent employed, the concern of microbial drug resistance is a real phenomenon and is the main criticism of such an approach.

Bladder irrigation

Finally, to reduce encrustation on urethral catheters a variety of bladder washouts have been investigated and comprise either washouts of saline, various antiseptics or weak acidic solutions. Through the manipulation of urinary pH, catheter encrustation may be minimized. Urine collected from 64 patients with long-term indwelling urinary catheters demonstrated a difference in urinary pH between those who suffered from recurrent catheter blockage and those who did not.[12] 'Non-blockers' had a significantly more acidic voided urine pH as compared to 'blockers' and did not have a urinary infection. To provide further support to the concept of urinary pH manipulation as a possible therapeutic strategy, Getliffe et al. showed that it is possible to dissolve urinary catheter encrustations using small volumes of acidic bladder washout solutions.[65] In another study, the daily instillation of the acidic Suby G solution demonstrated efficacy in controlling encrustation in vitro,[66] and dissolved struvite crystals in suspension but was ineffective in removing crystals entrapped within the biofilm,[67] and in vivo.[68] As urease-producing bacteria are routinely the cause of elevated urinary pH and subsequent encrustation, Morris and Stickler have evaluated the use of urease inhibitors to control encrustation.[69] It was observed that acetohydroxamic acid and fluorofamide restricted the increase in pH of *Proteus mirabilis*-infected urine from 9.1 to 7.6. Significant reductions in the deposition of calcium and magnesium salts were also observed.

Future directions

Prevention of biofilm formation and encrustation requires a detailed understanding of the events and processes involved. As the physicochemical mechanisms become elucidated, novel approaches will be gained. Surface modification techniques will continue to improve and will include the immobilization of biomolecules and more potent antimicrobials designed to penetrate biofilm. Prevention of surface fouling will involve the tailoring of molecular interactions between urinary proteins and the biomaterial surface. Continued progress in molecular genetic approaches and scanning microscopic techniques will further advance into biofilm research and understanding. It will be imperative that clinicians, microbiologists, molecular biologists and surface scientists continue a collaborative, multidisciplinary approach to provide answers to these many questions.

References

1. Mardis H K, Kroeger R M. Ureteral stents. Materials. Urol Clin North Am 1988; 15(3): 471–479
2. Bitschay J, Brodny M L. A history of urology in Egypt. New York: Riverside Press, 1956
3. Schierholz J M, Yucel N, Rump A F, Beuth J, Pulverer G. Antiinfective and encrustation-inhibiting materials – myth and facts. Int J Antimicrob Agents 2002; 19(6): 511–516
4. Mulhall A B, Chapman R G, Crow R A. Bacteriuria during indwelling urethral catheterization. J Hosp Infect 1988; 11(3): 253–262
5. Slade N, Gillespie W A. The urinary tract and the catheter: infection and other problems. Chichester, UK: Wiley, 1985
6. Kohler-Ockmore J, Feneley R C. Long-term catheterization of the bladder: prevalence and morbidity. Br J Urol 1996; 77(3): 347–351
7. Keane P F, Bonner M C, Johnston S R, Zafar A, Gorman S P. Characterization of biofilm and encrustation on ureteric stents in vivo. Br J Urol 1994; 73(6): 687–691
8. Reid G, Denstedt J D, Kang Y S, Lam D, Nause C. Microbial adhesion and biofilm formation on ureteral stents in vitro and in vivo. J Urol 1992; 148(5): 1592–1594
9. Reid G, Tieszer C, Denstedt J D, Kingston D. Examination of bacterial and encrustation deposition on ureteral stents of differing surface properties, after indwelling in humans. Coll Surf B: Biointerfaces 1995; 5: 171–179
10. Schierholz J M, Lucas L J, Rump A, Pulverer G. Efficacy of silver-coated medical devices. J Hosp Infect 1998; 40(4): 257–262
11. Reid G, Busscher H J. Importance of surface properties in bacterial adhesion to biomaterials, with particular reference to the urinary tract. Int J Biodetergents and Biodegradation 1992; 30: 105–122
12. Choong S, Wood S, Fry C, Whitfield H. Catheter associated urinary tract infection and encrustation. Int J Antimicrob Agents 2001; 17(4): 305–310
13. Davies D G, Parsek M R, Pearson J P, Iglewski B H, Costerton J W, Greenberg E P. The involvement of cell-to-cell signals in the development of a bacterial biofilm. Science 1998; 280(5361): 295–298
14. Reid G, Tieszer C, Bailey R R. Bacterial biofilms on devices used in nephrology. Nephrology 1995; 1: 269–275
15. Kulik E, Ikada Y. In vitro platelet adhesion to nonionic and ionic hydrogels with different water contents. J Biomed Mater Res 1996; 30(3): 295–304
16. Liedl B. Catheter-associated urinary tract infections. Curr Opin Urol 2001; 11(1): 75–79
17. Mobley H L, Warren J W. Urease-positive bacteriuria and obstruction of long-term urinary catheters. J Clin Microbiol 1987; 25(11): 2216–2217
18. Stickler D, Ganderton L, King J, Nettleton J, Winters C. *Proteus mirabilis* biofilms and the encrustation of urethral catheters. Urol Res 1993; 21(6): 407–411
19. Jones B D, Mobley H L. Genetic and biochemical diversity of ureases of Proteus, Providencia, and Morganella species isolated from urinary tract infection. Infect Immun 1987; 55(9): 2198–2203
20. Stickler D, Hughes G. Ability of *Proteus mirabilis* to swarm over urethral catheters. Eur J Clin Microbiol Infect Dis 1999; 18(3): 206–208
21. Falkinham J O, III, Hoffman P S. Unique developmental characteristics of the swarm and short cells of *Proteus vulgaris* and *Proteus mirabilis*. J Bacteriol 1984; 158(3): 1037–1040
22. Sidhu H, Holmes R P, Allison M J, Peck A B. Direct quantification of the enteric bacterium *Oxalobacter formigenes* in human fecal samples by quantitative competitive-template PCR. J Clin Microbiol 1999; 37(5): 1503–1509
23. Verkoelen C F, Schepers M S. Changing concepts in the aetiology of renal stones. Curr Opin Urol 2000; 10(6): 539–544
24. Sofer M, Denstedt J D. Encrustation of biomaterials in the urinary tract. Curr Opin Urol 2000; 10(6): 563–569
25. Mardis H K, Kroeger R M, Morton J J, Donovan J M. Comparative evaluation of materials used for internal ureteral stents. J Endourol 1993; 7(2): 105–115
26. Thornhill J A, Mardis H K, Lennon G. Patient tolerance of ureteral stents. In: Smith A D (ed). Controversies in endourology. Philadelphia: W B Saunders, 1995: 287
27. Marx M, Bettmann M A, Bridge S, Brodsky G, Boxt L M, Richie J P. The effects of various indwelling ureteral catheter materials on the normal canine ureter. J Urol 1988; 139(1): 180–185
28. Culkin D J, Zitman R, Bundrick W S, Goel Y, Price V H, Ledbetter S et al. Anatomic, functional, and pathologic changes from internal ureteral stent placement. Urology 1992; 40(4): 385–390
29. Korhonen P, Talja M, Ruutu M, Andersson L C, Alfthan O. Comparison of two different cell culture methods in evaluation of biocompatibility of latex urinary catheters. Urol Res 1991; 19(2): 127–130
30. Pariente J L, Kim B S, Atala A. In vitro biocompatibility assessment of naturally derived and synthetic biomaterials using normal human urothelial cells. J Biomed Mater Res 2001; 55(1): 33–39
31. Pariente J L, Kim B S, Atala A. In vitro biocompatibility evaluation of naturally derived and synthetic biomaterials using normal human bladder smooth muscle cells. J Urol 2002; 167(4): 1867–1871
32. Kirkpatrick C J. New aspects of biocompatibility testing: where should it be going? Med Device Technol 1998; 9(7): 22–29

33. Lifshitz D A, Winkler H Z, Gross M, Sulkes J, Baniel J, Livne P M. Predictive value of urinary cultures in assessment of microbial colonization of ureteral stents. J Endourol 1999; 13(10): 735–738

34. Franco G, De Dominicis C, Dal Forno S, Iori F, Laurenti C. The incidence of post-operative urinary tract infection in patients with ureteric stents. Br J Urol 1990; 65(1): 10–12

35. Watterson J D, Cadieux P, Stickler D, Hughes G, Reid G, Denstedt J. Ability of *Proteus mirabilis* 296 to swarm over ureteral stents: a comparative assessment (abstr). J Endourol 2001; 15 (suppl 1): A12

36. Choong S K, Whitfield H N. Urinary encrustation of alloplastic materials. J Endourol 2000; 14(1): 19–23

37. Choong S K, Wood S, Whitfield H N. A model to quantify encrustation on ureteric stents, urethral catheters and polymers intended for urological use. Br J Urol 2000; 86(4): 414–421

38. Reid G, Busscher H J, Sharma S, Mittelman M W, McIntyre S. Surface properties of catheters, stents and bacteria associated with urinary tract infections. Surf Sci Rep 1995; 21(7): 251–274

39. Denstedt J D, Reid G, Sofer M. Advances in ureteral stent technology. World J Urol 2000; 18(4): 237–242

40. Merchant M, Weinberger S R. Recent advancements in surface-enhanced laser desorption/ionization-time of flight-mass spectrometry. Electrophoresis 2000; 21(6): 1164–1177

41. Cadieux P, Beiko D T, Watterson J D, Burton J, Howard J, Gan B S et al. Surface-enhanced laser desorption/ionization-time of flight-mass spectrometry (SELDI-TOF-MS): a simple and novel urinary screening test for patients with urolithiasis (abstr). J Endourol 2002; 16 (suppl 1): A14

42. Denstedt J D, Wollin T A, Reid G. Biomaterials used in urology: current issues of biocompatibility, infection, and encrustation. J Endourol 1998; 12(6): 493–500

43. Dankert J, Hogt A H, Feijem J. Biomedical polymers: bacterial adhesins, colonization, and infection. Crit Rev Biocompat 1986; 2(3): 219–301

44. Holmes S A, Cheng C, Whitfield H N. The development of synthetic polymers that resist encrustation on exposure to urine. Br J Urol 1992; 69(6): 651–655

45. Tieszer C, Reid G, Denstedt J. XPS and SEM detection of surface changes on 64 ureteral stents after human usage. J Biomed Mater Res 1998; 43(3): 321–330

46. Olweny E O, Landman J, Andreoni C, Collyer W, Kerbl K, Onciu M et al. Evaluation of the use of a biodegradable ureteral stent after retrograde endopyelotomy in a porcine model. J Urol 2002; 167(5): 2198–2202

47. Laaksovirta S, Talja M, Valimaa T, Isotalo T, Tormala P, Tammela T L. Expansion and bioabsorption of the self-reinforced lactic and glycolic acid copolymer prostatic spiral stent. J Urol 2001; 166(3): 919–922

48. Lumiaho J, Heino A, Tunninen V, Ala-Opas M, Talja M, Valimaa T et al. New bioabsorbable polylactide ureteral stent in the treatment of ureteral lesions: an experimental study. J Endourol 1999; 13(2): 107–112

49. Isotalo T, Tammela T L, Talja M, Valimaa T, Tormala P. A bioabsorbable self-expandable, self-reinforced poly-l-lactic acid urethral stent for recurrent urethral strictures: a preliminary report. J Urol 1998; 160(6 Pt 1): 2033–2036

50. Talja M, Valimaa T, Tammela T, Petas A, Tormala P. Bioabsorbable and biodegradable stents in urology. J Endourol 1997; 11(6): 391–397

51. Ratner B D, Hoffman A S. Synthetic hydrogels for biomedical applications. In: Anrade JD (ed). Hydrogels for medical and related applications. Washington, DC: American Chemical Society, 1976

52. Riedl C R, Witkowski M, Plas E, Pflueger H. Heparin coating reduces encrustation of ureteral stents: a preliminary report. Int J Antimicrob Agents 2002; 19: 507–510

53. Zupkas P, Parsons C L, Percival C, Monga M. Pentosanpolysulfate coating of silicone reduces encrustation. J Endourol 2000; 14(6): 483–488

54. Senthil D, Malini M M, Varalakshmi P. Sodium pentosan polysulphate – a novel inhibitor of urinary risk factors and enzymes in experimental urolithiatic rats. Ren Fail 1998; 20(4): 573–580

55. Norman R W, Scurr D S, Robertson W G, Peacock M. Sodium pentosan polysulphate as a polyanionic inhibitor of calcium oxalate crystallization in vitro and in vivo. Clin Sci (Lond) 1985; 68(3): 369–371

56. Sidhu H, Schmidt M E, Cornelius J G, Thamilselvan S, Khan S R, Hesse A et al. Direct correlation between hyperoxaluria/oxalate stone disease and the absence of the gastrointestinal tract-dwelling bacterium *Oxalobacter formigenes*: possible prevention by gut recolonization or enzyme replacement therapy. J Am Soc Nephrol 1999; 10 (suppl 14): S334–S340

57. Lung H Y, Baetz A L, Peck A B. Molecular cloning, DNA sequence, and gene expression of the oxalyl-coenzyme A decarboxylase gene, oxc, from the bacterium *Oxalobacter formigenes*. J Bacteriol 1994; 176(8): 2468–2472

58. Watterson J D, Cadieux P, Beiko DT, Cook A, Burton J, Harbottle R et al. Oxalate-degrading enzymes from *Oxalobacter formigenes*: a novel device coating to reduce urinary tract biomaterial-related encrustation. J Endourol 2003; 17(5): 269–274

59. Johnson J R, Roberts P L, Olsen R J, Moyer K A, Stamm W E. Prevention of catheter-associated urinary tract infection with a silver oxide-coated urinary catheter: clinical and microbiologic correlates. J Infect Dis 1990; 162(5): 1145–1150

60. Subramanyam S, Yurkovetsiky A, Hale D, Sawan S P. A chemically intelligent antimicrobial coating for urologic devices. J Endourol 2000; 14(1): 43–48

61. Darouiche R O. Infection-resistant alloplasts. J Endourol 2000; 14(1): 33–37

62. Burrows L L, Khoury A E. Issues surrounding the prevention and management of device-related infections. World J Urol 1999; 17(6): 402–409

63. Darouiche R O, Smith J A, Jr., Hanna H, Dhabuwala C B, Steiner M S, Babaian R J et al. Efficacy of antimicrobial-impregnated bladder catheters in reducing catheter-associated bacteriuria: a prospective, randomized, multicenter clinical trial. Urology 1999; 54(6): 976–981

64. Williams J F, Worley S D. Infection-resistant nonleachable materials for urologic devices. J Endourol 2000; 14(5): 395–400

65. Getliffe K A, Hughes S C, Le Claire M. The dissolution of urinary catheter encrustation. BJU Int 2000; 85(1): 60–64

66. Hesse A, Nolde A, Klump B, Marklein G, Tuschewitzki G J. In vitro investigations into the formation and dissolution of infection-induced catheter encrustations. Br J Urol 1992; 70(4): 429–434

67. McLean R J, Lawrence J R, Korber D R, Caldwell D E. *Proteus mirabilis* biofilm protection against struvite crystal dissolution and its implications in struvite urolithiasis. J Urol 1991; 146(4): 1138–1142

68. Kennedy A P, Brocklehurst J C, Robinson J M, Faragher E B. Assessment of the use of bladder washouts/instillations in patients with long-term indwelling catheters. Br J Urol 1992; 70(6): 610–615

69. Morris N S, Stickler D J. The effect of urease inhibitors on the encrustation of urethral catheters. Urol Res 1998; 26(4): 275–279

17

Bacterial adherence to hydrophilic-coated polymer stents

B. Jansen, W. Kohnen and D. Filippas

Introduction

The use of various indwelling stents in urology has led to major progress in the therapy of patients with genitourinary diseases. However, stent colonization by bacteria (mainly *Pseudomonas* and other Gram-negative bacilli) and fungi, as well as encrustation by precipitation of urine salts, may limit their use.[1] Colonization increases with increasing stenting duration, with a high rate of bacterial colonization in long-term stenting.[2] Furthermore, stent material properties influence bacterial adhesion and colonization of stents.[3] In addition, in endoscopic biliary stenting, which is a useful method in the palliation of malignant obstructive jaundice,[4,5] it is estimated that up to one-third of all stents are blocked after a period of 3–5 months, independent of the plastic material used.[6] Stent blockage is usually managed by exchange of the blocked stents. Despite improvements in the manufacturing of stent materials (e.g. the development of modified polymers or self-expandable metal stents) clogging remains a major problem, considerably limiting the lifetime of stents.

Today it is generally believed that, in the pathogenesis of stent blockage, adherence of bacteria, formation of a biofilm and deposition of urine salts or biliary sludge are the main contributory factors.[6–8] Bacterial adherence is regarded as the first important step in the pathogenesis of stent occlusion and depends on the physicochemical properties of the material surface and on surface-adsorbed proteins acting as adhesion mediators. The reduction of bacterial adherence and biofilm formation by modification of stent materials is a promising approach in preventing stent blockage. In this chapter, the basic mechanisms of bacterial adhesion to polymers are discussed, with regard to physicochemical surface properties; further, an overview on microbial adherence to hydrophilic polymer stents is given.

Bacterial adhesion to polymers

Basic considerations

Bacterial adherence to solid surfaces is a naturally occurring phenomenon. Many bacterial species live and grow under conditions in which they are attached to natural surfaces,[9] often growing embedded in their own organic polymer matrix as biofilms. Adherence of bacteria to, and subsequent biofilm formation on, synthetic surfaces such as industrial or medical material surfaces is also well known but may have undesirable effects. For example, marine bacteria can readily adhere to solids and thus cause fouling.[10] Industrial polymers susceptible to bacterial adherence may undergo changes in their properties and degrade following enzymatic attack by microorganisms.[11] In medicine, bacterial adherence to and colonization of devices, usually associated with biofilm formation, play an important role in the development of dental plaque and of device- or implant-related infections.[12,13]

Adhesion of microorganisms to mammalian cells is assumed to be the first important step in the development of an infectious disease. There is also evidence from many investigations that bacterial adherence to medical devices (mostly synthetic polymers) is the first and most important step in the pathogenesis of infections associated with foreign bodies. Subsequent colonization, production of extracellular substances ('slime', 'glycocalyx') and involvement of host factors (cells, proteins) lead to the formation of a compact matrix (biofilm) on a biomaterial surface. Generally, biofilm formation protects embedded microorganisms, for example against host defence mechanisms and antibiotic attack,[14,15] and can lead to their undesirable persistence and survival on industrial polymers such as pipes and tubes and, even more importantly, on medical devices and implants. Biofilm formation may, therefore, explain the difficulties in treatment of most foreign-body infections and their chronic, long-lasting nature, as well as the the phenomenon of stent occlusion.

From the physicochemical point of view, bacterial adhesion to a polymer can be regarded as the adhesion of a colloid particle to a solid surface in a liquid environment. Beside the hydrodynamic conditions (in the liquid environment) that regulate the transport of the particle to the surface, the adhesion is governed by attractive or repulsive physical interactions including electrostatic, van der Waals', dipole–dipole and hydrophobic interactions.[16] If only electrostatic and van der Waals' interactions are considered, the DLVO theory of lyophobic colloid stabilization can be applied to bacterial adhesion.[17,18] For example, in the case of adhesion of a negatively charged bacterial cell to an (also) negatively charged surface (e.g. a mammalian cell), adhesion can be described as a balance between electrostatic repulsion and van der Waals attraction. Depending on the electrolyte concentration of the liquid medium, a secondary and a primary minimum in total energy are observed, at which interactions between bacteria and surface are possible (Fig. 17.1). The secondary minimum is located at a longer range, typically at a distance of 5–8 µm, while primary minimum is at a much shorter range, thus allowing more specific interactions once a particle has reached

the primary minimum. As was shown by Hogt and colleagues[19] and others, the DLVO theory can be applied for a qualitative description of bacterial adhesion to polymers in vitro; quantitative calculations are difficult to obtain because the necessary magnitudes are not easily measurable in practice.[19] For situations in vivo the DLVO model is not suitable, owing to other interactions (e.g. specific interactions between protein structures) that may occur and that are not considered in the DLVO theory (Table 17.1).

Another physicochemical model for the description of biological adhesion processes is based upon thermodynamic considerations and was developed by Neumann et al.[20] Provided that electrostatic interactions can be neglected, adhesion is regarded to be controlled by a change in the free energy of adhesion (ΔG), which is a function of the interfacial tensions between solid and bacteria (χ_{sb}), solid and liquid medium (χ_{sl}) and bacteria and liquid medium (χ_{bl}).

Adhesion is thermodynamically favoured if ΔG becomes negative. Like the DLVO model, the thermodynamic approach can be applied only to situations in vitro. Both models are based upon non-specific interactions occurring between particles (cells) and solid surfaces.

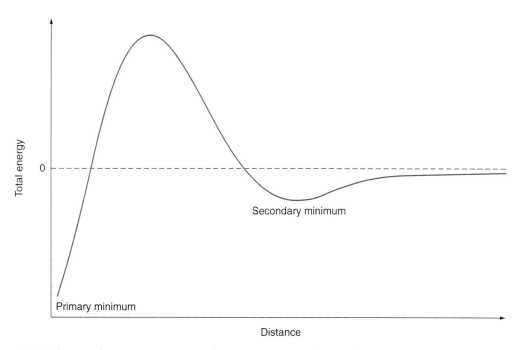

Figure 17.1. *DLVO theory predicts two energy minima where strong interactions between bacteria and biomaterial are possible.*

Table 17.1. *Interactions involved in bacterial adhesion to polymers*

Non-specific interactions	Electrostatic attraction or repulsion Van der Waals' interactions 'Hydrophobic' interactions
Specific interactions	Adhesin–receptor interactions Lectin-like interactions Interactions with proteins

The authors have recently used the glow discharge technique to modify a wide range of different polymers used for medical devices. With the aid of contact angle measurements of both the modified materials and of the bacterial cell surface (in this case *Staphylococcus epidermidis* KH6), it was possible to calculate surface interaction parameters and the free enthalpy of adhesion, ΔG.[21] Attempts were made to find a correlation between physicochemical surface parameters and bacterial adherence in order to draw conclusions as to how anti-adhesive surfaces could be manufactured.

Is adherence thermodynamically favoured if the free enthalpy of adhesion is negative and decreases with increasing free enthalpy values? Results obtained with polymer samples having negative enthalpy values gave

an answer to this question. No adherence should occur if the free enthalpy of adhesion is positive (the bacterium needs energy to adhere). In contrast to this, the authors found that *S. epidermidis* strain KH6 showed a constant adhesion value of about $1\%*ml/cm^2$ on modified polymers with positive values of adhesion enthalpy (Fig. 17.2). These results suggest that, in vitro, there appears to be a certain minimum number of adherent bacteria, independent of the free enthalpy of adhesion and the nature of the polymer surface.[21]

As most of the bacteria in a liquid medium are negatively charged, a negatively charged polymer surface should repel bacterial cells. This could be demonstrated for negatively charged, modified polymers, which showed less bacterial adherence than uncharged modified polymers. However, all negatively charged samples showed a minimum number of adherent bacteria of about $1\%*ml/cm^2$. These observations may have implications for the development of strategies to avoid bacterial adhesion and biofilm formation on polymers, since it might be impossible to create a polymeric surface on which bacterial adherence will definitely not take place.[21]

Nevertheless, some materials in this study showed very low adherence, e.g. negatively charged surfaces. Such polymers, with a reduced tendency for bacterial

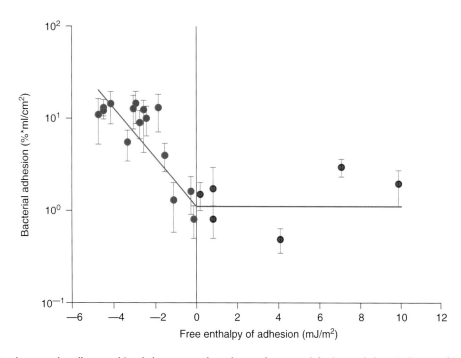

Figure 17.2. *Correlation between the adhesion of Staphylococcus epidermidis to polymers and the free enthalpy of adhesion, ΔG.*

Table 17.2. *Studies of the influence of hydrophilicity on the adhesion of microorganisms to synthetic materials*

Microorganism	Biomaterial	Reference
Staphylococci	Hydrophilic-coated polyurethane, polyurethane	26
Staphylococci	Polystyrene modified with poly(ethylene oxide) and poly(propylene oxide)	27
Staphylococci	Teflon, polyethylene, polycarbonate	28
Staphylococci	Teflon, polyethylene, polypropylene, polyethylene terephthalate, silicone, polycarbonate, cellulose acetate	29
Staphylococci, *Lactobacillus* sp., *Escherichia* sp.	Polystyrene, sulfonated polystyrene, polyethylene terephthalate, silicone, glass, FEP	30
Pseudomonas sp.	Silicone, copper, steel, glass	31
Escherichia sp.	Polymethylmethacrylate	32

adherence, might be useful materials with regard to the prevention of adhesion, colonization and biofilm formation, since, in practice, the bacterial load is much less than in these experiments in vitro. Thus, very few bacteria should adhere to such modified surfaces in comparison with currently used materials.

Under conditions more closely related to the situation in vivo, specific interactions are likely to occur. Such specific interactions have been shown to mediate adhesion between bacteria and natural substrates (e.g. adhesion of streptococci to dental enamel[12] and adhesion of *Escherichia coli* to urothelial cells.[23] Although they have not been clearly demonstrated for bacterial adhesion to synthetic polymers, it is highly possible that specific interactions also play an important role. Gristina et al.[23] have extended the DLVO model by considering additional specific interactions in the bacteria/polymer adhesion process, suggesting that, initially, adhesion is governed mainly by non-specific forces and that, at a later stage, specific interactions may occur nearer to the surface, involving protein-, sugar- and lectin-like interactions.[23] It is now known that specific surface-adsorbed proteins, such as albumin, fibrinogen, fibronectin, vitronectin and collagen, will have an influence on bacterial adhesion: thus, surface-adsorbed albumin leads to a reduction in bacterial adherence, whereas fibrinogen and fibronectin may enhance adherence of *Staphylococcus aureus* and *S. epidermidis*, respectively.[24] Further, certain structures on the bacterial surface, such as proteins and polysaccharides (PS/A), play a role in mediating adhesion to and colonization of polymer surfaces.[25]

Both types of interactions, non-specific and specific, are determined by the specific properties of the structures that are involved in the adhesion process. From this it is evident that a single model will not be sufficient to describe all the complex events of bacterial adhesion.

Hydrophilic surfaces

As the hydrophilicity of a polymer surface can be determined easily by means of contact angle measurements, a number of investigators have tried to find a correlation between (surface) hydrophilicity and bacterial adhesion. The matter appears somewhat controversial, as some, but not all, authors found a correlation (Table 17.2).[26–32] In the present authors' studies on glow-discharged polymers, the free enthalpy of adhesion, ΔG, was found to be a better parameter to describe bacterial adherence than (surface) hydrophilicity. In former studies, the same authors had shown that hydrophilic polymers adsorb much albumin and less fibrinogen, depending on their capability to absorb water.[33] Such polymers had a very low interfacial tension against water and appeared to be more blood compatible in terms of low platelet adhesion than more hydrophobic, non-expansible materials; in addition bacterial adherence to such surfaces is significantly reduced.[34,35] For example, it was shown that adhesion of *S. epidermidis* to polyurethane modified with 2-hydroxyethylmethacrylate, acrylamide or other hydrophilic monomers is greatly reduced, compared with adhesion to unmodified polyurethane. Hydrophilic surfaces, therefore, seem to be of special interest if low bacterial adherence is anticipated.

Bacterial adherence to hydrophilic polymer stents

As previously stated, stent colonization, encrustation and clogging still remains a major problem in urological and endoscopic biliary stenting. Typical complications associated with the use of certain stents include encrustation, stent migration, infection and breakage.[2] In biliary stenting, clogging of stents occurs in one-third of all patients, after a mean interval of approximately 5 months. In several studies it was shown that stent clogging is mainly due to the deposition of biliary sludge on the luminal stent surface.[6–8] Microscopic examination revealed that, in the deposited sludge, bile pigments, cholesterol crystals, bacteria and proteins are found, whereas in urological stents crystals from struvite, apatite and fibrin and bacteria may be present.[36,37] Mixed microcolonies of cocci and bacterial rods embedded in an amorphous matrix are seen on the inner and outer surface of stents.[7] The organisms most often found are members of the common enteric and urethral flora, e.g. Gram-negative bacteria such as E. coli, Klebsiella spp. and others and, on the other hand, Pseudomonas, Enterococcus and also Candida albicans. It is now generally believed that bacterial adherence and formation of microcolonies with subsequent biofilm development are the main inital events in stent blockage, whereby the extent of bacterial colonization is assumed to be a significant parameter in the determination of the onset of stent encrustation and clogging.[6] The phenomenon of stent colonization and encrustation is observed with almost all plastic materials used for the manufacture of stents (e.g. polyethylene, polyurethane, silicone, Teflon polymers, rubber). In biliary stents, deposition of biliary sludge may be greatly dependent on the flow rate, the friction coefficient of the material, and the diameter and wall thickness of the stent, which may thus greatly influence the amount and onset of stent clogging.[38] Therefore, stents with a large diameter, thin walls with no side-holes and a small friction coefficient may decrease the rate of sludge deposition.

Several approaches have been taken for the prevention of stent colonization, encrustation and clogging by reducing bacterial adherence to the stent material. First, aseptic procedures during stent insertion and the use of prophylactic antibiotics may be of benefit in the prevention of early bacterial adherence. However, for the long-term patency of stents, other concepts have to be developed. The coating or incorporation of antimicrobial substances into stents has been proposed, in order to reduce bacterial adherence over a longer period.[6] This strategy (which is already commercially used in the form of antimicrobial intravascular catheters) has the disadvantage of possible induction of microbial resistance and an unpredictable effect on the balance of microbial flora. In recent studies it has been demonstrated that silver-containing polyurethane is able to reduce bacterial adherence to gastrointestinal stents over a limited period, this effect being more pronounced in the presence of bile.[39] Sung et al.[40] have investigated the effects of bile salts such as deoxycholate and taurodeoxycholate on bacterial adhesion, demonstrating a reduction in adherence by 100- to 1000-fold.[40] Incorporation of such hydrophobic bile salts into stent materials might help to increase the lifetime of biliary stents. Ultrasmooth and hydrophilic materials might be promising candidates to reduce the possibility of stent occlusion, by reduced bacterial adhesion. McAllister et al.[41] have reported the excellent performance in vitro of an ultrasmooth polymer (Vivathane), which had few, if any, microorganisms adherent to its surface after challenge with infected bile in a perfusion model.[41]

For urological stents, modified material, and also acidification of urine, have been used in an attempt to avoid microbial colonization and deposition of urine salts.[36,42] In a recent review of the management of ureteric injuries, the performance of various stenting materials was discussed, with polyurethane being the worst and silicone and Hydro-plus™ (a hydrogel-coated C-Flex polymer) being the best materials investigated.[3]

As bacterial adherence to polymers is greatly enhanced by prior adsorption of proteins such as fibronectin and vitronectin,[43] the use of hydrophilic surface-modified polymers seems to be a promising approach to reduce bacterial adherence and thus stent clogging. It has long been known that hydrophilic surfaces with a low surface tension against water tend to adsorb less proteins (especially fibrinogen) than more hydrophobic polymers.[33] The authors have investigated the adherence of various common microorganisms to hydrophilic polyurethane stents (Hydromer®-coated), in order to assess their ability to resist bacterial adherence.[44] The Hydromer® coating consists of the hydrophilic polymer poly-N-vinylpyrrolidone (PVP, Hydromer®) which gives the inner surface of the stents a smooth texture. Hydrogels such as PVP have been shown to exhibit excellent biomedical properties, e.g. reduced thrombogenicity, reduced bacterial adherence and a good tissue compatibility.[45] However, in the pure state they are mechanically weak, so their use is limited. Surface modification using PVP, however, offers the advantage of combining the beneficial biocompatible properties of PVP with good mechanical properties of other polymers, e.g. polyethylene or polyurethane. In the past, several investigations have demonstrated the benefit of surface-modified polymers using PVP coatings: thus, studies on Hydromer®-coated silicone wound drains,[46] and Hydromer®-coated silicone cardiac pacing leads[47] have indicated the biocompatibility and lowered thrombogenicity of such modified devices. In the present study it has been shown that bacterial adherence, especially in perfusion experiments, is greatly reduced in polyurethane stents with a Hydromer® coating. After perfusion of the stents with a bacterial suspension of a high inoculum (10^8 colony-forming units/ml), a reduction in adherence of 1 log (perfusion in phosphate-buffered saline) and 2–3 logs (perfusion in human bile) was observed, compared with non-coated polyurethane control stents. This effect was observed with E. coli and enterococci, microorganisms typically found in infections of the genitourinary and biliary tracts and in encrustation and sludge material from clogged stents. Even in perfusion experiments with mixtures (K. oxytoca/enterococci and E. coli/ enterococci), reduced adherence of both micro-organisms was observed for the Hydromer®-coated stents (Fig. 17.3). In the stationary adherence experiment, however, the effect of reduced adherence was not as great. This can be explained by the fact that bacteria adhering to a solid surface have a greater tendency to produce a biofilm if stress factors such as a permanent flow are present.[48] The observed reduction in bacterial adherence to the Hydromer®-coated polyurethane stents may be explained by the fact that, owing to the low interfacial energy of the hydrophilic Hydromer®-coating, adherence of cells and adsorption

of proteins is far less than that to hydrophobic surfaces.[33,49]

The results reported here suggest that hydrophilic coating of stents may be a useful tool in preventing or reducing the rate of stent colonization, encrustation and clogging and thus may increase the long-term patency of the hydrophilic stents. Further, undesirable effects of the release of toxic components from modified stents (e.g. antibiotics, metal salts such as silver) are avoided. The stents tested were Hydromer®-coated on the inner lumen only; because Hydromer® is a very lubricious material, the stents are deliberately uncoated on the outer surface, in order to avoid stent migration after implantation.

Conclusions

Bacterial adhesion, colonization and encrustation of stents used in urology are limiting factors, decreasing the lifetime of stents by causing mechanical or infectious complications. In addition, biliary stent blockage by the adherence of bacteria and formation of biofilm is a major problem in endoscopic stenting procedures. Hydrophilic polymers have been shown to be materials with low protein adsorption and low bacterial adherence, thus representing good candidates for stenting devices.

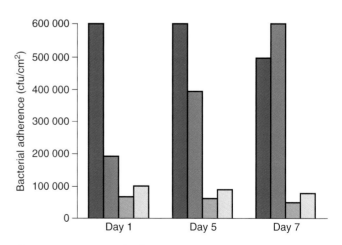

Figure 17.3. Bacterial adherence of a mixture of E. coli and E. faecalis (initial inoculum 10^8 cfu/ml) in human bile: to Hydromer®-coated and non-coated polyurethane (PU) stents: bacterial adherence to the internal stent surface was determined by ultrasonication. (From ref. 44 with permission). ■ PU (E. coli); ■ PU (E. faecalis); ▦ Hydromer® (E. coli); ▫ Hydromer® (E. faecalis).

References

1. Farsi H M, Mosli H A, Al-Zemaity M F et al. Bacteriuria and colonization of double-pigtail ureteral stents: long-term experience with 237 patients. J Endourol 1995; 9(6): 469–472

2. El Faqih S R, Shamsuddin A B, Chakrabarti A et al. Polyurethane internal ureteral stents in treatment of stone patients: morbidity related to indwelling times. J Urol 1991; 146(6): 1487–1491

3. Cormio L. Ureteric injuries. Clinical and experimental studies. Scand J Urol Nephrol Suppl. 1995; 171: 1–66

4. Cotton P B. Endoscopic methods for relief of malignant obstructive jaundice. World J Surg 1984; 8: 854–861

5. Huibregtse K, Katon R M, Coene P P, Tytgat G N J. Endoscopic palliative treatment in pancreatic cancer. Gastrointest Endosc 1986; 32: 334–338

6. Coene P L O. Endoscopic biliary stenting. Thesis, Amsterdam, 1990

7. Speer A G, Cotton P B, Rode J et al. Biliary stent blockage with bacterial biofilm. A light and electron microscopy study. Ann Intern Med 1988; 108: 546–553

8. Leung J W C, Ling T K W, Kung J L S, Vallance-Owen J. The role of bacteria in the blockage of biliary stents. Gastrointest Endosc 1988; 34: 19–22

9. Marshall K C, Stout R, Mitchell R. Selective sorption of bacteria from seawater. Can J Microbiol 1971; 17(11): 1413–1416

10. Fletcher M, Marshall K C. Are solid surfaces of ecological significance to aquatic bacteria? In: Marshall K C (ed) Advances in microbial ecology, Vol.6. New York: Plenum Press, 199–220

11. Kaplan A M. Microbial deterioration of polyurethane systems. Dev Ind Microbiol 1968; 9: 201

12. Gibbons R J, van Houte J. Bacterial adherence and the formation of dental plaques. In: Beachey E H (ed) Bacterial adherence, receptors and recognition, Series B, Vol. 6. London: Chapman and Hall, 1980: 61–000

13. Sugarman B, Young E J. Infections with prosthetic devices. CRC Press: Boca Raton, 1984

14. Evans R C, Holmes C J. Effect of Vancomycin Hydrochloride on Staphylococcus epidermidis biofilm with silicone elastomer. Antimicrob Agents Chemother 1987; 31: 889–894

15. Hoyle B D, Costerton J W. Bacterial resistance to antibiotics: the role of biofilms. Progr Drug Res 1991; 37: 91–105

16. Rutter P R, Vincent B. In: Berkeley R C W, Lynch J M, Melling J, Rutter P R, Vincent B (eds) Microbial adhesion to surfaces. Chichester: Ellis Horwood, 1980: 79–95

17. Derjaguin B V Landau L D. Theory of the stability of strongly charged lyophobic sols and of the adhesion of strongly charged particles in solutions of electrolytes. Acta Phys Chim USSR 1941; 14: 633

18. Verwey E J W, Overbeek J T G. Theory of stability of lyophobic colloids. Amsterdam: Elsevier, 1948

19. Dankert J, Hogt J A H, Feijen J. Biomedical polymers: bacterial adhesion, colonization and infection. In: Williams D F (ed) CRC Critical Reviews in Biocompatibility. Boca Raton: CRC Press, 1986; 2(3): 219

20. Absolom D R, Francis D W, Zingg W et al. Phagocytosis of bacteria by platelets: surface thermodynamics. J Colloid Interfac Sci 1982; 85: 168–177

21. Kohnen W, Jansen B. Prevention of biofilm formation by polymer modification. J Ind Microbiol 1995; 15: 391–396

22. Svanborg-Eden C, Ericksson B, Hanson L A. Adhesion of E.coli to human urothelial cells in vitro. Infect Immun 1977; 18: 767

23. Gristina A G, Hobgood C D, Barth E. Biomaterial specificity, molecular mechanisms and clinical relevance of S. epidermidis and S. aureus infections in surgery. In: Pulverer G, Quie P, Peters G (eds) Pathogenicity and clinical significance of coagulase-negative staphylococci. Stuttgart: Gustav Fischer Verlag, 1987; 143–158

24. Vaudaux P, Suzuki R, Waldvogel F A et al. Foreign body infection: role of fibronectin as a ligand for the adherence of Staphylococcus aureus. J Infect Dis 1984; 150: 546–553

25. Tojo M, Yamashita N, Goldmann D A, Pier G B. Isolation and characterization of a capsular polysaccharide adhesin from Staphylococcus epidermidis. J Infect Dis 1988; 157: 713–730

26. Tebbs S E, Elliott T S J. Modification of central venous catheter polymers to prevent in vitro microbial colonisation. Eur J Clin Microbiol Infect Dis 1994; 13: 111–117

27. Bridgett M J, Davies M C, Deneyer S P. Control of staphylococcal adhesion to polystyrene surfaces by polymer surface modification with surfactants. Biomaterials 1992; 13: 411–416

28. Ferreirós C M, Caballo J, Criado M T et al. Surface free energy and interaction of Staphylococcus epidermidis with biomaterials. FEMS Microbiol Lett 1989; 60: 89–94

29. Caballo J, Ferreirós C M, Criado M T. Factor analysis in the evaluation of the relationship between bacterial adherence to biomaterials and changes in free energy. J Biomater Appl 1992; 7: 130–141

30. Reid G, Hawthorn L-A, Eisen A, Beg H S. Adhesion of Lactobacillus acidophilus, Escherichia coli and Staphylococcus epidermidis to polymer and urinary catheter surfaces. Coll Surf 1989; 42: 299–311

31. Mueller R F, Characklis W G, Jones W L, Sears J T. Characterization of initial events in bacterial surface colonization by two pseudomonas species using image analysis. Biotechnol Bioeng 1992; 39: 1161–1170

32. Harkes G, Feijen J, Dankert J. Adhesion of Escherichia coli on to a series of poly(methacrylates) differing in charge and hydrophobicity. Biomaterials 1991; 12: 853–860

33. Jansen B, Ellinghorst G. Modification of polyetherurethane for biomedical application by radiation induced grafting. II. Water sorption, surface properties, and protein adsorption of grafted films. J Biomed Mater Res 1984; 18: 655–669

34. Jansen B. Bacterial adhesion to medical polymers — use of radiation techniques for the prevention of materials-associated infections. Clin Mater 1990; 6: 65–74

35. Jansen B, Schareina S, Steinhauser H et al. Development of polymers with anti-infectious properties. In: Gebelein C G (ed) Applied bioactive polymeric materials. New York: Plenum, 1988: 97–113

36. Fuse H, Ohkawa M, Nakashima T, Tokunaga S. Crystal adherence to urinary catheter material in rats. J Urol 1994; 151: 1703–1706

37. Hukins D W L, Hickey D S, Kennedy A P. Catheter encrustation by struvite. Br J Urol 1983; 55: 304

38. Speer A G, Cotton P B, MacRae K D. Endoscopic management of malignant biliary obstruction: stents of 10 French gauge are preferable to stents of 8 French gauge. Gastrointest Endosc 1988; 34: 412–417

39. Leung J W C, Lau G T C, Sung J J Y, Costerton J W. Decreased bacterial adherence to silver-coated stent material: an in vitro study. Gastrointest Endosc 1992; 38: 338–340

40. Sung J J Y, Shaffer E A, Lam K et al. Hydrophobic bile salts inhibits bacterial adhesion on biliary stent material. Dig Dis Sci 1994; 39(5): 999–1006

41. McAllister E W, Carey L C, Brady P G et al. The role of polymeric smoothness of biliary stents in bacterial adherence, biofilm deposition, and stent occlusion. Gastrointest Endosc 1993; 39(3): 422–425

42. Bibby M, Hukins D W L. Acidification of urine is not a feasible method for preventing encrustation of indwelling urinary catheters. Scand J Urol Nephrol 1993; 27: 63–65

43. Yu J L, Andersson R, Ljungh A. Protein adsorption and bacterial adhesion to biliary stent materials. J Surg Res 1996; 62: 69–73

44. Jansen B, Goodman L P, Ruiten D. Bacterial adherence to hydrophilic polymer-coated polyurethane stents. Gastrointest Endosc 1993; 39: 670–673

45. Bruck S D. Aspects of three types of hydrogels for biomaterial applications. J Biomed Mater Res 1973; 7: 387

46. Edlich R, Rodeheaver G T et al. Evalutions of a new hydrogel coating for drainage tubes. Am J Surg 1984; 146: 687–691

47. McArthur W A et al. Povidone as an implant aid for cardiac pacing leads. Proceedings of the International Symposium on Povidone, University of Kentucky, April 1983.

48. Costerton J W, Gessey G G, Cheng K J. How bacteria stick. Sci Am 1978; 238: 86–95

49. Lee R G, Kim S W. Adsorption of proteins onto hydrophobic polymer surfaces; adsorption isotherms and kinetics. J Biomed Mater Res 1974; 8: 251–259

18

Bacterial adhesion to biodegradable stents
A. Pétas

Introduction

Infection is one of the most common complications of the use of stents in urology and can range from asymptomatic bacteriuria to clinical urinary tract infection (UTI) with dysuria, discomfort, frequency and nocturia. Management may require several courses of antibiotics and may call for removal of the stent for definitive eradication of the infection. These problems can, therefore limit the usefulness of stents. In a report by Williams on the Urolume® stent, infection was detected in 15 of 96 patients at 12 months, and was associated with encrustation in seven patients and with non-epithelialization of the intravesical portion of the stent in two patients.[1]

Bacterial adherence to the implant surface and urothelium is known to be a crucial mechanism in the initiation of the process. Pathogens must bind to the epithelial surface to cause disease.[2,3] Chemical inertness is one of the properties of an ideal implanted biomaterial. In terms of urology, it involves the property of not inducing stone formation, infection or irritation of the urinary tract.

Biodegradable spiral stents, which have been introduced recently in clinical trials, have been made of self-reinforced polyglycolic acid (SR-PGA) or poly-DL-lactic acid (SR-PLA). Polyglycolic acid and polylactic acid, which are both polymers of poly-alpha-hydroxy acids, have been used as surgical suture material, in bone surgery and for drug delivery for several years with good biocompatibility. However, the use of a temporary biodegradable device in the urinary tract is a new concept.

Bacterial factors

Uropathogens originate mainly in the intestine, colonize the periurethral region and ascend into the urethra and the urinary bladder, where they can cause symptomatic UTI, depending on host factors and bacterial virulence. Bacteria can adhere to almost any surface. The mechanism by which bacteria adhere to tissues or implant surfaces is mediated by bacterial adhesins (Table 18.1) that are located either on filamentous appendages called fimbriae (Fig. 18.1) or directly on the bacterial surface.[4] Adhesion permits the bacteria to resist being washed away by the flow of urine in the urinary tract and is a necessary prerequisite to growth, colonization and subsequent infection. Many examples of the role of bacterial adherence to host tissues have been reported in the literature, and specific bacterial adherence to host tissues has been shown to be characteristic of many pathogenic microorganisms.[5] Guzman et al.[6] reported on the adherence of *Enterococcus faecalis* in UTI and endocarditis: they concluded that adhesive properties were important virulence factors in the pathogenesis of these conditions and also suggested that UTI strains showing the highest invasion and adhesive potential invaded the kidneys, caused bacteraemia and colonized the heart.[6] Adherence was mediated by hair-like pili projecting

Table 18.1. *Adhesion of uropathogenic types of* E. coli

Adhesin type	Role in UTI	Fimbriae present
Mannose resistant		
P fimbriae		
P	+++	+
F	++	+
ONAP	+/–	+
X adhesins (X fimbriae)		
Dr blood group related		
Dr	++	–
AFA-I, AFA-III	+	–
S, G fimbriae	+/–	+
M adhesin, NFA-1, NFA-2	+/–	–
Mannose sensitive role in UTI		
Type 1 fimbriae (pili)	++	+
Miscellaneous	+/–	–
Other		
F1C	+/–	+

ONAP = O-negative, A-positive;
AFA = afimbrial adhesin;
NFA = non-fimbrial adhesin.

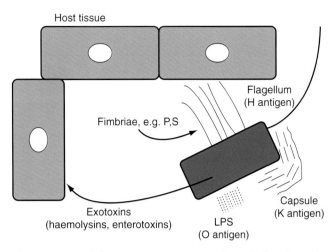

Figure 18.1. *Schematic representation of an Escherichia coli bacterium with host tissue. (Reproduced from ref. 4, with permission.)*

from the surface of the cells. Production of these pili is controlled by a specific plasmid. Antibody to the pilus antigen prevents adherence of the piliated organisms.[7]

In addition, bacterial receptor sites have been demonstrated on urothelial surfaces. There is evidence of natural anti-adherence mechanisms in humans, as well as possible increased susceptibility to UTI when these mechanisms are defective and when receptor density on urothelial cells is altered.[8]

Extensive bacterial biofilms have been found on a large number of medical devices made of a variety of biomaterials.[9] However, there is not uniform correlation between biofilm formation and clinical infection. Although clinical infection can be treated, the bacteria remain embedded inaccessibly in the biofilm and can subsequently give rise to recurrent bacterial colonization. Bacterial contamination of stents or implants differs from that of implanted prostheses that are not in contact with urine: the majority of the latter are infected by *Staphylococcus epidermidis*, whereas the most frequent bacterium in UTI is *Escherichia coli*.

Studies on bacterial adherence

Bacterial adherence to SR-PGA and SR-PLA 96 has been evaluated in vitro. Gold-plated metal wire (Prostakath®), polyurethane (Intraurethral catheter-IUC®) and latex were used as reference materials. To imitate the situation in vivo and to characterize the effect of degradation and

encrustation, the test materials were incubated for 3 h, and for 7, 14 and 28 days in synthetic urine. The bacterial strains selected for the assay were *Proteus mirabilis*, *Pseudomonas aeruginosa*, *Enterococcus faecalis*, and four strains of *Escherichia coli*. Bacterial adherence was studied by incubating the materials and bacteria together to allow adherence. The unattached bacteria subsequently were removed by repeated washing, and the numbers of adherent bacteria were determined using either microscopy, radiometric studies or determination of colony-forming units (CFU).[10]

The results are shown in Figures 18.2–18.5. Adhesion was relatively stable at various time points of incubation. There were obvious differences between the adherence of different bacteria: in general, the adhesion of *P. aeruginosa* to SR-PGA, SR-PLA 96, polyurethane and gold-plated wire was greater than that of any other bacterium. None of the study materials was superior to the other, in terms of resisting bacterial adhesion. The degradation of SR-PGA and SR-PLA 96 is apparently so slow that it does not have any significant effect on detaching the adherent bacteria from the surface. The adhesion of bacteria without P-fimbriae was significantly lower. A scanning electron microscopy (SEM) study was performed using parallel samples after incubation and bacterial exposure: the results showed the pattern of fragmentation of the biodegradable material and figures of bacterial adherence were similar for each test material. It was concluded that bacterial properties are as important as, or more important than, material properties in the adhesion process.[11]

Cormio et al.[12] studied bacterial adhesion and biofilm formation on various indwelling double-J stents in vivo and in vitro to determine whether they were dependent on the stent material, but those authors did not find any significant difference in bacterial adherence on the various stent materials. However, they did find a statistically significant difference in adhesion among the bacterial test strains, and concluded that bacterial adhesion on the biomaterials used for ureteric stents may depend on the properties of the bacteria rather than on the biomaterials.[12]

Barton et al.[13] have described a method of determining the growth rates of bacteria on polyorthoester, poly-L-lactic acid and polysulphone, using a new videomicroscope system and a mathematical model. They observed the

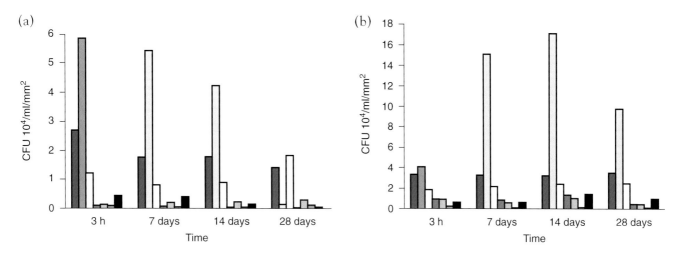

Figure 18.2. *Bacterial adherence to (a) SR-PGA and (b) SR-PLA 96:* ■ Proteus mirabilis;   Pseudomonas aeruginosa; □ Enterococcus faecalis; ■ Escherichia coli *P-negative;* ■ E. coli *P-positive;* ■ E. coli *P-negative;* ■ E. coli *P-positive.*

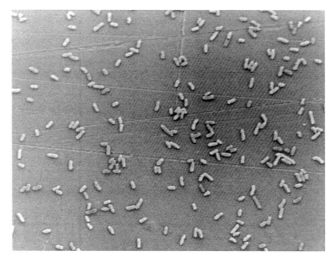

Figure 18.3. *Scanning electron microscopic image of SR-PGA after 3 h preincubation time and exposure to* Proteus mirabilis *suspension. The adherent bacteria are clearly visible. Magnification X 2000.*

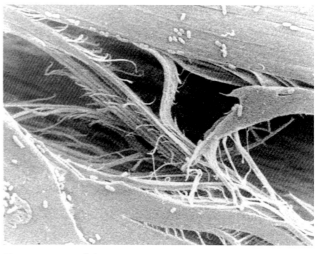

Figure 18.4. *A cleft on SR-PLA 96 is shown, with microfibrils of the stent material.* Proteus mirabilis *bacteria are attached to the outer surface of the stent, but not in the cleft, which is an artefact due to the dehydration process. Magnification X 2000.*

rates of bacterial adhesion, desorption and growth, and showed that, under the experimental conditions, the generation time of adherent bacteria is longer than that of planktonic bacteria. No correlation was found between growth rate, adhesion or desorption, and whether the substrate biomaterial had a stable or degradable surface. Barton et al.[13] regarded their new method as preferable to simple adhesion experiments because, in clinical infections, the polymer is usually

contaminated with a few bacteria that subsequently grow in situ until they form a biofilm.[13]

Discussion

P-fimbriae are important in the pathogenesis of UTI, permitting bacterial colonization and stimulating inflammation. Knowledge of bacterial adherence mechanisms may permit alternative methods of

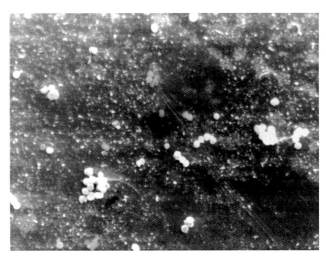

Figure 18.5. Enterococcus faecalis *bacteria and minor encrustations are visible on the gold-plated metal wire after 14 days preincubation. Magnification X 3000.*

prevention and management of urinary infection, including the use of vaccine and non-immune inhibition of bacterial adhesins and receptor sites.[14] It may be possible to affect the biofilm so that bacteria cannot be enveloped in it. In an experimental study, biofilm on the bacterial surface can be disrupted by using substances, such as quaternary amines or protamine sulphate, known to adhere to the mucus and prevent its ability to control permeability.[15–17] It has been found in vitro that S. *epidermidis* is easily destroyed by a combination of protamine and vancomycin, which is more effective than either compound alone.[18]

In the future, surface properties of the stents must be improved to resist bacterial adherence. Hydrophilic covering surfaces have already been shown to reduce bacterial adherence and new types of molecules could be attached to the implant surface to have an antibacterial ionic effect. Antibiotic or bactericidal molecules could be incorporated within the temporary implant to overcome the adherent bacteria.

References

1. Williams G, Coulange C, Milroy E J G et al. The Urolume, a permanently implanted prostatic stent for patients at high risk for surgery. Br J Urol 1993; 72: 335–340
2. Fowler J E Jr, Stamey T A. Studies on introital colonization in women with recurrent urinary tract infections. J Urol 1997; 117: 472
3. Mulholland S G. Lower urinary tract defence mechanisms. Invest Urol 1979; 17: 93
4. Siitonen A. What makes Escherichia coli pathogenic? Ann Med 1993; 26: 229–231
5. Schaeffer A J. The role of bacterial adhesion in urinary tract infections. Urologe A 1993 Jan; 32(1): 7–15
6. Guzman C A, Pruzzo C, LiPira G, Calegari L. Role of adherence in pathogenesis of Enterococcus faecalis urinary tract infection and endocarditis. Infect Immun 1989; 57(6): 1834–1838
7. Schaeffer A J. The role of bacterial adhesion in urinary tract infections. Urologe A 1993; 32(1): 7–15
8. Reid G, Sobel J D. Bacterial adherence in the pathogenesis of urinary tract infection: a review. Rev Infect Dis 1987; 9(3): 470–487
9. Costerton J W, Cheng K J, Geesey G G et al. Bacterial biofilms in nature and disease. Ann Rev Microbiol 1987; 41: 435–464
10. Johnson J R. Virulence factors in Escherichia coli urinary tract infection. Clin Microbiol Rev 1991; 4: 80–128
11. Pétas A, Vuopio-Varkila J, Siitonen A et al. Bacterial adherence to self-reinforced polyglycolic acid and self-reinforced polylactic acid 96 spiral stents in vitro. Biomaterials: in press
12. Cormio L, Vuopio-Varkila J, Siitonen A et al. Bacterial adhesion and biofilm formation on various Double-J stents in vivo and in vitro. Scand J Urol Nephrol 1996; 30: 19–24
13. Barton A J, Sagers R D, Pitt W G. Measurement of bacterial growth rates on polymers. J Biomed Mater Res 1996; 32: 271–278
14. Reid G, Sobel J D. Bacterial adherence in the pathogenesis of urinary tract infection: a review. Rev Infect Dis 1987; 9: 470–487
15. Lilly J D, Parsons C L. Bladder surface glycosaminoglycans in human epithelial permeability barrier. Surg Gynecol Obstet 1990; 171: 493–496
16. Parsons C L, Lilly J D, Stein P C. Epithelial dysfunction in non-bacterial cystitis (interstitial cystitis). J Urol 1991; 145: 732–735
17. Teichman J M H, Stein P C, Parsons C L. Quaternary amine (protamine sulphate) is bactericidal to Staphylococcus epidermidis. J Infect Dis 1993; 167: 1500–1501
18. Teichman J M H, Abram V E, Stein P C, Parsons C L. Protamine sulphate and vancomycin are synergistic against Staphylococcus epidermidis. J Urol 1994; 152: 213–216

19

Urinary tract infection in patients with urethral stents

D. Hassin, V. Istomin, B. Shohat, M. Kaufstein and D. Yachia

Introduction

Urinary tract infection (UTI) is the most common infection among hospitalized patients. Catheterization of the bladder causes approximately 40% of nosocomial UTI.[1] The bacteria reach the bladder through the lumen of the catheter or move up by pericatheteral route within 24–72 hours.[2] Urinary catheterization results in the colonization of uropathogens in the urethra and bladder, and bacteriuria. In addition, the catheter induces an inflammatory reaction in the urethra and the bladder because of mechanical and chemical irritation and depresses the response of polymorphonuclear cells.[3] Factors predisposing symptomatic UTI in patients with an indwelling catheter (IC) are duration of bladder catheterization, recurrent catheterizations, underlying disorders (diabetes mellitus, renal insufficiency), absence of prophylactic antibiotic treatment and nosocomial infection. About 100 000 residents of nursing homes and hospitals for chronic patients in the United States have IC.[4] The main indications for IC insertion in this population are bladder outlet obstruction (BOO) and urinary incontinence. Clinically, most catheter-associated infections are asymptomatic with leukocyturia and positive urinary culture. Apart from the infectious complications, patients with longstanding IC can develop obstruction, urolithiasis, renal insufficiency and rarely squamous cell carcinoma of the bladder.[5,6]

In the past two decades urethral stent insertion was introduced into medical practice as an alternative treatment of urethral obstruction due to benign prostatic hypertrophy (BPH), carcinoma of the prostate (CaP) and urethral strictures. To date, limited data are available concerning the association between urethral stent and UTI. A study was conducted in our institution to determine the frequency and bacteriology of symptomatic and asymptomatic UTI among patients with a urethral stent (US) and compared it to the patients with IC, all having BOO.

Patients and methods

In this study, three groups of patients were compared:

1. Patients with more than 6 months of indwelling urethral stent for benign prostatic hypertrophy (BPH), carcinoma of the prostate (CaP) and urethral stricture.
2. Patients with bladder outlet obstruction (BOO) due to benign prostatic hypertrophy (BPH) waiting for surgery.
3. Patients with a longstanding (more than 6 months) indwelling catheter (IC).

The patients were interviewed and their outpatient and hospital files were screened for previous and present symptomatic and asymptomatic UTI. The patient's urinary sediment was examined for leukocyturia by microscope and the urine was cultured. Bacteriuria is defined as $\geq 10^5$ CFU (colony-forming units)/ml. Leukocyturia is defined as more than 10 white blood cells per field ($\times 400$). To increase the significance of the bacteriological results we added six additional positive cultures from patients with urethral stents after the study was concluded.

The stents used were the ProstaCoil (PC-50, PC-60, PC-70) and Prostakath (PK-65) which were inserted to the prostatic urethra for BPH or CaP, and the UroCoil stents (UC and UC-S 40, 50, 60, 70, 80, UC-T 40-40, 50-50) which were inserted to the anterior urethra for urethral strictures.

The PC, UC, UC-S and UC-T stents are made of a nickel and titanium alloy (Nitinol) (Fig. 19.1) and the PK is made of gold-plated stainless steel. All the patients received ofloxacin as antibiotic prophylaxis one day before and five days after stent insertion.

Statistical analysis

The Pearson chi-square test was used for comparison of all three groups, two-tailed Fisher exact test for comparison of each pair of groups. The probability value

(a)

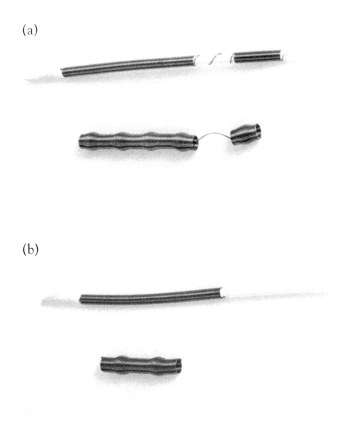

(b)

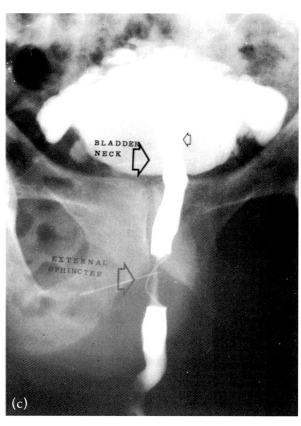

Figure 19.1. *(a) The ProstaCoil and (b) UroCoil stents. (c) The ProstaCoil in place in a patient with benign prostatic hypertrophy.*

of ≤0.05 was considered significant (SAS G.Software, procFreq).[7]

A total of 76 patients (age: 18–98 years, median 75) with urethral stents were studied. The time range since the urethral stent insertion was from 6 to 24 months. The indication for stent insertion were BPH in 42 patients, CaP in 9 patients and urethral stricture in 25 patients. The control groups included 60 patients with BOO due to BPH (age: 57–93 years, median 77) and 36 patients with long-term IC (age: 26–98 years, median 79). Historical data were collected from all patients with a urethral stent and current evaluation was possible in 41 of those patients. In 35 of the patients with a urethral stent in the past, current evaluation was impossible because the stents were taken out before the beginning of the study. All patients from the control groups were evaluated historically and currently.

Results

Previous urinary tract infection
Symptomatic infection occurred in 31.5% of the urethral stent (US) patients compared with 73.5% of

the indwelling catheter (IC) patients ($p = 0.001$) and 23.3% of the bladder outlet obstruction (BOO) patients ($p = 0.19$). Severe UTI necessitating hospitalization occurred in 10.5% of the US group compared with 64.7% of the IC group ($p = 0.001$) and 23.3% of the BOO group ($p = 0.04$). Previous positive urine cultures were 55.3% of the US as compared to 79.4% of the IC group ($p = 0.04$) and 16.6% of the BOO group ($p = 0.001$). Evidence of previous leukocyturia (mostly 20–100 leukocytes per field) was significantly higher in the IC group than in the US group (100% vs 60.5%, $p = 0.001$), but in both of the groups it was significantly higher than in the BOO group (28.3%, $p = 0.001$). Dysuria was less common complaint in the US group compared to the IC group and similar to the BOO group (35.5% vs 79.4%, $p = 0.001$ and 26.7%, $p = 0.18$, respectively) (Table 19.1).

Current urinary tract infection
Symptomatic UTI was reported by 19.5% of the US group as compared to 64% of the IC patients ($p = 0.001$) and 13% of the BOO patients ($p = 0.29$). Leukocyturia (mostly 20–100 leukocytes per field) was

Table 19.1. *Data concerning previous urinary tract infection (UTI) in patients with a urethral stent (US) compared to control groups*

	US group N (%)	BOO group N (%)	IC group N (%)
No. of patients	76	60	36
Dysuria	27 (35.5)	16 (26.7) $p = 0.18$	27 (79.4) $p = 0.001$
Clinical UTI	24 (31.5)	14 (23.3) $p = 0.19$	25 (73.5) $p = 0.001$
Hospitalization due to UTI	8 (10.5)	14 (23.3) $p = 0.04$	22 (64.7) $p = 0.001$
Positive urine culture	42 (55.3)	10 (16.6) $p = 0.001$	27 (79.4) $p = 0.04$
Leukocyturia	46 (60.5)	17 (28.3) $p = 0.001$	36 (100) $p = 0.001$

Table 19.2. *Evidence for current urinary tract infection (UTI) in patients with a urethral stent (US) compared to control groups*

	US group N (%)	BOO group N (%)	IC group N (%)
No. of patients	41	60	36
Clinical UTI	8 (19.5)	8 (13) $p = 0.29$	23 (64) $p = 0.001$
Leukocyturia	30 (73)	17 (28) $p = 0.001$	34 (94) $p = 0.02$
Positive urine culture	24 (58.5)	8 (13) $p = 0.001$	25 (69) $p = 0.22$

present in 73% of the US group, in 98% of the IC patients ($p = 0.02$) and in 28% of the BOO patients ($p = 0.001$). Bacteriuria was found in 58.5% of the US group compared to 69% of the IC group ($p = 0.22$) and only 13% of the BOO group ($p = 0.001$) (Table 19.2).

Bacterial culture profile of the patients

This is detailed in Table 19.3. Bacteriology of the urethral stent (US) group was similar to that of the indwelling catheter (IC) group, polymicrobial infection was found in 53% of the US group as compared to 36% in the IC group ($p = 0.16$) and 12.5% in the bladder outlet obstruction (BOO) group ($p = 0.002$).

The most common bacteria in the urethral stent group compared to IC group were: *Escherichia coli* (36.7% vs 40%), Proteus (20% vs 24%), *Pseudomonas aeruginosa* (20% vs 24%) and Enterococcus species (20% vs 24%)

Table 19.3. *Bacterial isolates in urine culture from all patients' groups*

	US group (N = 30) N (%)	BOO group (N = 8) N (%)	IC group (N = 25) N (%)
Polymicrobial infection	16 (53)	1 (12.5) $p = 0.002$	9 (36) $p = 0.16$
Escherichia coli	11 (36.7)	4 (50)	10 (40)
Proteus	6 (20)	3 (37.5)	6 (24)
Pseudomonas aeruginosa	6 (20)	1 (12.5)	6 (24)
Enterococcus sp.	6 (20)	1 (12.5)	6 (24)
Klebsiella pneumoniae	4 (13.4)	0	3 (12)
Enterobacter	3 (10)	1 (12.5)	0
Acinetobacter	3 (10)	0	2 (8)
Providencia	1 (3.3)	0	3 (12)
MRSA	2 (6.7)	0	0
Candida	0	0	2 (8)

MRSA, *methicillin-resistant* Staphylococcus aureus.

Discussion

Impediment to the free flow of urine in the urethra by stricture, prostatic hypertrophy or tumor results in stasis of urine in the bladder and increased frequency of urinary tract infection.

The increased incidence of UTI in men aged 50–70 is mostly due to bladder outlet obstruction.[8] About 15–20% of all hospitalized patients undergo urinary tract catheterization.[1] Placing a urinary catheter in a hospitalized patient results in 10–15% incidence of urinary tract infection. Duration of bladder catheterization and underlying diseases are important factors predisposing to UTI in these patients. The risk of infection is about 3–5% per day of catheterization.[1,9] All patients catheterized for longer than 30 days eventually develop bacteriuria, usually resistant to treatment.[1,4] In the past few years the knowledge of bacterial biofilm development explains facts observed in catheter-associated UTI.[10,11] The bacteria colonize the catheter surface with biofilm that protects the microorganisms from host defense and antibacterial agents and explains the difficulties in the treatment of foreign-body infections.[12] The most common bacteria associated with IC infection are *E coli*, Proteus, Pseudomonas, Enterococcus species and *Providencia stuartii*.[1,4,7,8,13] Polymicrobial bacteriuria is characteristic in patients with a permanent indwelling catheter.[14] Most of the urinary infections in patients with IC are asymptomatic or have a subclinical course. In the past two decades urethral stent insertion was introduced into the medical practice as an alternative treatment of urethral obstruction. Stent colonization with biofilm formation, encrustation by precipitating urine salts and clogging still remains a major problem in urological stenting. The incidence of colonization and bacteriuria in patients with ureteral stents is 28–90% and 7–34%, respectively. A negative urine culture did not rule out colonization of ureteral stent.[15] As in catheterization of the urethra, the risk of ureteral stent colonization increases with increasing stenting duration. Current publications on urethral stenting are aimed at urological aspects, are retrospective, relating only to symptomatic UTI, without control groups or bacteriologic data. Studies on urethral stents found 0–26% of symptomatic UTI.[16–22] Asymptomatic UTI was not studied rigorously. It was claimed that the UTI in patients with a urethral stent is due to the fact that permanent urinary catheters were common before urethral stent insertion.[22] Anidjar et al.[23] mention infectious complications of patients with a US but did not detail the clinical presentation and frequency of them. Thomas et al.[19] report 10% symptomatic UTI among 64 patients with Prostakath. Similar results were also reported by Yachia et al. in one of the largest studies on urethral stents which involved 117 patients with ProstaCoil and Prostakath. Yachia found no differences between the type of stents.[16] Nissenkorn et al.[18] have found only 15.4% of bacteriuria and 4% of symptomatic UTI in 78 patients with long-term stents in the prostatic urethra. Morgentaler et al. have reported 2 of 25 US patients with clinical infection.[21] In contrast, Yachia et al.[22] in another study and Yasumoto et al.[24] did not report any case of symptomatic UTI after urethral stent insertion among 27 and 32 patients, respectively.

The present study analyses retrospectively and prospectively the frequency and the different manifestations of UTI in patients after urethral stent insertion compared to patients with a permanent IC and bladder outlet obstruction without catheter before surgery. In contrast to previous reports the present study found that the frequency of UTI in patients with a US is high, around 60%, it is mostly asymptomatic, but 30% of the patients experienced symptomatic UTI in the past while 73% of patients with an IC had symptomatic UTI in their past, most of them severe, necessitating hospitalization. The occurrence of clinical UTI in patients with a urethral stent and BOO is the same with 31% and 23% in the past and 19% and 13% current symptomatic UTI, respectively. However, asymptomatic UTI was significantly less in patients with BOO compared to urethral stent (55% vs 16% in the past and 58% vs 13% current). The lowest rate of hospitalizations was in urethral stent patients. Despite the significant frequency of bacteriuria in IC patients it was less frequent than that described in literature (69–79.4% vs 100%). This difference may be related to prophylactic antibiotic treatment. Among those with positive urinary cultures, polymicrobial infection was frequent in the US group (53%) and in the IC patients (36%) and significantly less in the BOO patients. The urethral stent and IC groups revealed the same spectrum of bacteria. The bacteriology was consistent with the literature on UTI in IC patients.[1,4,8,9,13] Some of the patients with a urethral stent without bacteriuria complained about dysuria or had leukocyturia, possibly due to an inflammatory reaction to the foreign body in the urethra.

Conclusions

The present study confirmed that urinary tract infection is a significant problem in patients with a urethral stent but still less frequent and severe than in patients with an indwelling catheter. This advantage of the urethral stent over the indwelling catheter, in addition to the patient's obvious preference, makes the urethral stent an important mode of management for patients with bladder outlet obstruction. Further studies are needed to lower the frequency of urinary tract infection in urethral stent patients by modifications of the stents with biological substances, antiseptics or antibiotics.

References

1. Sant G R, Meares E M Jr. Urinary tract infections. In: Sant G R (ed) Pathophysiologic principles of urology. Oxford: Blackwell Scientific 1994: 271

2. Schaeffer A J, Chiniel J. Urethral meatal colonization in the pathogenesis of catheter-associated bacteriuria. J Urol 1983; 130: 1096

3. Zimmerly W, Lew P D, Waldvogel F A. Pathogenesis of foreign body infection: Description and characteristics of an animal model. J Infect Dis 1982; 146: 487

4. Kunin C M, McCormack R C. Prevention of catheter-induced urinary tract infections by sterile closed drainage. N Engl J Med 1966; 274: 1155

5. Chin Q F, Chambers S. Formation of encrustations of indwelling catheters in the eldery. J Urol 1987; 138: 899

6. Rocke J R, Hill D E, Walzer Y. Incidence of squamous cell carcinoma in catheter drainage. J Urol 1985; 133: 1034

7. SAS Institute Inc SAS/STAT user's guide, Version 6. 4th edn, Vol. 1. Cary, NC: SAS Institute, 1989: 943 pp

8. Cox A J et al. Infection of catheterized patients. Urol Res 1989; 17: 349

9. Stamm W E, Hooton T M. Catheter-associated urinary tract infections: Epidemiology, pathogenesis, prevention. Am J Med 1991; 91(suppl 3B): 655

10. Morris N S, Stickler D J, McLean R J C. The development of bacterial biofilms on indwelling urethral catheters. World J Urol 1999; 17: 245

11. Costeron J W. Introduction to biofilm. Int J Antimicrob Agents 1999; 11: 217

12. Leidl B. Catheter-associated urinary tract infections. Curr Opin Urol 2001; 11: 75

13. Warren J W. *Providencia stuartii*: A common cause of antibiotic-resistant bacteriuria in patients with long-term indwelling catheters. Rev Infect Dis 1986; 8: 61

14. Warren J W, Tenney J H, Hoopes J M. A prospective microbiologic study of bacteriuria in patients with chronic indwelling urethral catheters. J Infect Dis 1982; 146: 719

15. Lifshitz D A, Winkler H Z, Gross M et al. Predictive value of urinary cultures in assessment of microbial colonization of ureteral stents. J Endourol 1999; 13: 735

16. Yachia D, Aridorgan I A. Comparison between first-generation (fixed-caliber) and second-generation (self-expanding, large caliber) temporary prostatic stents. Urol Int 1996; 57: 165

17. Williams G, Coulange C, Milroy E J et al. The Urolume, a permanently implanted prostatic stent for patients at high risk for surgery. Br J Urol 1993; 72: 335

18. Nissenkorn I, Richter S. Intra-urethral catheter (IUC) in the treatment of prostatic obstruction. In: Yachia D (ed) Stenting the urinary system, 1st edn. Oxford: ISIS Medical Media 1998: 291

19. Thomas P J, Britton J P, Harrison N W. The Prostakath stent: Four years experience. Br J Urol 1993; 71: 430

20. Petas A, Talja M, Tammela T et al. Randomized compare biodegradable self-reinforced polyglycolic acid spiral stents to suprapubic and indwelling catheters after visual laser ablation of the prostate. Editorial comment. J Urol 1997; 157: 184

21. Morgentaler A, Dewolf W C. A self-expanding prostatic stent for bladder outlet obstruction in high risk patients. J Urol 1993; 150: 1636

22. Yachia D, Arigodan I A. The use of a removable stent in patients with prostate obstruction. J Urol 1996; 155: 1956

23. Anidjar M, Teillac P. Non-surgical instrumental treatment of benign hypertrophy of the prostate. Presse Med 1995; 24: 1477–1480

24. Yasumoto R, Yoshihara, Kawashima H et al. The use of metallic stent in 32 patients with benign prostatic hypertrophy. Nippon Hinyokika Gakkai Zasshi Apr. 83: 473, 1992

20

How to prevent encrustations on metallic stents
Z. Markovic

Introduction

The state of the art approach to patients with severe urinary tract obstruction and who are unfit for definitive surgery is to consider metal stent insertion. However encrustation of stents — which leads directly to further urinary obstruction — is a characteristic complication of this procedure. Accumulating experience with the use of stents in different types of urinary obstruction has shown that different clinical aspects may directly determine the possibility of stent encrustation, which may occur early in the post-procedural course or several months later. Prevention of stent encrustation starts with pre-procedural evaluation and selection of the stent type and insertion technique, and is subsequently continued virtually permanently after the insertion (by infection control, promotion of diuresis and maintenance of normal urodynamics).

Indications

Well-established indications for the application of a metal endoprosthesis are very important for prevention of stent dysfunction.[1,2] This particularly applies to the ureter, where experience is fairly limited and where various aetiopathogenic causes create urinary stasis. Surgical evaluation, understanding of the stricture aetiology, evaluation of the vascularization of the stricture, the general condition of the patient, renal function, morphology of the ureter/urethra and the possibility of stricture recanalization by interventional uroradiological methods (balloon dilatation and different types of catheter stents) are only some of the important issues that require consideration in the planning of the therapeutic strategy. The accepted attitude is that insertion of a permanent endoprosthesis is the last resort in the therapeutic algorithm for the management of urinary obstruction,[3,4] especially in the ureter.

Choice of stent

The technique of metal stent insertion is fairly simple. The calibre of the 'preliminary' dilatation before stent insertion is open to debate from the encrustation point of view. Most authors advocate that, for sufficient dilatation, the calibre should be almost equal to the calibre of the expanded stent. If the dilatation is wider than the stent, encrustation can start from the external wall of the stent with fast propagation into the lumen; this is seen particularly in bedridden patients. On the other hand, insufficient preliminary dilatation causes greater reaction of the urothelium after insertion, increasing the possibility of obstruction by this reactive proliferative tissue. Biocompatibility of the stents used in the urinary tract should be appropriate for the chemical environment of the urinary tract.[5]

Selection of a stent can be one of the factors determining subsequent encrustation. The number and types of stents available commercially, particularly the intraprostatic endoprostheses, are continuously increasing. At the ureteral level, balloon-expandable or self-expandable stents of different designs that are not specifically designed for the urinary tract are starting to be used. From the point of view of the prevention of encrustation/obliteration, ureteral stent dimensions are important. For the ureter, the stent calibre should not be less than 7 mm in adults and 5 mm in children. Stents longer than 4 cm placed in the ureter exponentially increase the risk of encrustation.[6] The calibre of the intraprostatic and urethral stents should not be less than 1.0 cm. Compared with permanent stents, the possibility of easy replacement of an encrusted stent with a new one favours the use of one of the UroCoil stents for recanalization of urethral strictures.[7,8]

Complications, including encrustation, and their prevention

Transitory haematuria, as a consequence of per-cutaneous renal manipulation in conditions where ureteral peristalsis is impaired and chronic stasis is present, may precipitate stent obstruction as an early post-procedural complication. Post-procedural percutaneous nephrostomy is very important for the prevention of ureteral stent encrustation. Percutaneous nephrostomy facilitates frequent irrigation of the collecting system and ureter with different solutions for reducing urine crystallization or for direct litholysis. The period of indwelling of the percutaneous nephrostome after stent insertion varies and depends on the condition of the urinary system, but it is usually 2–3 weeks. Before removal of the nephrostomy, ureteral (stent) patency should be controlled by closing the nephrostomy catheter for several days.

Urinary infection, reduced renal function and associated metabolic disorders can affect urine composition which may be of primary importance in initiating encrustation and calcification of a metallic stent, either ureteric or urethral.[9–11] Additionally, for the prevention of encrustation, pre-procedural and post-procedural antibiotic cover should be given according to urine culture, which should take place at least 3-month intervals after stent insertion.

Each episode of catheter manipulation or instrumentation in the canalicular system results in post-procedural local oedema of different degrees. This particularly applies to cases of periprocedural iatrogenic lesions of the ureteral or urethral walls. In interventional radiology, minor lesions of the wall usually result from repeated or forced placement of the guidewire. Chronic oedema and altered local biochemical reactions associated with changes in urodynamics may induce faster crystallization and stent encrustation. The use of corticosteroids immediately after stent insertion has proved effective for prevention of oedema.

Increased diuresis reduces the risk of stent encrustation. However, since these patients are usually severely ill with renal failure, support of renal function after stent insertion by urological and nephrological therapy is advised.

Prevention of encrustation of intraprostatic and urethral stents is achieved by the increase in the quality of micturition obtained by the stent insertion itself.[12,13] In conditions of chronic retention in elderly patients with a long-standing indwelling catheter, who have a bladder with thick walls and poor tonus, improving the quality of micturition may be decisive for the overall success of the inserted intraprostatic or urethral stent and prevention of its obstruction by the contents of the urine. Simple exercises help patients with urethral stents to reduce the frequency of voiding and to increase the volume voided, thus increasing the flow of urine after stent insertion. Weakening of the stream suggests that stent obstruction may be developing. A number of ready-made preparations for dissolving crystals in the urine can be applied repeatedly by retrograde irrigation. In more severe cases, temporary placement of an indwelling catheter for continuous irrigation through the stent and frequent laboratory follow-up can also be decisive for preventing stent encrustation.

References

1. Milroy E J G, Chapple C R, Cooper J E et al. A new treatment for the urethral strictures. Lancet 1988; I: 1424–1427
2. Reinberg Y, Ferral H, Gonsales R et al. Intraureteral metallic self-expanding endoprosthesis (Wallstent) in the treatment of difficult ureteral strictures. J Urol 1994; 151: 1619–1622
3. Castaneda-Zuniga W R, Tadavarthy S M, Hunter D W et al. Recanalization in nonvascular interventional radiology. In: Castaneda-Zuniga W R, Tadavathy S M (eds) Interventional radiology, 2nd edn. Baltimore: Williams and Wilkins, 1992: 777–989
4. Lang E K. Interventional radiology of the lower urinary tract. In: Mueller P R (ed) A categorial course in diagnostic radiology — interventional radiology. Chicago: RSNA Publication, 1991: 49–55
5. Donald J J, Rickards D, Milroy E J G. Stricture disease: radiology of urethral stents. Radiology 1991; 180: 447–450
6. Markovic Z, Goldner B, Masulovic D, Bozovic Z. Recanalization of postoperative ureteral stricture with metal stent. Cardiovasc Intervent Radiol 1996; 19(suppl 2): 139
7. Yachia D, Beyar M. Temporarily implanted urethral coil stent for the treatment of recurrent urethral strictures: a preliminary report. J Urol 1991; 146: 1001–1004
8. Yachia D, Beyar M. New, self-expanding, self-retaining temporary coil stent for recurrent urethral strictures near the external sphincter. Br J Urol 1993; 71: 317–321
9. McLoughlin J, Jager R, Williams G. Case Report. Stone formation on a self-expanding metallic stent. Br J Urol 1992; 69: 430–438
10. Holmes S A V, Miller P D, Crower P R, Kirby R S. Encrustation of intraprostatic stents — a comparative study. Br J Urol 1992; 69: 383–387
11. Wright K C, Dobben R L, Magal C et al. Occlusive effects of metallic stents on canine ureters. Cardiovasc Intervent Radiol 1993; 16: 230–234
12. Ashken M H, Coulange C, Milroy E J, Sarramon J P. European experience with the Wallstent for urethral strictures. Eur Radiol 1991; 19: 181–185
13. Chapple C R, Rickards D, Milroy E J G. Permanently implanted urethral stents. Semin Intervent Radiol 1991; 8: 284–294

Ureteral stents: urological disease

21

Optimal drainage of the obstructed kidney: stent versus nephrostomy

M. S. Pearle and G. M. Watson

Introduction

Indications for drainage of the obstructed kidney include relief of pain, preservation of renal function, prevention of urinary extravasation and treatment of infection associated with obstruction. Drainage can be accomplished in a minimally invasive fashion with either retrograde ureteral catheterization by means of a ureteral stent or with percutaneous nephrostomy. Both drainage modalities have proven efficacy in renal decompression and are associated with high success rates and low complications rates. In general, stent placement is performed in the operating room by a urologist while percutaneous nephrostomy falls under the purview of the interventional radiologist; however, antegrade stent placement may be accomplished percutaneously by an interventional radiologist, and at some centers percutaneous nephrostomy is performed by urologists.

The choice of optimal drainage modality depends on a variety of factors, including experience and availability of the operator, patient and physician preference, indication for drainage, patient characteristics and cost. For example, at some centers, percutaneous nephrostomy is precluded by lack of availability of interventional radiology. Likewise, operating room availability may be at a premium at some busy trauma centers, thereby favoring percutaneous nephrostomy in the angiography suite rather than intraoperative stent placement. Patient characteristics may favor one modality or the other; a morbidly obese patient may undergo stent placement more expeditiously than percutaneous nephrostomy due to an unfavorable body habitus for percutaneous puncture, or it may be easier for a nursing home patient to maintain an internal ureteral stent than an external nephrostomy tube that requires additional care.

In this chapter, we explore the advantages and disadvantages of the two forms of drainage with the goal of providing guidelines for drainage selection in particular patient circumstances.

Ureteral stents

Although stent placement is generally performed in the operating room under general or regional anesthesia, office stent placement using local anesthesia and a flexible cystoscope is an attractive alternative in select cases. After cystoscopic placement of a guidewire, an 8/10 Fr coaxial dilator is passed into the ureter under fluoroscopic guidance and the 8 Fr catheter is removed, leaving the 10 Fr sheath in place. A 6 Fr or 7 Fr stent is passed over the guidewire, through the 10 Fr sheath, and positioned using a metal-tip pusher that can be viewed fluoroscopically. Using this technique, a stent can be placed as effectively with the patient in the supine as in the dorsolithotomy position.

Among the advantages of internal stent placement is that the treating urologist can perform the procedure without the need for an additional consultant, and there is no external tube or cumbersome collection bag. Because the stent is placed endoscopically rather than percutaneously there is minimal risk of bleeding, and the procedure can be performed safely in anticoagulated patients or in those with uncorrected bleeding disorders.

Physiologic consequences of stent placement

While nephrostomy drainage occurs almost exclusively through the lumen of the tube and flow is guided by a simple pressure gradient, renal dynamics and flow characteristics in response to an indwelling ureteral stent are more complex. Ramsey and colleagues performed in vivo pressure-flow studies in a porcine model to determine the effect on renal dynamics and ureteral flow characteristics with and without a ureteral stent in place.[1] Indwelling 5 Fr or 6 Fr ureteral stents were associated with a rise in intrapelvic pressure, dilation of the ureter, vesicoureteral reflux and thickening of the ureteral wall. Other investigators have also demonstrated an increase in intrapelvic pressure in the presence of an indwelling unreteral stent and additionally showed that ureteral peristalsis is impaired in the stented ureter. Ryan and associates assessed the acute and chronic effects of stent placement in a canine model using pressure flow studies.[2] Although an initial rise in intrapelvic pressure was observed acutely, it resolved within a week; however, a decrease in renal pelvic and ureteral peristalsis persisted throughout the duration of stenting. Futhermore, the transit time for an inserted model ureteral calculus to pass from the proximal ureter into the bladder was shorter in a de-stented porcine ureter that had previously undergone prolonged stenting compared with the contralateral still-stented ureter or a never-stented ureter. Although mechanical obstruction from the stent may have contributed to the slower transit time in the stented ureter, the decreased peristalsis associated with prolonged stenting is likely a prominent factor in impeding calculus passage.

The flow characteristics of the stinted ureter have also been investigated to determine the relative contribution of intraluminal and extraluminal flow. Mardis and associates constructed a mock urinary system and determined that urine flow rates increased with stent diameter and with the addition of side holes along the stent, suggesting preferential flow through the stent.[3] In contrast, Ramsey and colleagues concluded that urine flow occurs preferentially around, rather than through, an indwelling stent as a consequence of ureteral dilation due to the stent. Olweny and co-workers at Washington University performed a series of in vivo studies in minipigs and determined that urine flow in the stented ureter is comprised of both intraluminal and extraluminal flow.[4,5] Although luminal and total flow varied directly with the internal diameter of a standard-shaped stent similar to the findings of Mardis, the flow characteristics of variably shaped stents were unpredictable likely as a result of unknown relative contributions of the luminal and extraluminal components.

Based on these observations, it may be difficult to predict the flow capabilities of stents in vivo; however, in the case of extrinsic ureteral obstruction where extraluminal flow is prohibited due to compression of the ureter around the stent, overall urine flow might be optimized by the use a stent with a large internal diameter.

Outcomes
Success
The outcomes of stent placement, including success rates and complication rates, have been well documented in the literature. However, stratification of results by obstructive etiology or indication for stent placement is less common. The success of ureteral stent placement was reviewed by Smedley and colleagues who reported 90% success among 132 attempts at cystoscopic stent placement performed for a variety of obstructive etiologies or urinary fistulas.[6] In a more contemporary series, Yossepowitch and associates prospectively evaluated 92 consecutive patients undergoing 100 retrograde stent placements and achieved a 94% success rate for cases of intrinsic ureteral obstruction, but only 73% success for extrinsic obstruction.[7] Improvements in stent and guidewire design aimed at facilitating bypass of stones and strictures have contributed to the high success rates of stent insertion.

Complications
Complications associated with stent placement and indwelling stents include urinary tract infection and sepsis, stent encrustation, stent obstruction and stent migration. The incidence of urinary infection in patients with ureteral stents increases with the duration of stenting. Kehinde and co-workers found a 16.8% incidence of positive urine cultures in 250 patients with ureteral stents indwelling for a mean of 27 days; among 44 patients with stents in place for <30 days, only 6.8% of patents had a positive urine culture at the time of stent removal compared with 31% of patients when the stent was left indwelling for longer than 90 days.[8] Likewise, el-Faqih and colleagues reported a 9% incidence of new urinary tract infections in 290 patients undergoing stent placement in association with shock wave lithotripsy or endoscopic procedures for stones, including 3% among 65 patients with a stent in place <6 weeks, 4% in 120 patients stinted for 6–12 weeks, 14% in 79 patients stented for 13–24 weeks and 23% in 35 patients with stent in place for >25 weeks.[9] Farsi and associates noted an even higher incidence of bacteriuria (30%) among 266 patient with indwelling ureteral stents, with a strong positive correlation between bacteriuria and dwell time; for stents removed at <1 month, 1–3 months and >3 months, the incidence of

bacteriuria was 15%, 21% and 38%, respectively.[10] Although in many cases, bacteriuria does not cause symptoms, the incidence of clinical pyelonephritis has been reported at 3.5% in one series of 255 patients.[11]

Stent encrustation poses a risk by potentially occluding the stent and often preventing simple stent removal. In cases of severe encrustation, adjuvant shock wave lithotripsy or endourologic procedures may be necessary to fragment the adherent stone and remove the stent. In one series of 146 patients (157 renal units) stented for a mean of 101 days to relieve obstruction or facilitate stone management, stent encrustation was the most commonly encountered complication of stent placement (22%).[12] El-Faqih and co-workers noted that the incidence of encrustation increased with stent dwell times, occurring in 9%, 48% and 76% of patients with stents indwelling for <6 weeks, 6–12 weeks and >12 weeks, respectively.[9] Other investigators have found that the incidence of encrustation also varied with stent composition.[13,14]

Stent migration has been reported to occur in 3–10% of patients, more commonly occurring as downward displacement rather than upward.[6,9,11,12] Although downward stent migration can be managed with simple stent removal with or without stent replacement, upward migration often requires ureteroscopic or percutaneous intervention for stent retrieval.

Stent occlusion or failure may necessitate stent replacement or salvage percutaneous nephrostomy. Alsikafi and colleagues prospectively evaluated 22 patients with 29 chronically obstructed renal units managed with indwelling ureteral stents in whom plain abdominal radiographs, serum creatinine and renal and bladder sonography were performed to determine the durability of stent function.[15] Stent replacement was prompted by radiographic demonstration of encrustation, an increase in serum creatinine or sonographic evidence of an increase in hydronephrosis or absence of ureteral jets. Stents exchange was required in 28%, 52%, 76%, and 92% of patients at 3, 6, 9 and 12 months, respectively. Yossepowitch and associates also prospectively evaluated 92 patients (100 renal units) with ureteral obstruction in whom retrograde stent placement was attempted and found that extrinsic ureteral obstruction was associated with a significantly higher likelihood of functional stent failure than intrinsic ureteral obstruction; at 3 months after initial stent placement, stents remained patent in all patients with intrinsic obstruction but in only 56% of patients with extrinsic obstruction.[7]

Patient tolerance

The morbidity associated with indwelling stents also relates to patient symptoms and tolerance of the stent. Joshi and associates evaluated 120 patients with indwelling ureteral stents using a variety of quality of life questionnaires and determined that 80% of patients experienced bothersome stent-related symptoms and/or pain.[16] Urinary symptoms were most commonly related to problems with urine storage and incontinence. Pain was also common and typically involved the flank, suprapubic area, groin and penis. In addition, 30–40% of patients experienced sexual problems that they attributed to the stent.

A number of investigators have attempted to correlate stent symptoms with the type or size of the stent. McDougall and co-workers, comparing polyurethane pigtail, polyurethane J, silicone figure four and silicone pigtail stents, found that silicone composition and a short intravesical stent segment were associated with the least irritative symptoms, and stents with a long renal pelvic component were most commonly associated with flank pain.[17] Rane and associates also evaluated 60 patients in whom stents were placed for treatment of renal or ureteral calculi and concluded that stents crossing the midline of the bladder were associated with more frequency and urgency, and stents with an incomplete distal coil were associated with more pain, hematuria and frequency.[18] Lennon and colleagues performed a prospective, randomized trial comparing soft versus firm double pigtail stents and found that firm stents were associated with significantly more dysuria, flank pain and suprapubic pain than soft stents.[19] On the other hand, Candela and Bellman found that stent size and composition had no effect on patient symptoms in a prospective randomized trial of 60 patients undergoing stent placement; no difference in irritative voiding symptoms, hematuria, pain or incontinence was observed among patients with 6 Fr Percuflex™, 6 Fr HydroPlus™ or 4.8 Fr HydroPlus™ stents.[20]

Percutaneous nephrostomy

Percutaneous nephrostomy is typically performed in the interventional radiology suite using a combination of conscious sedation and local anesthesia. In most cases, the procedure is performed under fluoroscopic guidance often with the aid of intravenous contrast to facilitate localization of the collecting system. Alternatively, sonographic guidance may be used in cases of contrast allergy or renal insufficiency. An 8–12 Fr self-retaining catheter is generally placed via a posterior calyx, into the renal pelvis. The size of the drainage catheter is dictated by the indication for drainage and the appearance of the fluid at initial aspiration; larger caliber drainage catheters are usually reserved for purulent or bloody urine.

Outcomes
Success
The success of initial percutaneous nephrostomy is uniformly high (92–100%).[21–27] Lee and colleagues reviewed their series of 160 emergency percutaneous nephrostomies performed under fluoroscopic guidance and reported successful tube placement in 98% of patients.[21] Likewise, Farrell and Hicks reported a 99% technical success rate for 454 consecutive percutaneous nephrostomies performed in 303 patients.[22]

Complications
Mortality rates for percutaneous nephrostomy are low. Although Farrell and Hicks reported a 3% 30 day mortality rate among 303 patients undergoing the procedure, none of the deaths was attributable to the procedure, and the high mortality rate reflected the relatively large number of patients in poor health or with advanced malignancy requiring percutaneous drainage.[22] Major complication rates range from 4% to 7%, and include hemorrhage requiring transfusion, sepsis, pleural complications and bowel transgression.[23–25,27–30] The transfusion rate for percutaneous nephrostomy is generally 4% or less, and the need for embolization is less than 1%.[21–25,30] Farrell and Hicks identified a baseline platelet count of <100 000/mm^3 as a significant risk factor for hemorrhage, despite the administration of platelets pre-procedure.[22] Minor complications include catheter displacement or occlusion, which occurs in up to 18% of patients.[21–26] In the largest series of percutaneous nephrostomies in the literature to date, Farrell and Hicks reported a complication rate of 6.5%, including a transfusion rate of 2.8%, sepsis in 4%, pneumothorax in 1% and catheter-related complications in 2.6%.[22]

The choice of stent or nephrostomy

The choice of optimal drainage modality, stent versus nephrostomy, depends on a variety of factors, including the indication for the procedure, physician experience, patient and physician preference, patient characteristics and cost. Proponents of stent placement cite the low morbidity of the procedure, the lack of external urine collection device and the seemingly greater patient comfort with an internal tube. On the other hand, advocates of percutaneous nephrostomy note the presumed superior drainage obtained with a larger caliber tube, the ability to monitor ongoing urine drainage and the potential to irrigate the tube if it becomes occluded (Table 21.1).

Obstruction associated with infection
In the setting of obstruction with associated urinary infection, such as obstructive pyelonephritis associated with a ureteral calculus, prompt drainage of the collecting system is nearly uniformly advocated because of the high risk of life-threatening urosepsis. Interestingly, Klein in 1983 conservatively treated 16 patients with fever and obstructing ureteral stones with hydration and broad spectrum antibiotics according to a planned treatment regimen and noted that all patients responded favorably, 11 passing their stones within 48 hours.[31] However, this approach is not widely accepted and this retrospective, uncontrolled study should be viewed with caution.

The most severe manifestation of obstructive pyelonephritis, pyonephrosis, is associated with a high mortality and the risk of renal loss. Historically, pyonephrosis was initially managed with surgical nephrostomy followed by nephrectomy. With the development of percutaneous drainage procedures, percutaneous nephrostomy replaced surgical nephrostomy, and subsequent nephrectomy was performed only in cases where renal salvage was deemed unlikely.[32,33] Percutaneous nephrostomy now commonly constitutes first line therapy for pyonephrosis. Ng and colleagues

Table 21.1. *Advantages and disadvantages of ureteral stent vs percutaneous nephrostomy for drainage of the obstructed kidney*

Ureteral stent		Percutaneous nephrostomy	
Advantages	Disadvantages	Advantages	Disadvantages
No external bags	High incidence of patient symptoms	Able to monitor urine drainage	External tube and collection bag
Easy insertion	High failure rate for extrinsic obstruction	Able to irrigate in case of occlusion	Greater risk of bleeding
Low risk of injury	Unable to monitor urine drainage	Able to place a larger drainage tube	Higher rate of complications
Coagulopathy not a contraindication	No access to unobstruct stent	Local anesthesia/i.v. sedation	Requires interventional radiologist
No need for radiologist	Requires manipulation of obstructed ureter	No manipulation of ureter	

reviewed their series of 92 patients undergoing percutaneous nephrostomy for pyonephrosis due to a variety of obstructive etiologies and found a 2% mortality and 14% morbidity rate.[34] Of interest, only 30% of bladder cultures were positive prior to drainage while nephrostomy cultures were positive in an additional 39% of patients, thereby providing valuable microbiological information that impacted antibiotic treatment.

The routine use of internal stenting for drainage of the obstructed, infected system occurred only with advances in the design of ureteral stents that improved stent placement, maintenance and drainage. However, few reports actually address the use of indwelling stents to relieve obstruction in this clinical scenario. St Lezin and associates treated 23 patients with pyonephrosis with percutaneous drainage, among whom 30% had failed a previous attempt at retrograde stent placement.[33]

Many investigators favor nephrostomy drainage for relief of obstruction in the face of suspected infection because the percutaneous approach avoids manipulation of the obstructed ureter with the associated potential for perforation and bacteremia.[35] Furthermore, the viscous, infected urine may drain better through a large caliber nephrostomy tube compared with the standard 6 Fr or 7 Fr double pigtail ureteral stent, and a nephrostomy tube can be irrigated and unobstructed in case of occlusion. On the other hand, ureteral stent drainage is effectively utilized in other circumstances for relief of obstruction, and stent placement can be performed successfully and expeditiously in most cases. However, few studies have assessed the clinical outcomes of

patients undergoing stent placement for this indication. Despite arguments on both sides of the controversy, only two prospective, randomized trials have directly compared the efficacy of the two drainage modalities for decompression of the obstructed, infected collecting system.

Pearle and co-workers prospectively randomized 42 consecutive patients presenting to the emergency department with obstructing renal or ureteral stones and clinical signs of infection (temperature >38°C and/or white blood count >17 000/mm³) to undergo retrograde ureteral stent placement in the operating room (n = 21) or percutaneous nephrostomy in the interventional radiology suite (n = 21).[36] The two groups were comparable with respect to patient, stone and clinical characteristics, including age, body mass index, initial white blood count and temperature, stone size and degree of hydronephrosis. The sole treatment failure occurred in the percutaneous nephrostomy group and was salvaged with subsequent stent placement. Procedure and fluoroscopy time were significantly shorter in the ureteral stent group compared with the nephrostomy group (by 16.5 min and 2.6 min, respectively), but there was no significant difference between groups in the time to clinical improvement (time to normalization of temperature or white blood count) or length of hospital stay: time to normal temperature, time to normal white count and length of stay were 2.6, 1.7 and 3.2 days, respectively, for the stent group and 2.3, 2 and 4.5 days, respectively, for the nephrostomy group. A cost analysis of the two procedures revealed that stent placement was twice as costly as percutaneous nephrostomy, largely because of the higher operating room overhead costs. Based on the comparable clinical outcomes achieved with the two forms of drainage, the authors suggested that the choice of diversion be left to the discretion of the treating physician.

Mokhmalji and associates also prospectively randomized 40 patients with obstruction due to stones to either percutaneous nephrostomy or ureteral stent placement.[37] In their series, however, only 65% of the 20 stent patients and 55% of the 20 nephrostomy patients had clinical signs of infection. Successful drainage was achieved in 100% of nephrostomy patients but only 80% of stent patients all of whom subsequently underwent successful nephrostomy drainage; of note, only local anesthesia was used in both groups. The duration of tube drainage was significantly shorter in the nephrostomy group compared with the stent group, although the endpoint of diversion was somewhat arbitrarily defined as the time to successful stone removal or passage and resolution of infection; over half the stented patients and only 20% of the nephrostomy patients maintained an indwelling tube for longer than 4 weeks. Although the duration of antibiotic use was longer in the stent group than in the nephrostomy group, the difference did not reach clinical significance. Based on their findings, these authors favored percutaneous nephrostomy over ureteral stent placement in patients with obstructing stones, with or without infection, but particularly with infection because of the higher success rates, shorter diversion time and presumed more rapid resolution of infection.

Patient satisfaction with the two procedures was assessed in both studies. Pearle and colleagues used a visual analog pain questionnaire immediately after the procedure to assess patient tolerance of the procedure, and additionally measured the amount and duration of pain medication used post-procedure. Flank pain was perceived to be greater in the nephrostomy versus the stent group. Although the duration of pain medication was not significantly different between the two groups, more nephrostomy patients (38%) used parenteral or intramuscular narcotics than did stent patients (4.8%).[36] In contrast, Mokhmalji and associates detected a 7% higher quality of life index after percutaneous nephrostomy compared with stent placement which was particularly pronounced in male

patients and in patients <40 years of age, although the differences were not statistically significant.[37]

Joshi and co-workers prospectively compared patients undergoing percutaneous nephrostomy or stent placement for relief of obstruction using a common single health index (EuroQoL EQ-5D) and procedure-specific questions to assess pain, urinary symptoms and inconvenience.[38] Patients in the stent group experienced significantly more irritative voiding symptoms and pain for a longer period of time than patients in the nephrostomy group; however, based on the EuroQoL assessment, there was no significant difference in the impact of the drainage modalities on the quality of life between the two groups.

These studies suggest that both drainage procedures are effective in relieving obstruction and facilitating resolution of infection, and patient tolerance of the procedure and drainage tube is comparable between the two modalities. Success rates are uniformly high for percutaneous nephrostomy, but successful stent placement may be enhanced with the use of intravenous sedation or general anesthesia. In these studies, both forms of diversion provided adequate short-term drainage needed to relieve obstruction and clear infection prior to definitive therapy without the need for tube replacement due to occlusion or displacement. Consequently, the choice of treatment may be left to the discretion of the treating physician. If a large, obstructing stone might ultimately require percutaneous nephrostolithotomy, judicious placement of a nephrostomy tube in a location that will facilitate stone removal may be preferable. On the other hand, if a ureteral stone will likely be treated with shock wave lithotripsy or ureteroscopy, stent placement may be a reasonable choice.

Extrinsic obstruction

Decompression of the obstructed collecting system in cases of extrinsic ureteral obstruction often requires long-term or permanent diversion, particularly in cases of obstruction due to non-urologic malignancy. Several retrospective studies have suggested that internal ureteral stenting is associated with a high rate of failure in cases of extrinsic obstruction. Docimo and Dewolf reported a 43% incidence of stent failure within 30 stays of stent placement in 46 patients with extrinsic ureteral obstruction.[39] Hyppolite and colleagues reviewed 34 patients with gynecologic malignancy associated with hydronephrosis and renal insufficiency and found that among 7 patients managed with an indwelling ureteral stent, 6 developed urosepsis resulting in death in 3 patients.[40] Yossepowitch and associates prospectively evaluated 92 patients with 100 obstructed renal units in whom retrograde ureteral stent placement was attempted in all cases.[7] Among 39 patients with extrinsic ureteral obstruction stent placement failed in 27% of cases, and at 3 month follow-up, only 44% of patients had a functionally patent stent. In contrast, stent placement was successful in 94% of 61 patients with intrinsic ureteral obstruction, and among the stents still in place at 3 month follow-up all were patent.

The high rate of failure among patients with extrinsic ureteral obstruction treated with stent placement may be attributed to the fact that urine flow in this case necessarily occurs intraluminally because extraluminal flow is prohibited by coaptation of the ureter around the stent. Consequently, the use of a firm, large diameter stent could prove efficacious in promoting optimal urine drainage. Indeed, Hübner and co-workers determined that 'hard' stents, that are more compression-resistant, prevent the increase in flow resistance that is seen with softer stents in situations of external compression.[41] If internal stent diversion is performed, close monitoring for urinary infection and stent occlusion is recommended. Further studies will be necessary to ascertain whether particular stents may be better suited to relieve extrinsic obstruction. On the other hand, percutaneous nephrostomy may be the preferred form of urinary diversion for patients with extrinsic ureteral compression causing severe, long-standing hydronephrosis.[42]

Obstruction and urinary diversion

Management of the patient with ureteral obstruction and a urinary diversion, such as an ileal conduit or neobladder, typically involves initial percutaneous nephrostomy drainage. Although it is tempting to subsequently place an internal stent by the antegrade percutaneous route and remove the external nephrostomy tube, occlusion of the stent by mucus produced in the bowel segment may result in life-threatening sepsis. Walther and colleagues reported two case of fatal urosepsis in patients with an ileal conduit in whom internal ureteral stents were placed for relief of obstruction.[43] The use of external stents with drainage holes positioned only in the renal pelvis portion of the stent prevents mucus plugging along the stent. Consequently, patients with urinary diversions containing a bowel segment are best served by percutaneous nephrostomy or by an externalized ureteral stent that lacks side holes along the shaft of the stent and in which the distal end of the stent exits the stoma.

Obstruction in patients with bleeding disorders

For patients with a coagulopathy, correction of the underlying disorder or normalization of coagulation parameters with blood products may allow either drainage procedure to be safely performed. However, Farrell and Hicks found that even correction of a low platelet count (<100 000/mm^3) is associated with a higher rate of blood transfusion when performing percutaneous nephrostomy.[22] On the other hand, although no studies have directly assessed the safety of cystoscopic stent placement in patients with bleeding disorders, Watterson and colleagues safely treated 29 patients with uncorrected bleeding disorders with ureteroscopy and Holmium:YAG laser lithotripsy.[44] By extrapolation, simple stent placement in this patient population can likely be performed safely with or without correction of the underlying bleeding disturbance.

Conclusions

Both percutaneous nephrostomy and internal ureteral stent placement provide adequate short-term urinary drainage in most cases, although patients with extrinsic ureteral obstruction may be better managed with percutaneous nephrostomy. While the mechanism of nephrostomy drainage is almost exclusively via intraluminal flow, the mechanism of ureteral stent drainage is more complex and likely involves both intraluminal and extraluminal urine flow. The predominant component may depend on the characteristics of the stent as well as the properties of the ureter and the etiology of the obstruction. In most cases, the choice of drainage modality will depend on the availability and experience of the urologist or radiologist, the preference of the patient and physician, the etiology of the obstruction, patient characteristics, and the plan for definitive treatment and cost.

References

1. Ramsey J W, Payne S R, Gosling P T, Whitfield H N, Wickham J E, Levion D A. The effects of double J stenting on unobstructed ureters. An experimental and clinical study. Br J Urol 1985; 57: 630–634
2. Ryan P C, Lennon G M, McLean P A, Fitzpatrick J M. The effects of acute and chronic JJ stent placement on upper urinary tract mortility and calculus transit. Br J Urol 1994; 74: 434–439
3. Mardis H K, Kroeger R M, Hepperlen T W, Mazer M J, Kammandel H. Polyethylene double-pigtail ureteral stents. Urol Clin North Am 1982; 9: 95–101
4. Olweny E O, Portis A J, Afane J S, Brewer A V, Shalhav A L, Luszczynski K et al. Flow charcteristics of 3 unique ureteral stents: investigation of a Poiseuille flow pattern. J Urol 2000; 164: 2099–2103
5. Brewer A V, Elbahnasy A M, Bercowsky E, Maxwell K L, Shalhave A L, Kahn S A et al. Mechanism of ureteral stent flow: a comparative in vivo study. J Endourol 1999; 13: 269–271
6. Smedley F H, Rimmer J, Taube M, Edwards L. 168 double J (pigtail) ureteric catheter insertions: a retrospective review. Ann R Coll Surg Engl 1988; 70: 377–379
7. Yossepowitch O, Lifshitz D A, Dekel Y, Gross M, Keidar D M, Neuman M et al. Predicting the success of retrograde stenting for managing ureteral obstruction. J Urol 2001; 166: 1746–1749
8. Kehinde E O, Rotimi V O, Al-Awadi K A, Abudul-Halim H, Boland F, Al-Hunayan A et al. Factors predisposing to urinary tract infecion after J ureteral stent insertion. J Urol 2002; 167: 1334–1337
9. el-Faqih S R, Shamsuddin A B, Chakrabarti A, Atassi R, Kardar A H, Osman M K et al. Polyurethane internal stents in treatment of stone patients: morbidity related to indwelling times. J Urol 1991; 146: 1487–1491
10. Farsi H M, Mosli H A, AL-Zemaity M F, Bahnassy A A, Alvarez M. Bacteriuria and colonization of double-pigtail ureteral stents: long-term experience with 237 patients. J Endourol 1995; 9: 469–472
11. Wu W J, Chen M T, Huang C N, Huang C H, Chiang C P, Chang LL. Experience in the morbidity associated with double-J catheter indwelling and its management. Gaoxiong Yi Xue Ke Xue ZA Zhi 1993; 9: 532–539
12. Damiano R, Oliva A, Esposito C, De Sio M, Autorino R, D'Armiento M. Early and late complications of double pigtial ureteral stent. Urol Int 2002; 69: 136–140
13. Cormio L, Talja M, Koivusalo A, Makisalo H, Wolff H, Ruutu M. Biocompatibility of various indwelling double-J stents. J Urol 1995; 153: 494–496
14. Mardis H K, Kroeger R M, Morton J J, Donovan J M. Comparative evaluation of materials used for internal ureteral stents. J Endourol 1993; 7: 105–115
15. Alsikafi N F, O'Connor R C, Kuznetsov D D, Dachman A H, Bales G T, Gerber G S. Prospective evaluation of ureteral stent durability in patients with chronic ureteral obstruction. Urology 2002; 59: 847–850
16. Joshi H B, Stainthorpe A, Keeley F X Jr, MacDonagh R, Timoney AG. Indwelling ureteral stents: evaluation of quality of life to aid outcome analysis. J Endourol 2001; 15: 151–154
17. McDougall E M, Denstedt J D, Clayman R V. Comparison of patient acceptance of polyurethane vs. silicone indwelling ureteral stents. J Endourol 1990; 4: 79–91
18. Rane A, Saleemi A, Cahill D, Sriprasad S, Shrotri N, Tiptaft R. Have stent-related symptoms anything to do with placement technique? J Endourol 2001; 15: 741–745
19. Lennon G M, Thornhill J A, Sweeney P A, Grainger R, McDermott T E, Butler M R. 'Firm' versus 'soft' double pigtail ureteric stents: a randomised blind comparative trial. Eur Urol 1995; 28: 1–5
20. Candela J V, Bellman G C. Ureteral stents: impact of diameter and composition on patient symptoms. J Endourol 1997; 11: 45–47
21. Lee O J, Patel U, Patel S, Pillari G P. Emergency percutaneous nephrostomy: results and complications. J Vasc Interv Radiol 1994; 5: 135–139
22. Farrell T A, Hicks M E. A review of radiologically guided percutaneous nephrostomies in 303 patients. J Vasc Interv Radiol 1997; 8: 769–774
23. Sim L S, Tan B S, Yip S K, Ng C K, Lo R H, Yeong K Y et al. Single centre review of radiologically-guided percutaneous nephrostomies: a report of 273 procedures. Ann Acad Med Singapore 2002; 31: 76–80
24. von der Recke P, Nielsen M B, Pedersen J F. Complications of ultrasound-guided nephrostomy. A 5-year experience. Acta Radiol 1994; 35: 452–454
25. Mahaffey K G, Bolton D M, Stoller M L. Urologist directed percutaneous nephrostomy tube placement. J Urol 1994; 152: 1973–1976
26. Kehinde E O, Newland C J, Terry T R, Watkin E M, Butt Z. percutaneous nephrostomies. Br J Urol 1993; 71: 664–666
27. Vehmas T, Kivisaari L, Mankinen P, Tierala E, Somer K, Lehtonen T et al. Results and complications of percutaneous nephrostomy. Ann Clin Res 1988; 20: 423–427
28. Stables D P, Ginsberg N J, Johnson M L. Percutaneous nephrostomy: a series and review of the literature. AJR 1978; 130: 75–82
29. Nielsen O S, Grossmann E. Ultrasonically guided percutaneous nephrostomy. Scand J Urol Nephrol 1990; 24: 219–221
30. Ramchandani P, Cardella J F, Grassi C J, Roberts A C, Sacks D, Schwartzberg M S et al. Quality improvement guidelines for percutaneous nephrostomy. J Vasc Interv Radiol 2001; 12: 1247–1251
31. Klein L A, Koyle M, Berg S. The emergency management of patients with ureteral calculi and fever. J Urol 1983; 129: 938–940
32. Camunez F, Echenagusia A, Prieto M L, Salom P, Herranz F, Hernandez C. Percutaneous nephrostomy in pyonephrosis. Urol Radiol 1989; 11: 77–81
33. St Lezin M, Hofmann R, Stoller M L. Pyonephrosis: diagnosis and treatment. Br J Urol 1992; 70: 360–363
34. Ng C K, Yip S K, Sim L S, Tan B H, Wong M Y, Tan B S et al. Outcome of percutaneous nephrostomy for the managment of pyonephrosis. Asian J Surg 2002; 25: 215–219
35. Zagoria R J. In the management of a patient with nonmalignant obstructive uropathy and known infection, isn't it safer and more prudent to attempt retrograde placement of a ureteral stent before percutaneous nephrostomy? AJR 1997; 168: 1616
36. Pearle M S, Pierce H L, Miller G L, Summa J A, Mutz J M, Petty B A et al. Optimal method of urgent decompression of the collecting system for obstruction and infection due to ureteral calculi. J Urol 1998; 160: 1260–1264
37. Mokhmalji H, Braun P M, Martinez Portillo F J, Siegsmund M, Alken P, Kohrmann K U. Percutaneous nephrostomy versus ureteral stents for diversion of hydronephrosis caused by stones: a prospective, randomized clinical trial. J Urol 2001; 165: 1088–1092
38. Joshi H B, Adams S, Obadeyi O O, Rao P N. Nephrostomy tube or 'JJ' ureteric stent in ureteric obstruction: assessment of patient perspectives using quality-of-life survey and utility analysis. Eur Urol 2001; 39: 695–701
39. Docimo S G, Dewolf W C. High failure rate of indwelling ureteral stents in patients with extrinsic obstruction: experience at 2 institutions. J Urol 1989; 142: 277–279
40. Hyppolite J C, Daniels I D, Friedman E A. Obstructive uropathy in gynecologic malignancy. Detrimental effect of intraureteral stent placement and value of percutaneous nephrostomy. ASAIO J 1995; 41: M318–323

41. Hübner W A, Plas E G, Stoller M L. The double-J ureteral stent: in vivo and in vitro flow studies. J Urol 1992; 148: 278–280

42. Park D S, Park J H, Lee Y T. Percutaneous nephrostomy versus indwelling ureteral stents in patients with bilateral nongenito-urinary malignant extrinsic obstruction. J Endourol 2002; 16: 153–154

43. Walther P J, Robertson C N, Paulson D F. Lethal complications of standard self-retaining ureteral stents in patients with ileal conduit urinary diversion. J Urol 1985; 133: 851–853

44. Watterson J D, Girvan A R, Cook A J, Beiko D T, Nott L, Auge B K et al. Safety and efficacy of holmium:YAG laser lithotripsy in patients with bleeding diatheses. J Urol 2002; 168: 442–445

22

Double-J (JJ) stents versus nephrostomy tube drainage
G. M. Watson

Introduction

The kidney is at risk of permanent damage when it is obstructed and this is particularly true when there is infection; expeditious treatment of renal obstruction is therefore one of the most important duties of the urologist. This chapter is concerned with the techniques of relieving the obstruction in the acute and chronic setting. The choice of nephrostomy tube or JJ stent is discussed for a variety of clinical problems, together with the developments in both modalities.

Drainage using a ureteric stent

A JJ stent is a self-retaining stent that traverses the entire ureter. It was developed from the temporary stents used after open surgery, such as the Gibbons stent.[1] JJ stents, however, have preformed curved sections that are sufficiently flexible to straighten out when placed over a guidewire but with sufficient memory to form a curve in the renal pelvis and bladder that prevents migration. The stents are hollow tubes with side-holes at regular intervals throughout their length. They are sited by inserting a guidewire up the ureter under cystoscopic visual control or, more rarely, by manipulating it down the ureter via a nephrostomy; the JJ stent is advanced over the guidewire and the position confirmed radiologically. The procedure is therefore most commonly performed by a urologist in an endoscopic suite. The stent insertion can easily be combined with a retrograde X-ray examination of the ureter and this is important because the obstruction is much more difficult to define once a JJ stent has been inserted. Furthermore, the retrograde contrast gives greater confidence about the correct placement of the stent.

It is possible to dissect out of the ureter into a subepithelial plane, even using a guidewire. A useful test is to place an open-ended ureteric catheter over the guidewire into the obstructed pelvicalyceal system. After removal of the guidewire, free drainage of urine down the catheter confirms that the guidewire has been placed correctly. The guidewire can then be replaced and the ureteric catheter exchanged for a JJ stent. A pusher is used to advance the JJ stent over the static guidewire, taking care not to form a loop within the bladder and not to kink the guidewire.

The most commonly used stent is a 7 Fr stent 24 cm long but this cannot be considered a universal stent because incorrect sizing does make the stent more likely to migrate up the ureter (if too short) or to irritate the trigone excessively (if too long). Unless variable length stents are used, it is still necessary to measure the length between the renal pelvis and the bladder on the intravenous urogram (IVU). The stent has a series of markings to help with cystoscopic placement of the stent. The operator is warned how far the stent has been inserted and is therefore less likely to push the stent completely into the ureter (which would make retrieval awkward). Any kinking of the guidewire may make it impossible to advance the stent over the guidewire, in which case the stent should be removed and a ureteric catheter placed over the guidewire so that the latter can be exchanged.

Problems associated with stent placement

The problems associated with stent placement and some possible solutions are detailed below:

- The patient may not tolerate cystoscopy without a general or spinal anaesthetic. In females the procedure can be performed more easily under local urethral anaesthesia alone and the discomfort of JJ stent placement is equivalent to that of nephrostomy tube placement.
- Spinal or hip deformity may obviate rigid cystoscopy. The solution is to use a flexible cystoscope.
- The prostate, if enlarged, may obscure the ureteric orifices. A rigid cystoscope can be used to level the middle lobe sufficiently for the ureteric orifices to be seen. A large prostate might be good reason for a

nephrostomy placement, because of the risk of failure.

- Oedema or cancer may obscure the ureteric orifices. The solution is to resect the abnormal tissue until the proximally dilated ureter is exposed. A guidewire can then usually be advanced up the ureter and a JJ stent placed. However a covering nephrostomy with the possibility of a 'rendezvous procedure' is recommended. The rendezvous procedure is where access is both via cystoscopy and a nephrostomy. Either a guidewire or methylene blue or even a flexible ureteroscope is used to help establish continuity with the bladder.

- A hooked ureter usually associated with a moderately enlarged prostate may make it difficult to advance a guidewire. A small-calibre ureteroscope will provide a solution by showing the true lumen from a false passage and will allow placement of the guidewire under vision. A curved Cobra catheter combined with retrograde ureterography can help in directing the guidewire around the curve of the ureter.

- The guidewire may not pass by the obstruction. As a solution, it may be possible to pass a ureteroscope, to visualize the obstruction and then treat it, thereby allowing the guidewire to pass. If this is contraindicated, as for example in the presence of sepsis, then a hydrophilic-coated guidewire such as the Glidewire or the Roadrunner will, after wetting, become so slippery that it can be manoeuvred past the obstruction. If a very fine slippery guidewire is used, then it can be exchanged for a stiffer guidewire using a retrograde ureteric catheter as described before.

- If a kink has been made in the guidewire, as soon as this is recognized and, if possible, before placing a JJ stent over the guidewire, it should be exchanged for a new guidewire using the ureteric catheter technique. Stiffer guidewires and guidewires made from Nitinol are less likely to kink.

- If a guidewire can be manoeuvred past the stone but a JJ stent will not pass, a polyurethane or Percuflex stent passed over a stiff guidewire may be used in preference to using a silicone or similar soft stent. If this cannot be passed, then a ureteric catheter may be passed over the guidewire and then secured to a urethral catheter. After a minimum of 48 hours it is generally possible to exchange the ureteric catheter for a stent.

- There may be a pronounced kink in the ureter that cannot be negotiated with the guidewire, in which case a combination of a hydrophilic-coated guidewire and a curved catheter (such as the Cobra catheter) may be used in order to manoeuvre the guidewire past the kink. Once the outer catheter has been positioned above the kink, either it can be left to drain for 48 hours, or the guidewire can be replaced by a stiff guidewire and a polyurethane or Percuflex stent can be passed.

- The JJ stent may form its upper curve in a dilated upper ureter when there is a dilated ureter or an awkward pelvi-ureteric junction (PUJ). Dilute contrast introduced just prior to stent insertion will show the anatomy clearly, and use of a stiffer guidewire will stop the stent forming a curl below the renal pelvis. An awkward PUJ can be negotiated using a hydrophilic-coated guidewire in virtually all instances.

Advantages and disadvantages of JJ stents

The obvious advantage of a JJ stent is that it is completely enclosed within the body but there are a number of inherent disadvantages, which are discussed below.

The stent may not disobstruct the system as certainly as would a nephrostomy

Fine et al.[2] examined patients with indwelling JJ stents, using contrast X-ray studies. They noted that all patients refluxed contrast via the centre of the stent during micturition, but that drainage was predominantly by peristaltic ureteric activity with flow around the stent.

The effect of placing a JJ stent in a normal pig ureter was investigated by Ramsay et al.[3] The normal control ureter was capable of drainage during normal urine production and during a diuresis without the renal pressure rising above 10 cmH$_2$O. The acute effect of insertion of a 5 Fr or 6 Fr polyurethane stent was to cause a rise in intrapelvic pressure to approximately 30 cmH$_2$O at normal urine production and this pressure rose to approximately 50 cmH$_2$O with a diuresis. The effect persisted for 1 week but by 3 weeks had partially resolved, with pressure rises of 10–30 cmH$_2$O during a diuresis. Simply inserting a urethral catheter reduced the level of the acute pressure rise in the kidney by about 50%. In clinical cases these authors studied the pressure rise in the kidney during perfusion of the pelvicalyceal system via a nephrostomy tube at a rate of 10 ml/min: the subtracted renal pelvic minus bladder pressure rose by 16 cmH$_2$O. The total renal pelvic pressure was reduced significantly by urethral catheterization.

Hubner et al.[4] studied intrarenal pressures in patients who had JJ stents and nephrostomy tubes in place: 20 studies were performed in 14 patients. Drainage to the bladder was achieved in 17 of the 20 studies at an average pressure of 19.9 cmH$_2$O. Reflux was noted in 17 studies at an average pressure in the bladder of 20 cmH$_2$O; three stents neither drained nor refluxed.

In in vitro modelling of extrinsic compression of the ureter, polyurethane stents had far better pressure–flow characteristics than soft silicone stents. Mardis and colleagues[5] have shown the same phenomenon in a model in vitro, but the clinical results may be less favourable for the use of JJ stents in extrinsic compression of the ureter. Docimo and Dewolf[6] looked at the rate of stent occlusion within 30 days of insertion. At one institution, silicone stents were used virtually exclusively: 23 stents were placed for intrinsic obstruction (stones, PUJ obstruction) and were uniformly successful; 24 stents were placed for extrinsic compression (ureteric stricture and retroperitoneal tumour) with 11 failures. At the second institution, where polyurethane stents were preferred, 21 were placed for intrinsic obstruction, with uniform success, and 22 were placed for extrinsic obstruction, with nine failures. The authors did not know why there was such a reduced efficacy for extrinsic obstruction, but suggested that a length of aperistaltic ureter resulted in reduced drainage alongside the stent.

Hyppolite et al.[7] performed a retrospective review of 41 patients over a 5-year period who had obstructive uropathy secondary to gynaecological malignancy: 14 patients were treated by open operation, 17 patients were treated by nephrostomy, seven by JJ stent and three by a combination of the latter two. Of seven patients treated by JJ stenting, six developed urosepsis, which was fatal in three cases; this did not occur in the nephrostomy group.

Jenkins and Marcus[8] reported on ten patients with lower third ureteric obstruction, secondary to malignancy in eight of the ten cases. Antegrade placement of the stent via a nephrostomy was successful in 10/11 attempts, with cystoscopic assistance in three. The stents were patent for an average of 20 months without replacement and without complications.

The ileal conduit may represent a particularly unfavourable environment for stenting. Walther et al.[9] reviewed four patients who had had an ileal conduit plus stenting for obstruction. One patient was lost to follow-up; of the three remaining patients, all had septic shock, which was fatal in two patients. In the one remaining patient, a permanent nephrostomy drain was substituted.

Even in the conventional situation where the patient has not undergone urinary diversion, regular changing of JJ stents is a more generally accepted approach nowadays. Provided that the stents are changed every 3–6 months, they are much less prone to obstruction.

An interesting variation on this theme of stenting for tumours is the use of the Wallstent, reported by Flueckiger et al.[10] This is a stainless steel fine-wire expandable stent that is inserted after dilatation of the stenosed segment. Flueckiger et al. implanted one stent in nine ureters and two stents in four ureters. Drainage was achieved in all cases at first, but within 2 weeks, four of the 13 ureters were obstructed by epithelial hyperplasia growing into the lumen of the stent, and a JJ stent was required. One ureter required a further stent placement because of tumour spread. The remaining stents remained patent for the period of follow-up, which was a mean of 5.8 months.

The stent causes pathological changes to the ureter

Cormio et al.[11] studied the effect of JJ stents on pig ureters: they found that polyurethane stents were associated with the most pressure changes and the greatest epithelial reaction. Hydrogel-coated stents and silicone stents provoked the least epithelial reaction, and the hydrogel-coated stent had the least tendency to encrustation.

Selmy et al.[12] looked at the effect of JJ stenting on the traumatized pig ureter. The right ureterovesical junction and lower third of the ureter were dilated to three times the normal calibre in 12 pigs and, of these 12 ureters, six were stented. All the renal units with stented ureters showed grade 3 reflux 7 weeks later but none of the dilated non-stented ureters refluxed. The stented ureters were found to have significant bacteriuria with *Pseudomonas* and also had a reduced creatinine clearance compared with the dilated, non-stented side. Histological examination of the dilated segment showed a muscular defect with signs of muscular regeneration by 4 weeks, which was equivalent in the stented and non-stented groups. By 7 weeks, the stented group showed pronounced metaplasia and chronic pyelonephritis. The JJ stent therefore had a pronounced negative impact on the kidney and on renal function. In this study there was not a noticeable improvement in ureteric repair after stenting.

Davis[13] has shown that ureteric strictures and PUJ obstruction can be treated effectively by incision and stenting. The ureter re-forms a complete layer of epithelium and muscle around the stent, as Davis subsequently showed in animal experiments. Clearly, this situation differs from that in which a normal diameter ureter is then traumatically dilated. This finding of Davis' is the basis of the endopyelotomy procedure for PUJ obstruction.

In clinical practice the stent is not associated with such an obvious decline in renal function. This is presumably because any negative effect is counteracted by the positive effect of overcoming any obstruction and because in Selmy's study a major cause of renal damage was the urinary tract infection associated with the refluxing.[12] Urinary tract infection is less common in clinical practice than it appeared to be in Selmy's study. Franco et al.[14] looked at the incidence of urinary tract infection in 36 paediatric patients with ureteric stents after surgery: only three patients developed urinary tract infection (8.3%).

Renal impairment resulting from infection and reflux might be corrected by using a non-refluxing stent. This hypothesis has been tested in the dog ureter ex vivo by Hubner et al.[15] The antireflux stent has a plastic membrane like an open bag over the intravesical loop of the JJ stent that prevents transmission of the intravesical pressure to the stent lumen without obstructing drainage out of the stent. The authors found that, in normal stents, 90% of the intravesical pressure was transmitted to the renal pelvis; using antireflux

stents, the pressure rise in the renal pelvis was less marked and reflux was delayed or absent in all cases. In their clinical series reflux was not detectable on fluoroscopy in any case.

The stent has an adverse effect on ureteric peristalsis

Ryan et al.[16] have looked at the effect of JJ stenting on the canine ureter. In an acute study, one ureter was stented with a 3.8 Fr JJ stent and one ureter was left unstented. Both ureters were then presented at their proximal portion with a model calculus, which was a stainless steel ball 3 mm in diameter. The stainless steel balls traversed the control (unstented) ureters in 3.4 ± 1.6 days; the mean time to traverse the stented ureter was 16.5 ± 2.2 days. In a chronic study, the authors looked at the renal intrapelvic pressure, peristaltic rate and peristaltic amplitude. Prior to stent insertion the mean intrapelvic pressure was 2.8 mmHg with a peristaltic amplitude of 3.7 mmHg at a rate of 10.8/min. The ureter had a peristaltic amplitude that peaked at a mean of 48.6 mmHg and the rate was 11.0/min. Some 24 hours after stent insertion the intrapelvic pressure rose significantly and renal pelvic motility was reduced in some and absent in others. After 1 week the renal pelvic pressure fell to baseline. At 30 days the mean renal pelvic peristaltic rate was only 1.9/min and the amplitude was 1.4 mmHg. Ureteric peristaltic amplitude was reduced from 48.6 to only 15.3 mmHg and the rate was reduced from 11.0 to 2.7 contractions/min. The authors then removed one stent and presented both ureters with the model stones. The ureters were noted to be markedly dilated. The destented ureters passed the calculus after a mean of 7.2 days, whereas the stented ureters passed the calculus in a mean of 24.1 days. Twelve weeks after stent removal the peristaltic rate had reached 7.5/min and the mean amplitude peak was 37.25 mmHg. Histological examination showed persistent muscular hypertrophy and collagen deposition.

JJ stent design

Mardis et al.[17] have produced a comparative analysis of the materials used in stents. The authors have identified a number of design features of the stent that promote drainage, as follows:

- A high internal/external diameter ratio.
- Numerous side-holes along the length of the stent.
- Reinforcement of the polymer with a wire spiral, which makes the stent stronger and thus allows wide side-holes with a wider internal diameter.

Silicone stents have the lowest internal/external diameter ratio and the smallest side-holes; C-Flex (Concept Polymer Technologies, Clearwater, FL, USA), polyurethane and Percuflex (Boston Scientific Corporation, Watertown, MA, USA) have a serially greater strength, allowing greater ratios and larger side-holes.

Other design features that are important for insertion include the following:

- A closed-end stent for easy insertion in the traditional retrograde catheter technique when used with a guidewire as a stylet. Making the tip soluble in urine (as in the Fader-tip) allows greater drainage and the possibility of exchanging over a guidewire.
- Constructing the stent of a low-friction material so that it will slide easily over the guidewire. Silicone and Silitek have a high coefficient of friction, with hydrogel-coated stents having the least coefficient of friction.
- Having a stent of sufficient strength to avoid any tendency to buckle on the guidewire.
- Having a relatively large-calibre guidewire, to avoid buckling of the guidewire itself.
- Other innovations include collars on the shaft of the stent to take pushers that are placed over the soft bladder coil, as with the J-Maxx stent of Microvasive.

Design features that promote retention of the coil of the stent revolve around the memory of the material. The longer the segment that is involved in the coil, the greater is the retentive strength of the stent, irrespective of the material. Thus, the J stent has been largely replaced by the cross-coil (i.e. spiral) design. A coiled strength of 20 g is sufficient to minimize the problem of migration. On this basis all stents made of silicone or Silitek with a cross-coil (spiral) or hook design at the renal pelvis fall below this coil strength value. All stents made of C-Flex or Percuflex have sufficient retentive strength, irrespective of coil type. The renal segment

should be relatively firm but should unravel easily. The pigtail occasionally may not unravel, whereas the cross-coil (spiral) stents tend to uncoil more consistently. The bladder coil is less critical in terms of unravelling but rigidity may make the stent more uncomfortable. The cross-coil design, perhaps with a variable-length stent, is popular.

Radiopacity of the stent is important for localization. Usually, metallic salts are added to the polymer mix prior to extrusion of the stent. Different stents vary widely in the percentage of metals added; the more metal added, the greater is the radiopacity. Unfortunately, these metals can leach out of the stent and may be relatively toxic (at least in theory) to the ureter. There is a 20-fold difference between the radiopacity of a Cook double-pigtail silicone stent (more radiopaque) and a Surgitek Finney double-J stent (less radiopaque).

The material from which a stent is manufactured will affect not only its mechanical properties but also its biodurability and biocompatibility. A stent will adsorb onto its surface proteins and crystals, leading to calcification and possibly bacterial colonization. Chemicals in the urine will start to degrade polymers and reduce their strength and flexibility. Some stents are constructed from a basic polymer for their mechanical properties but with a coating of a more biocompatible material. The first stents were made from latex, which produces a great deal of tissue reaction. The next generation of stents were made from silicone and polyurethane. Silicone has poor mechanical strength but is moderately biodurable, in that it does not lose its flexibility, and is moderately biocompatible, in that it encrusts less than polyurethane. Polyurethane, on the other hand, has good mechanical strength but does biodegrade and does calcify. The 'forgotten stent' may be removed easily if made of silicone but may break into multiple pieces if made of polyurethane.

New materials may prove to have better mechanical properties and biocompatibility. C-Flex is a silicone-modified thermoplastic polymer that is relatively cheap. It is less strong than polyurethane or Silitek, but it does function well when formed into a stent of calibre 7 Fr or larger. It is marketed currently with a hydrogel coating; hydrogels are giant polymers that have the property of absorbing water and swelling. C-Flex retains the hydrogel coating powerfully and the hydrogel surface becomes extremely slippery when wet. This favours stent insertion and increases its biocompatibility. Percuflex is a thermoplastic block polymer with excellent mechanical and biocompatible properties. It has a smooth surface that resists degradation and calcification. Its strength makes it function efficiently, even at stent sizes of less than 7 Fr, with good coil strength properties.

Marx et al.[18] looked at the effect of stenting on the dog ureter using polyurethane, Silitek and C-Flex stents (Percuflex was not available at that time). Polyurethane stents were frequently associated with epithelial ulceration, which was rare with other materials. Silitek caused more oedema than silicone, C-Flex or polyurethane. C-Flex was considered the most suitable material, in Marx's study.

Percuflex may represent a further improvement in terms of its mechanical and biocompatible properties. The development of these materials does seem to be associated with less encrustation than is seen with silicone and particularly with polyurethane. However, no material has zero risk of encrustation and all stents will need regular changing, but perhaps less frequently.

Nephrostomy tube drainage

Nephrostomy tube insertion was originally performed using a trochar and cannula and was therefore possible only for drainage of markedly hydronephrotic kidneys. The development of the Seldinger technique for angiography was adapted for drainage of the pelvicalyceal system: a needle is used to insert a guidewire; dilatation of the track over the guidewire then allows a drainage cannula to be inserted that is wider than the original needle. Thus, nephrostomy drainage of minimally dilated systems is now possible.

Advantages
The advantages of nephrostomy drainage are as follows:

- The kidney is drained directly.
- The output from the kidney can be monitored.
- The nephrostomy tube can be inserted and removed without recourse to cystoscopy; general anaesthesia is not required.
- Any pathology at the trigone can be avoided.
- The nephrostomy can be used to stent the ureter antegradely or as part of a 'rendez-vous' procedure.

The track can be dilated for antegrade ureteroscopy or for percutaneous stone surgery.

Disadvantages
The disadvantages of nephrostomy tube drainage are as follows:
- The patient has an external bag to collect urine.
- The nephrostomy is easily displaced.
- There is often some leakage of urine around the nephrostomy tube.
- Any side-holes outside the kidney can lead to perinephric collections.
- The needle puncture and any dilatation of the track is through the renal cortex; there is, therefore, a risk of haemorrhage and of some leakage of potentially infected urine into the bloodstream.
- There may be a distortion of the ultrasound image by staghorn calculus or by emphysematous pyelonephritis.
- The pelvicalyceal system may be undistended, making the puncture more difficult.
- The patient may be tachypnoeic or confused and therefore the puncture is on a moving target.
- The nephrostomy tube may become obstructed with debris, necessitating changing the tube possibly to one of a larger calibre.
- The patient can easily kink the outlet tubing between the nephrostomy tube and the bag and can completely obstruct the drainage.

Clinical experience
The published series suggest a 98% success rate in terms of nephrostomy tube placement. Failures were due to small pelvicalyceal systems and staghorn calculi. Success in terms of achievement of a stated goal was achieved in 90–95% of cases. Stables[19] has reviewed 1207 nephrostomy tube attempts at his institution: mortality was 0.2% and was always due to haemorrhage in the presence of a coagulopathy (either pre-existing or secondary to uraemia). Significant haemorrhage was the most important complication, occurring in 1.3%. Only one patient required embolization and eight patients required transfusion. Septic complications occurred in 1.9%, including failed drainage in 15 patients and exacerbation by antegrade pyelography in five patients. (Contrast injection into the pelvicalyceal system should be avoided until the urine is sterile and the patient no longer pyrexial. If a nephrostomy tube ceases to drain

then it is safer to exchange the tube with a larger, stiffer drain than to flush the nephrostomy tube. Fluid flushed into the pelvicalyceal system under pressure can enter the lymphatic and even the venous system.) Urine leak into the retroperitoneum occurred in 0.6%. Other complications were pneumothorax in one patient and catheter fracture in one patient. These complications relate to the insertion rather than the continued function of the drain.

Premature nephrostomy tube displacement is a much more common event than any complication of insertion. Nephrostomy tubes used to have Malecot tips or balloons for stability within the collecting system. Premature displacement occurred in up to 15%.[20] Securing the tube at the skin may result in displacement when the patient is obese. The most secure stent is the single J traversing the pelvicalyceal system and the entire ureter to the bladder where a coil retains it. However, this produces the bladder discomfort one would usually hope to avoid with a stent and it is not always possible to place this stent.

The self-locking coiled stents such as the Cope loop have been a considerable advance (Fig. 22.1). The stent is easier to pass than the Malecot or balloon tips. The multiple side-holes drain better than the balloon, which can obstruct calyces proximal to it. Finally, the improvements in materials have led to drains with larger inner/outer diameter ratios and to tubes that are less likely to kink.

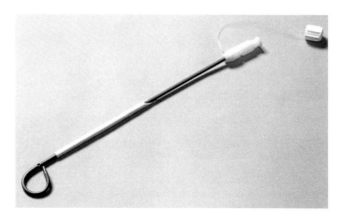

Figure 22.1. *The Cope loop nephrostomy. Traction on the thread forms a loop on the nephrostomy tube. A Luer locking device holds the thread and prevents displacement.*

Choice of JJ stent versus nephrostomy

When deciding whether to drain a pelvicalyceal system by inserting a JJ stent cystoscopically or a nephrostomy tube, the urologist always considers the best way to drain the system and the subsequent strategy for the pathology involved. The issues are therefore discussed below for a variety of pathologies.

Impending pyonephrosis

When a patient presents with an infected, obstructed kidney, the overriding principle is to secure certain drainage of the collecting system. A nephrostomy tube gives a more certain drainage than a JJ stent, as evidenced by the pressure studies of Ramsay et al. Furthermore, attempted JJ stent insertion might fail, and certainly a general anaesthetic or even a spinal anaesthetic would not seem advisable for a patient with threatening septic shock. If the patient had a haemorrhagic disorder or a pelvic kidney, then it would be reasonable to try JJ stenting as a first attempt; a ureteric catheter might be left to drain the system before converting to a JJ stent a few days later; if a JJ stent was used, a urethral catheter should be left in situ for a few days in order to maximize the drainage of the upper tracts.

Having opted for a nephrostomy tube, it is important to avoid any flushing or antegrade X-ray study until the patient is apyrexial and the urine sterile. The tube should be anchored securely, making sure that the tubing is not kinked. If at any stage the drainage is unsatisfactory, then the tube should be replaced with a larger-calibre nephrostomy tube.

Once the infection has been controlled, then an antegrade study will identify the likely cause of the obstruction and the nephrostomy access might prove useful in any subsequent endoscopy.

Obstructing ureteric calculus

Clinical practice has moved more towards direct intervention without stenting for the calculus in the absence of infection. On occasions, however, a JJ stent or nephrostomy is used to aid stone passage. A stent does dilate a ureter and this may aid the passage of a ureteroscope subsequently if the original ureter was narrow. The animal data of Ryan et al.[16], however, do cast doubt on the notion that a stone is more likely to pass with (or even after) a stent. Nephrostomy tube insertion, however, can aid stone passage when there is hydronephrosis above the stone. This is because the ureter regains useful peristalsis when the walls of the ureter coapt.

Injured ureter

After ureteric trauma it is important to stent the ureter as well as to control urinary extravasation. O'Sullivan et al. reported on 11 patients who had a nephrostomy tube before or after ureteroscopy, of whom eight developed a ureteric stricture[24]. In seven patients who had a JJ stent after ureteroscopy, or a nephrostomy tube that was clamped so that flow was maintained down the ureter, there were no cases of stricture formation. Therefore a JJ stent (possibly with temporary catheterization or nephrostomy drainage until the extravasation is controlled) is the ideal management.

Obstructed solitary kidney

The solitary kidney might be thought of as a relative contraindication to a nephrostomy tube placement in case any trauma led to injury to the kidney. However, the very good safety record of nephrostomy tube placement in centres of excellence shows that the risk of losing a kidney from the nephrostomy placement is virtually nil. The risk in this situation is probably not too dissimilar to the risk of injury to the ureter from JJ stent insertion. The chosen mode of action should therefore depend on the experience of the radiologist and the underlying pathology.

Obstructed kidney in pregnancy

In the first trimester of pregnancy the management of an obstructed kidney is problematic, from the point of view of both diagnosis and treatment. X-rays and intervention pose severe risks to the foetus. Fortunately, most ureteric calculi pass spontaneously but in some cases intervention is necessary. Placement of a JJ stent would be possible under local anaesthesia but the stent would possibly have to stay in for the length of the pregnancy and causes extra irritation to the bladder on top of the normal frequency as pregnancy progresses. The risk of urinary tract infection increases. A nephrostomy tube has the disadvantage of not being contained within the body, but the advantage that the track can be used for flexible ureteroscopy without need of anaesthesia. If a nephrostogram is performed, then the diagnosis can be suspected with less exposure to X-rays than with a limited IVU. These arguments favour the use of a nephrostomy tube in early pregnancy.

Antegrade ureteroscopy is well tolerated by the expectant mother, especially if performed with the patient sitting leaning over the back of a chair. If the obstruction is due to a stone, then this can be fragmented and the fragments chased down into the bladder. As pregnancy continues, so a simple attempt a JJ stent insertion might be increasingly favoured because idiopathic hydronephrosis of pregnancy becomes increasingly likely and because the stent would be in situ for only a relatively short period. A nephrostomy tube placement also is acceptable in this situation. Once the pregnancy has been successfully completed, the stent can be removed or a nephrostogram performed.

The literature shows ambivalence as to how best to manage the obstructed kidney in pregnancy. Quinn et al. advocate nephrostomy insertion on the basis that JJ stent insertion may result in damage to the ureter, requiring reconstruction, and because of infection secondary to reflux.[25] Kavoussi et al. reported on six patients with obstruction secondary to stones during pregnancy, all of whom were managed by nephrostomy placement.[26] One patient went on to have percutaneous surgery for a large pelvic stone while still pregnant; the remaining five patients all required nephrostomy tube changes because of obstruction from debris; urine was kept sterile. On the other hand, Loughlin and Bailey reported eight patients who were managed throughout pregnancy with JJ stent insertion without mishap.[27]

There may be a theoretical increased risk of encrustation because of physiological hypercalciuria. Fabrizio et al.[21] reported on the insertion of JJ stents using simple ultrasound to verify the position of the stent. Clearly, JJ stents in pregnancy can be inserted without any irradiation and with minimal complications. A stent can even be inserted in a severely symptomatic patient without any clear diagnosis as to the cause of the obstruction. Once pregnancy is completed, then the stent can be removed and the cause diagnosed and treated, if appropriate.

Extrinsic compression

The results of drainage using JJ stents in the presence of external compression, such as in retroperitoneal malignancy, suggest that this is an ineffective modality. However, the importance of regular changing of JJ stents on a 3- or 6-monthly basis, depending on the stent material and the patient's pathology, is now known. JJ stenting is more effective than one might suppose from the literature. Certainly, however, a relatively firm stent, such as the Percuflex stent, should be selected. A nephrostomy tube is less acceptable as a long-term solution and should be selected only if the ureter is impassable. There is always the possibility of passing a stent subcutaneously from a nephrostomy puncture around the flank to the anterior abdominal wall and thence into the bladder.[22,23]

Pelvic kidney

This is an example of a situation where nephrostomy tube placement is difficult or impossible and JJ stent placement is preferred.

Patient with a haemorrhagic disorder

Nephrostomy tube placement is relatively contraindicated in the presence of a haemorrhagic disorder because of the risk of serious bleeding. Either the disorder should be reversed, if possible in the time available, or a stent should be opted for in the first instance.

Patient with an ileal conduit

The risk of a patient with an ileal conduit is that the patient may present with fatal urosepsis at first presentation, as described by Walther et al.[9] A nephrostomy tube drainage followed by definitive correction of the obstruction is preferred.

Impassable ureterovesical junction

There are many possible reasons for failure to negotiate the ureter from the bladder. If the ureter has been reimplanted, or if there is severe pathology infiltrating the trigone, then the orifice cannot be negotiated with a guidewire. A nephrostomy tube can be used to gain access to the ureter for stenting directly or in combination with a cystoscopic procedure as part of a rendezvous procedure.

Conclusions

JJ stenting and nephrostomy drainage are complementary procedures that are both important modalities in the management of the obstructed urinary tract. Both modalities have benefited from the development of new materials, but this is particularly true of the JJ stent. Even the design of the JJ stent has undergone modifications, with improved retaining devices. When selecting which modality to use, the urologist must consider the short-term drainage of the kidney and his optimum access for resolution of the pathology. An example of adjusting the approach to the problem is given in the following case history.

Case history

An elderly, frail lady presented with severe urosepsis and circulatory collapse. Ultrasonography (Fig. 22.2) showed a dilated left kidney with probable hydronephrosis. A 6 Fr nephrostomy tube was inserted and several hundred millilitres of pus drained over the next 12 hours, but then stopped draining. The patient improved only slightly and remained tender in the left loin. A plain X-ray (Fig. 22.3) showed the presence of air in the collecting system and that the nephrostomy tube was draining the perirenal space. There was a possible ureteric stone at the lower border of L3. The perinephric drain was exchanged over a guidewire with a wider-bore Van Sonnenberg sump drain, and a ureteric catheter was passed under local anaesthetic to drain the collecting system (Fig. 22.4): the patient's condition then improved considerably. A few days later a

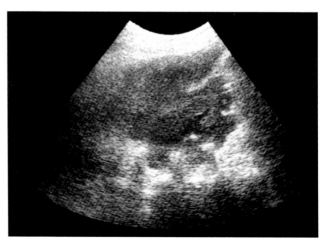

Figure 22.2. *Ultrasound of the left kidney showing a distended system with some echogenic areas.*

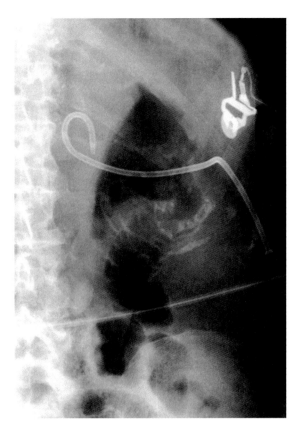

Figure 22.3. *Air is seen in the collecting system and the nephrostomy tube is outside the collecting system.*

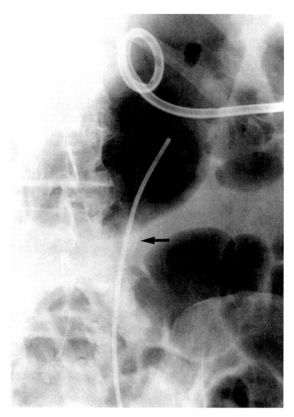

Figure 22.4. *A ureteric catheter has been passed beyond a calculus (arrow) into the pelvicalyceal system.*

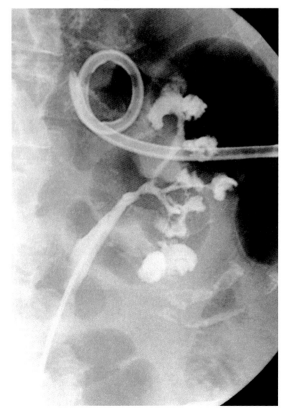

Figure 22.5. *A retrograde ureterogram showing a collapsed collecting system and no communication with the perinephric collection.*

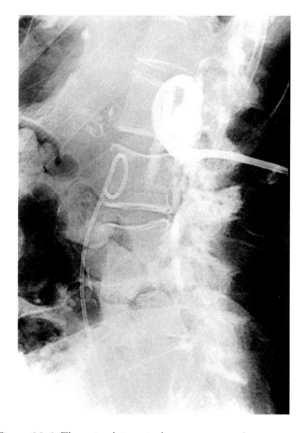

Figure 22.6. *The perinephric cavity has now contracted.*

retrograde study was performed via the ureteric catheter (Fig. 22.5). The collecting system had collapsed and contrast filled the ureter down to the stone. The ureteric catheter was removed over a guidewire and replaced with a JJ stent. Figure 22.6 shows the perinephric abscess cavity, now very much contracted and not communicating with the pelvicalyceal system, which contains a 6 Fr polyurethane stent. Definitive management by nephrectomy is being delayed indefinitely because of the physical state of the patient.

References

1. Gibbons R P, Correa R J Jr, Cummings K B, Mason J T. Experience with indwelling ureteral stent catheters. J Urol 1976; 115: 22

2. Fine H, Gordon R L, Lebensart P D. Extracorporeal shock wave lithotripsy and stents: fluoroscopic observations and a hypothesis on the mechanisms of stent function. Urol Radiol 1989; 11: 37

3. Ramsay J W A, Payne S R, Gosling P T et al. The effects of Double J stenting on unobstructed ureters. An experimental and clinical study. Br J Urol 1985; 57: 630–633

4. Hubner W A, Plas E G, Stoller M L. The double-J ureteral stent: in vivo and in vitro flow studies. J Urol 1992; 148: 278–280

5. Mardis H K, Kroeger R M, Hepper len T W et al. Polyethylene double-pigtail ureteral stents. Urol Clin North Am 1982; 9: 95

6. Docimo S G, Dewolf W C. High failure rate of indwelling ureteral stents in patients with extrinsic obstruction: experience at 2 insititutions. J Urol 1989; 142: 277–279

7. Hyppolite J C, Daniels I D, Friedman E A. Obstructive uropathy in gynecologic malignancy. Detrimental effect of intraureteral stent placement and value of percutaneous nephrostomy. ASAIO J 1995; 41: 318–323

8. Jenkins C N, Marcus A J. The value of antegrade stenting for lower ureteric obstruction. J R Soc Med 1995; 88: 446–449

9. Walther P J, Robertson C N, Paulson D F. Lethal complications of standard self-retaining ureteral stents in patients with ileal conduit urinary diversion. J Urol 1985; 133: 851–853

10. Flueckiger F, Lammer J, Klein G E et al. Malignant ureteral obstruction: preliminary results of treatment with metallic self-expandable stents. Radiology 1993; 186: 169–193

11. Cormio L, Koivusalo A, Maksalo H et al. The effects of various indwelling JJ stents on renal pelvic pressure and renal parenchymal thickness in the pig. Br J Urol 1994; 74: 440–443

12. Selmy G I, Hassouna M M, Begin L R et al. Long-term effects of ureteric stent after ureteric dilatation. J Urol 1993; 150: 1984–1989

13. Davis D M. Intubated ureterotomy. Surg Gynecol Obstet 1943; 76: 513–523

14. Franco G, De Dominicis C, Dal Forno S et al. The incidence of post-operative urinary tract infection in patients with ureteric stents. Br J Urol 1990; 65: 10–12

15. Hubner W A, Plas E G, Trigo-Rocha F, Tanagho E A. Drainage and reflux characteristics of antireflux ureteral double-J stents. J Endourol 1993; 7: 497–499

16. Ryan P C, Lennon G M, McLean P A, Fitzpatrick J M. The effects of acute and chronic JJ stent placement on upper urinary tract motility and calculus transmit. Br J Urol 1994; 74: 434–439

17. Mardis H K, Kroeger R M, Morton J J, Donovan J M. Comparative evaluation of materials used for internal ureteral stents. J Endourol 1993; 7: 105–115

18. Marx M, Bettman M A, Bridge S. The effects of various indwelling ureteral catheter materials on the normal canine ureter. J Urol 1988; 139: 180

19. Stables D P. Percutaneous nephrostomy: techniques, indications and results. Urol Clin North Am 1982; 9: 15–29

20. Cope C. Improved anchoring of nephrostomy catheters: loop technique. AJR 1980; 135: 402–403

21. Fabrizio M D, Gray D S, Feld R I, Bagley D H. Placement of ureteral stents in pregnancy using ultrasound guidance. Techn Urol 1996; 2: 121–125

22. Ahmadzadeh M. Clinical experience with subcutaneous urinary diverison: new approach using a double pigtail stent. Br J Urol 1991; 67: 596–599

23. Lingam K, Paterson P J, Lingam M K et al. Subcutaneous urinary diversion: an alternative to percutaneous nephrostomy. J Urol 1994; 152: 70–72

24. O'Sullivan D C, Lemberger R J, Bishop M C et al. Ureteric stricture formation following ureteric instrumentation in patients with a nephrostomy drain in place. Br J Urol 1994; 74: 165–169

25. Quinn A D, Kusuda L, Amar A D. Das S. Percutaneous nephrostomy for treatment of hydronephrosis of pregnancy. J Urol 1988; 139: 1037–1038

26. Kavoussi L R, Albala D M, Basler J W et al. Percutaneous management of urolithiasis during pregnancy. J Urol 1992; 148: 1069–1071

27. Loughlin K R, Bailey R B. Internal ureteral stents for conservative management of ureteral calculi during pregnancy. N Engl J Med 1986; 315: 1647–1651

23

Tricks for stenting the obstructed ureter
D. Eiley and A. D. Smith

Introduction

Ureteral obstruction is a common cause of urological morbidity, requiring rapid and effective treatment. Prolonged obstruction can cause pain, infection and eventual loss of renal function. Few would argue that initial drainage or bypassing of the obstruction is favourable initial management; however, urologists are often faced with technically difficult cases not responsive to the standard operative manoeuvres.

In recognizing the diversity of pathology and the potential complicating issues, urologists should have in their armamentarium a systematic approach, or algorithm, for dealing with these common dilemmas, as well as an understanding of various 'tricks of the trade'. This will prevent heightened anxiety at the time of surgery and will ensure the availability of the proper operative equipment. In this chapter, an approach is outlined and the obstacles and options in stenting the obstructed ureter are discussed.

Procedures

The cause of the obstruction is investigated and can be classified as either intrinsic or extrinsic (i.e. arising from either within or from outside the ureteral wall — see Table 23.1). Once the diagnosis is established, informed consent is obtained for a retrograde urogram, stent placement, ureteroscopy, percutaneous nephrostomy tube placement, and general anaesthesia. The patient is taken to the operating room.

The patient is positioned on a radiolucent table in the dorsal lithotomy position. If ureteroscopy becomes necessary, the authors prefer to flex the contralateral hip and keep the ipsilateral hip in a neutral position. In addition to the standard equipment, the operating-room staff should have access to hydrophilic guidewires in different sizes, hydrophilic stents, various angiography catheters, peel-away catheters (Cook Urological, Spencer, IN, USA), rigid or semi-rigid dilators and a nephrostomy tube set.

Table 23.1. *Classification of ureteral obstruction*

Intrinsic	Extrinsic	Congenital
Calculus	Arterial obstruction,	Ureteropelvic junction obstruction
Transitional cell carcinoma	e.g. aneurysm, crossing vessels	Ureterovesical junction obstruction
Benign tumour	Benign pelvic mass,	e.g. primary megaureter
e.g. inverted papilloma	e.g. pregnancy, fibroids	
Stricture	Pelvic inflammation	Ureterocoele
Blood clots	e.g. Pelvic inflammatory disease	Retrocaval ureter
Sloughed papillae	Endometriosis	Valves
Inflammation	Iatrogenic	
e.g. Tuberculosis, ureteritis	e.g. ligature	
Trauma	Gastrointestinal inflammation,	
	e.g. diverticulitis, appendicitis	
	Retroperitoneal fibrosis	
	e.g. idiopathic, radiation induced	
	Retroperitoneal inflammation	
	Retroperitoneal haemorrhage	
	Retroperitoneal mass	
	• Benign, e.g. lipoma, neurofibroma	
	• Malignant – primary, e.g. lymphoma	
	– secondary, e.g. cervix, prostate	
	bladder	
	Pelvic lipomatosis	

An intra-operative retrograde urogram will delineate the ureteral anatomy distal to the obstruction, as well as the exact location, degree and, sometimes, length of the obstruction. Generally, the retrograde approach is first attempted for stenting; if this is unsuccessful the antegrade approach is then tried. If both approaches fail to bypass the obstruction, a percutaneous nephrostomy tube is left in place to achieve drainage as a temporizing measure. After adequate decompression (several days), another attempt at stenting is often successful; this is because the system is less dilated, straighter and less oedematous, thus making it easier to negotiate an obstruction. There are extenuating circumstances in which definitive patient management involves either a chronic percutaneous nephrostomy tube for drainage or use of a stent meant to bypass the ureter altogether (see later discussion).

The first step in stenting the ureter involves passing a guidewire beyond the obstruction. This can be achieved by either blind, fluoroscopic or endoscopic manipulation. This chapter first addresses the routine stent insertion with several common problem spots. Special anatomical concerns will then be considered. Different techniques to negotiate the obstructed ureter are then discussed, followed by stent passage in certain special situations. Finally, an orderly approach to stenting the ureter in the face of obstruction is outlined.

Routine stent passage

Stent placement is a common urological procedure; nevertheless, a seemingly easy '5 minute case' can be the source of tremendous frustration and anxiety. A subtle miscalculation in one step can offset the cascade of steps in an otherwise uncomplicated stent insertion (see Table 23.2). To begin with, all the materials should be set up on the sterile field in an orderly fashion. This will allow for an orderly approach and prevent later time delays.

The stent chosen should be of an appropriate length (e.g. ureteral length on X-ray minus 10% plus 2 cm) and should have tapered tips to allow for smoother placement. The authors routinely use double-pigtail stents as opposed to Double-J stents, owing to their increased retention (and decreased migration) properties.[1] Retrograde stents should be passed and positioned with the help of an assistant and under fluoroscopic control.

Table 23.2. *Summary of tips for routine stent placement*

Materials
    Stent
        Double-pigtail design
        Tapered tips
    Guidewire
        Teflon coated
        Proper size for stent
Procedure
    Prepare and arrange sterile field before beginning
    Proper cystoscope size for stent
    Do not overdistend the bladder
    Fluoroscopy
    Avoid coils in wire
    Beak of cystoscope abutting ureteral orifice
    Maintain wire taut as stent is advanced

The ureteral orifice should be catheterized in an atraumatic manner in order to avoid excessive oedema and creation of a false passage. The bladder should not be overdistended. The cystoscope chosen should be of adequate size to accommodate the selected stent diameter (i.e. to avoid excessive friction and binding of the stent). The guidewire should be Teflon coated to reduce the friction of the stent sliding over the wire. It should also be the appropriate size for the given stent, an important consideration if a complete stent set is not being utilized (see Table 23.3). Care should be taken not to coil the guidewire in the bladder. The cystoscope beak is positioned adjacent to the ureteral orifice in order to prevent buckling. The wire is held taut by the assistant and both the ureteral orifice and the fluoroscopy monitor should be watched as the stent is being advanced, its position verified and the wire subsequently removed. The preferred positions for the proximal coil is in the renal pelvis (i.e. not in a calyx).

Table 23.3. *Maximum wire diameter for most double-pigtail stents*

Stent size (Fr)	Maximum wire diameter [inches (mm)]
3	0.018 (0.46)
4	0.025 (0.64)
5	0.038 (0.97)
6	0.038 (0.97)
7	0.045 (1.14)
8	0.045 (1.14)

When the stent fails to advance and its distal tip is not yet in the bladder, this is often due to coiling of the wire in the renal collecting system, thereby preventing further advancement. The proximal wire should be straightened by withdrawing slightly under fluoroscopic control, thus allowing the stent to be advanced.

Anatomical considerations

Tricks and tools for difficult wire or stent passage

Hydrophilic guidewires

Several manufacturers produce wires with hydrophilic coatings that, when in contact with fluid, bind to water to create a lubricious coating with greatly diminished friction. The wires are composed of an alloy core, a polyurethane jacket, and a thin hydrophilic polymer coating as the outermost layer. The tips can be straight, curved, floppy or stiff and are available in various sizes.

These wires can often be passed through stenotic segments of ureter, and even past impacted calculi. This can be accomplished under fluoroscopic guidance or ureteroscopic vision. Often, several gentle prods at the level of the obstruction are required for success. This wire is more effective when placed through an open-ended ureteral catheter. This will help straighten the distal ureter and will provide support for the wire (i.e. prevent more distal buckling). With the floppy-tipped wires, ureteral perforation is extremely unlikely. Once it is properly past the obstruction, the ureteral stent can be placed over this wire or, preferably, an open-ended ureteral catheter can be advanced over this slippery wire, and the wire can then be exchanged for a stiffer wire (Teflon coated). Stent placement can then proceed. The use of this type of guidewire constitutes the first step when faced with a difficult wire passage.

Hydrophilic stents

Two main sources of friction exist when considering stent placement: one is between the guidewire and the stent, and the other is between the stent and the ureteral wall. Both forms of friction, and particularly the latter, can be somewhat diminished by the use of a more lubricious stent (see Table 23.4). Like the hydrophilic guidewire, these stents are coated with various polymers that will bind water in their lattice.

Table 23.4. *Surface coefficient of friction for various stent materials*

High	Medium	Low
Silicone	Polyurethane C-Flex Percuflex	Hydrogel coated

These stents are manufactured by several companies, and are available in various sizes (see Table 23.4). Although they are often used for initial stent placement in the setting of ureteral strictures, these stents may not be required upon changing the stent in the future. Passive dilatation with prolonged stent placement in the face of strictures may allow for easier stent changes compared with the initial attempts.

Balloon catheters

When a tapered-tip stent will not pass over a wire because of extrinsic compression or stricture, a ureteral balloon dilator can be passed over the wire to the site of pathology and inflated to 15 to 20 atm ($\approx$1.52–1.72 MPa) according to the manufacturer's recommendations. Fluoroscopy will confirm disappearance or diminution of a 'waist'. Dilatation can be safely performed to 18 Fr (6 mm), and the balloon should remain inflated for several minutes. In the case of a long stricture, where several balloon dilatations will be necessary, it is preferable to begin with the most proximal area and work distally. After the initial use, it is easier to pull the collapsed balloon distally than to advance it proximally.

Peel-away sheaths

A 9/11 Fr peel-away catheter set (Cook Urological) or, alternatively, an 8 Fr Amplatz coaxial introducer with a 10 Fr sheath, can be placed over a guidewire and through the narrowed ureter by use of a gentle, steady rotational force. Care must be taken to ensure that the tapered introducer is leading, and that a pushing action is not applied; these errors could avulse the ureter. Once it is past the obstruction, the introducer is removed and a ureteral stent is placed through the sheath's lumen. The sheath is then removed by peeling it open and away (Fig. 23.1).

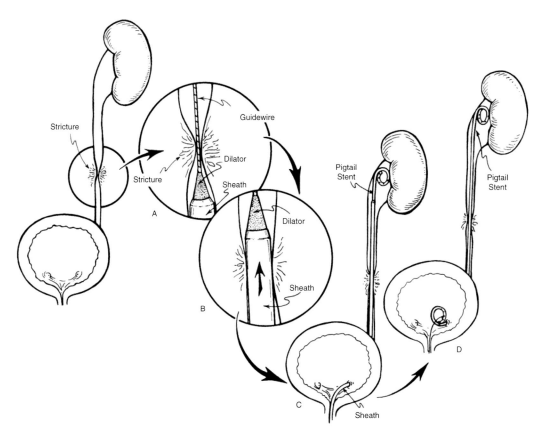

Figure 23.1. *Stenting a strictured ureter. In (A) an 8/10 or 9/11 coaxial sheath set is advanced over a guidewire to the level just distal to the mid-ureteral stricture. The set is advanced through the stricture in (B) with care to ensure that the tapered end is leading. When the proximal tip is advanced beyond (proximal to) the stricture, the inner catheter is removed, leaving the outer 10 or 11 Fr sheath (C). A double pigtail ureteral stent is placed through the lumen of the sheath and the guidewire is partially withdrawn revealing the proximal coil properly positioned in the renal pelvis (D). The outer sheath is then removed, followed by removal of the guidewire. The ureteral stent is in proper position. Note the string at the distal tip of the stent, which may serve as a safety in the event that the stent has to be further withdrawn distally.*

Use of ureteral catheters

As mentioned above, straight open-ended ureteral catheters (5 or 6 Fr) can aid in wire passage by positioning the wire just distal to the ureteral obstruction. The use of 3 Fr or 4 Fr spiral-tipped ureteral catheters (with no wire) has also been described in one paper with success in 24/30 (80%) patients with malignant strictures.[2] In addition, angiography catheters with preformed tips of various sizes can be used. The common tip configurations used include straight, curved, shepherd's tip and cobra catheters. The catheter is positioned just distal to the obstruction and, by extracorporeal catheter rotation, the internal wire can be advanced in many directions in an attempt to bypass the obstruction (see Fig. 23.2).[3]

Stone displacement

An impacted stone that can not be bypassed with a wire can sometimes be displaced proximally. This is a common adjunct to extracorporal shock-wave lithotripsy (ESWL). The technique involves placement of a 5 or 6 Fr ureteral catheter just distal to the stone and gently injecting a 1:1 mixture of lignocaine (lidocaine) jelly and contrast material[4] or saline.[5] This is monitored by fluoroscopy. The ureter proximal to the stone is often capacious (secondary to obstructive hydroureter) and the stone can be dislodged. As it is difficult to inject with force through a ureteral catheter (it will buckle), a 9/11 Fr peel-away stent set can similarly be positioned just distal to the stone, thus allowing for a larger lumen in which to inject the lubricant and dislodge the stone. A guidewire and stent can then be passed.

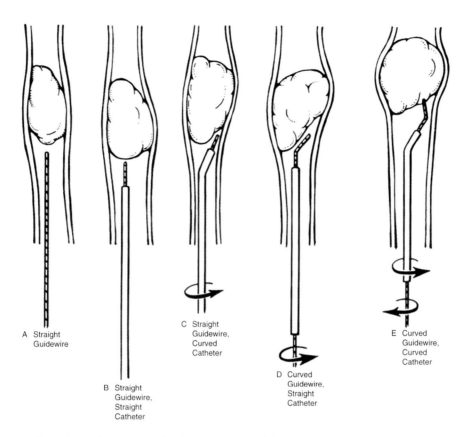

A Straight Guidewire

B Straight Guidewire, Straight Catheter

C Straight Guidewire, Curved Catheter

D Curved Guidewire, Straight Catheter

E Curved Guidewire, Curved Catheter

Figure 23.2. *Use of straight- and curved-tip wires and catheters. Rotation of the guidewire and/or catheter allows for a multitude of directional combinations in an attempt to bypass a ureteral obstruction. Performed under fluoroscopic control both wire and catheter can be rotated a full 360° extracorporeally. Several torque control devices are commercially available to aid in rotation of the guidewire.*

Single-step stent insertion

Several ureteral stents exist that can be inserted over a guidewire in one step (i.e. obviating the need to put up a guidewire alone as the first step). One such system uses a stent with a closed proximal tip (Surgitek, Racine, WI, USA). Another variation involves a mechanism to lock the wire at the proximal tip (opened tip) and the whole unit is advanced as one (Cook Urological). The wire is removed after proper position is confirmed.

Closed-tip stents cannot be changed over a guidewire and are more cumbersome when performing percutaneous surgery, as the tip has to be cut off before passing a wire down its lumen. The authors therefore favour open-ended double-pigtail stents for routine use.

Ureteroscopy

Direct visualization can often be helpful when passing a guidewire up a ureter. The ureteroscope should be well lubricated prior to its insertion. In the case of a false passage, ureteroscopic visualization can be utilized to direct the wire into the true lumen.[6] In the case of ureteral stenosis or stricture, the ureteroscopic view might delineate a pinhole opening that can be catheterized. Intravenous injection of furosemide (frusemide) or indigo carmine may aid in identifying a jet of urine. Similarly, an impacted calculus can be passed if a passage is seen; if not, directing the guidewire medial to the stone is more likely to be met with success.[7] An open-ended ureteral catheter placed at the level of obstruction will allow for better irrigation return and hence improved visualization.[7]

Definitive relief of obstruction

Before performing ureteroscopic surgery, it is recommended that a safety guidewire is placed past the obstruction. The use of a working guidewire is highly recommended to increase the margin of safety and control and to allow for easier post-procedural stent placement. If the procedure is started without such a wire and the ureter cannot subsequently be stented, stenting via a percutaneous antegrade route is then inevitable.

Unstentable strictures may be treated by endo-ureterotomy in order to open up the passage and stent the ureter. The success of this procedure is variable, averages approximately 79% and depends mostly on the length of the stricture, with strictures of less than 1 cm portending the best prognosis.[8] An incision down to periureteral fat is made by cold knife, electrocautery or laser, and is orientated in different directions depending on the level of the stricture. Strictures of the ureteropelvic junction (UPJ) and proximal ureter down to the level of the iliac vessels are incised in a posterolateral direction. Strictures at the iliac bifurcation are incised at 12 o'clock (i.e. anterior), more distal strictures are incised medially (i.e. at 9 o'clock on the left side and 3 o'clock on the right side) and UVJ strictures at 12 o'clock, or in the direction of the submucosal tunnel, thereby marsupializing the ureter into the bladder. Balloon dilatation for the treatment of ureteral strictures has a poorer success rate, ranging from 50 to 57%.[9,10]

Calculi — particularly distal stones, ESWL failures and *steinstrasse* — can similarly be treated in order to afford stenting and definitive management. A working guidewire is required at all levels, except perhaps for the impacted stone in the intramural ureter. Intracorporeal lithotriptors with different energy sources, including electrohydraulic, ultrasonic, electromechanical, laser and ballistic, have been safely used in the ureter. Impacted proximal and middle calculi can also effectively be managed by nephrostomy tube drainage followed by ESWL with X-ray localization.

Antegrade stent placement

The antegrade approach to stenting the ureter usually follows unsuccessful retrograde stenting attempts. Although, in most institutions, this task is performed by the interventional radiologist, in the authors' opinion urologists should be able to perform their own percutaneous renal access and hence should be familiar with several techniques to stent the ureter in an antegrade manner. Success with this approach is high, with Lu and colleagues[11] reporting 88% overall success in 50 consecutive patients, including 35/37 (95%) successful stent placements in the setting of malignant strictures.

The most critical step in antegrade stenting is the access site. The renal puncture should be of a posterior calyx, in either the middle or upper pole. This angle will provide easier access to the ureter and avoid undue torque on the renal parenchyma and collecting system.

Techniques similar to retrograde placement are used for antegrade stenting, including hydrophilic guidewires, angiographic catheters,[12] balloon dilatation,[13] and peel-away sheaths.[14,15] An important addition to these techniques is the transurethral retrieval of the guidewire (placed in the bladder by antegrade means) to obtain through-and-through access.[16] This is performed either by using a transurethral snare under fluoroscopic guidance, or by simultaneous cystoscopy. This technique allows for simultaneous pushing and pulling forces when introducing the stent.

Proper positioning of a ureteral stent placed in an antegrade fashion can be troublesome. Assurance of correct positioning of the proximal and distal pigtails can be accomplished by several means. A stent pusher with a metal tip (i.e. radiopaque marker) can allow for improved proximal positioning when using fluoroscopic guidance. As a precaution, a long nylon thread can be looped around the most proximal tip of the stent. If the stent is advanced too far distally, the nylon can be pulled through the flank wound, thereby properly repositioning the stent. In addition, the nephroscope can be used as an adjunct to confirm the position of the proximal stent, and to modify its position accordingly.

An alternative means to final stent placement is to pass a 9/11 Fr peel-away catheter in a retrograde manner over the through-and-through wire. The 9 Fr obturator is removed and a second wire is passed through the 11 Fr catheter in a retrograde manner. Fluoroscopy will confirm the position of this wire in the renal pelvis. The stent is then passed over this second wire in a retrograde manner, using standard techniques.

Bypassing the obstructed ureter

Lingeman and colleagues have described a combined antegrade and retrograde approach to bypass the ureteral obstruction.[17] Antegrade flexible ureteroscopy is performed to the level of obstruction; the ureter is then intentionally perforated with a guidewire at this level. A rigid ureteroscope is passed up to the distal obstruction and forceps placed through the scope intentionally perforate the ureter at this level and retrieve the anteriorly placed guidewire. Through-and-through access is thus achieved and a stent is placed. In the same report, the combined antegrade and retrograde approach is used to achieve 'cutting to the light', with an antegrade flexible ureteroscope and a retrograde ureteroresectoscope. Alignment of the two ureteroscopes is confirmed by fluoroscopy prior to the incision. After ureteral patency is achieved, a stent can be passed over a wire.

A subcutaneous urinary diversion stent (Cook Urological) is passed subcutaneously from the renal collecting system to the bladder.[18] It is available in 8.5 and 10.2 Fr sizes with lengths of 60–70 cm. It can be changed through a 2 cm skin incision and represents another minimally invasive means of bypassing the obstructed ureter that is useful in patients for whom reconstructive surgery is not indicated. Its use is described in Chapter 62 of this volume.

The ureterovesical junction (UVJ)

Difficulties encountered at the level of the ureteral orifice usually are caused by an iatrogenic false passage (from a prior ureteroscopy), by a ureteral stone or a by a stenotic orifice. The use of a small ureteroscope (miniscope) can identify the true ureteral lumen (i.e. normal mucosa) in most cases of a false passage. It should be kept in mind that ureteral perforations of this nature are most often located posteriorly. In the case of a calculus, an obstructing UVJ stone can be bypassed with a hydrophilic guidewire after adequate balloon dilatation. Alternatively, a ureteral catheter over a guidewire can sometimes be manipulated to dislodge an impacted stone more proximally and permit wire passage.

Situations involving narrow or stenotic ureteral orifices can be managed by balloon dilatation, by graduated rigid or semi-rigid dilators, or by increasing the pressure of irrigation flow though a ureteroscope. This last objective can be accomplished by raising the height of the irrigant, by having a ureteroscope with a dedicated channel for irrigation, or by exerting high positive pressure, either manually (e.g. with a Pathfinder™: Microvasive, Natick, MA, USA), or machine driven (e.g. Ureteromat™: Storz, Charlton, MA, USA). Alternatively, a movable core guidewire may be used: first, the most distal stenosis is punctured

with the rigid tip; then the inner core can be withdrawn to allow the floppy tip to lead the wire up to the renal pelvis.[19]

Occasionally, a ureteral meatotomy (12 o'clock) with a cold knife, electrocautery or laser, is required to negotiate this most distal area. Success is uniformly satisfactory with all methods.[20–22] Transurethral resection or incision of the ureteral orifice can also be accomplished by electrocautery with an Orandi knife onto a ureteral occlusion balloon tip placed at the UVJ from an antegrade approach.[8] In addition, resection of the orifice can be performed with a standard resectoscope onto a ureteral catheter placed at the UVJ from an antegrade approach. The resectoscope loop should always be cutting directly onto the catheter and not straying. The proper position can be confirmed by direct vision, by 'feel' at the tip of the loop and by fluoroscopy. A metal wire should not be used in place of an insulating substance as it may conduct to other areas of the ureter in contact with the wire, resulting in thermal injury.

Transcatheter electrocautery of a rigid guidewire placed at the UVJ by an antegrade access has also been shown to negotiate the stenotic ureteral orifice.[23] This technique involves applying electrocautery cutting current to a guidewire insulated by a 7 Fr ureteral catheter while applying moderate forward pressure on the wire. Using another technique, Mygind and colleagues[24] have reported the creation of an internal ureter-to-bladder fistula for an obstructing lesion in the intramural ureter, by an antegrade transureteral bladder puncture that was then stented. This was accomplished using a puncture needle-catheter assembly, originally designed for puncturing the atrial septum in transvenous trans-septal left heart catheterization. The inner cannula is pushed in an anterior direction into the bladder wall and its final position is confirmed by instillation of contrast material via the needle into the bladder, with fluoroscopic confirmation. After a wire has been threaded through the assembly into the bladder, the assembly is removed and a stent is placed.

The iliac bifurcation

The posterior impression on the ureter by the bifurcating common iliac artery can at times cause an apparent obstruction of the ureteral passage. Care must be taken not to cause intussusception of the ureter at this level. If a hydrophilic wire is unsuccessful in negotiating this angle, a movable core guidewire or Benson guidewire may be used. A ureteral catheter placed over a wire may allow for easier passage and, occasionally, a curved-tip angiography catheter orientated anteriorly will enable negotiation of the angle. If this is unsuccessful, rigid ureteroscopy (with inversion of the scope) or use of an actively deflecting flexible ureteroscope may be helpful. Of note is that the angulation at this level is accentuated in those with more developed psoas muscles (males, in general). A greater degree of torque is also maintained in the more proximal ureter in these patients.

Proximal and middle ureter

The mid-ureter can be the site of a wide variety of pathological conditions, including stricture, extrinsic tumour or nodal tissue compressing the ureter, and calculi. This section of the ureter can be highly mobile and is associated with the highest complication rate for ureteroscopic manipulation. A flexible, actively deflecting, small-calibre ureteroscope is usually recommended for use at this level. Hydrophilic wire placement under fluoroscopic or ureteroscopic guidance should be attempted. Often, an antegrade approach is mandated for easier wire passage, as it is easier to pass a wire from the larger-calibre to the smaller-calibre ureter. Once a dense stricture has been bypassed with a soft wire, the wire can be exchanged for a stiffer guidewire (e.g. Amplatz superstiff) or it can be managed by a 'cut to the light' technique with combined antegrade and retrograde approaches. Stiff wires should not be burrowed blindly past strictured areas, as ureteral perforation is highly likely.

The ureteropelvic junction (UPJ)

The UPJ is more easily passed by a retrograde approach. Lubricious or stiff guidewires are sometimes necessary. When a tortuous area (or kink) exists just distal to the UPJ, it can be straightened with a wire to allow for easier stent passage or ureteroscopic visualization.

Special considerations

Tortuous ureter

The ureter may be tortuous as a variation of normal (e.g. in pregnancy) or secondary to obstruction and hydro-ureter. Several techniques are useful to help 'straighten' the ureter and thus allow easier instrumentation. One manoeuvre is to place the patient in the Trendelenberg position. Also described is the use of a 7 Fr occlusion balloon-tip catheter distal to the tortuosity, which can be gently pulled distally once inflated.[25,26] If these techniques are unsuccessful, a fixed-tip angiography catheter (e.g. Cobra catheter) or a J-tipped guidewire can help to negotiate the ureteral curves under fluoroscopic guidance. These materials can be rotated extracorporeally in order to attempt advancement in a myriad of pathways, thereby bypassing each curve. Similarly, a Bentson wire can be passed through a straight ureteral catheter for each curve sequentially, thereby straightening the ureter in a stepwise manner.[27] Once a wire has been placed successfully, straightening often occurs. This should allow for successful ureteroscopy or stent placement.

Malignant strictures

Malignant strictures represent one of the most challenging types of obstruction for retrograde passage. If the stricture can be traversed with a hydrophilic guidewire, balloon dilatation can be carried out to 8–10 Fr. If the ureteral catheter (or balloon catheter or stent) binds, the authors attempt to pass a 9/11 Fr peel-away catheter through the stricture. This tapered, stiff catheter can often be twisted (not pushed) past the stricture. A double-pigtail stent can then be placed through the 11 Fr sheath. If this is unsuccessful, obtaining through-and-through access (i.e. retrieving the proximal wire by a percutaneous nephrostomy tract with stabilization of both ends) can provide the leverage required for successful stent passage.

Other techniques can be used for these strictures. A coaxial cancer dilator (Cook Urological) may be used as a single-step dilation technique.[28] This semi-rigid 6–12 French coaxial system is placed over a wire and left traversing the stricture for 30–60 minutes. Van Andel catheters have also been used with success,[29] as have flexible fascial dilators and straight ureteral catheters of gradually increasing sizes.[30]

In their study looking at stent failure rates, Docimo and Dewolf[31] noted a 49% incidence of clinical occlusion in the 41 stented patients with a diagnosis of extrinsic obstruction versus a 0% failure in the 43 patients stented for intrinsic obstruction. Of the parameters analysed, the only reliable predictor of stent failure in the extrinsic obstruction group was stent size: 6 Fr stents were most common in the group that failed, whereas every stent in the successfully stented group was 7 Fr.

An ideal stent for this situation would be sufficiently stiff to prevent intraluminal compression from the extrinsic pressure, and long lasting in order to prolong the interval between stent changes. To take advantage of the extraluminal drainage, and with the intention of preventing stent engulfment by the extrinsic process, the authors often place two double-pigtail stents (e.g. 5 Fr) next to each other.[32]

Changing the obstructed stent

Stented patients with a new diagnosis of hydronephrosis or flank pain are assumed to have an obstructed stent (i.e. secondary to encrustation, biofilm) that necessitates stent replacement. The authors' first approach is to pass a wire next to the existing obstructed stent. An open-ended ureteral catheter placed over the wire often helps to guide the wire. If this proves to be impossible, the distal tip of the stent is pulled out of the urethra and an attempt is made to thread a Teflon-coated wire through its lumen. If this does not work, the tip of the stent can be sutured to the tip of the introducer (9 Fr component) of a 9/11 Fr peel-away catheter. The 11 Fr outer sheath is then advanced up the ureter, over both the 9 Fr introducer and the stent. The introducer and stent are then withdrawn completely through the 11 Fr sheath and a new double-pigtail stent is placed through the sheath under fluoroscopic control; the sheath is then removed. Alternatively, the stent can be pulled out completely and a new wire inserted, followed by the new stent. This may, however, cause loss of retrograde access if the wire cannot then be passed up the ureter.

Conclusions

The urologist should have an understanding of the options available for negotiating the obstructed ureter, as for other therapeutic dilemmas often encountered. More minor, less-invasive techniques should precede more advanced and involved manoeuvres in order to achieve the desired results with maximal efficiency (see Table 23.5).

The new lubricious guidewires and stents have been a tremendous advance in this area and the majority of difficult obstructions can now be bypassed with their use. Similarly, balloon dilatation can be safely applied throughout the course of the ureter, thereby affording a more capacious ureteral lumen for both stent placement and endoscopy. Also, as urologists become trained in achieving percutaneous renal access and familiar with the techniques and materials used by the interventional radiologist, a whole new realm of treatment options becomes available (e.g. antegrade stenting). The urinary system thus becomes fully accessible and the ability of the treating physician to utilize a full management plan becomes complete.

Table 23.5. *Tools used to accomplish difficult wire passage**

Advance guidewire through ureteral catheter
Hydrophilic guidewire
Hydrophilic stent
Fixed-tip angiography catheter
Balloon dilator catheter
Ureteroscopy
Inject furosemide (frusemide), indigo carmine
Treat underlying pathology
Calculus
• fragment if distal
• push up if proximal
• ESWL
Stricture
• balloon dilatation
• peel-away sheath
• endoureterotomy (e.g. Acucise™ catheter)[†]
Antegrade stenting
Nephrostomy drainage

*Sequence of steps will depend on aetiology and location of obstruction.
[†]Applied Medical Technology (Laguna Hills, CA, USA).

References

1. Mardis H, Kroeger M, Morton J, Donovan J. Comparative evaluation of materials used for internal ureteral stents. J Endourol 1993; 7(2): 105–115

2. Matu J, Cullin J, Venable D. Techniques for bypassing and stenting ureteral obstructions. J Urol 1994; 152: 917–919

3. Patterson D. Access to the difficult ureter. In: Smith A, Badlani G et al. (eds) In: Smith's Textbook of Endourology. St. Louis: Quality Medical Publishing, 1996: 420–434

4. Steinbock G, Bezirdjian L. Technique for retrogade ureteral stone displacement. Urology 1988; 31(2): 160–161

5. Danuser H, Achermann D, Marth D et al. Extracorporeal shock wave lithotripsy in situ or after push-up for upper ureteral calculi: a prospective randomized trial. J Urol 1993; 150(3): 824–826

6. Kraebber D, Torres S. Use of ureteroscope to avoid distal ureteral false passages. Urology 1988; 31(1): 80

7. Huffman J. Ureteroscopic surgery. Course, AUA annual meeting. AUA Office of Education, Orlando, Florida, May, 1996.

8. Clayman R, Kavoussi L. Endosurgical techniques for noncalculous disease. In: Walsh P, Retik A, Stamey T, Vaugn E Jr (eds) Campbell's Urology, 6th ed. Philadelphia: Saunders, 1992: 2281–2282.

9. Netto N R, Ferreira U, Lemos G. Endourological management of ureteral strictures. J Urol 1990; 144: 631

10. O'Brien W, Maxted W, Pahira J. Ureteral stricture: experience with 31 cases. J Urol 1988; 140: 737

11. Lu D, Papanicolaou N, Girard N et al. Percutaneous internal ureteral stent placement: review of technical issues and solutions in 50 consecutive cases. Clin Radiol 1994; 49: 256–261.

12. Gray R, Rooney M, Grosman H. Indwelling angiographic catheters to facilitate placement of ureteric stents. Can Assoc Radiol J 1991; 42(2): 127–129

13. Asch M, Jaffer N. Antegrade placement of a ureteric stent by a pull-through technique. Can Assoc Radiol J 1995; 46(6): 465–467

14. Mercado S, Hawkins J, Herrera M et al. Simplified method of introducing Double J stent catheters using a coaxial sheath system. American Journal of Roentgenology 1985; 145: 1271–1273

15. Gray R, St Louis E, Grosman G. Use of Amplatz introducer sheath to facilitate ureteral stent placement. Journal of Canadian Association of Radiologists 1987; 38: 120-121

16. Mitty H A. Ureteral stenting facilitated by antegrade transurethral passage of guidewire. AJR 1984; 142: 831–832

17. Lingeman J, Wong M, Newmark J. Endoscopic management of total ureteral occlusion and ureterovaginal fistula. J Endourol 1995; 9(5): 391–396

18. Paterson P, Lingam V, Forrester A. Extra anatomical diversion as an alternative to nephrostomy. First International Symposium on Urological Stents, Jerusalem, Israel, 27–31 October 1996. Abstract 010.5

19. Schmeller N, Overbeck H. Steerable guidewire for insertion of ureteric stent into tortuous ureter. Br J Urol 1985; 57(5): 595

20. Strup S, Bagley D. Endoscopic ureteroneocystostomy for complete obstruction at the ureterovesical junction. J Urol 1996; 156: 360

21. Lusaya D, David F, Parreno F. Ureteral meatotomy with local-prototype urethrotome in the management of lower ureteral stones. J Endourol 1994; 8(3): 207–211

22. Vijayan P. Optical urethrotome for ureteric meatotomy. Br J Urol 1987; 59(6): 597

23. Horowitz M, Feigenbaum L. Transcatheter electrocautery as an aid in the percutaneous insertion of a ureteral stent. J Urol 1984; 132: 111–112

24. Mygind T, Dorph S, Nielson H et al. New techniques for stenting severely strictured or occluded ureters. Eur J Radiol 1985; 5(4): 321–324

25. Fraser K. A technique for stenting tortuous ureters. J Urol 1987; 138: 831

26. Clayman R. Editorial comment. In: Fraser K (ed) A technique for stenting tortuous ureters. J Urol 1987; 138: 831

27. Thomas R. Catheterizing a tortuous ureter. J Urol 1988; 140: 778–779

28. Cardella J, Castaneda-Zuniga W et al. Coaxial cancer dilator. Radiology 1985; 157(3): 820

29. Alexander R, Thompson N, Pockaf B, Chang R. Dilation of lower ureteral strictures with Van Andel catheters. J Urol 1994; 152: 68–69

30. Segura J. Editorial comment. In: Alexander R, Thompson N, Pockaf B, Chang R Dilation of lower ureteral strictures with Van Andel catheters. J Urol 1994; 152: 69

31. Docimo S, Dewolf W. High failure rate of indwelling ureteral stents in patients with extrinsic obstruction: experience at 2 institutions. J Urol 1989; 142: 277–279

32. Gupta M, Tuncay O, Smith AD. Video: Tips and tricks of placing guidewires and stents. New York: Long Island Jewish Medical Center, 1996

Non-refluxing ureteral stents
M. Ahmadzadeh

24

Brief history of stent development

Internal and external ureteral catheters have, for many years, been used to establish urinary drainage, mainly to bypass ureteral obstruction in chronic urinary diseases. The initial concern with such ureteral stents was how to prevent their migration; even when the catheter was placed endoscopically and fixed outside the body, it could migrate into the bladder.[1] However, in recent years, investigations of the pathophysiology of the upper urinary tract have furnished valuable information with regard to the phenomenon of stent migration. It has been shown that stent migration is not a simple event caused by gravity but occurs as the result of multifactorial changes that determine the actual position of the stent in the upper urinary tract. Historically, in 1961 Brown and Harrison[2] reported the efficacy of plastic ureteral catheters for constant drainage and in 1967 Zimskind et al.[3] described the use of indwelling silicone rubber stents for long-term drainage.[3] Gibbons et al.,[7] in 1976, introduced a stent with side-wings and a proximal flange to prevent upward migration and downward expulsion, but technically the insertion and removal of this stent was very difficult.[4] Mardis et al.[5] subsequently described a technique using a single-pigtail angiographic catheter as a ureteral stent. He reported that the upper end of the pigtail stent acts as an anchoring device in the renal pelvis, preventing its downward migration.[5] A better stent was not produced until 1978, when Finney[6] presented the first double-pigtail stent. In his report he defined an ideal stent as follows: it should be made of silicone elastomer; it should be radiopaque; it should be of uniform diameter; it should not migrate in either direction. In his initial study he used such a stent in 51 patients with excellent results. Control cystograms 3 weeks after insertion revealed a vesicorenal reflux, which could detect not only the eventual (possibly) persisting extravasation but also the vesicostent reflux could be useful to control the localization of the stent.[6]

Modern stent materials and design have improved the safety and tolerance of these stents. Internal urinary drainage using an indwelling double-pigtail stent is now routine in urological practice; this allows patients greater mobility and social acceptance. Although the double-pigtail stent is widely used to relieve ureteral obstruction secondary to benign and malignant diseases, it is also very useful in the treatment of ureteral fistulas, and as an adjunct to extracorporeal shock-wave lithotripsy and ureterorenoscopic procedures.[7] Complications associated with chronic indwelling ureteral catheters have been well described.[8–10] Serious complications due to ureteral stenting are very rare. One of the major problems in stented patients is flank pain and discomfort during voiding;[11–13] this is the result of sudden vesicorenal reflux. Normally, the vesico-ureteral junction in the non-stented ureter prevents such reflux. The intramural segment of ureter passes in an oblique direction through the bladder wall. Lengthening and compression of the distal ureter during the filling phase and during detrusor contraction play a major role in reflux prevention. In an attempt to minimize episodes of flank pain during micturition, which are related to transluminal vesicorenal reflux and, more importantly, to the development of reflux nephropathy, in 1988 new types of ureteral stents with an antireflux mechanism were designed and, subsequently, the new Mono-J stent with a reflux-prevention system was introduced for clinical use.[14] This chapter describes functional and technical aspects of reflux-preventing stents.

Basic clinical investigation

The value of stents for internal drainage is generally accepted. In order to have a better understanding of the function of an internal ureteral stent and of reflux-preventing stents, it is useful to be familiar with ureteral physiology and the rules that can affect prevention of vesicorenal reflux. The electrical activity of the urinary tract is located at the pacemaker site, which is in the proximal portion of the collecting system. There are also other areas in the ureter that possesses latent pacemaker properties. The ureteral peristaltic contraction waves transport the bolus of urine from the kidney to the bladder, at a rate of 2–6 times per minute. The peristaltic contraction pressure is 20–60 cmH$_2$O and baseline pressure in the ureter is 0–5 cmH$_2$O. In contrast to multi-unit smooth muscles, in which each smooth muscle fibre is innervated separately, the smooth muscle fibres in the ureter do not have such a system; this suggests that the ureter can function without innervation.

The role of the autonomic nervous system in the control of ureteral peristalsis is under investigation. The ureter contains both alpha- and beta-adrenergic receptors. Clinical data also suggest that the parasympathetic nervous system minimally affects the ureter. The peristaltic wave can be initiated not only by internal electrical activity but also as the result of intrinsic or extrinsic mechanical stretching,[15] by such agents as a urine bolus, stones, or foreign bodies. Stenting changes the ureter to an open tube. In such circumstances vesicorenal reflux may occur not only because of higher bladder pressure, which pumps urine through the stent, but also because the stent causes mechanical stretching, resulting in retrograde peristalsis and urine reflux. Under normal conditions, and at the usual physiological flow rates, the antegrade ureteral peristaltic pressure is higher than the intravesical pressure, forcing urine to enter the bladder.

In a ureter obstructed owing to extra- or intra-ureteral factors, or following elevation of intravesical pressures, an initial increase in ureteral peristaltic frequency may be noted.[16] After stenting, the ureter becomes an open tube and the bladder affects the transport of urine through the ureteral stent, by active and passive changes of detrusor pressure or by changes in bladder wall tension which result in vesicorenal reflux.[17] The flow rate of urine through the stent is dependent on the following hydrostatic forces: intrarenal pressure; internal diameter of the stent; stent length; intravesical pressure; and urine density.

Finney,[6] and Ramsay et al.[7] have shown that urine flow is not only through but also around the stent.[6,7] In cases of intrinsic ureteral obstruction (ureteral stenosis and congenital and acquired ureteral obstruction) or extrinsic ureteral compression (retroperitoneal tumours, endometriosis, retroperitoneal fibrosis), the urine flows mandatorily through the stent rather than around the stent. In some reported series vesicorenal reflux may be seen in up to 90% of stented patients.[8,11,13] Despite a normal voiding cystogram, it is possible to detect vesicorenal reflux. This may result from higher pressures in the pyelo-ureteral system. In a higher percentage of patients, vesicorenal reflux can be expected if the intrarenal pressure declines or the internal lumen of the stent suffices for the flow of urine. Generally, after acute obstruction and stenting, an increase in intrarenal pressure is noted. The extent of this increase has been well documented;[16] however, the pressure gradually reverts to the baseline level after 3 weeks because of the hydrostatic changes that take place after stent insertion. The ureteral dilatation seen after stenting is of unknown origin. Drake et al.[18] hypothesized that this phenomenon may be related to the cytotoxic effect of foreign bodies on the ureter;[18] but infection or urodynamic interaction also may play a role. In 1988 the present author started to experiment with different types of stents that could prevent vesicorenal reflux.

Materials and methods

It has long been recognized that stenting of the ureter is associated with vesico-ureteral or vesicorenal reflux,[6,11,19] but it is not known how far this vesicorenal reflux, which increases intrarenal pressure during voiding, affects the upper urinary system, and what is its clinical impact on patients' well-being. Clinical data over the last three decades have demonstrated that vesicorenal reflux is associated with urinary tract infection, and can cause pyelonephritis and renal scarring;[20] however, vesicorenal reflux in stented patients has not been well studied. Presumably it produces minor renal damage in those patients in whom the stent is kept in place for short periods (stenting for 7–10 days is most usual after ureterorenoscopy to prevent obstruction secondary to early post-procedural oedema). In patients in whom a chronic ureteral stent is needed, there is already some degree of renal damage caused by the chronic obstruction. Therefore, there are no data regarding the grade of pathological changes that are merely related to the reflux caused by stenting, which leads to false interpretation of the harmful effects of chronic ureteral stenting on the urinary system. Another type of morbidity after stenting is the flank discomfort felt by the patient during voiding, which is attributed to reflux of urine into the renal collecting system during an increase in intravesical pressure. Bregg and associates[12] have reported that 20% of stented patients who underwent extracorporeal shock-wave lithotripsy therapy developed chills and fever, possibly because of vesicostent reflux. Thus, a stent with an antireflux system not only may prevent flank pain but also, in cases of bacterial cystitis, may minimize the transmission of infected urine from the bladder to the renal collecting system. Another criterion in the construction of an antireflux stent was the prevention of the reflux of urine, which contains the end products of cytotoxic agents during systemic or intravesical chemotherapy. Such a stent may also be useful in patients with ureteral or calyceal leakage; in such cases, reflux prolongs the healing process. Ramsay et al.[7] have emphasized the importance of the reduction of hydrostatic pressure at both ends of the stent by placement of an ipsilateral nephrostomy tube and a transurethral catheter. A reflux-preventing stent can improve healing by minimizing urine extravasation in the damaged section.

A reflux-preventing stent can be constructed at the three levels of the upper urinary system:

1. Above the ureterovesical junction;
2. Within the ureterovesical junction;
3. Below the ureterovesical junction (intravesical).

We have designed, for each level, one stent that prevents vesicorenal reflux, as described below.

Stent type 1

In 1979, some authors reported that upper migration of a stent is not very harmful and can even prevent vesicostent reflux.[21] To investigate this, a short mono-J polyurethane stent (Angiomed, Karlsruhe, Germany) was designed. To prevent stent migration into the collecting system and also to allow its removal, a nylon pull thread was attached to the lower end of the stent. The stent was inserted cystoscopically; fluoroscopy was required for safe insertion. The stent was tested in four patients; the stent length being approximately half the length of the ureter, as estimated radiographically. The stents were inserted endoscopically after open ureteral surgery in three patients, and in one patient because of ureteral stricture following surgery for retroperitoneal fibrosis.

Stent type 2

This stent was designed for prevention of reflux at the level of the ureterovesical junction. It was constructed from a double-pigtail stent with a transparent thin-walled segment also of polyurethane (polyetherurethane) (Fig. 24.1). The valve segment had the same diameter as the other parts of the stent. The aim was to locate this portion in the ureterovesical junction, with the hope that this part would remain at this level and that its walls could be compressed together and thus prevent reflux during voiding. The length of this portion was about 2 cm, and the double-pigtail stent and valve segment were both 7 Fr in diameter. Insertion was carried out cystoscopically.[22]

Stent type 3

This stent was constructed of polyurethane and possessed a double pigtail at both ends (Willy Rüsch AG, Kernen, Germany). A valve system made of two thin transparent Wiruthane membranes was attached at its bladder end (Fig. 24.2). The two layers of the valve simply coapted to a closed position when the external pressure in the bladder rose during voiding. Since the valve was designed to be wider (15 mm) than the ureteral orifice, it also served as an additional mechanism against upward migration. The selected stents were 26–28 cm (7 Fr) in diameter. Initially, these stents were used in 10 patients[22] and then in all patients.[23] Up to February 1996, over 200 patients underwent insertion of a reflux-preventing type 3 stent cystoscopically (Fig. 24.3).

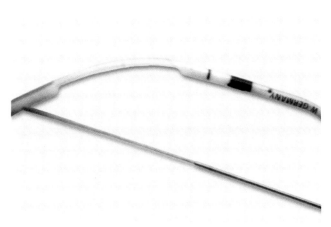

Figure 24.1. *Lower part of a double-pigtail type 2 stent with a valve system.*

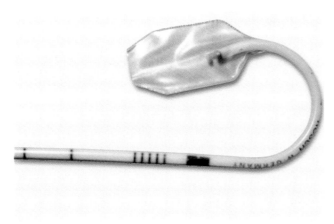

Figure 24.2. *Valve system at the lower part of a type 3 stent. The flap valve is 25 mm long and 15 mm wide. It is constructed from two thin Wiruthan membranes and is able to prevent reflux during increased intravesical pressure.*

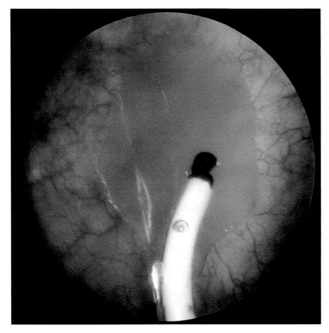

Figure 24.3. *Appearance of the valve in the bladder after insertion of a type 3 stent.*

Results with experimental stents

Stents, types 2 and 3, were investigated in vitro simulating the intravesical pressure transmitted through the stent to the renal pelvis. Experimentally, the distal part of the type 2 stent was tightly fitted to the chamber of a 50 ml syringe filled with water. To this system was connected the pressure transducer of a cystomanometer. On manually increasing the pressure by pushing the piston, it was observed that the valve of the type 2 stent could prevent reflux up to pressures of 150 cmH$_2$O. The

flow of water through the upper part of the stent demonstrated the loss of capability of its valve system at higher pressures.

The ability of the intravesical (type 3) valve to prevent reflux was examined in the same way and was found to be more effective. The valve system failed to prevent reflux when the pressure exceeded 250 cmH$_2$O (Fig. 24.4). The difference between these two stents in preventing reflux was attributable to the difference in the valve design concept. The valve system in the type 2 stent could not close tightly because both ends of the valve were attached to the rigid parts of the stent, whereas in the type 3 stent the valve was attached only at one end to the stent and its other end could move freely. To evaluate the flow rate through the stent, a 7 Fr common pigtail stent, a type 2 stent and a type 3 stent all 7 Fr in calibre, were used. A 10 cm length of the lower part of the stents was cut and connected through a three-way stopcock adapter to a transducer and infusion pump (Fig. 24.5). The perfusion rate varied between 1 and 6 ml/min. The relationships between flow rate and pressure that were produced in the lower part of the stents (type 2, type 3, and common stent) showed that the type 3 valve increases flow resistance (R) to a lower degree at a flow rate of 1 ml/min (flow resistance = pressure in stent in cmH$_2$O / flow rate in ml/min = 0.16/1 = 0.16) and to a higher degree at a flow rate of 6 ml/min, when the pressure increases up to 1.09 cmH$_2$O (R = 0.18). For the common stent the pressure was 0.1 cmH$_2$O at a flow rate of 1 ml/min. (R = 0.1) and at a flow rate of 6 ml/min the pressure was 0.62 cmH$_2$O (R = 0.10). The same flow resistance was measured in the type 2 stent, but this resistance was lower than that with the type 3 stent. This indicates that the elevation of flow resistance in the type 3 stent is negligible compared with that in the common and type 2 stent (Fig. 24.6).

The valve was not found to interfere significantly with urine transport but was capable of preventing reflux.

Clinically, after type 1 stent insertion, patients reported moderate to severe dysuria. These discomforts can be explained by the division of the ureter into two parts — the non-stented lower half, with normal urodynamic activity, and the upper half, where the hydrostatic balance is disrupted by ureteral intubation. Despite the nylon pull thread at the lower end of the

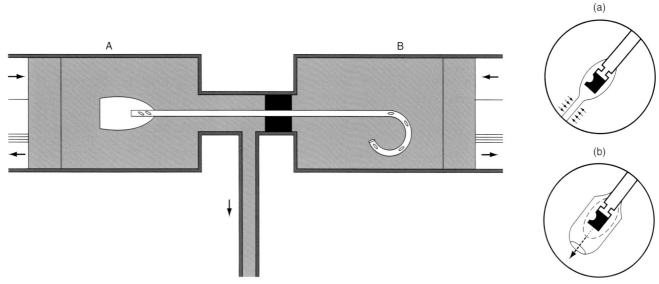

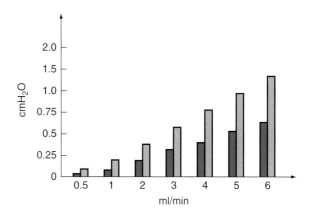

Figure 24.4. *The reflux-preventing stent is located in the chamber of two syringes. The chambers are filled with water and the pressure in chamber A can be transmitted additionally to a transducer. By increasing the pressure in chamber A, the valve is capable of preventing reflux up to 250 cmH$_2$O: (a) during increasing the pressure in chamber A, the membranes of the flap valve coapt and prevent reflux; (b) in the decompression phase the valve allows fluid transmission from chamber B to chamber A.*

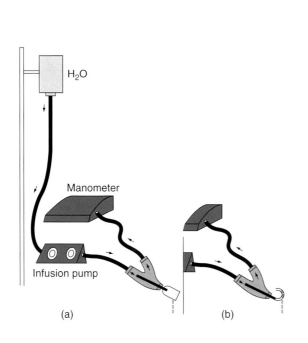

Figure 24.5. *An appropriate system for flow study in two different stents:*
(a) the valve affects the flow rate through the stent by increasing the flow resistance;
(b) the flow rate through a common stent is minimally higher than that in a reflux-preventing stent.

Figure 24.6. *Pressure–flow study in common (■) and reflux-preventing (■) stents (26 cm, 7 Fr), demonstrating that the valve at the lower portion of stent increases flow resistance, but that such increases at low flow rates (up to 6 ml/min) are negligible.*

stent, upward migration was observed in one case; this is the result of antiperistaltic waves originating from the lower ureter pushing the stent into the collecting system.

In vivo, the type 2 stent could drain urine but was incapable of preventing reflux. The thin transparent segment, which should stay in the intramural part of the ureter, retracted backwards during micturition and returned to its intramural position after bladder emptying, remaining in place during the filling phase of the bladder.

The type 3 stent drained the urine effectively and also could prevent vesicorenal reflux. Vesicorenal reflux was evaluated by filling of bladder with 200–500 ml diluted (30%) contrast medium through a Foley catheter or cystoscope. With active increase of the detrusor pressure or manual compression of the bladder, intravesical pressures could be increased up to 100 cmH_2O (Fig. 24.7). It was observed that, in vivo, type 1 and type 3 stents could effectively prevent reflux.

As previously mentioned prevention of reflux through the stent is important in ureteral healing, especially when a ureteral fistula is present. A high-pressure reflux interferes with the healing process. It is important to know that reflux alongside the stent in cases of ureteral obstruction (extrinsic and intrinsic aetiologies) does not follow the hydrostatic changes that take place in an unobstructed ureter. In obstructed cases the urine can pass only through the stent at the site of obstruction (Fig. 24.8); therefore, a reflux-preventing stent can prevent transmission of the intravesical pressures to the kidney and the ureter.

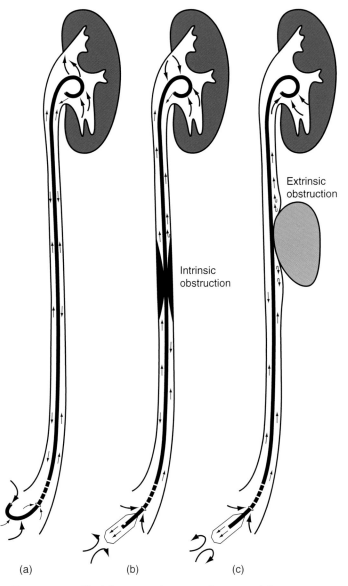

Figure 24.8. *Fluid dynamics after ureteral stenting: (a) a common double-pigtail stent in an unobstructed ureter; (b) reflux-preventing stent in an intrinsically obstructed ureter; (c) reflux-preventing stent in a ureter with extrinsic compression.*

Complications

Encrustation

After clinical testing, the reflux-preventing stents were removed endoscopically. The stents were cut in half longitudinally to examine both the outer and the inner surfaces. All parts were examined for encrustation, and were then cut into small pieces for bacteriological culture. Encrustation was very minor; only in two cases was encrustation moderate, and in one case, where the stent remained in the ureter for over a year encrustation

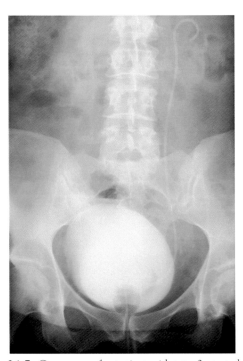

Figure 24.7. *Cystogram of a patient with type 3 stent shows the absence of vesicorenal reflux.*

was severe. Encrustation on stents is a complex phenomenon, since it depends on the stent material and on changes in urine composition. The presence or absence of urinary infection probably plays a significant role in this matter. Studies have shown that the harder the stent, the more likely it is to induce reactive changes such as mucous metaplasia and crystallization of urine on the surface of the stent.[24] Patients receiving cancer chemotherapy also tend to develop mucous dysplasia, which accelerates crystalloid deposition on the stent. The author's clinical observations have shown that encrustation on the valve system of a reflux-preventing stent is minimal; this may be because of a greater degree of mucous metaplasia in a narrow interior passage of the stent, and not in the valve which is 15 times wider than the internal lumen of a 7 Fr stent.

Infection

The first and second series of patients in this study had urine culture tests before and after stent insertion. No patient was treated for asymptomatic urinary tract infection during the period of study. Some authors have recommended administration of low doses of antimicrobial agents:[25] Mosli and associates[11] recommend the use of antimicrobial agents in children until the stent is removed. Only in 11% of patients (25 male and 21 female, ages ranging from 28 to 79 years, median age 55) has urine culture before stent insertion been positive (more than 100,000 bacteria/ml); urine culture after stent removal has been positive in 21% of patients. The author's data have shown that the indwelling period does not increase bacterial colonization and encrustation per se, but that this may play a role in biofilm formation over the surface of the stent.

The following microorganisms were isolated from stents: *Escherichia coli.*, *E. faecalis*, cocci, *Streptococcus* spp., *Staphylococcus* spp., *Streptococcus epidermis*, *Proteus mirabilis* and *Staphylococcus haemolyticus*. *P. mirabilis* was the most adherent microorganism found in biofilm formation.

How important is bacterial colonization on the stent surface in an asymptomatic patient? The study in vitro has shown that *P. mirabilis* and some other bacterial species tend to colonize and adhere to the surface of the stent and this may lead to biofilm formation, resulting in encrustation and obliteration of the lumen.[8,26]

Dilute, acidified urine may reduce the rate of encrustation on the stent; however, this remains a problem with some patients. Bacterial colonization on the surface of the stent was also examined in four patients who underwent radical prostatectomy. In these patients a reflux-preventing stent was inserted in one ureter and a common double-pigtail stent was inserted in the other, before the operation. After 3 weeks the stents were removed and both stent pieces were cultured. The bacteriological studies demonstrated no significant differences on the surface of the stents.

Migration

Since the lower part of the stent is supplied with valves that cannot pass easily through the ureteral orifice, upward stent migration was not observed in these patients.

After the three different types of reflux-prevention stents had been tested clinically, the distal valve stent (type 3) was found to be the nearest to the ideal ureteral stent.

New type of reflux-preventing (valve) stent

The distal portions of all stents protrude into the bladder and irritate the bladder mucosa. Cystoscopically, it was observed that the length of the section protruding into the bladder varies during inspiration and expiration and advancing ureteral peristalsis. To reduce bladder irritation caused by the double-J valve stent, a new mono-pigtail reflux-preventing ureteral stent was designed (Fig. 24.9). The primary consideration was how the length of the lower stent portion could be shortened; during increased intravesical pressures, such as in voiding, the stents tend to retract into the ureteral orifice. The incidence of upward migration of a simple mono-J stent is presumably much higher than that with the double-pigtail stent because the straight lower part lacks resistance against retraction into the ureter, compared with curved lower parts. This reflux-preventing stent is a Mono-J stent but possesses a Malecot-like flanged segment (in the valve mechanism) that also prevents upward migration of the stent.

Another aim of this new stent was to reduce bladder irritation by producing a stent with a more elastic segment at the lower end. Functionally, this stent is comparable with other stents; because of its design, it reduces flank discomfort during micturition, and bladder

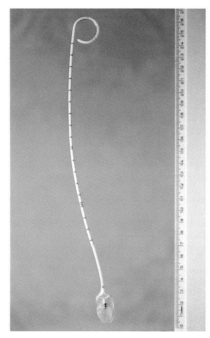

Figure 24.9. *Mono-J reflux-preventing stent.*

part is approximately 3.5 cm and this is retained in the bladder. The interior lumen of this part of the stent is smooth, so the risk of encrustation is not higher in this segment than in any other part. The valve at the lower end of the stent and the Malecot segment in it provide

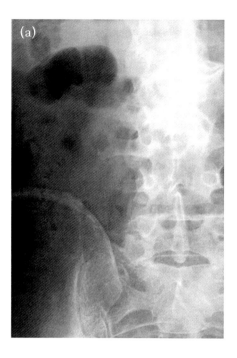

irritation and erosive trigonitis. The stent is constructed in three parts: its upper part is a single J with side-holes and the length of its middle part is selected to fit the approximate length of the ureter; the lower part of the stent is composed of two sections — the spiral and valve parts (Fig. 24.10). The spiral section is designed to bend into the bladder without disturbing urine flow through the stent. It has semiflexible and highly flexible parts, both of which have a spiral contour with different gradients on the axial length. The length of the flexible

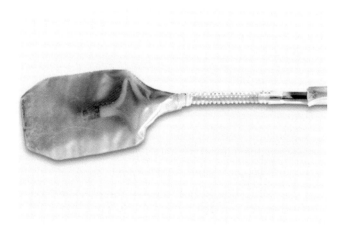

Figure 24.10. *Lower part of a mono-J reflux-preventing stent, showing the smooth lumen. The spiral segment allows the catheter to bend in either direction without kinking.*

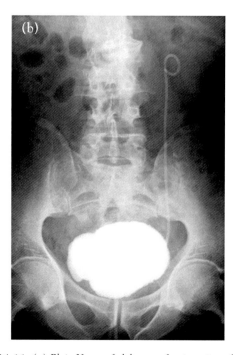

Figure 24.11. *(a) Plain X-ray of abdomen after insertion of a mono-J reflux-preventing stent; (b) cystogram shows no vesicorenal reflux through the stent.*

enough anchorage in the bladder and prevent upward migration. The stent is inserted cystoscopically like any other double-J or pigtail stents (Fig. 24.11a). This type of stent was tested in 40 patients.[14] The results showed that this stent was better tolerated than the common double-pigtail stent in the bladder. A urethrocystogram showed the absence of vesicorenal reflux (Fig. 24.11b). The indwelling period varied from 1 to 6 months. No significant encrustation was observed on the valve and spiral segment, or even on the stent itself. In 60% of patients, urethrocystoscopy revealed slight hyperaemia and oedema of the ureteral orifices, probably attributable to irritation by the stent material.

Conclusions

In the author's opinion, despite possible complications following insertion of the ureteral stent (migration, crystalloid encrustation, reflux and flank pain, haematuria and trigonal erosion), the advantages of this method are very great and they can be improved further with new technology. However, the use of long-term stenting should be limited to patients with clinical situations that justify the risk of these complications. A reflux-preventing stent in selected cases, especially when long-term ureteral stenting is indicated, is very desirable. In the past, ureteral stenting was indicated for patients at great surgical risk; however, today, in modern urology, the ureteral stent is probably one of the most commonly used devices for a variety of endo-urological interventions.

References

1. Marmar J L. The management of ureteral obstruction with silicone rubber splint catheters. J Urol 1970; 104: 386–389
2. Brown H P, Harrison J H. The efficacy of plastic ureteral and ureteral catheters for constant drainage. J Urol 1951; 66: 85–93
3. Zimskind P D, Fetter T R, Wilkerson J L. Clinical use of long-term indwelling silicone rubber ureteral splints inserted cystoscopically. J Urol 1967; 97: 840–844
4. Gibbons R P, Correa R J Jr, Cummings K B, Tate Mason J. Experience with indwelling ureteral stents catheters. J Urol 1976; 115: 22–26
5. Mardis H K, Hepperlen T W, Kammandel H. Double pigtail ureteral stent. Urology 1979; 14: 23–26
6. Finney R P. Experience with new double J ureteral catheter stent. J Urol 1978; 120: 687–681
7. Ramsay J W A, Payne S R, Gosling P T et al. The effects of double stenting on unobstructed ureters. Br J Urol 1985; 57: 630–634
8. Reid G, Denstedt J D, Kang Y S et al. Microbial adhesion and biofilm formation on ureteral stents in vitro and in vivo. J Urol 1992; 148: 1592–1594
9. Benoit G, Blanchet P, Eschwege P et al. Insertion of a double pigtail ureteral stent for the prevention of urological complications in renal transplantation: a prospective randomized study. J Urol 1996; 156: 881–884
10. Marx M, Bettmann M A, Bridge S et al. The effects of various indwelling ureteral catheter materials on the normal canine ureter. J Urol 1988; 139: 180–185
11. Mosli H A, Farsi H M A, Fawzi Al-Zimaity M, Saleh T R. Vesicoureteral reflux in patients with double pigtail stents. J Urol 1991; 146: 966–969
12. Bregg K, Riehle R A Jr. Morbidity associated with indwelling internal ureteral stents after shock wave lithotripsy. J Urol 1989; 141: 510–512
13. Hübner W A, Plas E G, Trigo-Rocha F, Tanagho E M. Drainage and reflux characteristics of antireflux ureteral double-J stents. J Endourol 1993; 7: 497–499
14. Ahmadzadeh M. Velvet Uretersplint, Erste klinische Erfahrungen. Urologe (B) 1995; 35: 95–98
15. Weiss R M. Clinical implications of ureteral physiology. J Urol 1979; 121: 401–413
16. Payne S R, Ramsay J W A. The effects of double J stents on renal pelvic dynamics in the pig. J Urol 1988; 140: 637–641
17. Bäcklund L, Reuterskiöld A G. The abnormal ureter in children. Scand J Urol 1969; 3: 219–223.
18. Drake W M, Bartone C J, Cottone F et al. Evaluation of materials used a ureteral splints. Surg Gynecol Obstet 1962; 114: 47–51
19. Camacho M F, Pereiras R, Carrion H et al. Double-ended pigtail ureteral stent: useful modification to single end ureteral stent. Urology 1979; 13: 516–520
20. McLorie G A, McKenna P H, Jumper B M et al. High grade vesicoureteral reflux: analysis of observational therapy. J Urol 1990; 144: 537–540
21. Oswalt G C Jr, Bueschen A J, Lloyd L K. Upward migration of indwelling ureteral stents. J Urol 1979; 122: 249–250
22. Ahmadzadeh M. Die Wirksamkeit der Doppel-J-Ureterschiene mit Ventilmechanismus als antirefluxive Schiene im Ureter. Urologe (B) 1990; 30: 235–237
23. Ahmadzadeh M. Flap valve ureteral stent with an antireflux function: a review of 46 cases. Urol Int 1992; 48: 466–468
24. Ramsay J W A, Miller R A, Crocker P R et al. An experimental study of hydrophillic plastics for urological use. Br J Urol 1986; 58: 70–74
25. Pocock R D, Stower M J, Ferro M A et al. Double J stents: a review of 100 patients. Br J Urol 1986; 58: 629–633
26. Docimo S G, Dewolf W C. High failure rate of indwelling ureteral stents in patients with extrinsic obstruction: experience at 2 institutions. J Urol 1989; 142: 277–279

Use of pyelo-ureteral DD stents in children
U. Friedrich and R. Vetter

Introduction

Postoperative results after reconstruction of a malformed supravesicular urinary tract in children are influenced essentially by the pathomorphology of the renal pelvis and ureter, as well as by the primary partial function of the kidneys, which is sometimes clearly impaired. Current extensive statistics, provided by Duckett et al.[1] and Hohenfellner et al.,[2] have revealed that the reoperation rate after pyeloplasty is 6.1% and after traditional terminal ureter reconstruction due to reflux or obstruction the chances of success are about 90%. Devascularization of the ureter and ureteral tension with secondary ischaemia, as well as anastomotic failure, are regarded as being responsible for the complications.

Disorders of the ultrastructural muscle syncytium, with distension and rupture of the intercellular nexus as a result of fibrosis,[3–5] are also particularly important as they, too, can cause postoperative damage to the pyelo-ureteral pacemaker activities and ureteral peristaltic processes (Figs. 25.1 and 25.2). Ransley et al.[6] conducted a trial on 142 hydronephrotic kidneys in early childhood and also prospectively assessed partial function. They found no postoperative improvement in function in 39% of the moderate (group II) patients, whereas nephrectomy had to be performed in 67% of the poor (group III) patients. Pyelo-ureteral junction obstruction has an incidence of nearly 1 per 1000 births. Whereas the surgical techniques used to eliminate supravesical flow impairment are standardized to a great extent and are chosen according to a generally recognized system of indications, conventional external stents are applied in very different ways as an accompanying anastomotic splint or nephrostomy. These external stents are associated with many disadvantages and complications. The risk of infection, urodynamic malfunction, long hospitalization times for the children and lack of variability of use are some of the problems involved (Table 25.1). This is why the trend towards closed internal stenting has been a main topic of discussion in paediatric urology for many years now; however, an ideal solution to these problems has not been found to date.

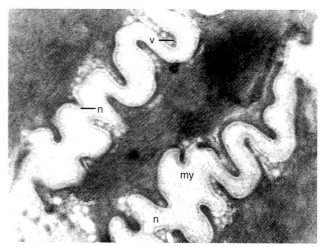

Figure 25.1. *Normal intercellular bridges ('nexus close contacts') in the intravesical express regular cell functions. X 55,000. n = nexus; v = pinocytic vesicles; my = myofilaments.*

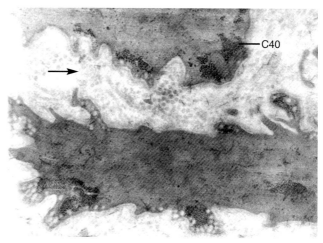

Figure 25.2. *Rupture of the nexus. Arrow indicates increased pinocytosis. Many 'dense bodies' (db) are situated near the cell periphery and collagen fibrils fill up the intercellular space. X 27,000.*

Table 25.1. *Disadvantages and risks associated with the use of conventional external renal and anastomotic stents in paediatric urology*

- Risk of infection
- Urodynamic disruption
- Prolonged hospitalization
- Lack of variability of use of anastomotic stent
- Necessity of surgical placement

Pyelo-ureteral valve DD stent

The risk of encrustation and fear of vesicorenal reflux has restricted the use of pyelovesical stents as a routine in many centres.

In order to help improve the generally unsatisfactory situation in the area of ureteral stenting for children with urological disorders, a new type of directable and disconnectable ureteral stent with coupling and a membrane valve, termed the valve DD ureteral stent (Rush AG, Kernen, Germany), has been developed. This polyurethane ureteral catheter features a membrane valve made of soft Wiruthan® at the bladder end, which automatically closes with increasing bladder pressure, preventing urinary backflow from the urinary bladder into the renal pelvis (Fig. 25.3). In addition, the wide valve prevents the stent end at the bladder side from migrating through the ureteric orifice, and thus ensures the position of the catheter in the ureter. This device has established itself in clinical practice owing to its ease of handling. However, it must be ensured that the membrane valve is not turned inside out when removing the instrument from the original packaging and when withdrawing it during endoscopic use.

The use of conventional lubricants facilitates passage of the stent through the working channel of the

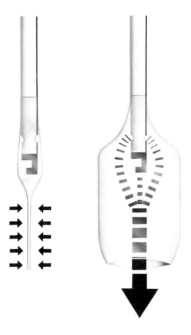

Figure 25.3. *Function of the antireflux valve with increasing urinary bladder pressure in the DD valve stent.*

cystoscope and a final check on the position of the stent in the urinary bladder is required. Different types (3–6 Fr) of DD valve stents for neonates, infants and schoolchildren are available.

Experimental model and results

Initial urodynamic experiments in animals were required to justify the use of such stents in children. The main areas of interest were pressure in the renal pelvis and the behaviour of pyelo-ureteral peristalsis when the stent was inserted.

All investigations were performed at the Institute of Experimental and Clinical Research at Åarhus University, Denmark. In-depth studies demonstrated that the animals used (five female Danish Landrace pigs) were particularly suitable for such investigations. There is a clear similarity between these animals and the human organism in respect of macroscopic and microscopic architecture, alpha-receptor distribution, pressure conditions and electrophysiological characteristics in normal and dilated urinary tract systems.[7–14]

The trial design corresponded to the standards published by Djurhuus et al.[15] and Mortensen.[16] The peristaltic processes of the renal pelvis and the mean pressure in the renal pelvis were registered continuously using a 6 Fr ureteral catheter inserted through a cystostomy using a retrograde approach. A second ureteral catheter inserted in the same way was used to vary perfusion from 1 to 10 ml/min with or without an applied Double-J stent. In order to prevent the results being influenced by changes in intravesical pressure a free draining cystostomy tube was inserted. This was easily done as the bladder had to be opened anyway in order to insert the measuring catheter into the renal pelvis.[17]

The baseline values of the renal pelvis of the animals investigated were initially checked without the stent. With an increase in pelvic flow rate of up to 10 ml/min, the increase in pressure in the renal pelvis was practically the same as that found by Mortensen.[16] Baseline pressure was 7 cmH$_2$O and peristaltic frequency was five to six pyelocontractions per minute. The four-phase behaviour of this pressure–flow relationship is depicted in Figure 25.4. The pelvic perfusion rates were chosen in this range because correlation was to be encouraged and expected, particularly from the point of view of clinical requirements. After the pyelo-ureteral stent had been inserted, the parameters measured were found to be changed fundamentally. Initially constant baseline values of 8 cmH$_2$O increased transiently at a perfusion flow rate of 1 ml/min to 10 cmH$_2$O with constant peristaltic frequency. Subsequently, the renal pelvic pressure remained almost constant up to a maximum perfusion rate of 10 ml/min. This limit was reached via a pressure–flow relationship of 9 cmH$_2$O at a renal pelvis perfusion rate of 2 ml/min, 8 cmH$_2$O at a rate of 5 ml/min and 9.1 cmH$_2$O at a flow rate of 8 ml/min. This constancy in values was caused by an increase in the frequency of pyelocontraction from 8 to 15 per minute and to increasingly stronger peristaltic amplitudes (Figs. 25.4–25.7). Such phenomena were also unaffected by the use of a valve at the bladder end of the ureteral stents.

The experimental results proved without doubt that the antireflux DD valve ureter stent could protect the kidneys from excessive pressure increases despite a constant transluminal flow rate with increasing perfusion of the renal pelvis and physiological baseline conditions. Pyelo-ureteral peristaltic function not only is maintained but also receives an additional stimulus. To date, there have only been a few investigations on this point in the literature. In 1992, Yamaguchi et al.[18] tested a similar antireflux Double-J stent manufactured by Create Medic Co. They showed that the flow resistance of the valve could be ignored from a urodynamic point of view because

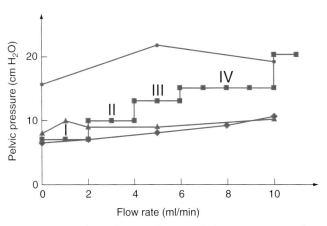

Figure 25.4. *Relation between the normal phasic increase in pelvic pressure (cmH$_2$O) and ureteral stenting with different pressure–flow relationships (PFR; ml/min): pHd (■) physiological pelvic hydrodynamics of the pig; S, (▲) ureteral stenting; oMu (●), obstructive megalo-ureter; oMu-S (◆), obstructive megalo-ureter after DD valve stent insertion.*

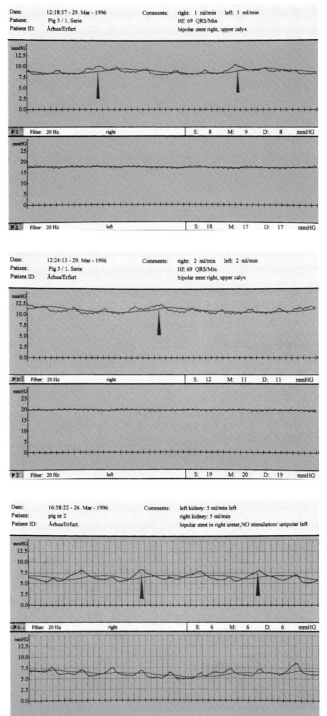

Figures 25.5–25.7. *Decreasing pelvic pressure, increasing peristaltic activity and contraction amplitudes with increasing PFR in the stented urinary system.*

urinary flow increased both through the stent openings and paraluminally.[19,20] Thus the trials conducted to date show excellent correlation with the results shown here.

In addition to studies of the behaviour of the stented ureter under physiological conditions, urodynamic investigations in obstructive megalo-ureters as a result of bilateral ectopia of the ureters could also be performed on one Danish Landrace pig. The high baseline pressure of the renal pelvis of 15.6 cmH$_2$O without stent or perfusion increased to 21.6 cmH$_2$O at a perfusion rate of 5 ml/min and to 18.9 cmH$_2$O at a perfusion rate of 10 ml/min. Peristalsis at a frequency of 3–4 pyelocontractions/min began only with above-moderate flow rates. With stent implantation, peristaltic activity of the ureter occurred immediately, with a fall in baseline pressure in the renal pelvis to 6.5 cmH$_2$O, although the normal baseline value for renal pelvic pressure for these animals of 10.4 cmH$_2$O was achieved again with a sharp increase in peristaltic intensity at 10 ml/min (Figs. 25.4 and 25.8–10). The

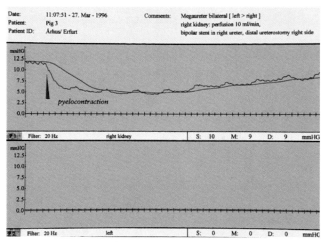

Figure 25.10. *Powerful pyelocontractions and low pressure conditions in the stented megalo-ureter system.*

results in distal ureter obstruction are comparable to those found in trials published by Hanna et al.[21] and Mortensen.[16]

Overall, all the data measured with regard to antireflux ureter stenting and presented here justify the clinical use of such a stent in children, as the urodynamic in vivo criteria and requirements were fulfilled completely.

Clinical experience

From 1993 to 1996 the authors have gained clinical experience with the application of 340 pyelo-ureteral DD stents in 241 children. Whereas additional stents without a valve were used occasionally at the outset, now only DD valve stents are used to protect the children from the dangers of transluminal reflux. A total of 259 stents were inserted intra-operatively and 81

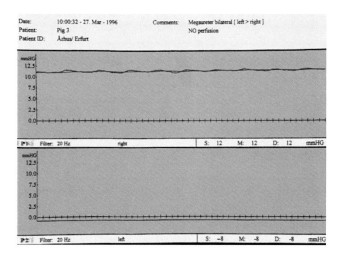

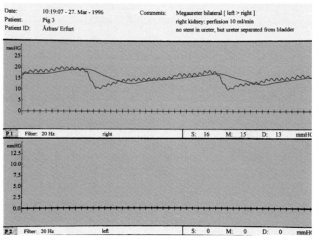

Figures 25.8–25.9. *Urodynamics of obstructive megalo-ureter with high baseline pressure in the pelvis and delayed peristalsis.*

Table 25.2. *Indications for 259 pyelo-ureteral DD stents applied surgically in children (1993–1996)*

Indication	No. of stents
Politano–Leadbetter procedure	70
Anderson–Hynes plastic surgery	81
Mega-ureter; folding/Hendren	50
Duplex kidney; en bloc UCNST	17*
Horseshoe kidney	5
Neurogenic bladder; ureteral dilatation	5
Ureteral hypoplasia	3
Cutaneous ureterostomy	11
Total no. of stents	259

* Both ureters stented.

Table 25.3. *Indications for 81 pyelo-ureteral DD stents applied endoscopically in children (1993–1996)*

Indications	No. of stents
Change of stents	38
Increasing postoperative pyelo-ureteral dilatation	26
SCIN; therapy; reduced renal function	17
Total no. of stents	81

SCIN = subureteral collagen injection in reflux.

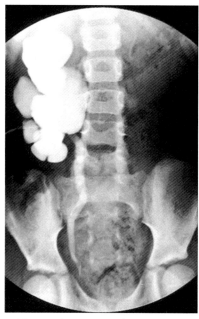

Figure 25.11. *Ureteropelvic junction obstruction in an 8-year-old girl with terminal long-distant ureterohypoplasia. Anderson–Hynes plastic surgery and endoscopic stenting with a special 3 Fr valve stent.*

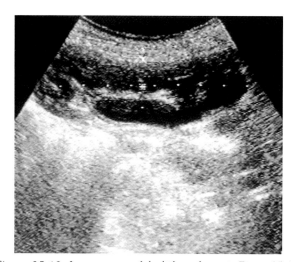

Figure 25.12. *Improvement of the kidney shown in Figure 25.11, 6 months later.*

stents were applied by endoscope. Tables 25.2 and 25.3 show the various indications.

During ureteral implantation it was very easy to insert the ureter catheter, as the route to the renal pelvis could be found easily with an open bladder. Intra-operative ultrasound control of the stent position in the kidney was necessary in every case. Ureteral kinks, compensated subpelvic stenosis or abnormal position of the kidneys were not an obstacle, owing to the easily directable soft stent tip and the large number of sizes available. However, applications of the valve stent in pyeloplasty still requires intra-operative cystoscopy as at present the valve can be inserted only using a retrograde transvesico-ureteral approach. However, the urodynamic advantages of such stenting particularly in the case of very poor baseline renal findings, appear to the authors to be of sufficient importance not to perceive this additional intervention as being a problem, as it does not involve additional risks. However, there should always be short-term nephrostomy after extensive interventions on the renal pelvis as the anastomoses can be endangered by peristalsis which starts at a very early stage. Particularly difficult situations, such as combined Hendren and folding plastic surgery, cranial and terminal ureter stenoses, ureteral dilatation in neurogenic urinary bladders and ureteral hypoplasia, may be overcome effectively on a long-term basis owing to the excellent properties of the stent in retaining function (Figs. 25.11–25.14).

It was particularly impressive that, secondarily, considerably reduced renal function could be regained and stabilized using long-term stenting, even in some older children with chronic supravesical ureteral obstruction (Figs. 25.15, 25.16). After uncomplicated routine operations, the stents were endoscopically removed 3–6 weeks postoperatively; the duration of application was, however, always based on the individual case. With a complicated course after several ureterovesical reconstructions, ureteral stents inserted on both sides could be left in place for 18 months without creating any difficulties.

Regardless of the primary surgical procedure, postoperative diagnostic procedures included ultrasound follow-ups 2, 3 and 4 weeks and 3 months after the child was discharged from hospital. Monitoring continued every 6 months until the child was 14. In order to be

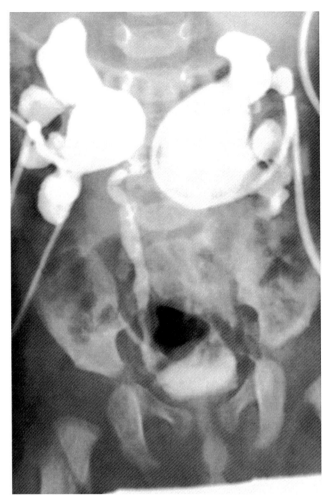

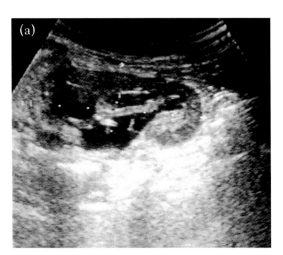

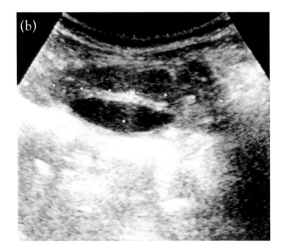

Figure 25.13. *Anterograde pyeloureterography of a 3-month-old boy with decompensated hydronephrosis on both sides. Surgery: Bilateral Anderson-Hynes plastic surgery and Politano-Leadbetter procedure; pelvic replacement by abdominal wall fascia because of extreme fibrosis and thickness (renal pelvis). Bilateral antireflux pyeloureteral stenting.*

Figure 25.14. *Postoperative ultrasound control after long-term stenting. Renal function could be maintained: (a) right kidney; (b) left kidney.*

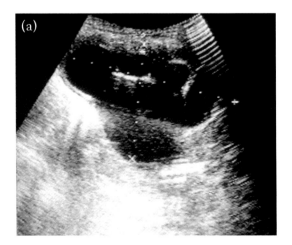

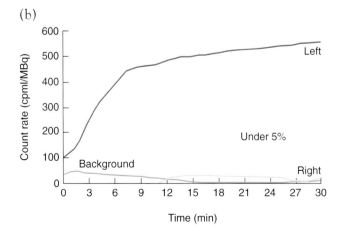

Figure 25.15. *(a) 6-year-old boy with decompensated hydronephrosis due to ureteropelvic junction obstruction; (b) 5% residual function of the kidney on the right side. Initial stenting with the DD valve stent.*

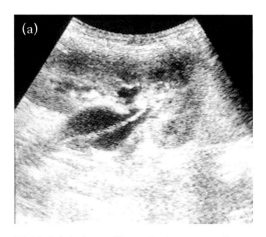 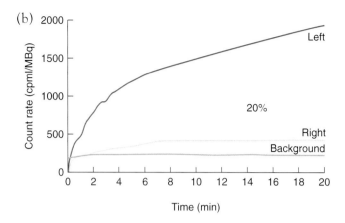

Figure 25.16. *(a) Anderson–Hynes plastic surgery and stenting for an additional 4 months; (b) 20% increase in renal function.*

able to assess ureteral urinary transport objectively using the jet phenomenon or staircase pattern in the ureterokinetogram, Doppler sonography and nuclear medicine investigations were included in the postoperative follow-up programme.[22,23] Thus, Doppler sonography and demonstration of an ostial and pigtail jet could be used in several children to demonstrate the maintenance of ureteral peristalsis and stent patency (Fig. 25.17). On the other hand, the ureterokinetogram also gave reliable information on ureteral function. Serious complications, such as stent dislocation with the possible consequence of reoperation, or serious infections, did not occur in the patient population. A few cases of transient haematuria disappeared after the patients increased their liquid intake; three older girls lost their stent, which was passed with the urine during forced urodynamic studies.

All children with an implanted antireflux pyelo-ureteral valve DD stent were discharged from hospital 7–10 days after surgery, with antibiotic cover. This routine decision was largely independent of the intra-operative baseline finding. Even after removal of the pigtail stents, no complications in supravesical reconstruction of the urinary tract in children have been observed to date. Thus, the favourable urodynamic effect of this stent as demonstrated in animal experiments was found also to be clinically relevant. In the authors' opinion, this particularly emphasizes the value of pyelo-ureteral peristalsis starting soon after surgery for a good long-term outcome.

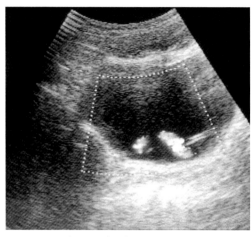

Figure 25.17. *Good ureteral and stent function can be shown by the ultrasound double-jet phenomenon after reconstructive surgery on a megalo-ureter.*

A total of 26 ureteral DD stents were applied endoscopically in cases of progressive postoperative pyeloureteral dilatation. In such cases, reoperations could be avoided by early stenting. In addition, this stent could maintain its position during treatment, by endoscopic injection, of vesicorenal reflux, particularly in parenchymally reduced kidneys (Table 25.3).

In smaller children, the stent was inserted over a previously inserted Teflon-coated guidewire. Cystoscopes of calibre from 14.5 Fr upwards were wide enough for stent insertion. All endoscopic interventions were monitored by ultrasound and the children were usually discharged the same day.

Although there is no similar extensive experience in the literature, these results tally with those of Yamaguchi et al.[18] in a smaller patient population using a similar antireflux Double-J stent. Work is ongoing to simplify stent retrieval avoiding the use of cystoscope and anaesthesia. The development of a magnetic stent is a first step in this direction, although it does not feature a valve at the bladder end.[24] Further development of this concept is awaited; it does, however, appear to be a logical approach, especially in children.

Conclusions

In the light of the many problems (e.g. the risk of infection, urodynamic malfunction and lack of variability of use) associated with the use of conventional external stents in supravesical reconstructive urinary tract surgery in children, the return to internal pyelo-ureteral stenting is a much-discussed topic in paediatric urology. To date, the clinical use of such double-J stents has been complicated, above all, by the dreaded transluminal vesicoureterorenal reflux. The development of a DD valve stent suitable for children could eliminate this risk and thus offer surgeons new possibilities. The excellent properties of these stents include their favourable urodynamic effects, reduced risk of infection and clear reduction in hospitalization times for children. In addition, early restoration of ureteral peristalsis clearly also brings about a general improvement in late results after interventions, some of which are extremely complicated. Using a few very poor baseline findings, the restitution of renal function that had been impaired by obstruction was particularly impressive with the use of these stents.

Although some minor technical details have to be clarified (such as simplification of stent retrieval and an antireflux valve stent design that can be applied using an antegrade approach), the DD valve stent used in this patient population for the reconstruction of a malformed supravesical urinary tract in children can be recommended without any reservations.

Acknowledgements

The authors would like to thank K. F. Schmitt and M. Muhr of Rusch International for their enormous support during the development of the ureteral stent and during the research project.

The authors would also like to thank J. C. Djurhuus and T. M. Jorgensen, Institute of Experimental and Clinical Research at Aarhus University in Denmark, for their invaluable ideas and advice.

References

1. Duckett J W, Howards S S, Grayhack J T, Gillenwater J Y. Adult and Pediatric Urology, 3rd edn, Vol 3. St Louis: Mosby Year Book, 1996: 2119–2255
2. Hohenfellner R, Thuroff J W, Schulte-Wiessermann H. Stenosen. Sekundareingriffe. In: Kinderurologie in Klinik und Praxis. Stuttgart: Georg Thieme Verlag, 1986: 284–306
3. Hanna M K, Jeffs J M, Sturges J M, Barkin M. Ureteral structure and ultrastructure. Part III. The congenitally dilated ureter (megaureter). J Urol 1977; 117: 24–27
4. Tokuneka S, Koyanagi T, Tsuji I. Two infantile cases of primary megaloureter with uncommon pathological findings: ultrastructural study and its clinical implications. J Urol 1980; 123: 214–217
5. Friedrich U, Schreiber D, Gottschalk E, Dietz W. Die Ultrastruktur des distalen Ureters bei kongenitalen Malformationen im Kindesalter. Z Kinderchir 1987; 42: 94–102
6. Ransley P G, Dhillon H K, Gordon I et al. The postnatal management of hydronephrosis diagnosed by prenatal ultrasound. J Urol 1990; 144: 584–587
7. Melick W F, Naryka J J, Schmidt J H. Experimental studies of ureteral peristaltic patterns in the pig. 1. Similarity of pig and human ureter and bladder physiology. J Urol 1961; 85: 145–148
8. Melick W F, Naryka J J, Schmidt J H. Experimental studies of ureteral preistaltic patterns in the pig. II. Myogenic activity of the pig ureter. J Uorll 1961; 86: 46–50
9. Constantinou C E, Djurhuus J C. Pyeloureteral dynamics in the intact and the chronically obstructed multicalyceal kidney. Am J Physiol 1981; 241: R398–R411
10. Satani Y. Histologic study of the ureter. J Urol 1919; 3: 247–267
11. Murnaghan G F. Experimental investigation of the dynamics of the normal and dilated ureter. Br J Urol 1957; 29: 403–409
12. Longrigg N. Autonomic innervation of the renal calyces. Br J Urol 1974; 46: 357–370
13. Djurhuus J C, Nerstrom B, Gyrd-Hansen N, Task-Andersen H. Experimental hydronephrosis. An electrophysiologic investigation before and after release of obstruction. Acta Chir Scand 1976; 472: 17–28
14. Djurhuus J C, Nerstrom B, Rask-Andersen H. Dynamics of upper urinary tract in man. Preoperative electrophysiological findings in patients with manifest or suspected hydronephrosis. Acta Chir Scand 1976; 472: 49–58

15. Djurhuus J C, Nerstrom B, Hansen R I et al. Dynamics of the upper urinary tract. I. An electrophysiologic in vivo study of renal pelvis in pigs: methods and normal pattern. Invest Urol 1977; 14: 465–468

16. Mortensen J. Hydrodynamics of the pyeloureter of the pig. Neurourol Urodyn 1986; 5: 87–117

17. Zimskind P D. The influence of bladder dynamics on ureteral dynamics. In: Lutzeyer W, Melchior H (eds) Urodynamics: upper and lower urinary tract. Berlin: Springer Verlag, 1973: 339–347

18. Yamaghuchi O, Yoshimura Y, Irisawa C, Shiraiwa Y. Prototype of a reflux-preventing ureteral stent and its clinical use. Urology 1992; 40: 326–329

19. Ramsay J W A, Payne S R, Gosling P T et al. The effects of Double-J stenting on unobstructed ureters: an experimental and clinical study. Br J Urol 1985; 57: 630–634

20. Finney R P. Double-J and diversion stents. Urol Clin North Am 1982; 9: 89–94

21. Hanna M K, Jeffs R D, Sturgess J M, Barkin M. Ureteral structure and ultrastructure. Part II. Congenital uretero-pelvic junction obstruction and primary obstructive megaureter. J Urol 1976; 116: 725–730

22. Friedrich U, Reid-Zimmermann G U, Endert G, Ritter E P. Die Urokinetographie in der Diagnostik und Verlaufsbeobachtung obstruktive Uropathien im Kindesalter. Z Kinderchir 1990; 45: 100–108

23. Woolfson R G, Hilson A J W, Lewis C A et al. Scintigraphic evidence of abnormal ureteric peristalsis following urological surgery. Br J Urol 1994; 73: 142–146

24. Mykalak D J, Herskowitz M, Glassberg K I. Use of magnetic internal ureteral stents in paediatric urology. Retrieval without routine requirement for cystoscopy and general anesthesia. J Urol 1994; 152: 976–977

26

Design faults in currently available ureteric stents

S. K. S. Choong, H. N. Whitfield and A. Petrik

Introduction

Ureteric stents, being placed within the urinary tract, are influenced by factors arising from the interaction between urine and the stent, leading to complications such as depolymerization, encrustation and bacterial adherence to biomaterials that are unique to the urinary system. The failure to recognize this, and the inadequacy of the standards for testing materials, which do not include performance tests for common clinical complications such as encrustation, bacterial adherence and depolymerization, have held back advancements in ureteric stent design and manufacture and have contributed to the perpetuation of these complications.

Ureteric stent design has made some progress since the 19th century, when Gustav Simon placed a tube in the ureter while performing an open cystostomy. In the early 1900s, Joaquin Albarrano created the first catheter for use in the ureter. The early ureteric catheters caused significant irritation to the bladder mucosa. Since they were connected to external drainage devices, infection of the urinary tract was common, leading to encrustation formation, poor drainage and patient discomfort, limiting their use to a few days. In 1967, Zimskind and associates[1] described the use of a long-term indwelling silicone stent that could be introduced cystoscopically. Without any proximal or distal features to hold them in place, these stents migrated in both directions. Out of necessity, several design modifications were developed to prevent migration. Gibbons,[2] in 1976, described a stent with multiple barbs along its shaft and a distal flange. The barbs made proper placement difficult and the distal flange failed to prevent migration of the stent towards the bladder. Marmar[3] and Orikasa[4] improved techniques for passing the stents in a retrograde manner. McCullough[5] initially described the use of a polyethylene stent with a 'memory' such that a shepherd's crook configuration re-formed after the tube was correctly placed with its proximal end in the renal pelvis. In 1978, Hepperlen et al.[6] developed

a single-pigtail configuration that could be straightened with a wire stylet and passed to the kidney. Effective placement was achieved and downward migration was greatly reduced, but it did not prevent upward migration.

To overcome this limitation, Finney[7] in 1978 saw the need for a stent to incorporate specific characteristics — uniform diameter, easy passage through an endoscope into the ureter, prevention of upward or downward migration, minimal trauma to the endothelial surfaces, and radiopacity. He described the double-J stent, which had coils in the shape of a J in the proximal and distal ends to prevent antegrade or retrograde migration. The Js formed in opposite directions so that the proximal J hooked into a lower calyx or the renal pelvis while the distal J curved out into the bladder, reducing trauma and inflammation to the bladder lining. Various stent configurations have been in common use at different times — the JJ stent, then the double pigtail and currently the multicoil, which is believed to have a lower incidence of migration; however, it has been reported that a knot can occur at the upper end and stent removal has had to be performed by the percutaneous route.[8]

To facilitate the passage of a ureteric stone or of *steinstrasse*, ureteric stents with a non-round cross-section have been described. Towers[9] designed a stent with a small central lumen for positioning over a guidewire and three grooves on the outside for increased drainage. Phan and Stoller[10] described a helix-like ridge along a thin central core. Fine et al.[11] observed that free fluid reflux from the bladder to the kidney triggered active peristalsis down the ureter and proposed that stents should have side-holes only at their proximal and distal ends, as side-holes in the shaft would dissipate the reflux pressure essential for the peristaltic action and allow entry of debris into the stent and cause blockage.

In order to prevent urinary reflux from the bladder to the kidney with the risk of pain and discomfort during micturition, and to reduce the risks of renal parenchymal lesions and upper urinary tract infections, ureteric stents with a distal flap valve to prevent transluminal vesicorenal reflux have been described.[12,13] Dauleh et al.[14] reported a non-refluxing minimal-irritation ureteric stent in which the lower J was replaced by a fine strong nylon loop that was attached to a fine radiopaque polyethylene tube anchor to prevent upward migration.

Despite this wide variety of design modifications, the JJ stent by Finney has remained the most widely used and has been adapted for passage cystoscopically[3–5,15–20] or percutaneously.[21–24]

Complications

The indications for stent placement and the conditions under which stents are placed are varied. Differing patient characteristics, such as pregnancy, ureteric trauma, recurrent stone formation, ureteric manipulation and urinary tract infection, have different effects on the function and dynamics of an indwelling stent and hence on the complications that may result. A stent may be needed for a few days, for several months or for life. Special stents have been developed to address the requirements of the varied indications for stent placement but there is no design that will perform optimally in all situations. Despite advances in the design and the materials used, the ideal stent does not exist and complications occur with the use of stents.

The complications that can occur may be classified into minor or major. Minor complications include loin discomfort and trigonal irritation, stent migration, urinary tract infection and encrustation. More serious complications include stone formation on the stent, ureteric erosion, stent fracture and uretero-arterial fistula, which may develop when the stent is left indwelling for an extended period.[25,26]

Smedley et al.[27] reviewed 168 JJ stent insertions in a 6-year period between 1981 and 1987. The mean length of time the stents were left in situ was 79 (range 5–180) days and the complications encountered were failure of cystoscopic stent insertion (14%), loin discomfort (19%), trigonal irritation (19%), stent migration (3%), stent obstruction due to encrustation (1%), urinary tract infection as documented by positive MSU (35%) and stent breakage (0.6%). Accidental perforation of a

ureter with the guidewire or stent occurred infrequently, but perhaps more frequently than is generally recognized. Hard stents were associated with a higher incidence of loin discomfort and trigonal irritation.

Stent hardness

Lennon et al.[28] conducted a prospective, randomized study to compare firm and soft stents regarding their ease of insertion, positional stability, biocompatibility and patient tolerance. A total of 155 patients were randomized to receive 'firm' (polyurethane) or 'soft' (Sof-Flex) stents and there was no significant difference in the ease of insertion, positional stability, degree of bladder inflammation or stent encrustation between the two groups. There was a significantly higher incidence of dysuria and renal and suprapubic pain in the firm stent group. The higher incidence of symptoms associated with firm stents appeared to be independent of the length of the stents and the duration of stent dwell-time. There was no significant difference in the incidence of urgency, frequency, nocturia or haematuria. The authors believed that the patient tolerance of the stent was directly related to the softness of the stent material. Both the 'soft' and 'hard' stents were constructed of polyurethane material. The majority of double-pigtail ureteric stents are now made of materials that can be softened by heating and demonstrate increased flexibility (thermoplastic elastomers). The hardness of the stent is reflected by the term durometer, which is a measure of the resistance of the material to a calibrated pin gauge under standard test conditions. The number increases with the hardness of the material and there is a wide range of durometers between 40 and 90 A, which are arbitrarily divided into 'soft' (40–64 A) and 'hard' (65–90 A) groups. The Sof-Flex stent used in the study by Lennon et al. had a durometer of 55 A (similar to silicone) compared with 80 A for the firmer polyurethane stent.

The optimal softness of a ureteric stent has not been achieved. The study by Lennon et al.[28] had suggested that soft stents migrated downwards so that the upper coil was out of the renal pelvis more often than was seen with hard stents, and 7% of patients with firm stents had some encrustation on the bladder coil compared with 14% of patients with soft stents ($p < 0.2$).

Stent hardness needs to be evaluated in a scientific manner by constructing stents with a range of hardness, such as a stepwise difference of 5 A, and these should then be evaluated in vitro and in vivo.

Stent fracture

Spontaneous fracture of stents is a major complication that demands unscheduled surgical interference to remove the broken parts. Retrieval of proximally migrated broken stents may require percutaneous nephroscopy, ureteroscopy or open surgery. El-Sherif[29] reported seven cases of spontaneous stent fracture in a 2-year period. Large polyurethane stents were found to bow and displace the upper ureter anteriorly, whereas small, soft stents conformed to the anatomical course of the ureter.

The majority of stents fractured at the upper third through the side-holes of the stent. The number of side-holes in currently available ureteric stents varies from 19 to 39 and the diameter of side-holes varies by a factor of four.[30] Stent material also plays an important part in the ability to maintain stent strength over time. Polyethylene material met all of the standards for tissue–implant biocompatibility but clinical experience within the urinary tract was adverse because polyethylene stents became brittle and fractured spontaneously. Analysis showed evidence of depolymerization, probably by free-radical and hydrolytic degradation, markedly reducing tensile strength and elasticity.[31] Device retrieval and analysis studies are an important technique in critical evaluation of all biomaterials.

Stent migration

The kidneys and upper ureter move, with respiration or body movements, up to 4 cm or more. The indwelling double-pigtail ureteric stent is retained within the kidney only by the J coil in the renal pelvis. Stents migrate in both the cephalad and caudal directions. Proximal migration of Double-J stents is uncommon (0.6–3.5% of cases) but usually requires general anaesthesia for stent removal. A shorter than ideal stent, inadequate distal curl of less than 180 degrees, a proximal curl in the upper calyx, inadequate technique and failure to monitor stent placement radiologically appear to be significant factors in the process of stent migration.[32]

Encrustation and biofilm

'Many foreign bodies have been taken from the bladder, uniformly encrusted with stone. I believe no foreign body was ever extracted from the bladder, which has remained long there, without having required a calculous encrustation.'

Austin, 1790.

Little has changed since that statement was made. Insufficient research has been carried out in this field and our understanding of the mechanism of encrustation is still incomplete. Poor biocompatibility has precluded successful development of any prosthesis that can be permanently placed within the urinary tract.

Encrustation is the process by which urinary crystalloids and colloids adhere to the surface of biomaterial surfaces. The appearance of crystalline encrustation on the surface of polymers can appear within hours of exposure to urine. Encrustation is a multifactorial phenomenon and the factors contributing to encrustation include urinary tract infection, differences in biomaterials and surface properties, and individual variations. There are two distinct types of encrustation that can form around a polymer in contact with urine: these are, first, the rapidly forming struvite stone that is a direct result of urine infection, urealysis, pH elevation and the precipitation of struvite; secondly, the more slowly forming encrustation, principally consisting of calcium phosphate, which forms in sterile urine and is independent of bacterial urease.

Bacterial infection and biofilm formation

Bacterial infection is known to be an important factor in the development of encrustation on ureteric stents and urethral catheters. The association between urinary infection and stone formation was first recognized by Horton Smith in 1897 and Brown in 1901. At that time, the structure, chemical composition and pathogenesis of stone formation was not understood. The mechanism of encrustation on biomaterials in the presence of urinary tract infection is now believed to involve the following steps: (1) protein adsorption on the biomaterial; (2) the formation of an organic conditioning film on the surface; (3) the adherence of the urease-producing bacteria to the biofilm; (4) the development of a bacterial biofilm community within a matrix of bacterial exopolysaccharide; (5) the elevation of the pH of urine and biofilm matrix by the action of urease on urea; (6) the attraction of calcium and magnesium ions into the gel of the matrix; (7) stabilization of the calcium and magnesium ammonium phosphate crystals by the biofilm matrix; (8) crystal formation in the alkaline urine and bacterial attachment to the surfaces of the biofilm, promoting aggregation and growth of the biofilm.

It is known that proteins are able to adhere to polymer surfaces. Adsorption of protein onto polymer surfaces is the net result of various interactions involving the surface, the protein and the solvent. The factors influencing the binding of proteins include the electrostatic and polarity forces between the molecules and the surface, and the temperature and solute composition of the fluid environment. The kinetics of adsorption in biological fluids depend on the amount and type of proteins present. Initially, the interface will accommodate mainly those protein molecules that are most abundantly present in solution. Later, the adsorbed molecules may be displaced by other molecules that have a stronger tendency to adsorb (sequential adsorption). This adsorbed layer may initiate the process of encrustation by attracting certain molecules. To prevent encrustation, it will be necessary to identify the adsorbing proteins and investigate further the interaction of urinary solutes and bacteria to this layer.

Desgrandchamps et al.[33] performed a comparative encrustation study in vitro of five different types of JJ stents in human urine and concluded that hydrogel-coated stents had a higher risk of encrustation than uncoated stents. Spirnak and Resnick[34] reported five cases of clinically significant stone formation associated with indwelling ureteric stents, two of which had no evidence of urinary tract infection. When stone formation occurs solely on the distal tip, patient morbidity usually will be limited to the need for stent replacement. However, when extensive proximal stone formation occurs, additional surgical intervention may be necessary to remove the stent and the associated stone(s) successfully. Keane et al.[35] examined ureteric stents from 40 patients and identified a profuse biofilm on 28% and encrustation on 58% of the stents; they concluded that newer materials must be sought if effective long-term stenting is to be achieved. Schulze et al.[36] reported severe encrustation and stone formation

on indwelling ureteric stents in two patients with a lithogenic history in the presence of sterile urine, both requiring surgical intervention. He observed that patients who are stone-formers are at an increased risk for stent encrustation. The problem of encrustation has been exacerbated by the increased use of extracorporeal shock-wave lithotripsy (ESWL) in combination with JJ stents. These stone-forming patients have been shown to develop encrustation rapidly.[36]

Reid et al.[37] examined 30 ureteric stents inserted for 5–128 days following ESWL and found that 90% had adherent pathogens, 45% of which were present in low numbers ($10^1 - 10^2$ per 1 cm^3 section) and 55% were in small and large microcolony biofilms ($>2 \times 10^2 - 10^7$). The organisms isolated were Gram-positive cocci (77%), Gram-negative rods (15%) and *Candida* sp. (8%), even though urine culture was positive in only 27% of patients and no blockage occurred. Experiments in vitro demonstrated the ability of *Escherichia coli*, *Proteus mirabilis*, *Staphylococcus epidermidis* and *Enterococcus faecalis* uropathogens to adhere and form biofilms on ureteric stents within 24 h. The ability of uropathogens to adhere to the surface of a prosthetic material is an important factor in the development of infection. Adherence may be influenced by factors such as cell surface properties,[38] biomaterial surface characteristics[39] and the clinical conditions presenting.[40] The biofilm resists host defences and treatment with antimicrobial agents,[41] and provides a reservoir of viable organisms that can continue to cause infection and encrustation leading to blockage of the stent. Gram-negative bacilli adhere differentially to catheter materials and bacterial colonization may be influenced by catheter surface properties.[42] The antibacterial properties of silver have been used in silver alloy-coated catheters that are associated with a reduced incidence of bacteriuria.[43] New developments in biomaterial coating could be directed towards limiting colonization by urease-producing microorganisms. Increased knowledge of the sequence of events and the precise mechanisms of encrustation formation will help better material to be developed, for example by interfering with protein adsorption or bacterial adhesion. Other potential sites of action at which the chain of events involved in encrustation could be broken need to be identified and exploited.

Surface properties

Encrustation is affected by such surface properties as roughness and irregularity, surface charge and zeta potential, surface hydrophobicity and wettability, polymer chemistry and surface coatings. Surface roughness of polymer materials was shown to be proportional to thrombogenicity[44] until the surface imperfections were smaller than the dimension of the platelets,[45] when blood flowed freely over the surface. Intravascular catheters of identical poly (vinylchloride) (PVC) composition but with different degrees of surface roughness showed increasing thrombus adhesion to the increasingly uneven surface.[44] In an aqueous environment such as urine, local effects on flow, including turbulence and impedance, will also contribute to any surface interactions. The surface composition and configuration of the stent may also influence any reactivity at the interface. Protein adsorption and adherence has been shown to be affected by surface composition in different materials with the same surface morphology.[46] The surface energy of a material may be related to its chemical composition and has been shown to influence protein adsorption. A high surface energy suggests that there are forces present on the surface that will favour attraction and thus adhesion of molecules or particles of a certain charge, size or structure. The nature of any particular molecules or particles that are attracted to adhere to the polymer is unknown and further research in this field is warranted.

Stent design

The manufacturing technique and design of a ureteric stent also play an important role in stent function and thus in any complications that result. A large variety of ureteric stents are commercially available that vary widely in a number of critical design characteristics.

Choong et al.[30] measured the urinary flow rates and identified the relative importance of the differing features in ten types of 6 Fr 26 cm ureteric stents (Cook, Angiomed and Microvasive). A urinary tract model in vitro simulating a complete circumferential obstruction of the upper, middle or lower ureter was designed and the flow rates measured three times in the ten types of stent to obtain the mean values. The tensile strength and elongation capacity were measured and the surface characteristics of the stents, radiopaque markers and

side-holes were examined by SEM. The flow rates ranged from 32 to 58 ml/min for upper, middle, and lower ureteric stent obstruction with the fastest in the stent with the highest tensile strength (varying from 10.59 to 28.70 N/mm^2) without any correlation to the number of side-holes, which varied from 19 to 39. The flow rates through the stents were dependent on the internal stent area and thickness of the stent wall, which were secondary to the tensile strength. The diameter of the side-holes varied from 0.58 to 2.33 mm (Figs. 26.1 and 26.2); the inner diameter of the stent varied from 0.96 to 1.41 mm and the outer diameter varied from 1.66 to 2.16 mm. SEM revealed widely

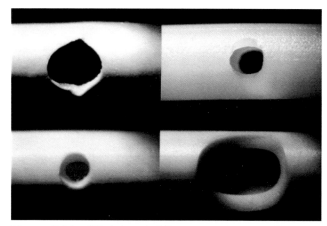

Figure 26.1. *Side-holes of different ureteric stents illustrating irregularity and differences in size and shape.*

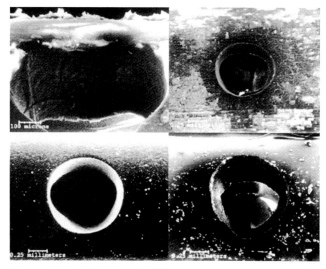

Figure 26.2. *Side-holes of different ureteric stents, as seen by electron microscopy, illustrating irregularity and differences in size and shape.*

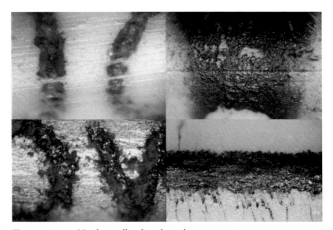

Figure 26.3. *Haphazardly placed markers on ureteric stents.*

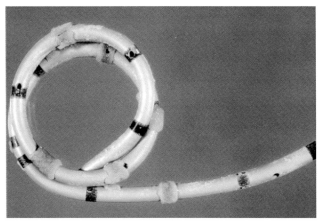

Figure 26.4. *Selective encrustation on the markers of this ureteric stent.*

varying irregularities at different sites on the surface, markers and side-holes. Markers haphazardly placed on the stents and irregular surfaces or side-holes can encourage encrustation deposition (Figs. 26.3 and 26.4). The ideal size and number of side-holes for each type of stent has not been determined.[30]

Individual variation

Encrustation of ureteric stents is influenced not only by the shape, surface properties and composition of the catheter but also by the physicochemical environment in which it is placed. Individual variations exist from one patient to another, irrespective of the type of material used. With identical ureteric stents, some patients show no evidence of encrustation and blockage whereas other patients show variable degrees of the phenomenon. This implies that encrustation is at least

partially dependent on the composition of the urine in which the stent dwells. Urinary pH and calcium are thought to be important determinants in catheter blockage.[47]

Langley and Fry[48] assessed the role of H^+ in determining the solubility of Ca^{2+} in urine from normal subjects and stone-formers to determine the conditions that cause the formation of crystalline products. Crystalline precipitates appeared in urine at a critical pH that was closer to the voided pH in stone-formers than in normal subjects and might explain the greater propensity of this group to form stones.

Choong et al.[49] studied the relationship between catheter blockage and the ionic composition of urine, in particular the relationship between pH and Ca^{2+}. Catheter 'non-blockers' were able to retain Ca^{2+} in solution over a wider range of pH values than catheter 'blockers' — the latter have a smaller safety margin in the variation of urinary pH before encrustation occurs.

Urine is generally supersaturated with respect to calcium, oxalate and phosphate and yet normal individuals do not form stones. Over the years, many different urinary constituents have been suggested as being responsible for the relative stability of normal urine to precipitation. The overall inhibitory action of crystallization in human urine is thought to come from low-molecular-weight molecules, high-molecular-weight protein macromolecules and glycosaminoglycans. Theoretically, these inhibitors could act by affecting nucleation, crystal growth or aggregation. However, the mechanism of action is unknown. The effect of various promoters and inhibitors of crystallization needs to be evaluated to discover which are the fractions in the urine that bind Ca^{2+}, affecting its dynamic characteristics and propensity to form stones and lead to encrustation. The question of whether it is beneficial to reduce the Ca^{2+} by increasing the concentration of anionic moieties, or whether it is these moieties themselves that help to generate precipitates, is as yet unanswered.[50] Further scientific research in this field is needed to examine the steps involved before therapeutic intervention can be effected.

Prevention of complications
Fracture

Small, soft stents that conform to the anatomical course and do not cause bowing of the upper ureter may be preferable. Currently available ureteric stents vary widely in the number of side-holes, from 19 to 39,[30] and their effect on stent function and complication needs further evaluation. The tensile strength of biomaterials for use in the urinary tract should be quantified prior to and following retrieval from urine in vitro and in vivo for the maximum period of time that the stent was recommended to dwell in the urinary tract.

Migration

Inadequate technique, failure to monitor stent placement radiologically, a shorter than ideal stent, a distal curl of less than 180 degrees and a proximal curl in the upper calyx appear to be significant factors in the process of stent migration.[32]

When a stent is inserted retrogradely, fluoroscopy is important to monitor the proximal position within the kidney and cystoscopy must confirm that the distal end of the stent is correctly positioned within the bladder. Simultaneous monitoring of the stent in the kidney and bladder avoids excessive placement of one end and inadequate length in the other.

Adequate tensile strength and memory of the coils is crucial in preventing migration. Currently available stents vary widely in the design, side-holes, types of biomaterials used and manufacturing process, which determine the tensile strength and memory of the stent. The optimal balance between tensile strength and memory of the coil must be evaluated by systematically varying the factors that influence them.

Encrustation and biofilm

The prevention of encrustation and biofilm formation requires a detailed and systematic examination of the processes of these multifactorial phenomena. Differences in the urinary constituents between 'stone-formers' and 'non-stone-formers' and their interaction with biomaterials that promote encrustation and biofilm formation need further studies. The optimum number, size and shape of side-holes have not been determined and — since these features may influence urinary flow and turbulence across the side-holes, hence influencing encrustation deposits — these are critical issues. There is marked surface roughness and irregularity on the surface of many currently available ureteric stents, which can be significantly improved. Radiopaque material and markers on the stents, which have led to

encrustation deposits on those uneven and raised markers, should be concealed. A higher standard of manufacturing technique and better quality control may improve surface roughness and irregularities. There are currently no standardized performance tests for encrustation and bacterial adherence, even though they are responsible for the majority of complications seen clinically.

A standardized method of quantifying encrustation on existing stents and newer biomaterials is an important step to reduce the morbidity and mortality associated with encrustation. Several studies in vivo and in vitro have attempted to compare the effect of different biomaterials on encrustation. However, the variability of human models in terms of diet, fluid intake and urinary constituents have impeded comparison between biomaterials. Animal models were less variable in terms of their breeding, diet and fluid intake but urinary constituents still varied between the animals and, therefore, in vitro models have been preferred. In vitro tests provide a means of determining the tendency of materials to encrust and so have an advantage over clinical trials: the results are not influenced by patient diet and medication or by metabolic differences between individuals.[51] As a result, in vitro tests provide a direct comparison of the propensity of the materials themselves to encrust.

In the past, human urine in vitro encrustation models were widely recognized as having several deficiencies — cross-contamination and turbulence within the model, inadequate polymer exposure and restricted polymer shape, disinfectant modifying polymer surface, cleaning difficulty and limited functions. Choong and Whitfield[52] have designed a new dynamic human urine encrustation model that has eliminated the shortcomings of the previous methods. It allows testing of polymers in their raw form (such as membranes) or as fully formed products (such as ureteric stents and urethral catheters). This model has overcome the problem of human urine variability by continuously passing urine from a single source to a test material and a reference material housed separately but simultaneously and under the same conditions. The amount of encrustation was quantified by calcium atomic absorption spectroscopy and expressed as an encrustation index, defined as the ratio of encrustation between the test and the reference materials. Any variation of urine from day to day or experiment to experiment will affect not only the test material but equally the reference material. Previously, Urolocide [benzyl (dodecylarbamylmethyl) di methyl-ammonium chloride] was used to sterilize the urine but, as was not known at that time, interacted with the polymer surface, which could have affected the deposition of encrustation. In this model, antibiotics, which have been shown not to affect the surface, were used to prevent urinary infection and allow the mechanism of encrustation in sterile urine to be studied.

This encrustation model will allow the propensity of biomaterials to encrust to be quantified using human urine, and also will enable the effect of biofilm and infection to be examined; it will also permit the effect of inhibitors and promoters of crystallization to be studied so that a greater understanding and therapeutic solution may be achieved.

Conclusions

Improvements in the design, manufacturing techniques and quality of ureteric stents could improve their performance and reduce complication rates. Appropriate standards for testing materials and devices in the urinary tract with regard to such factors as encrustation and bacterial adherence are vital to encourage the development of a ureteric stent with reduced complications.

Block et al.[53] have suggested eight desirable characteristics for synthetic biomaterials utilized in the urinary tract: these are (1) complete inertness, (2) durability, (3) partial flexibility, (4) partial rigidity, (5) resistance to encrustation, (6) workability, (7) sterilizability, and (8) permanence of physical characteristics. It may be useful to add a ninth characteristics — the ability to resist biofilm formation (protein adsorption and bacterial adhesion). There is a long way to go before a truly biocompatible ureteric stent becomes available. Indeed, more than one thousand years since Rhazes, a Persian scholar and physician in the ninth century, commented on the best type of material for catheter construction, there remains disagreement concerning the form and substance of endo-urological devices. Apart from the lack of a

completely inert biomaterial that is able to resist protein adsorption, bacterial adherence and encrustation formation and that causes no tissue reaction, the urinary system presents an unstable chemical environment, with supersaturation of uromucoids and crystalloids at the interphase between the material and urine, which creates a significant problem for long-term biocompatibility and biodurability of devices within this system. The design of the stent has room for improvement and further systematic research needs to be conducted, from the basic sciences level to device testing and clinical trial stages, to minimize the complications associated with the use of ureteric stents.

References

1. Zimskind P D, Fetter T R, Wilkerson J L. Clinical use of long-term indwelling silicone rubber ureteral splints injected cystoscopically. J Urol 1967; 97: 840
2. Gibbons R P, Correa R J Jr, Cummings K B et al. Experience with indwelling ureteral stent catheters. J Urol 1976; 115: 22
3. Marmar J L. The management of ureteral obstruction with silicone rubber splint catheters. J Urol 1970; 104: 386–389
4. Orikasa S, Tsuji I, Siba T et al. A new technique for transurethral insertion of a silicone rubber tube into an obstructed ureter. J Urol 1973; 110: 184–187
5. McCullough D L. 'Shepherds crook' self-retaining ureteral catheter. Urol Lett Club 1974; 32: 54–55
6. Hepperlen T W, Mardis H K, Kammandel H. Self-retained internal ureteral stents: a new approach. J Urol 1978; 119: 731–734
7. Finney R P. Experience with new double J ureteral catheter stent. J Urol 1978;120: 678–681
8. Kundargi P, Bansal M, Pattnaik P K. Knotted upper end: a new complication in the use of an indwelling ureteral stent. J Urol 1994; 151: 995–996
9. Towers R J. Design and use of externally-draining ureteral stent. Urology 1988; 32(6): 532–534
10. Phan C N, Stoller M L. Helically ridged ureteric stent facilitates the passage of stone fragments in an experimental porcine model. Br J Urol 1993; 72: 17–19
11. Fine H, Gordon R L, Lebensart P D. Extracorporeal shock wave lithotripsy and stents: fluoroscopic observations and a hypothesis on the mechanism of stent function. Urol Radiol 1989; 11: 37–41
12. Ahmadzadeh M. Flap valve ureteral stent with an antireflux function: a review of 46 cases. Urol Int 1992; 48: 466–468
13. Yamaguchi O, Yoshimura Y, Irisawa C, Shiraiwa Y. Prototype of a reflux-preventing ureteral stent and its clinical use. Urology 1992; 40(4): 326–329
14. Dauleh M I, Byrne D J, Baxby K. Non-refluxing minimal irritation ureteric stent. Br J Urol 1995; 76: 795–796
15. Camacho M F, Pereiras R, Carrion H et al. Double-ended pigtail ureteral stent: useful modification to single ureteral stent. Urology 1979; 13: 516
16. Drago J R, Royner T J, Chez R A. Management of urinary calculi in pregnancy. Urology 1982; 20: 578
17. Gibbons R P, Mason J T, Correa R J Jr. Experience with indwelling silicone rubber ureteral catheters. J Urol 1974; 111: 594
18. Kearney G P, Mahoney E M, Brown H P. Useful technique for long-term urinary drainage by inlying ureteral stent. Urology 1979; 14: 126

19. Mardis H K, Hepperlen T W, Kammandel H. Double pigtail ureteral stent. Urology 1979; 14: 23

20. Ortlip S A, Fraley E E. Indications for palliative urinary diversion in patients with cancer. Urol Clin North Am 1982; 9: 79

21. Bigongiari L R, Lee K R, Mebust W K et al. Transureteral conversion of a percutaneous ureteral stent to an indwelling stent. AJR 1978; 131: 1098

22. Mazer M J, LeVeen R F, Call J E et al. Permanent percutaneous antegrade ureteral stent placement without transurethral assistance. Urology 1979; 14: 413

23. Smith A D, Lange P H, Miller R P et al. Introduction of Gibbons ureteral stent facilitated by antecedent percutaneous nephrostomy. J Urol 1978; 120: 543

24. Smith A D, Miller R P, Reinke D B et al. Insertion of Gibbons ureteral stents using endourology techniques. Urology 1979; 14: 330

25. Saltzman B. Ureteral stents. Indications, variations and complications. Urol Clin North Am 1988; 15: 481

26. Reiner R J, Conway G F, Threlkeld R. Ureteroarterial fistula. J Urol 1975; 113: 24

27. Smedley F H, Rimmer J, Taube M, Edwards L. 168 double J (pigtail) ureteric catheter insertions: a retrospective review. Ann R Coll Surg Engl 1988; 70: 377–379

28. Lennon G M, Thornhill J A, Sweeney P A et al. 'Firm' versus 'Soft' double pigtail ureteric stents: a randomised blind comparative trial. Eur Urol 1995; 28: 1–5

29. El-Sherif A. Fracture of polyurethane double pigtail stents: an in vivo retrospective and prospective fluoroscopic study. Br J Urol 1995; 76: 108–114

30. Choong S, Whitfield H, Petrik A, Nicholas C. Current design faults in ureteric stents. Eur Urol 1996; 30(suppl 2): 181

31. Mardis H K. Evaluation of polymeric materials for endourologic devices; emerging importance of hydrogels. Semin Intervent Radiol 1987; 4(1): 36–45

32. Slaton J W, Kropp K A. Proximal ureteral stent migration: an avoidable complication? J Urol 1996; 155: 58–61

33. Desgrandchamps F, Moulinier F, Daudon M et al. An in vitro comparison of urease-induced encrustation on JJ stents in human urine. Br J Urol 1997; 79(1): 24–27

34. Spirnak J P, Resnick M I. Stone formation as a complication of indwelling ureteral stents: a report of 5 cases. J Urol 1985; 134: 349–351

35. Keane P F, Bonner M C, Johnston S R et al. Characterization of biofilm and encrustation on ureteric stents in vivo. Br J Urol 1994; 73: 687–691

36. Schulze K A, Wettlaufer J N, Oldani G. Encrustation and stone formation: complication of indwelling ureteral stents. Urology 1985; 25(6): 616–619

37. Reid G, Denstedt J D, Kang Y S et al. Microbial adhesion and biofilm formation on ureteral stents in vitro and in vivo. J Urol 1992; 148: 1592–1594

38. Jones D S, Gorman S P, McCafferty D F et al. A comparative study of the effects of three non-antibiotic antimicrobial agents on the surface hydrophobicity of certain microorganisms. J Appl Bacteriol 1991; 71: 218–227

39. Gorman S P, Mawhinney W M, Adair C G et al. Confocal scanning laser microscopy of CAPD catheter surface microrugosity in relation to recurrent peritonitis. J Med Microbiol 1993; 38: 411–417

40. Mawhinney W M, Adair C G, Gorman S P. Factors influencing the adherence of microbial pathogens to CAPD catheters. Pharmacotherapy 1992; 12: 253

41. Gorman S P. Microbial adherence and biofilm production. In: Denyer S P, Hugo W B (eds) Mechanisms and Actions of Chemical Biocides. Oxford: Blackwell Scientific Publications, 1991: 271–295

42. Sugarman B. Adherence of bacteria to urinary catheters. Urol Res 1982; 10: 37–40

43. Liedberg H, Lundeberg T. Silver coating of urinary catheters prevents adherence and growth of Pseudomonas aeruginosa. Urol Res 1989; 17: 357–358

44. Hecker J F, Edwards R O. Effects of roughness on the thrombogenicity of a plastic. J Biomed Mater Res 1981; 15: 1–7

45. Didisheim P, Tirrell M V, Lyons C S et al. Relative role of surface chemistry and surface texture in blood material interactions. Trans Am Soc Artif Intern Organs 1983; 29: 169–175

46. Cumming R D, Phillips P A, Singh P I. Surface chemistry and blood material interactions. Trans Am Soc Artif Intern Organs 1983; 29: 163–165

47. Burr R G, Nuseibeh I M. Blockage of indwelling urinary catheters: the roles of urinary composition, the catheter, medication and diet. Paraplegia 1993; 31: 234–241

48. Langley S E M, Fry C H. The influence of pH on urinary ionized $[Ca^{2+}]$: differences between urinary tract stone formers and normal subjects. Br J Urol 1997; 79: 8–14

49. Choong S, Fry C H, Whitfield H. The scientific basis of urinary catheter encrustation. J Endourol 1996; 10(suppl 1): S181

50. Resnick M, Gammon C, Sorrel M et al. Calcium binding proteins and renal lithiasis. Surgery 1980; 88 (2): 239–243

51. Cox A J, Hukins D W L, Sutton T M. Comparison of in vitro encrustation on silicone and hydrogel-coated latex catheters. Br J Urol 1988; 61: 156–161

52. Choong S, Whitfield H. A new model for quantification of encrustation on polymers, urethral catheters and ureteric stents. Eur Urol 1996; 30(suppl 2): 34

53. Block N L, Stover E, Politano V A. A prosthetic ureter in the dog. Trans Am Soc Artif Intern Organs 1977; 23: 367–370

27

Minimally invasive ureteric stent retrieval
W. Taylor

Introduction

Ureteric stents are indispensable to the practice of modern day adult and pediatric urology. When a stent has served its purpose it has to be removed, conventionally under direct vision with a grasping forceps through a cystoscope. This is invasive, time-consuming and expensive if done in the operating room with either sedation or general anesthesia, with its associated risk, albeit small. Retrieval of a stent is optimally performed in the ambulatory care setting using topical anesthesia and a flexible cystoscope with grasping forceps.[1–3] However, most children require a general anesthetic for stent retrieval. Flexible cystoscopy has made retrieval easier and more acceptable for adult stent retrieval, but it is still a costly procedure even in the outpatient setting.

Since stents have become part of everyday urological practise an easier method for stent retrieval has been investigated. Currently, the liberal indications for ureteral stenting are being questioned and re-evaluated but, nevertheless, ureteral stents continue to be used in large numbers.[4–6] Stents are no longer routinely used prior to extracorporeal shock-wave lithotripsy (ESWL) of ureteric calculi or after uncomplicated ureterorenoscopy. Despite these changing indications for the use of a stent, the need for less invasive and more cost-efficient removal is still pertinent and desirable.

Retrieval methods

Radiologists and urologists have developed innovative non-endoscopic methods for stent retrieval (Table 27.1).

The simplest non-endoscopic method for stent retrieval utilizes a length of suture, which is tied to the end of a stent and dangles from the urethra.[7] This suture is fixed to the skin of the penis or labia majora by means of adhesive tape. The stent is subsequently removed by traction on the dangling suture. The dangling suture method is short-term only, ideally for stents indwelling no more than 48 hours. Problems with these sutures are:

(1) accidental traction on them by the patient with dislodgement; (2) 'wicking' of urine around the suture, which causes a small degree of incontinence; and (3) an increased risk of retrograde nosocomial bladder infection along the suture. To overcome these problems a short intraurethral suture, which is later removed with a forceps at gas cystoscopy, has been described.[8] Patient tolerance of this intraurethral suture is excellent, accidental dislodgement does not occur, and gas cystoscopy retrieval by means of a bulb insufflator is economical and reliable. This short intraurethral dangling suture causes very little discomfort to the patient, and there is minimal discomfort with cystoscopic retrieval, as the urethral sphincter is not traversed by the cystoscope.

Retrograde radiological ureteric stent removal utilizing fluoroscopy is described.[9,10] In females, a small snare is inserted into the bladder per urethra, angulated towards the distal end of the stent, grasped and retrieved under fluoroscopic control. In males, up to an 8 Fr or smaller angiographic catheter is utilized to allow for similar passage of a snare into the bladder to grasp the distal portion of the stent. In the reported series, local anesthesia was used. This method of retrieval of a stent is more cost-effective than a cystoscopy with general anesthesia, but would seem to offer no advantages over flexible cystoscopic retrieval with topical anesthesia, which avoids the use of radiation.

Radiological retrieval of a stent from the renal pelvis or upper ureter was appropriate until the development of a flexible cystoscope allowed for a direct visual approach to the stent, which is the method of choice, as radiation is unnecessary.

Table 27.1. *Methods for stent retrieval*

- Cystoscopy
- Dangling suture
- Snail-head retriever
- Magnets
- Radiological
- Dissolving stents

Blind retrieval by means of a 'snail-head' or 'pigtail' catheter in females is reported.[11,12] A small 720° or 360° wire coil is inserted through the urethra and angulated towards the ureteric orifice. Rotation of this passive grasper blindly engages the distal end of the stent. The engagement is indicated by a feeling of resistance to gentle pulling of the grasper and then the stent is retrieved by traction on the inserted device. This procedure is limited to females and has minimal cost (Fig. 27.1).

Magnetic retrieval of a ureteric stent is an elegant concept and trials have been carried out in adults and children of both sexes.[13,14] A magnet attached to the end of a urethral catheter 'Magnetriever' is inserted under local anesthesia per urethra into the bladder where it makes contact with a magnet embedded into the end of the distal pigtail of the stent 'Magnetip'. Traction on the urethral catheter after the two magnets connected allowed for removal of the stent (Fig. 27.2).

A cylindrical magnet with a perforation for a guidewire (0.028 inches) was designed to fit into the distal end of a double pigtail stent. This stent with magnet was inserted cystoscopically, sometimes with difficulty (17% of patients), as the guidewire tended to buckle. The stent was later retrieved by insertion of a urethral catheter with a magnet attached to its tip. The magnets then connected and exerted enough attractive force to allow for retrieval of the stent in all females and 76% of adult males when the urethral catheter was withdrawn. In the pediatric study of seven patients, the stent was inserted antegrade and retrieved retrograde. In six out of seven children this was successful. The disadvantage of this device was the difficulty with insertion and high rate of retrieval failure in adult males.

Bioabsorbable stents are in current commercial use in the lower urinary tract as prostatic stents. These materials have been used in the lower ureter and are now being tested for use in the upper ureter. Their proposed use is to bridge a short span of the ureter or the ureteropelvic junction. The purpose of these stents is to

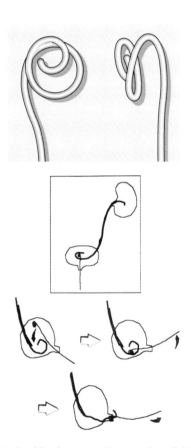

Figure 27.1. *Snail-head retriever. Rotating the coiled 'snail-head' captures the stent. From Yu D-S, Yang, Yang T-H, Ma C-P. Snail-head catheter retriever: a simple way to remove catheters from female patients. J Urol 1995; 154: 167–168. Reproduced with permission from Lippincott, Williams & Wilkins.*

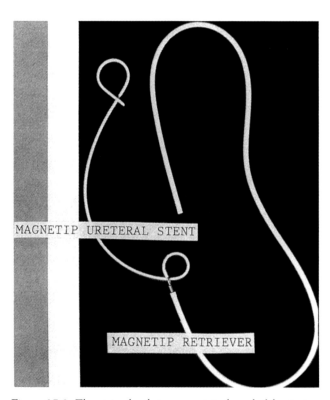

MAGNETIP URETERAL STENT

MAGNETIP RETRIEVER

Figure 27.2. *The retrieval catheter connects to the end of the stent. Mykulak D, Herskowitz M, Glassberg K. Use of magnetic ureteral stents in pediatric urology: retrieval without routine requirement for cystoscopy and general anesthesia. J Urol 1994; 152: 976–977. Reproduced with permission from Lippincott, Williams & Wilkins.*

make retrieval unnecessary.[15] An added advantage of these short stents is that they do not traverse the intramural ureter and therefore cause little or no bladder irritation and do not allow reflux of urine to the upper ureter. Different compositions of the stent may allow for rapid or slow dissolution of the stent in accordance with the time the stent is required. This pleasing idea shows promise and is under clinical evaluation.

None of these methods are reliable enough to replace cystoscopic retrieval under local anesthesia, particularly in male patients. The dangling suture method is a reasonable option if a stent is required for a short period of time only, particularly if it is not critical that the stent be accidentally dislodged.

Magnetic stent retrieval revisited

The concept of magnetic retrieval of a stent was revived utilizing advances in magnetics and the lower coefficients of friction of modern stents.[16] Rare earth magnets are more powerful than standard magnets and offer a better force of attractivity.

A biocompatible surgical grade stainless steel bead with a bore to accommodate a standard 0.038 inch guidewire for easy insertion was attached to the end of a double or single pigtail stent (Fig. 27.3).

A retrieval catheter with a rare earth magnet at its end and angulated at 30° was designed based on anatomical studies of the distances and angles from the bladder neck to ureteral orifice (Fig. 27.4).

The minimum force needed to retrieve a stent was determined by force gauge measurements in the retrieval of stents with dangling sutures. The holding force between a stainless steel bead and rare earth retrieval magnet provided a force three times higher than needed to retrieve a stent in females, and one and a half times in excess of that needed in males. The longer urethra and prostate account for the extra resistance to extraction of the stent.

A bead was designed to attach to the distal end of a stent by a tether, so as not to compromise the lumen and to allow for perfect alignment always with the retrieval magnet. The retrieval procedure was tolerated well using topical anesthesia only, allowing patients to return to normal activities immediately (Fig. 27.5).

This system was used in 30 consecutive patients

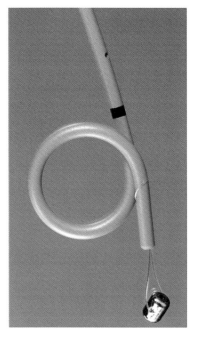

Figure 27.3. *The flail tether between the stainless steel bead and distal pigtail provides optimal end-to-end connection of the bead and retrieval magnet.*

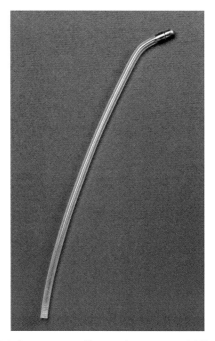

Figure 27.4. *Stent retriever. Rare earth magnet size 16 Fr.*

requiring stents.[16] Insertion through a standard 22 Fr cystoscope was easy and achieved in all patients (Fig. 27.6).

No adverse effects from the bead attached to the stent were noted in any of the patients. Retrieval was

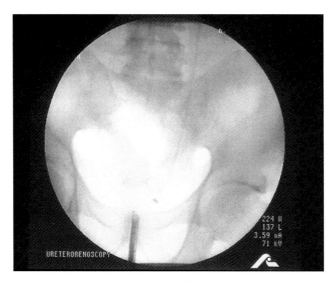

Figure 27.5. *Radiograph of stent with bead after insertion. The metallic band at the end of the pusher indicates the bladder neck.*

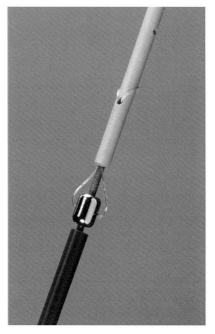

Figure 27.6. *Bead, between pusher and stent, is loaded onto the guidewire in preparation for insertion.*

successful in 29 of 30 patients, the single failure caused by a huge prostate with a large median lobe (Fig. 27.7).

In thin patients and most females an audible connecting 'click' was heard when the magnet and bead connected. An audio amplification system attached to the end of the catheter was used in some patients to confirm magnetic connection with the bead at the end of the stent. This concept is currently under development for pediatric patients.

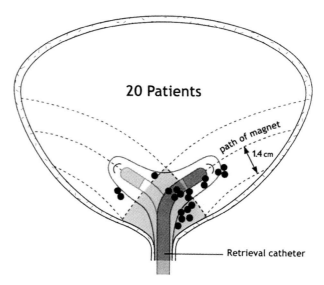

Figure 27.7. *Position of 20 successive left-sided stents with beads showing the 1.4 cm distance of attractivity on either side of the path of the magnet when inserted for a left stent and when rotated to capture a stent, which is longer than optimal. From Taylor W, McDougall I. Minimally invasive ureteric stent retrieval. J Urol 2002; 168: 2020–2023. Reproduced with permission from Lippincott, Williams & Wilkins.*

Conclusions

It remains pertinent and in the best interest of the patient to remove a stent without the need of anesthesia or intravenous sedation. An improved magnet retrieval system has been developed and provides a method to remove a stent in the outpatient setting with topical anesthesia. This device is minimally invasive, cost-efficient and very acceptable to the patient. Refinement of the magnetic retrieval system for pediatric use is under development and shows promise.

References

1. Blandy J, Fowler C. Removal of ureteric stents with a flexible cystoscope. Br Med Bull 1986; 42: 279–283
2. Evans J, Ralph D. Removal of ureteric stents with a flexible cystoscope. Br J Urol 1991; 67: 109
3. Smith A. Retrieval of ureteric stents. Urol Clin North Am 1982; 9: 109–112
4. Denstedt J, Wollin T, Sofer M, Nott L, Weir M, Honey J. A prospective randomized controlled trial comparing nonstented versus stented ureteroscopic lithotripsy. J Urol 2001; 165: 1419–1422
5. Hosking D, McColm S, Smith W. Is stenting following removal of distal ureteral calculi necessary? J Urol 1999; 161: 48
6. Borboroglu P, Amling C, Shenkman N S et al. Ureteral stenting after ureterorenoscopy for distal ureteral calculi: a multi-

institutional prospective randomized controlled study assessing pain, outcomes and complications. J Urol 2001; 166: 1651–1657

7. Siegel A, Altadonna V, Ellis D, Hulbert W, Elder J, Duckett J. Simplified method of indwelling ureteral stent removal. J Urol 1986; 28(5): 429

8. Naitoh J, Patel A, Fuchs G. A simplified method of ureteral stent removal using waterless rigid urethroscopy. J Urol 1997; 158: 2225–2226

9. Wetton C, Gedroyc W. Retrograde radiological retrieval and replacement of double-J ureteric stents. Clin Radiol 1995; 50: 563–565

10. Harding J. Fluoroscopically guided retrograde ureteric stent retrieval and replacement. Clin Radiol 1998; 53(7): 542

11. Alvaraz-Vijande R. Removal of ureteric stents in women without cystoscope. Br J Urol 1993; 72: 388–389

12. Yu D-S, Yang T-H, Ma C-P. Snail-headed catheter retriever: a simple way to remove catheters from female patients. J Urol 1995; 154: 167–168

13. Macaluso J, Deutsch J, Goodman J, Appell R, Prats L, Wahl P. The use of the Magnetip double-J ureteral stent in urological practice. J Urol 1989; 142: 701–703

14. Mykulak D, Herskowitz M, Glassberg K. Use of magnetic internal ureteral stents in pediatric urology: retrieval without routine requirement for cystoscopy and general anesthesia. J Urol 1994; 152: 976–977

15. Olweny E, Landman J, Andreoni C et al. Evaluation of the use of a biodegradable ureteral stent after retrograde endopyelotomy in a porcine model. J Urol 2002; 167: 2198–2202

16. Taylor W, McDougall I. Minimally invasive ureteric stent retrieval. J Urol 2002; 168: 2020–2023

28

Endo-urological evaluation and management of the 'forgotten' indwelling ureteral stent

R. J. Leveillee

Introduction

For over 30 years, ureteral catheters have been used to splint the urinary tract.[1,2] Their use has revolutionized the treatment of many disease processes affecting the upper urinary tract. However, with time, urologists and interventional radiologists have noted several complications associated with their use including bleeding, stone formation, uretero-arterial fistula formation, knotting, fracture and discomfort.[3–10] Problems pertaining to patient comfort, ease of insertion, and infection potential are addressed elsewhere in this textbook and are not elaborated on here. In this chapter, issues related to complications arising from chronic indwelling stents including the management of the forgotten, calcified, encrusted, or broken stent, are addressed.

The information contained herein should be both informative and useful, not only to the urologist in training but also to the practising urologist. The problems associated with patients harbouring a 'forgotten' stent can be frustrating. Several issues are discussed below, including:

- The recommended length of indwelling time for ureteral stents;
- Patients that are at risk for developing encrustation;
- The stents that are more prone to breakage;
- How to follow-up on stented patients;
- The best approach for removing complicated stents.

Recommended length of indwelling time

The recommended length of indwelling time is basically related to the material used and the milieu of the patient. In general, most manufacturers recommend that indwelling stents be exchanged at least every 3–6 months,[11] although some authors recommend that they be removed 'after serving their purpose', i.e. 6–8 weeks when wound healing is complete.[12] The first ureteral indwelling stents were made of silicone rubber;[1,13] however, owing to the high degree of 'friction'

associated with this material, other biocompatible materials were developed and instituted. These materials include polyurethane, polyethylene, C-Flex® (Concept Polymer Technologies, Inc., Clearater, FL, USA), Sof-Flex® (Cook Urological, Inc., Spencer, IN, USA), Percuflex™ (Boston Scientific Corporation, Microvasive, Medi-tech, Inc., Watertown, MA, USA), and Silitek™ (Medical Engineering Corporation, Racine, WI, USA).[11] These materials demonstrate a combination of biocompatibilty and biodurability commensurate with their intended use. They are all essentially giant molecules formed by polymerization of thousands of chemical monomers. They vary somewhat from each other in their specific co-linked molecules, which give each material specific physical properties. For those interested further, an excellent review is provided by Mardis et al.[11] Biodurability can be defined as the ability of the stent material (polymer) to resist absorption of biomolecules (proteins) on the surface, cellular interactions, encrustation, and surface penetration by chemicals within the urine. All of these can lead to degradation of the polymer and ultimately result in loss of critical physical characteristics, such as strength, flexibility and elasticity.

El-Faqih et al.[14] and Mardis and Kroeger[15] have described spontaneous breakage of polyethylene and polyurethane stents after several months (13–24 weeks). Mardis et al.[11] point out that clinical reports and device retrieval studies have shown that 'C-Flex® and Percuflex™ will not degrade significantly for as long as 2 years',[16,17] and, in fact, silicone rubber will retain most of its physical characteristics for up to 10 years. Encrustation, therefore, remains the most important limiting factor for prolonged stent function. All stents must be monitored for position and function at least every 3 months. It is well known that urine drains around indwelling stents as well as through them.[11] As discussed below, those patients with a history of urolithiasis (and especially those known to form stones rapidly on indwelling stents) should be evaluated and/or have their stents changed more frequently.

Patients at risk for developing encrustation

Hundreds of thousands of indwelling ureteral stents are placed annually worldwide, with relatively few serious complications. There are certain patients who anecdotally seem to be at increased risk for encrustation, although there has been relatively little experimental evidence to quantify this. It is generally believed that those patients with a lithogenic history are at increased risk for encrustation and subsequently for massive stone formation.[3,12,14,18] There is controversy as to whether infection plays a greater role than pre-existing metabolic abnormalities such as hypercalciuria or cysteinuria.[3,18–20] Encrustation, often associated with alkaline or infected urine, demonstrates a predominance of struvite and calcium phosphate deposits.[18–20] Encrustation by urinary mucoids and crystalloids is unpredictable. After a stent is placed, mucoproteins adhere to form a biofilm on the stent surface.[21–22] Progressive encrustation occurs in proportion to the degree of supersaturation in the urine. Infected urine, especially urine containing urea-splitting bacteria, can produce encrustation rapidly.[23] The author does not advocate the long-term use of prophylactic antibiotics to prevent encrustation, as some authors have done.[3,16] Choong and Whitfield[24] recently developed an ex vivo model utilizing various polymers percolated with fresh human urine at 0.5ml/min for 5 days at body temperature and pH. They measured calcium deposits by atomic absorption spectroscopy and were able to quantify encrustation indices of various compounds. Perhaps with more basic research such as this it will be possible to identify encrustation risk factors accurately and to minimize or eliminate them.

Stents that are more prone to breakage

It seems that the polyurethane stents and their copolymers have physical properties yielding greater tensile strength than silicone ones.[11] Albala notes that polyurethane stents are four times less likely to break than silicone stents but that microscopic 'irregularities can predispose them to encrustation'.[18,22] Once stents become encrusted they can become brittle; no material, therefore, is completely resistant to breakage. There are scattered reports in the literature confirming that,

during clinical use, both polyurethane and silicone stents will fracture.[23,25–27]

How to follow-up on stented patients

Although patient compliance cannot always be ensured, there are a few factors that may aid the practising urologist with regard to follow-up. In the author's institution it is routine practice to inform patients verbally and in writing that they are harbouring a temporary foreign body, which eventually must be removed/exchanged. Some commercially available stents (Boston Scientific Corporation, Microvasive, Medi-tech, Inc., Watertown, MA, USA) provide product identification stickers (much like those seen with implantable prostheses or cardiac pacemakers, including the device name, lot number, etc.) within the stent packaging material. These identification stickers are placed within the patient's hospital chart alongside the hand-written operative report, to become part of the permanent record. In addition, a generic wallet sized patient information card listing the physician, clinic/office phone number, date of insertion, follow-up, and scheduled removal date, are given to each patient at the time of discharge. At the author's institution, because of the cosmopolitan nature of the patient population, a locally produced card is provided, imprinted with the hospital name, appropriate contact phone numbers, date of scheduled removal, etc., in the patient's native language (Fig. 28.1). An alternative suggestion would be to provide a 'Stent Log Book' with demographics and appropriate follow-up listed.[25,28] This would then need to be checked on a monthly basis and patient contact provided. A computer database or scheduling sosftware would serve the same purpose (see also Chapter 37).

Best approach for removing complicated stents

Management of a retained stent is problematic and may require several ancillary procedures.[4,12] The method chosen is related in some degree to the overall stone burden as initially determined by plain radiography. Such methods include chemolysis, extracorporeal shock wave lithotripsy (ESWL), endoscopic cystolithalopaxy,

UM/JMH Department of Urology

Mr., Mrs., Ms. _____

**You have a plastic tube draining your
(Left Right Both) kidney(s).
It is important that you keep your appointment
on _____ to see the doctor. If you miss your
appointment, please call 585-5468 on Thursdays
only to reschedule your appointment.**

UM/JMH Departamento de Urología

Sr., Sra., Srta. _____

**Usted tiene un tubo plástico drenando su(s)
riñón(es)   (Izquierdo Derecho Ambos)
Es muy importante que no pierda su cita con el
médico el día _____. Si Ud. no puede asistir
a su turno, favor de llamar al 585-5468 los
jueves solamente y pedir un nuevo turno.**

Figure 28.1. Example of the wallet-sized card given to each patient who has placement of an indwelling stent at the author's hospital. Because of the cosmopolitan nature of the clientele, the card is written in the patients' native language to assist with compliance of follow-up. Key information imprinted on the card includes the following: hospital name; explanation that stent is temporary; date of insertion; key contact person(s) and telephone number(s); scheduled date of removal.

ureteroscopy, percutaneous nephrostolithotomy (PCNL), open surgery, and nephrectomy.[18,19,23,29–33]

There are basically three issues to consider when faced with the difficult question of managing the patient with the 'forgotten' stent. The first of the three major issues under consideration is whether the stent itself is encrusted or occluded. The second major issue pertains to overall stone burden in the bladder, kidney or ureter, and the last (and probably most important issue) is whether the affected renal unit retains any function. This discussion concentrates on those stents that have been indwelling for at least 6 months. Andriole et al.[34] have demonstrated a 10% incidence of obstruction due to encrustation in a series of 87 non-stone formers with a minimum of 2 months indwelling time. This rose to 47.5% between 6 and 12 weeks and was as high as 76.3% when stents were left indwelling for longer than 12 weeks![14]

Regarding encrustation/occlusion, it is generally accepted by most authorities that drainage of urine occurs both through the lumen of the stent and also by peristalsis around the stent. A functional study, either an intravenous urogram (IVU) or renal scintigram when combined with a plain abdominal film (KUB), is essential to determine the degree of encrustation, stone burden, and overall renal function of the affected kidney. An IVU is preferred over renal scintigraphy because it provides superior anatomical information (Fig. 28.2).

If no calcifications are noted and the stent does not appear to be fractured, then cystoscopic removal can be attempted. It is advisable to perform this under fluoroscopic imaging as often the proximal (renal) coil

will not unfurl. If it is noted that the encrusted stent is able to straighten, then gentle traction utilizing non-locking alligator-type grasping forceps can be tried. On the basis of the appearance of the vesical portion of the stent, it is also possible to predict the likelihood of successfully removing it without ancillary procedures (Fig. 28.3). Any vigorous pulling can result in stent fracture, ureteral or renal pelvis laceration, mucosal intussuception or, worst of all, ureteral avulsion. This would indeed be a surgical emergency!

When sizable stones are present, then the decision regarding management will be made according to the overall size, location, and number of calcifications. In the words of Abraham Maslow, 'If the only tool you have is a hammer... then you tend to see every problem as a nail'. A non-functioning or poorly functioning renal unit can occasionally be best managed by nephrectomy.[18] Somers advocates open procedures for those stents with more than 3 mm encrustation along the entire length.[29] Rembrink and Goepel have reported the case of an 81-year-old man with a multifractured stent who required both endoscopic and open techniques to clear the renal pelvis, ureter and bladder.[23] In almost all instances, minimally invasive endo-urological techniques can be utilized to remove the entire calcified stent under a single anaesthetic, thus relegating open surgery to the very rare instance.[19] Several authors have successfully utilized ESWL initially to manage calcified stents.[30–32,35] Many times, however, adjunctive measures such as electrohydraulic cysto-lithalopaxy are necessary to free the vesical end of the

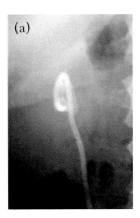

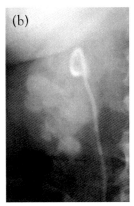

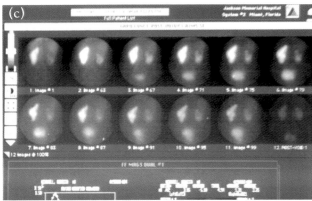

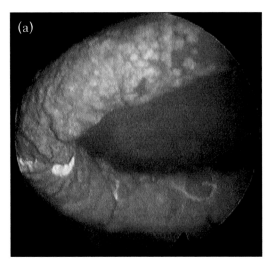

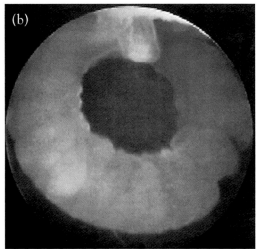

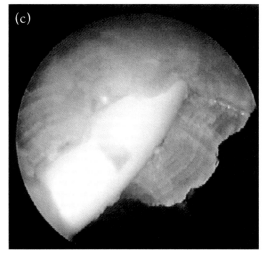

Figure 28.2. *(a) Scout film from intravenous urogram (IVU) demonstrating calcification involving proximal end of stent that had been in place for more than 24 months; (b) 60-minute close-up of the same patient as in (a), revealing the precise location of the stone and stent (i.e. upper pole calyx); this information is invaluable in planning a surgical approach; (c) a renal scintigram on the same patient reveals compromised function of the affected kidney due to the occlusive encrusted stents. No anatomical information can be gleaned from this study but it allows for accurate preoperative prediction of return of function. This is often helpful during patient counselling.*

Figure 28.3. *Cystoscopic view of a lightly encrusted stent on the left (a); compare with one that has a relatively thick coating (b) on its vesical portion. Simple extraction under fluoroscopic control could be attempted for the encrusted stent in (a); however, if the proximal end did not unfurl, then adjunctive measures would be necessary. (c) Note the overall thickness and laminations seen on stents (b) once electrohydraulic lithotripsy has cracked the outer shell.*

stent, making one-stage removal not possible.[18,31] In cases where the proximal end is so encrusted that it will not unfurl and/or there is a significant stone burden in the bladder, ureter or kidney precluding ESWL treatment the following procedure is currently favoured.

Surgical technique

Patients are evaluated preoperatively with standard blood chemistry assessments and must have sterile urine cultures. For those with infection (struvite) stones, antibiotic sensitivities are obtained from urine cultures and they receive at least 72 hours of appropriate oral antibiotics. Blood is made available at the blood bank, although transfusion is rarely necessary. Reported transfusion rates are between 3% and 11%.[36,37] General anaesthesia is given and patients are initially placed on the operating table in the dorsal lithotomy position. All endoscopic management takes place under videomonitoring and fluoroscopic control. Initially, after thorough bladder inspection, a floppy tipped (0.035 inch Bentsen type; Cook Urological, Spencer, IN, USA) or angled (0.035 inch Terumo Glide Wire; 44-1, 2-chrome, Hatagaya, Shibuya-ku, Tokyo 151, Japan) guidewire is placed alongside the calcified stent and negotiated retrograde to the kidney. Cystolithalopaxy can then be accomplished with any available intracorporeal lithotriptor. The author has successfully used electrohydraulic (EHL), ultrasonic (US) (Karl Storz, Culver City, CA, USA), pneumatic impaction (PI) (EMS Swiss Lithoclast, Boston Scientific/ Microvasive, Watertown, MA, USA; Calcusplit, Karl Storz) and laser lithotripsy (Holmium YAG-Versapulse; Coherent Medical Group, Palo Alto, CA, USA), each of which has certain advantages and disadvantages. The ultrasonic probe has the advantage of aspirating the stone fragments atraumatically and rapidly. It can also be used in the bladder. This technique is generally reserved for female patients utilizing the 24 Fr (8 mm) diameter rigid 'nephroscope', which can easily be placed transurethrally (see Fig. 28.4). The laser has several advantages, including the fact that it causes no bleeding and can be used to cut the intravesical end of the stent without the need to insert endoscopic scissors. Care must be taken not to cut the guidewire with the laser fibre, as has been reported.[38] Stone fragments are then evacuated with an Ellik evacuator or comparable device. The bladder

portion of the stent can then be excised using endoscopic scissors, although this is not a mandatory step. If significant calcifications exist along the ureteral portion of the stent, then a retrograde ureteroscopy along the stent with laser lithotripsy would be the next best step.

If direct access to the renal pelvis is required the previously placed guidewire is then replaced with an open-ended ureteral catheter. The bladder is drained with a Foley catheter and the patient is placed prone on the operating table on chest rolls in preparation for renal access, tract dilatation and percutaneous nephrolithotripsy.[39–41] In some cases, access may have been obtained previously following sepsis or high-grade obstruction. For those who do not obtain their own access, the assistance of an interventional radiologist is essential. In the author's institution, access is usually obtained by the urologist. Once the tract has been dilated and a working sheath has been placed, then stones are then removed from the renal portion of the

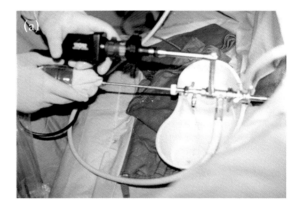

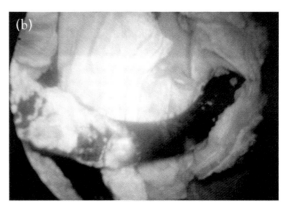

Figure 28.4. (a) Ultrasonic lithotriptor being placed transurethrally in a female patient via the 24 Fr (8 mm) rigid 'nephroscope'. This device has the advantage of aspiration of stone fragments atraumatically during cystolithalopaxy. (b) Endoscopic view of the retained calcified stent during ultrasonic cystolithalopaxy.

stent using various intracorporeal lithotriptors (e.g. EHL, US, PI, laser). The stent is then grasped with the rigid stone-removal forceps and withdrawn via the percutaneous nephrostomy tract.

Usually, gentle traction is all that is required; however, in some instances the stent will still resist removal. This is usually due to significant calciferous deposits along the midportion of the stent. An antegrade approach via the nephrostomy tract utilizing a flexible cystoscope or ureteroscope and laser fibre can then be performed. Visualization is facilitated utilizing a hand-pump syringe attached to the irrigation port of the flexible scope to flush small debris forward towards the bladder. The choice of the approach, whether retrograde or antegrade, depends on the stone location and the experience of the operator (Fig. 28.5). Large stone fragments can be removed with a standard four-wire ureteral stone basket. At this point the stent is usually sufficiently pliable to

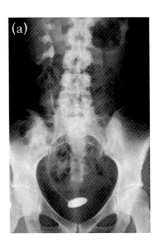

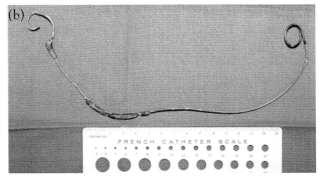

Figure 28.5. (a) Scout film of the abdomen, demonstrating large stone burden in the kidney as well as in the bladder. This patient was treated successfully utilizing a combined cystoscopic and percutaneous nephroscopic approach. (b) Note the amount of calcification along the ureteral portions that were not as obvious on the abdominal film.

allow retrograde removal. Once the stent has been removed via the nephrostomy tract and all the stone burden has been removed from the kidney, then a 22 Fr Council-tipped catheter and a 5 Fr ureteral 'safety' catheter are replaced. A nephrostogram is then performed at 48 hours and any adjunctive stone-removal procedures can then be planned.[36] Teichman et al.[19] have successfully treated 11 patients with 12 ureteral stents and large stone burdens left indwelling over 12 months. Eleven of the 12 stents (92%) were removed successfully under one anaesthetic, utilizing the technique described above. No patient required a blood transfusion, developed a postoperative urinary tract infection, or needed prolonged urinary drainage once the nephrostomy tube had been removed. The decision as to whether to leave a ureteral stent in place to prevent stricture formation is a difficult one to make, as these patients have already demonstrated poor compliance and lack of follow-up. In general, unless the ureter has been severely traumatized, once the stent and stones have been eradicated an indwelling long-term stent is not placed. It is important to document on follow-up, however, that no strictures have developed, by performing an IVU or renal scan. Stricture formation does occur, as noted in Figure 28.6. This particular patient was managed successfully with percutaneous endopyelotomy.

Conclusions

Bypassing obstructions within the urinary tract is a common function performed ubiquitously by urologists around the world. The advent of the indwelling ureteral stent has changed the way that many obstructive problems are handled by urologists and radiologists alike. Stents themselves, when left indwelling too long, are prone to complications of their own such as occlusion, encrustation and breakage. Endo-urological techniques have taken the management of many of these problems away from the open theatre and have replaced them with minimally invasive procedures. Total endoscopic management of the encrusted stent accomplishes safe, effective management of stone and stent, often under a single anaesthetic. Urologists may wish to consider this approach as an alternative to ESWL or open surgery when dealing with the complicated 'forgotten' stent associated with a large stone burden.

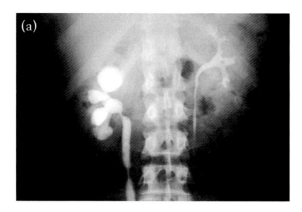

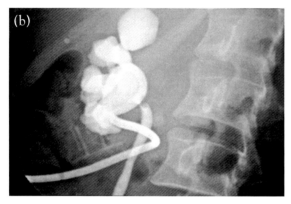

Figure 28.6. *(a) Preoperative intravenous urogram in a young woman with 24-month indwelling right ureteral stent. Note significant narrowing at ureteropelvic junction (UPJ). This patient is at great risk of forming a stricture following stent removal. (b) Postoperative nephrostogram demonstrating tight stricture at the UPJ. This patient was managed initially by a 22 Fr malecot nephro-ureteral re-entry catheter (Boston Scientific /Microvasive, Watertown, MA, USA) for 4 weeks. This was then changed to a pigtail catheter, which remained for an additional 2 weeks prior to this study. Ultimately she required antegrade percutaneous endopyelotomy.*

References

1. Zimskind P D, Fetter T R, Wilkerson J L. Clinical use of long-term indwelling silicone rubber ureteral splints inserted cystoscopically. J Urol 1967; 97: 840–844

2. Finney R P. Experience with new double J ureteral catheter stent. J Urol 1978; 120: 678–681

3. Shultze K A, Wettlaufer J N, Oldani G. Encrustation and stone formation; complication of indwelling ureteral stent. Urology 1985; 25(6): 616–619

4. Abber J C, Kahn R I. Pyelonephritis from severe incrustations on silicone ureteral stents: management. J Urol 1985; 130: 763–764

5. Lalude A O, Concry R M. Vascular complication of percutaneously placed pigtail ureteral stent. J Urol 1983; 130: 553–554

6. Bregg K, Riehle R A Jr. Morbidity associated with indwelling internal ureteral stents after shock wave lithotripsy. J Urol 1989; 141: 510-512

7. Toolin E, Pollack H M, McLean G K et al. Ureteroarterial fistula: a case report. J Urol 1984; 132: 553–554

8. Adams P S Jr. Iliac artery–ureteral fistula development after dilatation and stent placement. Radiology 1984; 153: 647–648

9. Flam T A, Thiounn N, Gerbaud P F et al. Knotting of a double pigtail stent within the ureter: an initial report. J Urol 1995; 154:1858–1859

10. Prashant K, Manish B, Pattnick P K. Knotted upper end: a new complication in the use of an indwelling ureteral stent. J Urol 1994; 151: 995–996

11. Mardis H K, Kroeger R M, Morton J J et al. Comparative evaluation of materials used for internal ureteral stents. J Endourol 1993; 7(2): 105–115

12. Spirnak J P, Resnick M I. Stone formation as a complication of indwelling ureteral stents: a report of 5 cases. J Urol 1985; 134: 349–351

13. Davis D M. Use of silicone rubber in urology. J Urol 1967, 97: 845

14. El-Faqih S R, Shamsuddin A, Chakrabarti A et al. Polyurethane internal ureteral stents in treatment of stone patients: morbidity related to indwelling times. J Urol 1991; 146:1487–1491

15. Mardis H K, Kroeger R M. Ureteral stents: materials. Urol Clin North Am 1988; 15 (3): 471–479

16. Cardella J F, Cateneda-Zuniga W R, Hunter D W et al. Urine compatible polymer for long-term ureteral stenting, Radiology 1986; 1612: 313–318

17. Rackson M E, Mitty H A, Lossef S V, et al. Biocompatible copolymer ureteral stent: maintenance of patency beyond six months. AJR 1989; 153: 783–784

18. Monga M, Klein E, Casteneda-Zuniga W S et al. The forgotten ureteral stent: a urological dilemma. J Urol 1995; 153: 1817–1819

19. Teichman J M, Lackner J E, Leveillee R J et al. Total endoscopic management of the encrusted ureteral stent under a single anaesthetic. Can J Urol 1997; 4 (4): 456–459

20. Kohri K, Yamate T, Amasaki N et al. Characteristics and usage of different ureteral stent catheters. Urol Int 1991; 4 (7):131–137

21. Reid G, Denstedt J D, Kang Y S et al. Microbial adhesion and biofilm formation on ureteral stents in vitro and in vivo. J Urol 1992; 148: 1592–1594

22. Albala D M. Complications of ureteral stents associated with extracorporeal shock wave lithotripsy. In: Smith A D (ed) Controversies of endourology. Philadelphia: W. B. Saunders, 1995: 177–178

23. Rembrink K, Goepel M. The forgotten double J stent. Case report of a multifractured ureter stent. J Urol 1992; 49(2): 119–120

24. Choong S, Whitfield H. A new standard for encrustation quantification on stents, catheters and polymers. J Endourol 1996; 10 (Suppl 1): S 57 (abstr BR1–10)

25. Ilker Y, Turkeri L, Dillioglugil O et al. Spontaneous fracture of indwelling ureteral stents in patients treated with extracorporeal shock wave lithotripsy: two case reports. Int Urol Nephrol 1996; 28 (1): 15–19

26. Benchekroun A, Chefchaouni M C, Marzouk M et al. Les complications rares des sondes urétérales double J. Ann Urol (Paris) 1995; 29(3): 163-166.

27. Witjes J A. Breakage of a silicone double pigtail ureteral stent as a long-term complication. J Urol 1993; 150(6): 1898–1899

28. Finney R P. Editorial comment in Spirnak JP Resnick MI. Stone formation as a complication of indwelling ureteral stents: a report of 5 cases. J Urol 1985; 134: 351

29. Somers W J. Management of forgotten or retained indwelling ureteral stents. Urology 1996; 47: 431–435

30. Cass A B, Kavaney P, Levine L et. al. Extracorporeal shock wave lithotripsy of calcified ureteral stent. J Endourol 1993; 7: 7–10

31. Lupu A N, Fuchs G J, Chaussy C G. Calcification of ureteral stent treated by extracorporeal shock wave lithotripsy. J Urol 1986; 136: 1297–1298

32. Cass A B, Kavaney P B, Smith C L. Multiple cysteine stone formations on an indwelling ureteral stent treated by extracorporeal shock wave lithotripsy. J Urol 1992; 147: 1076

33. LeRoy A J, Williams H J Jr, Segura J W et. al. Indwelling ureteral stents: percutaneous management of complications. Radiology 1986; 158: 219-222

34. Andriole G L, Bettmann M A, Garnick M B et al. Indwelling Double-J stents for temporary and permanent urinary drainage; experience with 87 patients. J Urol 1984; 131: 239–241

35. Smet G, Vandeursen H, Baert L. Extracorporeal shock wave lithotripsy for calcified ureteral catheter. Urol Int 1991; 46: 211–212

36. Segura J W, Preminger G M, Assimos D G et al. Nephrolithiaisis Clinical Guidelines Panel summary report on the management of staghorn renal calculi. The American Urological Association Nephrolithiasis Clinical Guidelines Panel. J Urol 1994; 151: 1648–1651

37. Segura J M, Patterson D E, LeRoy A J et al. Percutaneous removal of kidney stones: review of 1000 cases. J Urol 1985; 134: 1077–108l

38. Grasso M. Experience with the Holmium laser as an endoscopic lithotrite. Urology 1996; 48: 199–206

39. Reddy P K, Hulbert J C, Lange P H et al. Percutaneous removal of renal and ureteral calculi: experience with 400 cases. J Urol 1985; 134: 662–665

40. Casteneda-Zuniga W R. Establishing access: the percutaneous nephrostomy. In: Clayman RV, Casteneda-Zulliga WR (eds) Techniques in endourology: a guide to percutaneous removal of renal and ureteral calculi. Chicago: Year Book Medical, 1984: 73

41. Clayman R V, Castaneda-Zugina W R, Hunter D W et al. Rapid balloon dilatation of the nephrostomy tract for nephrostolithotomy, Radiology 1983; 147: 884–885

29

UPJ stenosis:
is surgery better than the endoscopic approach?
H. P. Beerlage and J. J. M. C. H. de la Rosette

Introduction

Since the first operative repair of ureteropelvic junction (UPJ) obstruction was described by Trendelenburg in 1886, a variety of surgical procedures have been developed, such as the advancement procedure (V–Y plasty) and the pelvic flap procedure. In 1949, Anderson and Hynes[1] described open dismembered pyeloplasty in a case of retrocaval ureter. In the following decades the 'Anderson–Hynes pyeloplasty' became the gold standard in the treatment of UPJ obstruction. It is considered a safe procedure with no major pitfalls and, although failures do occur, even many years after the operation,[2] in general the results are excellent.

Albarran[3] in 1903 performed the first open incision and stenting of the ureter, which was popularized by Davis et al.[4,5] in the 1940s and became known as the 'Davis intubation'. This was, however, still an open operation and it was not until decades later that an endoscopic technique became available.

Whereas, 50 years ago, transurethral resection of the prostate was the only endoscopic and minimally invasive operation replacing an open procedure (open prostatectomy), subsequently, as a result of major technical improvements in endoscopic equipment, more and more minimally invasive procedures started replacing open surgical procedures. In the 1970s, with the introduction of ureteroscopy a major breakthrough started in the treatment of ureteral stones and neoplasms; together with extracorporeal shock-wave lithotripsy, this procedure reduced the ureterolithotomy to the status of a historical operation that is very rarely performed nowadays. Diagnostic procedures of the ureter and renal pelvis, as well as stenting of the upper urinary tract, became routine procedures. In the 1980s, laparoscopy was added to the armamentarium of the urologist. Although laparoscopic operations take time to master, the advantages are obvious: smaller incisions significantly reduce the amount of intra- and postoperative pain medication required, only a very short hospital stay is necessary and convalescence time is markedly reduced, so normal daily activities and work can be resumed much earlier (Table 29.1).

Although the Anderson–Hynes pyeloplasty is an easy operation to perform, with good results, a (relatively large) flank incision is needed for performing the operation safely. In view of the above-mentioned developments in the field of minimal invasive therapy, it is not surprising that efforts have been made to replace the Anderson–Hynes pyeloplasty by less invasive procedures. In this chapter the pros and cons of the various endopyelotomy techniques and of the laparoscopic pyeloplasty are discussed, to ascertain whether there is still a place for open pyeloplasty.

Endoscopic treatment of ureteropelvic junction obstruction

Anatomical considerations

Before embarking on endopyelotomy the urologist should be informed about the exact anatomy of the

Table 29.1. *Characteristics of procedures*

Procedure	Operating time (minutes)	Postoperative stay (days)	Return to normal activities (days)
Open pyeloplasty (25 series)[26]	100	10	41.5
Endopyelotomy (antegrade)[7]	100	6.7	?
Endopyelotomy (antegrade)[9]	90	6.2	19.8
Balloon dilatation (retrograde)[18]	30	?	<21
Acucise[19]	60	1.6	?
Laparoscopic pyeloplasty[22]	270	3.5	21

operative field in order to avoid serious intraoperative problems and to prevent renal malfunction in the long term.

The first major concern is the vascular anatomical relationship to the UPJ in general and especially where there are aberrant lower-pole vessels that may cause the UPJ obstruction. Since the endopyelotomy should be performed through the stenotic wall into the periureteral fat, serious problems are to be expected in cases where there is a close relationship between a vessel and the UPJ. The aberrant vessel can be detected on angiography, spiral CT or with endoluminal ultrasonography.[6] It should also be mentioned that, in the study of Van Cangh et al.,[7] endopyelotomy was successful in no more than 42% of patients with aberrant lower-pole vessels. Sampaio and Favorito[8] studied the vascular anatomical relationship to the UPJ extensively in 146 kidneys in an autopsy study. They found a close relationship between a prominent vessel and the anterior surface of the UPJ in 65.1% of cases and in 6.2% they found a close relationship with the posterior surface. They demonstrated that the lateral wall of the UPJ is avascular and incisions are best made there.

In cases of severe hydronephrosis the pelvic wall is redundant and in open pyeloplasty the pelvic wall can be partially resected, thus creating a relatively normal renal pelvis. With an endopyelotomy this is, of course, not possible and although the obstruction has disappeared a redundant renal pelvis remains, causing some degree of urinary stasis and possibly leading to infection and/or stone formation.

More rare causes of UPJ obstruction are ureteral valves and fibroepithelial polyps. The ureteral valves can be destroyed by endopyelotomy but, in cases of fibroepithelial polyps, this will usually not be sufficient and resection is mandatory. With careful preoperative radiological imaging these diagnoses can be made and appropriate action can be taken.

Antegrade (percutaneous) endopyelotomy

Percutaneous nephrostomy was initially used only for decompression of the renal pelvis. Later, the tract was dilated to such an extent that endoscopic operations through this tract became feasible. Percutaneous nephrolitholapaxy has become a very popular first-choice treatment in cases of large stones in the renal pelvis, almost completely replacing open pyelolithotomy. From 1983 on, the same approach has been used for endopyelotomy procedures.

The procedure should be performed under general anaesthesia. With the patient in the lithotomy position, a retrograde ureteral catheter or a guidewire is inserted and advanced through the UPJ. It is mandatory to pass the UPJ. When the renal pelvis cannot be entered, the procedure should be aborted and an open pyeloplasty should be performed. Then the patient is placed prone on the table and after puncture the tract is dilated until an Amplatz sheath can be placed in position. The UPJ can now be identified easily by the retrogradely inserted ureteral catheter or guidewire. Several approaches are then possible.

In the technique of Smith,[9] the open end of the ureteral catheter is grasped and pulled out through the nephrostomy tract and a guidewire is inserted through the ureteral catheter; the wire is brought out at the urethral meatus and the ureteral catheter is removed. The guidewire is now in position from the flank through the urethral meatus. Then, under fluoroscopic guidance, a 16 Fr fascial dilator is advanced down the UPJ and the endopyelotome with the cold knifeblade is positioned. A full-thickness incision is made in a posterolateral position into the periureteral fat; a 14/8.2 Fr endopyelotomy stent is then positioned. This stent remains in place for 6 weeks.

Van Cangh[10] advances a second guidewire followed by a ureteral catheter through the UPJ and then literally railroads the ureterotome knife over the two stents. After the deep incision, a 6–8 Fr double-J stent is positioned and a second 4 Fr stent is also inserted through the UPJ. The separate nephrostomy tube is removed after a few days and both stents are removed in the outpatient department 6 weeks later.

It is possible to perform an antegrade balloon dilatation, as was reported by Kadir et al.[11] in 1982 for the first time, but this procedure is usually performed retrogradely and therefore is discussed later.

Retrograde endopyelotomy

Endoscopic retrograde procedures of the ureter are, as a result of major improvements in the endoscopic equipment, nowadays routinely performed in general urological practice. Stenting of the ureter with either ureteral catheters or double-J stents is currently done very frequently. Diagnostic and therapeutic procedures are possible and safe using the sophisticated instruments available today. The UPJ obstruction provides an interesting challenge for those who try to minimize the trauma of operation and approach it retrogradely, thereby avoiding the creation of a percutaneous tract with its possible complications.

Retrograde balloon dilatation of UPJ obstruction was first reported by O'Flynn et al.[12] in 1990. The procedure is carried out under fluoroscopic control with the patient in the lithotomy position under general anaesthesia. First, a guidewire is retrogradely introduced into the ureter and advanced through the UPJ. Over the guidewire a 7.5 Fr Olbert balloon catheter is introduced and the balloon is placed across the stenotic segment under fluoroscopic control. The balloon is then inflated to a maximum diameter of 1 cm (30 Fr) until rupture of the stenotic segment is observed. A 10 Fr double-J stent is inserted and left in place for 6 weeks.

In 1993, Chandoke et al.[13] for the first time reported on a retrograde endopyelotomy for UPJ obstruction using the so-called Acucise catheter, which is a 7 Fr catheter with an electrosurgical cutting wire 2.8 cm long and 150 μu wide mounted on an 8 mm balloon. All patients have a 7 Fr ureteral stent placed at least 1 week before operation. The patient is in the lithotomy position under general anaesthesia and the procedure is carried out under fluroscopic control. A guidewire is retrogradely introduced into the ureter and advanced through the UPJ. Over the guidewire the Acucise device is introduced and advanced until the area of obstruction is reached by the balloon. The cutting wire is placed laterally and, while the balloon is inflating, the cutting wire is activated with 75–100 W pure cutting current. When contrast extravasation is noted, the balloon is deflated and removed. A 7/14 Fr indwelling endopyelotomy stent is then introduced and a urethral catheter is placed for 24 h to prevent reflux in the early postoperative period. If no contrast extravasation is noted after activation of the cutting wire, a flexible ureteroscope is passed to inspect the UPJ and incise it if necessary. The ureteral stent is removed 4–6 weeks after the procedure.

Laparoscopic pyeloplasty

Laparoscopy has only recently been added to the urologist's armamentarium. Many urological operations can be performed laparoscopically, such as varicocoele correction, pelvic lymph node dissection and even nephrectomy. However, in general urological practice no dramatic shift towards laparoscopy has yet been observed comparable, for instance, to cholecystectomy, an operation nowadays routinely performed laparoscopically.

When compared with dismembered pyeloplasty the overall success rate of endoscopic procedures for UPJ obstruction is 10–20% lower. In an effort to combine the good results of dismembered pyeloplasty with the minimal invasive nature of endopyelotomy, since 1993 laparoscopic dismembered pyeloplasty has been performed, as first reported by Schuessler et al.[14] and by Kavoussi and Peters.[15] The laparoscopy is performed under general anaesthesia and a 7 Fr double-J stent is inserted. The patient is then placed in the lateral position and after pneumoperitoneum has been achieved three or four trocars are placed. The colon is then mobilized, as for laparoscopic nephrectomy, and the procedure is then completed as in normal open dismembered pyeloplasty, keeping the double-J stent in place. The ureteral stent is usually removed after 6 weeks.

More recently, the retroperitoneoscopic approach was developed for urological procedures.[16] This approach for pyeloplasty was reported by Puppo et al.;[17] the operative technique is similar to the transperitoneal laparoscopic pyeloplasty once the operative field has been established.

Results

As the antegrade endopyelotomy technique has been performed from 1983 onwards, a relatively long term follow-up is now available. Motola et al.[9] reviewed a large series of endopyelotomies, with a follow-up of more than 6 months in 189 patients and of more than 3 years in 102 patients. Patients were followed with intravenous pyelogram (IVP) postoperatively. Renal scans with furosemide (frusemide) were performed only in cases in which IVP was not definitive or in cases of allergy to contrast material. Whitaker tests were used only in cases with equivocal findings on renal scan. The overall success rate was 86%, with no differences between primary and secondary cases. Most failures (24/27) occurred in the first 6 months after the procedure, with only 2 of 27 after 1 year. A few major complications were encountered, such as severe haemorrhage in 2 patients, one of whom required immediate open exploration. This may be related to the fact that in this series the incision was made in the posterolateral plane and not in the avascular lateral plane as described by Sampaio and Favorito.[8] In one patient a ureteral avulsion occurred, also requiring immediate open exploration. UPJ stenosis was seen in two patients early in the series but, after introduction of a special endopyelotomy stent, this problem no longer occurred. In one patient requiring open pyeloplasty after failed endopyelotomy, microscopic examination of the UPJ revealed a transitional cell carcinoma! This again shows the importance of meticulous preoperative work-up.

Van Cangh et al.[7] reviewed 102 cases of endopyelotomy with a mean follow-up of 5 years (range 1–10 years). In 67 patients a preoperative angiogram was performed and in 26 (39%) a vessel was documented crossing the ureteropelvic region. Postoperative investigational studies performed as mentioned above showed an overall success rate of 73%. However, in patients with a crossing vessel and severe hydronephrosis, the success rate was only 39%, whereas it was 95% when neither factor was present. In this report no complications were mentioned but, in an earlier report of 47 cases,[10] three instances of bleeding requiring blood transfusion (posterolateral incision !), 3 of hydrothorax, 2 of stent migration and 1 of sepsis were observed. All patients could be managed conservatively.

McClinton et al.[18] reported on a series of 49 retrograde balloon dilatations for UPJ obstruction. Follow-up ranged from 3 to 48 months with a mean of 18 months. All patients were evaluated by IVP and diuresis renography preoperatively, and by clinical review and diuresis renography postoperatively. Clinical improvement, i.e. relief of pain, occurred in 80% of all cases and in 85% of primary cases. Improvement on renography occurred in 33 of 42 (79%) evaluable cases. These results could be achieved with a 10 Fr double-pigtail catheter only. Apart from stent migration, no intra- or postoperative complications occurred.

Nadler et al.[19] reported on the long-term durability of the Acucise endopyelotomy in 28 cases with a mean follow-up of 32.5 months (range 24–42 months). Preoperatively patients were assessed with an IVP, diuretic renal scan, Whitaker test and/or retrograde pyelogram. Failure in the first year occurred in four patients. Subjective improvement was found in 75% of cases. After 2 years, the objective success rate determined by diuretic renal scan was 81%. In this group there were no major complications, (probably) owing to the fact that a lateral incision of the ureteropelvic junction was performed. One patient developed an ileus and haematuria that could be treated conservatively. No (distal) ureteral stenoses were reported.

Faerber et al.[20] also reported on the Acucise device in 36 cases with practically the same results as Nadler; however, the follow-up was shorter, with a mean of 14 months (range 3–28 months). In this series the incision was made posterolaterally which resulted in significant bleeding in two of 36 cases that could be treated conservatively. All failures occurred early in the follow-up, the latest 2 months after stent removal. Here, also, no distal ureteral stenoses were reported.

Meretyk et al.[21] in 1992 compared antegrade and retrograde endopyelotomy in a prospective study with a total of 41 cases with a mean follow-up of 19.5 months (range 2–39 months). The success rate was similar in both groups — about 80% — but after the ureteroscopic approach the need for analgesics was significantly higher; in addition, in 20% of cases a late ureteral stricture occurred, so the authors concluded that the antegrade route is the preferred approach for endopyelotomy. These problems were attributable to the technique used: a 12 Fr rigid ureteroscope or a smaller flexible ureteroscope was used but the flexible scope was always used in combination with a 14 Fr ureteral access sheath. In the later series[18–20] no (large) ureteroscopes were used and no ureteral strictures were noted for.

After the initial publications on laparoscopic dismembered pyeloplasty,[14,15] Moore et al.[22] reported on 30 cases. Patients were evaluated by IVP or diuretic renal scan pre- and postoperatively. The mean operating time was 4.5 h (range 2.25–8 h); a Y–V pyeloplasty was performed in four cases and dismembered pyeloplasty in the remaining cases. In three patients a reduction of a large redundant renal pelvis was accomplished. One intraoperative complication occurred when a colonic diverticulum was clipped, and excised with a gastro-intestinal anastomosis (GIA) stapling device. Patients were followed for 4–73 months (mean 16.3 months). Only one failure occurred and this was probably due to problems related to a suturing device not used in the other cases; this patient refused reoperation and, later in the follow-up, an IVP demonstrated a patent ureteropelvic junction!

Puppo et al.[17] reported on the retroperitoneal approach for laparoscopic pyeloplasty. In their initial series with 11 patients with symptomatic ureteropelvic obstruction they reported excellent results in those patients who had a laparoscopic approach. Since, in five cases, they had to convert to open surgery, it was concluded that technical refinements are still necessary.

Discussion

The need for open surgery in the treatment of UPJ stenosis as an initial procedure of choice is nowadays being questioned. To address the question whether surgery is better than the endoscopic approach, several elements need to be considered — patient selection, complications, morbidity, success rate and durability.

Open pyeloplasty is the 'gold standard' against which all other modalities for the correction of UPJ obstruction are compared. Many series have shown that, in adults with primary and secondary UPJ obstruction, rates of success for endopyelotomy range from 75 to 100%, approaching those of open pyeloplasty.[7,9,12,19,20] Although a UPJ obstruction is often diagnosed and treated in children, experience with endopyelotomy is limited and a clear role in the management of UPJ obstruction in children has yet to be defined. Recently, Rodrigues Netto et al.[23] reported their experience in a group of nine children and compared success and morbidity with that in a series of adults treated similarly. It was concluded that percutaneous endopyelotomy can be performed safely and successfully in children with primary UPJ obstruction. However, in secondary stenosis the results were less than optimal. It was recommended that open pyeloplasty should be considered to be the first choice in the treatment of children, given its high rate of success and minimal morbidity.

Besides selection by age, patients may also be selected on the basis of anatomical features and of earlier procedures. Van Cangh et al.[7] were among the first to try to define rules for case selection. They showed that massive hydronephrosis and the presence of a crossing vessel at the UPJ are associated with a high failure rate. However, the exact role of crossing vessels in obstruction and the success of endopyelotomy in the presence of crossing vessels are yet to be determined.[24]

Major perioperative complications following an endoscopic approach are limited to conversion to open surgery and bleeding. The need for conversion to open surgery is usually related to the learning curve or, in rare cases, to major bleeding. The latter is often caused by injury of a (crossing) vessel near the UPJ. Keeping the anatomical vascular relationship in mind will minimize the risk of vascular damage. Moreover, intraluminal ultrasound may be used to visualize the vascular pattern and to guide the treatment device.[6] When applying balloon dilatation only, without a cutting wire, the risk of major bleeding is minimal.[18] Long-term complications may consist of the formation of a arteriovenous fistula in the case of a percutaneous approach. On the other hand, retrograde endopyelotomy might damage the distal ureter. The first complication is rare while the second has been prevented by using small sized instruments only (Table 29.2).

The rate of morbidity of this procedure is favourable when compared with open surgery. Brooks et al.[25] reported on the comparison of open versus endo-urological approaches to the obstructed UPJ. These data confirm the assumption of a lower morbidity following an endo-urological procedure, reflected in reductions in the use of analgesics, in hospital stay and in recovery time. This decrease in morbidity should be seen in the light of successful relief of obstruction. Overall, open pyeloplasty is still considered to be the 'gold standard' in the treatment of UPJ obstruction. However, the currently available minimally invasive modalities offer success rates close to those of open surgery but with diminished morbidity.[7,9,12,19,20] If an endoscopic treatment fails, an open procedure can still be performed easily, without jeopardizing the outcome of that procedure. In an era in which cost effectiveness is becoming more and more important, this will eventually

Table 29.2. *Complications following procedures*

Procedure	Ref	Percentage of complications			
		Haemorrhage	Sepsis	Stricture	Reoperation
Open pyeloplasty (25 series)	26	0.5	0.6	2.4	2.2
Endopyelotomy (antegrade)	17	5	2	0	11.7
Endopyelotomy (antegrade)	9	1.1	0	1.1	12.7
Balloon dilatation (retrograde)	18	0	2.3	0	20.9
Acucise	19	3.6	0	0	14
Laparoscopic pyeloplasty	22	0	0	0	3.3

Table 29.3. *Durability of procedures to treat UPJ obstruction*

Procedure	Ref	No. of patients	Mean follow-up (months)	Success rate (%)
Open pyeloplasty (25 series)	26	2856	?	90
Endopyelotomy (antegrade)	7	102	60	73
Endopyelotomy (antegrade)	9	189	48	86
Balloon dilatation (retrograde)	18	43	18	80
Acucise	19	26	32.5	81
Laparoscopic pyeloplasty	22	30	16.3	97

also influence the choice of treatment. In view of the success rate of the endo-urological approaches at a lower morbidity, this is definitely an argument for these techniques.

Finally, durability is important and in close relationship to the success of treatment (Table 29.3). The initial results of most procedures treating the UPJ obstruction appeared to be favourable but one awaits long-term results and substantiation of the outcome by other investigators. The latter especially concerns the most recently introduced techniques, such as the Acucise and laparoscopic approaches. When recommending such a technique, the choice will be affected not only by the above mentioned arguments but also by the simplicity of the technique. After all, the major breakthrough is supported not only by a high rate of success at low morbidity but also by applicability in the hands of the general urologist. Consequently, sophisticated procedures that can be performed easily by 'experts' only will not gain general acceptance by the urological community.

References

1. Anderson J C, Hynes W. Retrocaval ureter; case diagnosed preoperatively and treated successfully by a plastic operation. Br J Urol 1949; 21: 209
2. Scardino P T , Scardino P L. Obstruction at the ureteropelvic junction. In: Bergman H (ed) The ureter. New York: Springer Verlag, 1981: 697–716
3. Albarran J. Operations plastiques et anastomoses dans la traitment des retentions de veim. University of Paris, 1903.
4. Davis D M. Intubated ureterotomy: a new operation for ureteral and uretreopelvic strictures. Surg Gynecol Obstet 1943; 76: 513
5. Davis D M, Strong M and Drake W M. Intubated ureterotomy: experimental work and clinical results. J Urol 1948; 56: 851
6. Bagley D H, Conlin M J, Liu J. Device for intraluminal incision guided by endoluminal ultrasonography. J Endourol 1996; 10: 421–423
7. Van Cangh P J, Wilmart J F, Opsomer R J et al. Long-term results and late recurrence after endoureteropyelotomy: a critical analysis of prognostic factors. J Urol 1994; 151: 934–937
8. Sampaio F J B, Favorito L A. Ureteropelvic junction stenosis: vascular anatomical background for endopyelotomy. J Urol 1993; 150: 1787–1791
9. Motola J A, Badlani G H , Smith A D. Results of 212 consecutive endopyelotomies: an 8-year followup. J Urol 1993; 149: 453–456
10. Van Cangh P J, Jorion J L, Wese F X, Opsomer R J. Endoureteropyelotomy: percutaneous treatment of ureteropelvic junction obstruction. J Urol 1989; 141: 1317–1322
11. Kadir S, White R I Jr, Engel R. Balloon dilatation of ureteropelvic junction obstruction. Radiology 1982; 143: 263–264

12. O'Flynn K J, Hehir M, McKelvie G. Endoballoon rupture and stenting for pelviureteric junction obstruction: technique and early results. Br J Urol 1990; 64: 572–574

13. Chandoke P S, Clayman R V, McDoughall E M et al. Endopyelotomy and endoureterotomy with the Acucise ureteral cutting balloon device: preliminary experience. J Endourol 1993; 7: 45

14. Schuessler W W, Grune M T, Tecuanhuey L V, Preminger G M. Laparoscopic dismembered pyeloplasty. J Urol 1993; 150: 1795–1799

15. Kavoussi L R, Peters G A. Laparoscopic pyeloplasty. J Urol 1993; 150: 1891–1894

16. Gaur D D. Laparoscopic operative retroperitoneoscopy. J Urol 1992; 148: 1137

17. Puppo P, Perachino M, Ricciotti G et al. Retroperitoneoscopic treatment of Ureteropelvic junction obstruction. Eur Urol 1997; 31: 204–208

18. McClinton S, Steyn J H, Hussy J K. Retrograde balloon dilatation for pelviureteric junction obstruction. Br J Urol 1993; 71: 152–155

19. Nadler R B, Rao G S, Pearle M S et al. Acucise endopyelotomy: assesment of long-term durability. J Urol 1996; 156: 1094–1098

20. Faerber G J, Richardson T D, Farah N, Ohl D A. Retrograde treatment of ureteropelvic junction obstruction using the ureteral cutting balloon catheter. J Urol 1997; 157: 454–458

21. Meretyk I, Meretyk S, Clayman R V. Endopyelotomy: Comparison of ureteroscopic retrograde and antegrade percutaneous techniques. J Urol 1992; 148: 775–783

22. Moore R G, Averch T D, Schulam P G et al. Laparoscopic pyeloplasty: experience with the initial 30 cases. J Urol 1997; 157: 459–462

23. Rodrigues Netto N Jr, Ikari O, Esteves S C, D'Ancona C A L. Antegrade endopyelotomy for pelvi-ureteric junction obstruction in children. Br J Urol 1996; 78: 607–612

24. Gupta M, Smith A D. Crossing vessels at the ureteropelvic junction: do they influence endopyelotomy outcome. J Endourol 1996; 10: 183

25. Brooks J D, Kavoussi L R, Preminger G M, et al. Comparison of open and endourologic approaches to the obstructed ureteropelvic junction. Urology, 1995; 46: 791–795.

26. Scardino P T, Scardino P L. Obstruction at the ureteropelvic junction. In: Bergman H (ed) The ureter. New York: Springer Verlag, 1981; 697–716

30

Stenting after antegrade and retrograde endopyelotomy
R. Marcovich and A. D. Smith

Introduction

The introduction of percutaneous and retrograde endoscopic techniques in the 1970s and 1980s revolutionized the management of adult ureteropelvic junction (UPJ) obstruction. Endopyelotomy follows directly from the demonstration by Davis and co-workers in the 1940s that a sub-circumferential excision of the ureteral wall will heal adequately over a splinting tube by regeneration of muscle and epithelium.[1,2] Davis' group demonstrated in a dog model that rapid, early epithelial proliferation was followed by a slower restoration of the muscular layer, with almost complete regrowth of muscle by 6 weeks after incision. They further emphasized that a full thickness incision of the ureter, a large-bore splinting tube, and the maintenance of sterile urine were required for this process to succeed.

In 1983, Wickham and Kellett were the first to report what they termed 'percutaneous pyeloplasty', in which the principles of Davis' intubated ureterotomy were applied via a percutaneous antegrade approach.[3] Shortly thereafter, Badlani and associates introduced the moniker 'endopyelotomy' in a paper describing their technique and early results with the procedure.[4] Since then a variety of approaches to minimally invasive ureteropelvic incision have been introduced, including retrograde endoscopic and cautery balloon endopyelotomy. All of the approaches rely on preservation of the ureteral blood supply by avoiding transection of the ureter, maintenance of the adipose tissue surrounding the renal pelvis and ureter to promote healing, and insertion of a stent of appropriate size to maintain luminal patency and divert the urinary stream.

This chapter describes the technique of antegrade endopyelotomy, discusses principles of appropriate patient selection, and briefly compares outcomes of the various incisional approaches. The recently introduced technique of 'endopyeloplasty' will be reviewed. The final portion of the chapter will update the reader on stenting after endopyelotomy, touching upon stent design, composition, size, and duration of stenting.

Patient selection

As with most surgical procedures, proper patient selection is a major determinant in the ultimate success of endopyelotomy. Motola and associates demonstrated that patient age, sex, site of obstruction, and prior surgery for ureteropelvic junction obstruction do not affect the long-term results.[5] However, ureteral stricture length greater than 2 cm risks a high rate of failure and its presence should be considered a contraindication to performance of an endopyelotomy.[5–7] A high insertion of the UPJ into the renal pelvis has also been proposed as a contraindication to the procedure, since the redundant portion cannot be excised to create a funnel.[6,7] However, Shalhav and co-workers have obtained reasonable results (70% objective success) with both antegrade and retrograde approaches in patients with high insertion,[8] and Chow and associates found no difference in outcome after endopyelotomy for high versus low insertion.[9] Others have demonstrated renal pelvic decompression following endopyelotomy in patients with preoperative redundancy.[10,11]

Another issue with respect to patient selection for endopyelotomy is the potential for significant hemorrhage should a crossing vessel near the site of obstruction be injured. In a study of 146 cadaver kidneys, Sampaio and Favorito found that 65% of specimens were associated with an anterior crossing vessel and 6.2% were associated with posterior crossing vessels.[12] Based on these anatomical studies, the investigators advocated a direct lateral incision to prevent vascular injury. In the authors' experience, bleeding necessitating transfusion has been rare, indicating that the main issue concerning the crossing vessel is not hemorrhage, but rather its influence on outcome.

Up to 50% of patients with an obstructed UPJ can be shown to have extrinsic compression from a crossing vessel which, according to some, can lead to failure of the procedure.[11,13] Cassis suggested preoperative evaluation of all patients with angiography,[10] since an intravenous pyelogram (IVP) is a poor instrument for predicting the presence of crossing vessels.[14,15] Currently, spiral computed tomography following intravenous contrast administration is the modality of choice for uncovering the presence of crossing vessels. Intraluminal ureteral ultrasonography is also a viable alternative. In Van Cangh's series of 102 endopyelotomies, in which 67 patients underwent preoperative angiography, the long-term success rate was only 39% in patients who had both a crossing vessel and high grade hydronephrosis.[16] However, if these data were applied to the authors' series, failure would be expected in more than one-third of patients. This, however, has not been the case, and the authors have argued that an aberrant vessel alone does not seem to be a cause of obstruction or failure of the procedure.[17] In the authors' opinion, most primary UPJ obstruction is secondary to abnormal musculature at the UPJ that impedes passage of urine.[18,19] In patients with secondary obstruction, kinking of the ureter from fibrosis of the surrounding tissues impedes urinary flow. At the present time, the authors do not perform routine preoperative imaging owing to the overall rarity of significant postoperative hemorrhage, as well as to a conviction that the mere presence of a crossing vessel does not, in and of itself, portend a less successful prognosis.

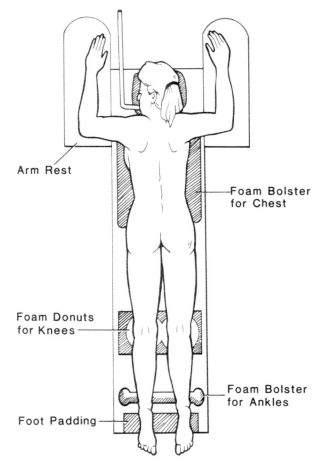

Figure 30.1. *Correct patient positioning for endopyelotomy.*

Technique

After induction of general anesthesia and intubation, the patient is placed in the dorsal lithotomy position. Cystoscopy and retrograde pyelography are performed to exclude ureteral stricture, stones or tumor, and to evaluate the position of the uteropelvic junction. A ureteral catheter is placed into the collecting system and secured to a Foley catheter. A glidewire or cobra catheter may facilitate passage of the ureteral catheter in cases of a tight UPJ.

The patient is then transferred to the prone position with care to pad all pressure points (Fig. 30.1). Biplanar fluoroscopy in the vertical and 30° projections is used to gain percutaneous access to the renal collecting system. An 18 gauge diamond-tipped needle is positioned into an upper pole or middle calyx, which allows direct access to the UPJ and facilitates passage of the nephroscope into the renal pelvis. Return of urine confirms appropriate needle position and a 0.038 inch

J-tip guidewire is passed through the needle and coiled in the renal pelvis. The tract is then dilated through a 1 cm skin incision to 30 Fr using either sequential fascial dilators or a balloon dilator under fluoroscopic guidance (Fig. 30.2). A 34 Fr working sheath is left in place. If necessary, stone extraction may be performed at this time.

Next, the previously positioned ureteral catheter is identified and its tip is grasped with forceps and brought out through the working sheath. A guidewire is threaded through the catheter and passed out the urethra, giving the surgeon through-and-through access to the urinary tract. Later in the procedure this can aid in positioning the endopyelotomy stent. A second, safety guidewire may also be placed.

In preparation for the incision, the UPJ is inspected for pulsations of the renal artery and accessory vessels. The incision should be directed towards the lateral aspect of the UPJ to avoid potential vascular injury.[12]

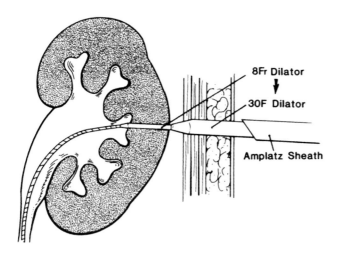

Figure 30.2. *Technique of endopyelotomy: access to the collecting system is obtained via a percutaneous nephrostomy and the tract is dilated to 30 Fr with Amplatz sheaths.*

Prior to making the incision, the UPJ is dilated to 14 Fr with Amplatz dilators to facilitate passage of the endopyelotome. The incision is then made using a hooked cold-knife (Fig. 30.3). The hook enables the surgeon to grasp and lift the tissue, which allows inspection of the mucosa prior to incision. It also allows multiple controlled cuts to the appropriate depth. The incision is performed by passing the knife alongside the guidewire and incising the UPJ in the lateral direction (Fig. 30.4). This avoids injury to the hilar vessels and ureteral vessels, as well as to any aberrant crossing vessels. The incision must be carried full thickness to

visualize periureteral fat and should extend to include healthy ureter distally. This might necessitate multiple passes of the knife, especially in a secondary procedure. Thermal incision of the UPJ has been used at some centers with satisfactory results. With increasing use of ureteroscopic endopyelotomy, the Holmium:YAG laser has also been shown to be an effective instrument for creating the incision.

At the authors' institution, stenting is accomplished with an endopyelotomy stent (Fig. 30.5), which is placed over the guidewire and its position confirmed by nephrostogram. The proximal stent protrudes from the flank, which allows access to the kidney for the duration of stenting. The stent is left to drain and a Foley catheter is placed. Alternatively, an internal double-pigtail endopyelotomy stent can be placed, along with a Councill catheter nephrostomy tube.

On postoperative day two, a nephrostogram is performed to confirm stent positioning and rule out persistent extravasation. If none is seen, the tube is clamped and, if no leakage occurs, the patient is discharged that day or the next. The patient returns 6 weeks later for tube removal. Flank drainage usually resolves within 24 hours of tube removal. At three weeks, an intravenous pyelogram is performed, and if improvement is noted over the preoperative state, the patient is followed. A renal scan is done if no improvement is seen on IVP. If asymptomatic, the patient is followed for 1 month, when a repeat IVP is performed to assess for resolution of edema of the UPJ.

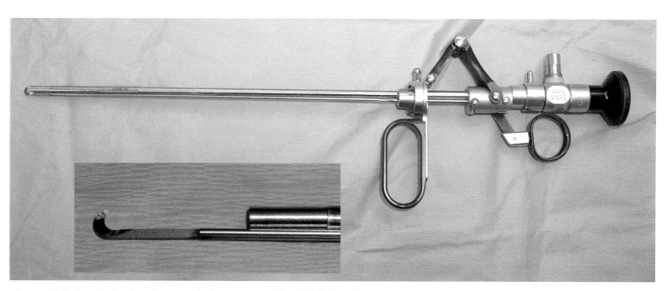

Figure 30.3. *Standard endopyelotome with close-up view of hook blade (inset).*

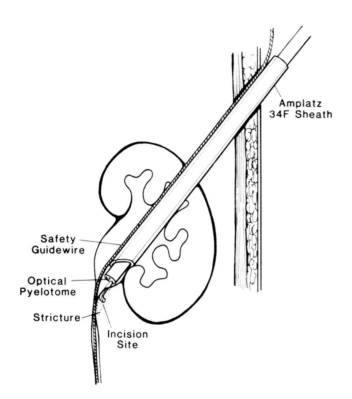

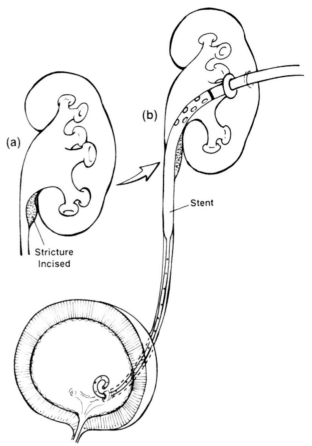

Figure 30.4. *An incision is made with the endopyelotome along the lateral aspect of the UPJ. The guidewire remains in place to maintain through-and-through control of the urinary tract.*

Figure 30.5. *After the stricture is incised (a), the endopyelotomy stent is placed; (b) the stent tapers from 14 Fr in the renal pelvis to 8 Fr in the mid-ureter.*

Results

The largest published series of endopyelotomies is by Gupta and associates, in which the results of 401 cases were reviewed.[20] These authors reported an 85% success rate at a mean follow-up time of 51 months. Other large series report success rates of 61% to 89% (Table 30.1). Although this rate is lower than the 95% success quoted for open pyeloplasty, the shorter hospital stay, decreased operative time, decreased morbidity, and quicker recovery[6] constitute a convincing argument for endopyelotomy as first line therapy for UPJ obstruction. Additionally, there is no difference in the outcome of open pyeloplasty after failed endopyelotomy compared to that of a primary pyeloplasty. The results of endopyelotomy are at least as good for secondary UPJ obstruction as they are for primary cases.[20]

Apart from failure, there are relatively few complications of endopyelotomy.[7,21] In the authors' series of 212 patients, only two patients experienced bleeding which required transfusion,[5] although others have reported rates as high as 10%.[22] Stent migration or leakage requiring repositioning can occur in up to 14% of patients.[5] Stricture of the distal ureter has been reported but seems to have been related to the use of a stent whose distal tip remains in the ureter. A relatively high stricture rate was reported in early series of retrograde endopyelotomy,[23] although the risk of this complication has been negligible in contemporary series in which smaller caliber ureteroscopes have been used. Pneumothorax is a known complication,[24] and the incidence increases with renal access above the 12th rib. Infection and sepsis may occur uncommonly and can be further minimized by using perioperative antibiotics and ensuring sterile urine.[22] Ureteral avulsion has been described in a single patient as a result of using a very large peel-away sheath to position a universal stent;[5] this technique is no longer employed.

Table 30.1. *Percutaneous endopyelotomy results (series with at least 50 patients)*

Series	No. renal units	Stent size (Fr)	Stent duration (wks)	Success rate (%)	Mean follow-up (mths)
Gupta et al.[20]	401	12 or 14/8	6	85	51
Kuenkel & Korth[24]	143	10–14	3–6	78	12
Van Cangh et al.[16]	123	–	–	71	62
Salhav et al.[8]	83	14/7	4–6	87	–
Danuser et al.[46]	80	12/7 or 4/8	6	86	26
Hatsuse et al.[47]	73	16/6*	3	89	24
Siegel et al.[48]	66	14/7	5	89	11
Szewczyck et al.[49]	64	–	–	61	4–20
Streitz et al.[50]	54	–	–	67	6–84
Kletscher et al.[38]	50	14/7 or 8–8.5	6	88	12

* *Percutaneous transhepatic cholangioscopy catheter.*

Retrograde techniques

There are numerous variations in the technique of incising the ureteropelvic junction, including cold-knife, electrocautery, and laser. In addition to the antegrade approach, retrograde endopyelotomy may be performed ureteroscopically or with a radiographically guided cautery balloon.

Retrograde endopyelotomy was introduced to decrease the morbidity of the procedure in comparison to the percutaneous approach, as well as to give urologists total control from the standpoint of obviating reliance on radiologists for gaining access to the upper urinary tract. Success rates for ureteroscopic and cautery balloon endopyelotomy are presented in Tables 30.2 and 30.3, respectively. Outcomes of antegrade and retrograde approaches are comparable. In a single-institution trial, Shalhav and associates found no statistically significant difference in success rates of antegrade or retrograde endopyelotomy.[8] Introduction of smaller caliber ureteroscopes and a thinner cautery balloon device have rendered the need to pre-stent the ureter obsolete. Endopyelotomy using the cautery balloon can be performed extremely rapidly, with minimal postoperative discomfort. Both ureteroscopic and cautery balloon endopyelotomy may be performed on an outpatient basis.

Despite these advantages, the retrograde approaches have some minor drawbacks. Both techniques necessitate postoperative placement of an internal stent, which risks stent migration through the incised ureter into the retroperitoneum. Additionally, access to the collecting system is not available in the event that the stent requires repositioning or a nephrostogram needs to be performed. Finally, if the stent were to become obstructed or malpositioned, another procedure would be necessary to remedy the situation.

Table 30.2. *Ureteroscopic endopyelotomy results*

Series	No. renal units	Stent size (Fr)	Stent duration (wks)	Success rate (%)	Mean follow-up (mths)
Thomas et al.[51]	39	14/7	6	90	15
Renner et al.[52]	34	9	6–8	85	18
Tawfiek et al.[53]	32	6–10 or 14/7	8	87.5	10
Savage & Streem[54]	29	14/7 or 10/7	4	83	14.1
Giddens & Grasso[55]	28	14/7 or 10	4–10	83	10
Gerber & Kim[56]	22	14/7 or 7–8	6	82	29
Conlin & Bagley[57]	21	8 or 10	6–10	81	23
Biyani et al.[58]	20	–	–	75	34
Meretyk et al.[23]	19	14/7	6	79	17

Table 30.3. *Cautery balloon endopyelotomy results*

Series	No. renal units	Stent size (Fr)	Stent duration (wks)	Success rate (%)	Mean follow-up (mths)
Kim et al.[59]	77	7 or 14/7	6–8	78	12
Shalhav et al.[8]	66	7 or 14/7	4–6	74	–
Preminger et al.[60]	66	6,7 or 14/7	1–9	77	7.8
Gelet et al.[61]	44	–	–	76	12
Lechevallier et al.[62]	36	9	6	75	24
Faerber et al.[63]	32	14/7	6–8	81	14
Nadler et al.[64]	26	14/7	4–6	81	32.9
Gill & Liao[65]	13	7	6–8	69	17.7

Endopyeloplasty

Recently, laparoscopic pyeloplasty has been introduced, and several series have demonstrated success rates higher than those of endopyelotomy. Recapitulation of open surgical techniques, combined with the decreased morbidity of laparoscopy, have made laparoscopic pyeloplasty an attractive alternative to endoscopic incision. However, the need for advanced laparoscopic suturing skills has precluded its widespread use.

In an attempt to apply some of the principles of pyeloplasty via an endoscopic approach, Oshinsky and colleagues reported eight cases of percutaneous endoscopic pyeloplasty in 1996.[25] In this technique, a percutaneous endopyelotomy was performed and then a suture was placed across the UPJ incision to close it in a Heinecke-Mikulicz fashion. The suture was introduced either through a separate nephrostomy tube in the retroperitoneum (3 cases) or through the nephrostomy tube in the renal pelvis (5 cases). Seven of the eight cases were successful after a mean follow-up time of 12 months. However, the procedure was abandoned because of difficulty suturing through the nephroscope.

Recently, the Cleveland Clinic group revived this technique with the assistance of a novel endoscopic suturing device, the SewRight SR-5 (LSI Technologies, Rochester, NY, USA) (Fig. 30.6 a, b). This device is introduced through a nephroscope and sequentially passes a suture through the distal and proximal leaves of the endopyelotomy incision. The suture is tied extracorporeally and cinched down with a knot pusher. One to three sutures are used (Fig. 30.7 a–d). After performing a feasibility study in pigs, Gill and co-workers reported their initial experience with the technique in nine patients.[26] The procedure was successful in all of the subjects at a short mean follow-up time of 4 months. The purported advantages of the endopyeloplasty technique include healing by primary intention with minimal urinary extravasation, increased luminal diameter from the Heinecke-Mikulicz closure which mimics a Fenger pyeloplasty, and decreased duration of postoperative stenting.[26] Stents were removed after 2 weeks in this study. Potential disadvantages of the technique include the added time and learning curve of nephroscopic suturing, the fact that the knots are tied on the inside of the urinary tract, and the need for a specialized suturing device.[26] Additionally, given the 80–85% success rate of endopyelotomy, a large number of endopyeloplasties will have to be performed in order to demonstrate improved outcomes over the former.

Stenting after endopyelotomy

Endopyelotomy stents have evolved with the procedure itself. Indeed, the changes in stent design and the question of duration of stenting have probably engendered as much controversy as the procedure itself. The importance of stenting after UPJ incision has long been appreciated. In his 1943 paper, Davis quotes Gibson: 'No matter how generous the surgeon is in the use of sutures in plastic repair, the outcome is likely to be failure unless he makes use of splinting; conversely, if he places his dependence on adequate splinting, the result will almost certainly be successful even though he uses no sutures at all'.[1] Nevertheless, stent design and the optimal duration of stenting have both been in question since Davis initially described the procedure.

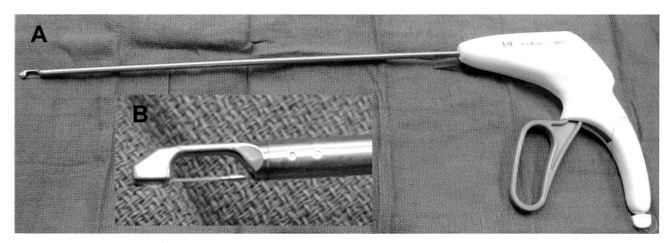

Figure 30.6. *(a) SewRight SR-5 (LSI Technologies, NY, USA) device for suturing through nephroscope. (b) Inset shows suturing tip of device.*

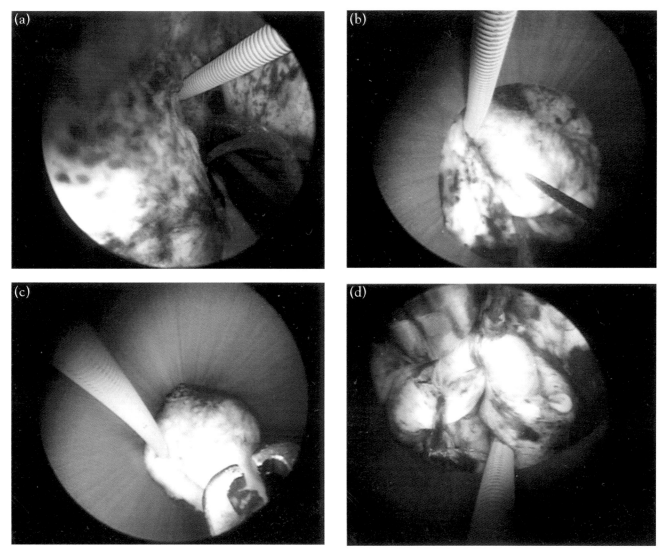

Figure 30.7. *Endopyeloplasty: after endopyelotomy incision is created in standard fashion, the SewRight is used to suture the incision in a Heinecke-Mikulicz closure. (a) First stitch being thrown. (b) Stitch across endopyelotomy incision. (c) Knot being tightened with knot pusher applied through nephroscope. (d) Two stitches have been placed across the UPJ incision.*

Davis was prophetic when he wrote: 'the size of the splint, its shape, and the length of time it is left in place are the most important points . . . It may well be that specially shaped splints . . . will prove to be useful'. The remainder of this chapter will address these 'specially shaped splints', addressing stent design, stent size, and duration of stenting.

Stent design

When Wickham and associates introduced percutaneous pyelolysis in 1983 they used a 10 Fr catheter with a pelvic nephrostomy tube.[3] Soon after, Smith began performing endopyelotomy in the United States, and he stented the ureter with his Universal stent.[27] This was an 8 Fr silicone rubber tube 90 cm in length with a 4 cm zone of drainage holes in the center of the stent, as well as drainage holes at the distal end, and a Luer-Lok adaptor at the proximal end (Fig. 30.8). This stent was

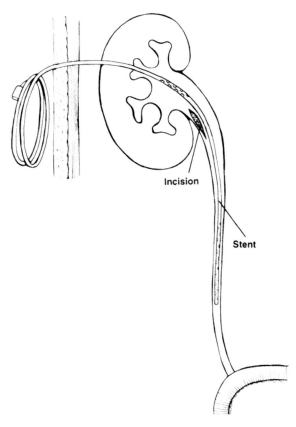

Figure 30.8. *The Smith Universal stent is a uniform 8 Fr along its length. The proximal end drains externally or is capped for internal drainage. The distal end was originally passed to the level of the pelvic brim, but ureteral stricture formation necessitated passage into the bladder. It is composed of silicone rubber and is placed with the aid of a Teflon peel-away introducer.*

intended to be useful for a wide array of indications and could be adapted for either internal or external drainage. Initially, the Universal stent was passed only to the level of the pelvic brim, but subsequently it was redesigned to pass into the bladder to avoid the risk of ureterovesical stenosis which occurred in a small percentage of cases.[28] The stent was composed of silicone, which has excellent biocompatibility and durability, but a low tensile strength, weak coil properties and a high coefficient of friction.[29] This required a relatively thick-walled stent which had to be placed using a Teflon peel-away sheath. The small lumen size prompted the increase of the stent to 12 Fr, necessitating the use of a 14–16 Fr peel-away introducer.[28] This size stent was difficult to pass down the ureter and caused concern over pressure effects on the lower ureter.

These issues led to the development of a stent designed specifically for endopyelotomy. The original endopyelotomy stent had a diameter of 14 Fr that tapered to 7 Fr with multiple coils distally. The multiple coils were supposed to allow the stent to be used in patients of any size: larger patients would have fewer coils enter the bladder. However, the additional coils in the bladder caused irritative symptoms, and in one case the coils knotted together. These problems soon led to the development of a new endopyelotomy stent, composed of polyurethane and with a single coil in the bladder (Fig. 30.9).[28] Current endopyelotomy stents are available in diameters ranging from 10/4.7 Fr to 22/7 Fr, and in lengths of 26 cm and 28 cm. They have greater tensile strength, a lower coefficient of friction and better coil retention than the older silicone stents.[29] The high tensile strength permits a greater internal diameter and larger drainage holes. The polyurethane stent may be introduced over a guidewire without the need for a peel-away introducer. Use of the external 14/8.2 endopyelotomy stent after antegrade endopyelotomy has been associated with an 85% success rate at the authors' institution.[20] This is the stent that the authors continue to use today.

An alternative to the external endopyelotomy stent is the internal double-pigtail stent developed by Clayman, which tapers from 14 Fr to 7 Fr, and which can be used for either antegrade or retrograde endopyelotomy. When used antegrade, a nephrostomy tube can be left in place in order to perform a nephrostogram later.[30] If satisfactory, the nephrostomy

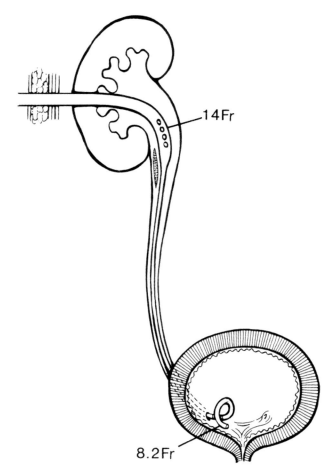

Figure 30.9. *The external endopyelotomy stent is 14 Fr proximally and tapers to 8.2 Fr with a single coil in the bladder. The proximal end can be capped for internal drainage or opened for external drainage.*

tube can be removed and the patient discharged home with only the internal stent. As originally described by Clayman, an 8 Fr pigtail nephrostomy tube was placed after retrograde endopyelotomy and removed when a nephrostogram confirmed absence of extravasation.[31] Success rates in cases in which this stent has been used after ureteroscopic or cautery balloon endopyelotomy are summarized in Tables 30.2 and 30.3.

The major advantage of an internal stent is the lack of external dressing or tube, while the main advantage of an external stent is the presence of two drainage outlets, one retrograde and one antegrade. Thus, the external stent can be capped for antegrade drainage, which is most convenient for the patient, but it can also be opened to external drainage if the patient develops flank pain or fever, or if a nephrostogram needs to be performed. If obstructed, it can be easily cleared by irrigation or by passing a guidewire through the lumen.

In contrast, stent malfunction with an internal stent may require changing the stent altogether or percutaneous nephrostomy. There is a small risk of the proximal end of an internal stent migrating out of the endopyelotomy incision, and this can lead to gross urinary extravasation and surgical failure. Furthermore, the internal stent requires cystoscopic removal while the external stent does not. Although an internal stent is unseen by the patient, the authors have found that the small loop of tubing under a dressing is well tolerated by patients who have externalized stents. For these reasons, the authors continue to use the external endopyelotomy stent.

Stent composition

Stent materials are chosen for a combination of properties, including biocompatibility, tensile strength, ability to retain a coil configuration at the ends and generation of a minimal amount of friction. The original 14/7 Fr internal stents were composed of silicone,[31] which has low tensile strength, weak coil properties and a high coefficient of friction. Currently, stents are composed of polyurethane, Percuflex or C-flex.[30] Percuflex is a proprietary block copolymer which exhibits medium to high tensile strength, good coil retention and, with the addition of hydrophilic coating, a very low coefficient of friction. C-flex is another proprietary block copolymer with good coil retention and intermediate coefficient of friction and tensile strength. Polyurethane exhibits the highest tensile strength of these materials, and has a moderate coefficient of friction and good coil retentive properties. Although the Percuflex stent with hydrophilic coating comes closest to the ideal, each of these materials represents an acceptable alternative for the four to six week stenting period after endopyelotomy. There have been no studies to date implying a difference in endopyelotomy outcome based on the stent material used.

As the search for the ideal endopyelotomy stent continues, the concept of a biodegradable stent has surfaced. A biodegradable stent would have the advantage of not having to be removed after the procedure and could potentially be engineered to deliver antimicrobials or biological response modifiers that could promote healing.[32] Olweny and co-workers tested such a stent in a recent animal study.[32] Nine pigs were randomized to postendopyelotomy stenting with either a poly-L-lactide-co-glycolide (PLGA) bioabsorbable stent or a standard 7 Fr stent. The PLGA stent is a 7 Fr diameter stent which expands to 12 Fr in an aqueous thermal environment and begins to degrade within 24 hours by hydrolysis. At 12 weeks postendopyelotomy there was no difference in average flow rate through the ureter between ureters stented with the PLGA stent versus the standard stent, nor was there a difference in flow rate between ureters stented with the bioabsorbable stents and ureters which had not been operated upon. However, the PLGA stent was incompletely reabsorbed at 12 weeks, and fragments of stent material were found embedded in the retroperitoneum and in the ureteral wall. The PLGA stents also generated a much more vigorous chronic inflammatory response than the standard stent, and impeded adequate regeneration of the muscular wall of the ureter. The investigators concluded that although feasible, biodegradable stenting needs further development in terms of biocompatibility, absorbability, and prevention of fragment migration. Despite these challenges, bioabsorbable endopyelotomy stents may provide an attractive alternative stent design in the future.

Stent size

One of the most controversial questions in endopyelotomy is whether stent size has any bearing on the outcome of the procedure. Is it necessary to have a large caliber stent across the endopyelotomy incision? In Davis' original description of the intubated ureterotomy he recommended use of a stent that would be 'as large as will enter the uncut, or presumably normal, part of the ureter without fitting so tightly as to cause ischemia . . .' and went as far as to suggest a conical shape for the ureteropelvic junction.[1] It was felt that: 'The splint is a mold upon which the tissues . . . re-form the ureteral channel. . . .'[1] Likewise, Smart suggested using the largest stent possible that would not cause ischemia of the ureteral wall, in other words, one that would slide down the ureter without drag.[33] In the development of the external endopyelotomy stent, a 14 Fr size was chosen to improve diversion of urine through the stent, rather than around it, in order to avoid urinary extravasation.

In the 1950s, several investigators began to experiment with smaller caliber stents.[34,35] Weaver used 3–5 Fr stents after partially excising a segment of ureter

in dogs. These were externally draining stents extending to just below the ureterotomy. He noted that larger stents were associated with increased stricture formation just distal to the end of the stent, and therefore recommended that they should not be used. More recently, Moon and colleagues compared use of the 14/7 Fr internal endopyelotomy stent with that of a 7 Fr Double-J stent in 20 pigs with experimentally induced strictures treated with cautery balloon endopyelotomy. Three months after stent removal, there was an equivalent 80% patency rate in both groups, with no difference in healing.[36]

A human study on 20 patients with primary strictures and 20 patients with secondary strictures treated with antegrade endopyelotomy compared use of the 6 Fr double-pigtail stent with that of the 14/7 Fr internal endopyelotomy stent. Overall success rate was 93% with the endopyelotomy stent and 84% with the 6 Fr double-pigtail stent. However, this difference did not reach statistical significance, and the secondary stricture group included patients with prior surgery, stones, tuberculosis and metastases.[37] Meretyk and associates performed 42 endopyelotomies (23 antegrade, 19 retrograde) using the internal endopyelotomy stent in 35 patients and a 7 Fr double-pigtail in seven patients. There was a 71% success rate in the 7 Fr double-pigtail group and a 79% success rate in the internal endopyelotomy group.[23] Kletscher and colleagues reported on 50 endopyelotomies in which 26 were stented with internal endopyelotomy stents and 23 were stented with double pigtail stents ranging from 6 Fr to 8.5 Fr: the 14/7 endopyelotomy stent group had three failures while the double-pigtail patients had two failures.[38] Unfortunately, all of these clinical studies have included only small numbers of patients. To date, there have been no randomized, controlled clinical trials addressing stent size after endopyelotomy.

Recently, a Swiss group presented the results of an intriguing study on stent size after endopyelotomy. These investigators assembled a 27 Fr external endopyelotomy stent by passing a 27 Fr wound drain over a 14/8.2 Fr endopyelotomy stent.[39] The wound drain extended to the region between the radiopaque marker and the caliber-decrease of the endopyelotomy stent, and the last 5–8 cm of the drain was perforated with multiple side holes. The wound drain was secured to the proximal end of the endopyelotomy stent with three sutures to prevent displacement of the outer drain from the inner stent. In addition, they extended the endopyelotomy 3–5 cm distally into the normal ureter, regardless of the stricture length, in order to prevent displacement of the 27 Fr portion back into the renal pelvis by the natural movement of the kidney in relation to the stent, which was fixed at the skin. The study compared two consecutive cohorts of patients, the first with 74 patients stented with the 14/8.2 Fr stent and the second with 55 patients in which the 27 Fr tube was used. At 2 years of follow-up for both groups, the 27 Fr group had a 93% success rate while the 14/8.2 Fr group experienced a 71% success rate. The aim of this technical modification was to create a funnel-shaped UPJ, which did occur in the patients in whom the 27 Fr stent was used. The authors also postulated improved fixation of the kidney-UPJ-ureter complex within a larger scar caused by the 27 Fr stent as a possible reason for the better outcome in this patient cohort. The only disadvantage of the larger stent was an increased requirement of postoperative analgesics, and the necessity of having to remove the 27 Fr stent early in three patients who had intercostal punctures. This interesting study requires confirmation by a prospective randomized trial, yet it adds some weight to the argument that a larger stent improves the outcome and durability of endopyelotomy.

Duration of stenting

The optimal duration of ureteral stenting has been in question since Davis first proposed the intubated ureterotomy. In 1943, he suggested a minimum of 3 weeks, but recommended 4 or 5 weeks.[1] In 1948, he tested his clinical impression in a dog study by removing two-thirds of the circumference of a 2 cm segment of ureter.[2] He found that the defect was bridged by granulation tissue and that epithelial proliferation was present after 4 days. At 6 weeks, a 90% regeneration of muscle had occurred. In 1955, Oppenheimer and Hinman performed a dog study in which one half of the circumference of 2 cm segments of ureter were removed. They concluded that the major factor in ureteral healing was smooth muscle regeneration and that healing was maximal by 6 weeks.[40] They also noted delayed healing and increased scar formation when urine was not maximally diverted. However, there was no histopathological examination prior to the 6 week

time point. In another dog study in 1960, McDonald and Calams performed ureterotomy on experimentally induced strictures.[41] Half the animals had nephrostomy tubes and were stented for 3, 7 or 12 weeks. Animals were sacrificed at the time of stent removal or 3 months later. Half the animals had no stent or nephrostomy, but had a Penrose drain positioned in the area of the stricture. In both groups, in the animals stented for 3 weeks, the ureteral defect was bridged by epithelium and fibrous tissue but muscle regeneration was absent. At 7 weeks, the smooth muscle layer completely encircled the ureter. After 12 weeks, mucosa, submucosa and muscle were completely formed. Unstented animals were noted to have increased periureteral fibrosis compared with animals killed 3 months after stent removal. Stented animals showed increased inflammation in the submucosa. It was concluded that stenting was important until the epithelium and regrowth pattern was established, but that after that point, the submucosal inflammatory reaction caused by the stent could delay healing.

More recently, Begin and associates examined pig ureters 4 and 7 weeks after balloon-induced rupture.[42] At 4 weeks there was restored mural continuity around a dilated lumen with a thin epithelium surrounded by a fibrous central zone. At 7 weeks the fibrous tissue was diminished with near-total muscular continuity. The epithelium appeared more normal, with formation of the lamina propria. The presence of a 6 Fr double-pigtail stent in half the animals did not affect muscular regeneration.

Kerbl and associates have evaluated the duration of stenting after cautery balloon endoureterotomy.[43] They experimentally induced strictures in pigs, then performed endoureterotomy and placed a 7 Fr double pigtail stent. Stents were removed at 1, 3 and 6 weeks and the animals were sacrificed 12 weeks after endoureterotomy. Ureteral specimens were graded based on a healing score that included urothelial resurfacing, degree of inflammation, lamina propria fibrosis, muscle layer fibrosis, and integrity of the musculature. No significant difference was noted in healing scores when mean values were compared.

Small clinical studies have also shown acceptable results with shorter stenting times. Abdel-Hakim performed antegrade endopyelotomy in seven patients stented with 7 Fr double-pigtail stents: five patients were stented for 4 days and two were stented for 5 weeks. All patients were considered cured without complications at 3–10 months.[44] Unfortunately, there has been no further follow-up reported on these patients. Kuenkel and Korth reported better results in 113 patients selected for 3 weeks of stenting compared with 30 patients stented for 6 weeks.[24] However, patients selected for 6 weeks of stenting were 'problem cases', with thick scarring and poor perfusion of the site of stenosis. Success was only 60% in those patients selected for 6 weeks of stenting and 78% for patients stented for 3 weeks. Kumar and associates performed a randomized study of 2 weeks versus 4 weeks of stenting in 26 patients.[45] The overall success rates in both groups was relatively low, possibly due to use of a less biocompatible polyethylene stent. However, at mean follow-up of 18 months, 70% of the 2 week group and 54% of the 4 week group were unobstructed on renal scanning. Although this difference did not reach statistical significance, the authors concluded that 2 weeks of stenting was at least as effective as 4 weeks.

A prospective randomized trial of 2, 4 and 6 week duration of stenting, using the same size and type of endopyelotomy stent for all patients involved, may one day definitively answer the question of how long to stent after endopyelotomy.

Conclusions

Endopyelotomy, in all its incarnations, is a procedure that has withstood the test of time. Many variations on the technique have been proposed, but the concept of a full-thickness incision with postoperative urinary diversion is common to all. Endopyeloplasty, should long-term results live up to the promise of the short-term outcomes, may one day become the procedure of choice for UPJ obstruction. However, until that time should arrive, endopyelotomy will remain the least invasive treatment.

Nevertheless, some very basic questions have not yet been satisfactorily answered. After 20 years, we still do not know definitively how large a stent to use, nor how long to keep it in. These questions are important because they impact both the success of the procedure as well as the patient's comfort during recuperation. Answering these questions, as well as improving the design of stents, particularly in terms of biodegradability and adding the capability for drug delivery, may at some point serve the dual goal of improving the outcome of endopyelotomy as well as decreasing the morbidity of convalescence.

References

1. Davis D M. Intubated ureterotomy: new operation for ureteral and ureteropelvic stricture. Surg Gynecol Obstet 1943; 76: 513–523
2. Davis D M, Strong G H, Drake W M. Intubated ureterotomy: experimental work and clinical results. J Urol 1948; 59: 851–862
3. Wickham J E A, Kellett M J. Percutaneous pyelolysis. Eur J Urol 1983; 9: 122–124
4. Badlani G H, Esghi M, Smith A D. Percutaneous surgery for ureteropelvic junction obstruction (endopyelotomy): technique and early results. J Urol 1986; 135: 26
5. Motola J A, Badlani G H, Smith A D. Results of 212 consecutive endopyelotomies: an 8-year follow-up. J Urol 1993; 149: 435–456
6. Karlin G S, Badlani G H, Smith A D. Endopyelotomy versus open pyeloplasty: comparison in 88 cases. J Urol 1988; 140: 476–478
7. Badlani G H, Karlin G S, Smith A D. Complications of endopyelotomy: analysis in series of 64 patients. J Urol 1988; 140: 473
8. Shalhav A L, Giusti G, Elbahnasy A M et al. Adult endopyelotomy: impact of etiology and antegrade versus retrograde approach on outcome. J Urol 1998; 160: 685–689
9. Chow G K, Geisinger M A, Streem S B. Endopyelotomy outcome as a function of high versus dependent ureteral insertion. Urology 1999; 54: 999–1002
10. Cassis A N, Brannen G E, Bush W H, Correa RJ, Chambers M. Endopyelotomy: review of results and complications. J Urol 1991; 146: 1492–1495
11. Brannen G E, Bush W H, Lewis G P. Endopyelotomy for primary repair of ureteropelvic junction obstruction. J Urol 1988; 139: 29–32
12. Sampaio F J B, Favorito L A. Ureteropelvic junction stenosis: vascular anatomical background for endopyelotomy. J Urol 1993; 150: 1787–1791
13. Van Cangh P J, Nesa S. Endoureteropyelotomy. Atlas Urol Clin North Am 1996; 4: 43
14. Hoffer F A, Lebowitz R L. Intermittent hydronephrosis: a unique feature of ureteropelvic junction obstruction caused by a crossing renal vessel. Radiology 1985; 156: 655–658
15. Bush W H, Brannen G E, Lewis G P. Ureteropelvic junction obstruction: treatment with percutaneous endopyelotomy. Radiology 1989; 171: 535–538
16. Van Cangh P J, Wilmart J F, Opsomer R J, Abi-Aad A, Wese F X, Lorge F. Long-term results and late recurrence after endoureteropyelotomy: a critical analysis of prognostic factors. J Urol 1994; 151: 934–937
17. Gupta M, Smith A D. Crossing vessels at the ureteropelvic junction: do they influence endopyelotomy outcome. J Endourol 1996; 10: 183–187
18. Gosling J A, Dixon J S. Functional obstruction of the ureter and renal pelvis: a histological and electron microscopic study. Br J Urol 1978; 50: 145–152
19. Hanna M K, Jeffs R D, Sturgess I M, Bark W M. Ureteral structure and ultrastructure: II. Congenital ureteropelvic junction obstruction and primary obstructive megaureter. J Urol 1976; 116: 725–730
20. Gupta M, Tuncay O L, Smith A D. Open surgical exploration after failed endopyelotomy: a 12-year perspective. J Urol 1997; 157: 1613–1618
21. Weiss J N, Badlani G H, Smith A D. Complications of endopyelotomy. Urol Clin North Am 1988; 15: 449–451

22. Gerber G S, Lyon E S. Endopyelotomy: patient selection, results, and complications. Urology 1994; 43: 2–10

23. Meretyk I, Meretyk S, Clayman R V. Endopyelotomy: comparison of ureteroscopic retrograde and antegrade percutaneous techniques. J Urol 1992; 148: 775–782

24. Kuenkel M, Korth K. Endopyelotomy: long-term follow-up of 143 patients. J Endourol 1990; 4: 109

25. Oshinsky G S, Jarrett T W, Smith A D. New technique in managing ureteropelvic junction obstruction: percutaneous endoscopic pyeloplasty. J Endourol 1996; 10: 147–151

26. Gill I S, Desai M M, Kaouk J H, Wani K, Desai M R. Percutaneous endopyeloplasty: description of a new technique. J Urol 2002; 168: 2097–2102

27. Smith A D. The universal ureteral stent. Urol Clin North Am 1982; 9: 103–107

28. Badlani G H, Smith A D. Stent for endopyelotomy. Urol Clin North Am 1988; 14: 445–448

29. Mardis H K, Kroeger M, Morton J J, Donovan J M. Comparative evaluation of materials used for internal ureteral stents. J Endourol 1993; 7: 105–115

30. Pearle M S. Use of ureteral stents after endopyelotomy. J Endourol 1996; 10: 169–176

31. Clayman R V, Basler J W, Kavoussi L R, Picus D D. Ureteronephroscopic endopyelotomy. J Urol 1990; 144: 246–252

32. Olweny E O, Landman J, Andreoni C et al. Evaluation of the use of a biodegradable ureteral stent after retrograde endopyelotomy in a porcine model. J Urol 2002; 167: 2198–2202

33. Smart W R. An evaluation of intubation ureterotomy with a description of surgical technique. J Urol 1961; 85: 512–524

34. Weaver R G. Ureteral regeneration: experimental and clinical: II. J Urol 1957; 77: 164–172

35. Boyarski S, Duque O. Ureteral regeneration in dogs: an experimental study bearing on the Davis intubated ureterotomy. J Urol 1955; 73: 53–59

36. Moon Y T, Kerbl K, Pearle M S et al. Evaluation of optimal stent size after endourologic incision of ureteral strictures. J Endourol 1995; 9: 15–22

37. Hwang T K, Yoon J Y, Ahn J H, Park Y H. Percutaneous endoscopic management of upper ureteral stricture: size of stent. J Urol 1996; 155: 882–884

38. Kletscher B A, Segura J W, LeRoy A J, Patterson D E. Percutaneous antegrade endoscopic pyelotomy: review of 50 consecutive cases. J Urol 1995; 153: 701–703

39. Danuser H, Hochreiter W W, Ackernmann D K, Studer U E. Influence of stent size on the success of antgrade endopyelotomy for primary ureteropelvic junction obstruction: results of 2 consecutive series. J Urol 2001; 166: 902–909

40. Oppenheimer R, Hinman F J. Ureteral regeneration: contracture vs. hyperplasia of smooth muscle. J Urol 1955; 74: 476–484

41. McDonald J H, Calams J A. Experimental ureteral stricture: ureteral regrowth following ureterotomy with and without intubation. J Urol 1960; 84: 52–59

42. Begin L R, Selmy G I, Hassouna M M, Khalaf I M, Elhilali M M. Healing and muscular restoration of the ureteral wall following balloon–induced rupture: an experimental animal model with light microscopic and ultrastructural observations. Exp Mol Pathol 1993; 59: 58–70

43. Kerbl K, Chandhoke P S, Figenshau R S, Stone A M, Clayman R V. Effect of stent duration on ureteral healing following endoureterotomy in an animal model. J Urol 1993; 150: 1302–1305

44. Abdel-Hakim A M. Endopyelotomy for ureteropelvic junction obstruction: is long-term stenting mandatory? J Endourol 1987; 1: 265–268

45. Kumar R, Kapoor R, Mandhani A, Kumar A, Ahlawat R. Optimum duration of splinting after endopyelotomy. J Endourol 1999; 13: 89–91

46. Danuser H, Ackernmann D K, Bohlen D, Studer U E. Endopyelotomy for primary ureteropelvic junction obstruction: risk factors determine the success rate. J Urol 1998; 159: 56–61

47. Hatsuse K, Ono Y, Kinukawa T et al. Long-term results of endopyeloureterotomy using the transpelvic extraureteral approach. Urology 2002; 60: 233–237

48. Siegel Y I, Lingeman J E, Newman D M. Endopyelotomy for ureteropelvic junction stricture: the Methodist Hospital of Indiana experience (abstr). J Urol 1993; 149 (Pt 2): 423A

49. Szewczyk W, Szkodny A, Noga A, Prajsner A, Szkodny G. Endopyelotomy for ureteropelvic junction stenosis. Int Urol Neph 1992; 24: 105–108

50. Streitz D, Hulbert J C, Hunter D. Long-term followup of the results of percutaneous treatment of strictures in the region of the ureteropelvic junction (abstr). J Urol 1992; 147 (Pt 2): 434A

51. Thomas R, Monga M, Klein E W. Ureteroscopic retrograde endopyelotomy for management of ureteropelvic junction obstruction. J Endourol 1996; 10: 141–145

52. Renner C, Frede T, Seamann O, Rassweiler J. Laser endopyelotomy: minimally invasive therapy of ureteropelvic junction stenosis. J Endourol 1998; 12: 537–544

53. Tawfiek E R, Liu J B, Bagley D H. Ureteroscopic treatment of ureteropelvic junction obstruction. J Urol 1998; 160: 1643–1647

54. Savage S J, Streem S B. Simplified approach to percutaneous endopyelotomy. Urology 2000; 56: 848–850

55. Giddens J L, Grasso M. Retrograde ureteroscopic endopyelotomy using the Holmium:YAG laser. J Urol 2000; 164: 1509–1512

56. Gerber G S, Kim J C. Ureteroscopic endopyelotomy in the treatment of patients with ureteropelvic junction obstruction. Urology 2000; 55: 198–203

57. Conlin M J, Bagley D H. Ureteroscopic endopyelotomy at a single setting. J Urol 1998; 159: 727–731

58. Biyani C S, Cornford P A, Powell C S. Retrograde endoureteropyelotomy with the holmium:YAG laser. Eur Urol 1997; 32: 471–474

59. Kim F J, Herrell S D, Jahoda A E, Albala D M. Complications of Acucise endopyelotomy. J Endourol 1998; 12: 433–436

60. Preminger G M, Clayman R V, Nakada S Y et al. A multi-center clinical trial investigating the use of a fluoroscopically controlled cutting balloon catheter for the management of ureteral and ureteropelvic junction obstruction. J Urol 1997; 157: 1625–1629

61. Gelet A, Combe M, Ramackers J M et al. Endopyelotomy with the Acucise cutting balloon device. Eur Urol 1997; 31: 389–393

62. Lechevallier E, Eghazarian C, Ortega J C. Retrograde Acucise endopyelotomy: long-term results. J Endourol 1999; 13: 575

63. Faerber G J, Richardson T D, Farah N, Ohl D A. Retrograde treatment of ureteropelvic junction obstruction using the ureteral cutting balloon catheter. J Urol 1997; 157: 454–458

64. Nadler R B, Rao G S, Pearle M S, Nakada S Y, Clayman R V. Acucise endopyelotomy: assessment of long-term durability. J Urol 1996; 156: 1094–1097

65. Gill H S, Liao J C. Pelvi-ureteric junction obstruction treated with Acucise retrograde endopyelotomy. Br J Urol 1998; 82: 8–11

31

Stenting after endopyelotomy for ureteropelvic junction stenosis in children

N. Rodrigues Netto Jr and M. Lopes de Lima

Introduction

Ureteropelvic junction (UPJ) stenosis is frequently found in children. The disease may be asymptomatic or diagnosed after a urinary tract infection or flank pain. In UPJ obstruction the diagnosis is based on pre- and postnatal ultrasonography, intravenous pyelogram (IVP) and/or renal scans.

Dismembered pyeloureteroplasty for the correction of the stenotic UPJ is the standard procedure with a success rate of over 90%.[1,2] The necessity of a large abdominal or lumbotomy incision and an inpatient stay of several days[3] has encouraged the search for alternative approaches in the treatment of UPJ stenosis.

Among the endo-ureteral procedures that have developed during the last 20 years, percutaneous incision of the UPJ stenosis (endopyelotomy) has significantly reduced morbidity in adults;[4] however, this technique has not been widely accepted for children.

Since Davis published details of the intubated ureterotomy in 1943,[5] the ureteral splint has been considered as a mold around which the regenerating tissue will proliferate after the incision of the UPJ stenosis, creating a ureteral channel of normal size and shape.

The relatively large calibre of the available nephroscopes and drainage tubes may explain the difficulties with percutaneous antegrade endopyelotomy and the limited enthusiasm for its use in children (Table 31.1). Retrograde endopyelotomy recently has been investigated as an alternative for reducing the morbidity of percutanous endopyelotomy in adults. The greater incidence of subsequent ureteral stricture appears to be the major disadvantage of the retrograde technique, probably secondary to prolonged ureteroscopic instrumentation.[6] Therefore, at present, the indication for such a procedure in children suffering from UPJ stenosis is very limited.[2]

Ideal ureteral stent for endopyelotomy

The ideal ureteral stent should be of a material entirely biocompatible with the internal ureteral environment. However, any foreign material placed in the ureter interacts with that environment and causes oedema, erosion, urothelial hyperplasia, and stent encrustation caused by the interface of the stent, urine and ureter.[7] The surface irregularity of the stent encourages deposits of uromucoids and crystalloids, leading to encrustation and stone formation.[8] The ideal stent should exhibit strong biodurability, retaining strength and elasticity after prolonged periods in situ. Several materials, such as polyethylene, C-Flex and silicone, are used to manufacture different types of stents.[7-9] Polyethylene has the roughest exterior and highest coefficient of

Table 31.1. *Published results of endopyelotomy in infants and children*

Reference	No. of patients	Age range	Success / total	Follow-up (months)
2	2	4–6 years	2/2	10
20	9	2 months – 15 years	7/9	18–56
19	8	4–15 years	7/8	2–32
21	2	1–4 years	1/2	18
22	4	6.5 weeks – 5.5 years	4/4	18–36
23	3	11–18 years	2/3	10–27
24	17	4 months – 16 years	13/17	3–36
25	5	11 months – 4 years	4/5	18–48
Totals	50		40/50 (80%)	

friction between these materials. Urine causes hydrolytic degeneration and depolymerization of polyurethane stents, making them brittle and prone to fracture if left indwelling for very long periods. Silicone is a biocompatible, biodurable, smoother and pliable biomaterial. C-Flex (Concept Polymer Technologies, Clearwater, FL, USA) is a biomaterial with a low coefficient of friction, but it permits stent encrustation with prolonged indwelling.[10]

Another feature of an ideal stent is biomechanical memory — the ability to return to a preset form after physical distortion.[11] This memory permits the stent to be retained without significant migration and is necessary to allow guidewire insertion, with return to its coiled configuration when the guidewire is removed. Silicone has a diminished memory; in contrast, polyurethane has the highest memory and tensile strength (referring to the force applied across a stent necessary to break it).[9]

According to Smith,[8] an ideal catheter should have a high ratio of internal to external diameter. This property refers to the facility with which the material can be manufactured into a stent. A silicone stent has a relatively small internal diameter, causing a decrease in the urinary flow rate though its lumen. On the other hand, polyurethane permits a larger ratio of internal to external diameter, with improved internal flow, and is easily manipulated and inserted.

Independent of the approach used to repair a ureteral stricture, stenting of the ureter is recommended in order to organize healing with an adequate lumen and to limit urinary extravasation. The stent is presumed to act as a scaffold around which the ureter regenerates, or a mould around which the ureter is restructured with a lumen of adequate calibre. Studies on incised ureters have shown that ureteric smooth muscle regenerates around a stent, and peristalsis has been shown to return after 6 weeks.[12]

Despite the extensive use of ureteral stents, the optimal stent size necessary to contribute to ureteral healing is unknown.[7,13,14] There has been little unanimity regarding either stent size or stenting duration;[15,16] however, it is accepted that the stent should be large enough to maintain urine flow and yet narrow enough to avoid ischaemia or pressure necrosis of the ureter.[13,17]

The effects of two sizes of stent (7 Fr and 14 Fr) were investigated in a model of ureteral stricture in vivo in female minipigs.[13] Healing of an endo-ureterotomy over a 7 Fr indwelling ureteral stent was compared with healing over a 14 Fr endopyelotomy stent. The objective of this investigation was to determine whether the larger stent provided any significant benefit over the smaller and more easily positioned stent. No statistical difference was found between the two groups with regard to such factors as the re-stricture rate and the overall healing scores measured by the degree of hydronephrosis, urinary tract infection, periureteral fibrosis or ureteral tortuosity.

Internal or external stent?

For antegrade or retrograde endopyelotomy, two general types of stents are available — the internal stent and the external stent. Most internal and external endopyelotomy stents used today are composed of polyurethane and thus have the same biomechanical advantages of memory, easy manipulation and favourable ratio of internal to external diameter.[7]

The adult lumbar ureter has an average calibre of 15 Fr whereas the pelvic ureter is narrowed to 8 Fr. This anatomy has led to the development of a stent with a 14 Fr/7 Fr taper, which is recommended following endopyelotomy.[7] The stent is large enough to promote wide regeneration of the incised UPJ, but not as large in its lower part, thus preventing pressure necrosis of the pelvic ureter.[18] This size of stent is inappropriate for children.[19]

The external endopyelotomy stent has the primary advantage of immediate and easy access.[7] If the stent becomes obstructed and the patient develops fever or pain, simply opening the nephrostomy tube solves the obstruction. Obstructed nephrostomy tubes can be cleared in the consulting-room with irrigation or by threading a guidewire without any anaesthesia, thus avoiding immediate interventions.

One disadvantage of the external endopyelotomy stent is the precision required for correct stent placement. An obstructed stent with renal pelvic holes excessively inside or excessively outside the pelvis may cause urinary leak around the stent.

The main advantage of an internal stent is that there is no external dressing or tube and it thus is more appropriate for children; on the other hand the renal pelvis coil of an internal stent may migrate out of the UPJ incision, causing extravasation of urine into the retroperitoneum and surgical failure, or causing pressure changes in the ureteral incision site. The obstruction of an internal stent mandates immediate interventions such as nephrostomy tube insertion or stent change, under anaesthesia. All these complications may contribute to subsequent surgical failure.

Stent after endopyelotomy in children

Experience with endopyelotomy in children is limited and a clear role in the management of primary and secondary UPJ obstruction in children has yet to be defined.[2,19,20] In the authors' experience,[20] nine children with primary (six) or secondary (three) UPJ obstruction underwent a one-stage cold-knife percutaneous antegrade endopyelotomy. Endopyelotomy was successful in five of the six with primary and two of the three with secondary UPJ obstruction. Failures were associated with high-grade hydronephrosis, the length of the stenotic segment (> 1.5 cm) and technical problems. One of the nine children had a complication caused by the dismemberment of the junction.

The lack of appropriate stents and drainage materials make endopyelotomy more difficult in children. To avoid this problem, the authors considered the Schneider endosplint (Angiomed, C.R. Bard, Karlsruke, Germany) (Fig. 31.1).

An orifice was made in the tip of a Foley catheter to its tip and a 5 Fr ureteral catheter was passed through it to drain the kidney and the ureter (Fig. 31.2). The distal end of the stent was placed in the distal ureter and the proximal end was brought out through the 18 Fr Foley catheter placed as a nephrostomy tube. The nephrostomy tube and, the ureteral catheter were left indwelling for 6 weeks (the nephrostomy tube was left to prevent accidental displacement of the ureteral stent, rather than for drainage). After 6 weeks, a nephrostogram was taken before the removal of both nephrostomy tube and ureteral catheter. This approach avoided the use of general anaesthesia for stent removal and did not cause a significant morbidity.

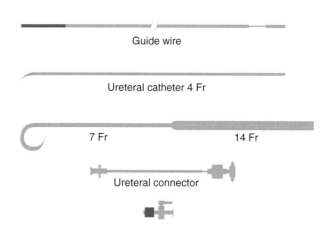

Figure 31.1. *Adaption of the Schneider endosplint.*

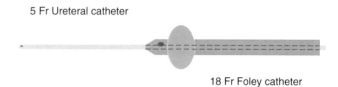

Figure 31.2. *Modification of the Foley catheter.*

Motola et al.[4] reported that the youngest patient in their series of 212 endopyelotomies was aged 33 months. In their opinion, the limiting factor for such a procedure is the size of the patient. A UPJ that cannot accommodate a 10/5 Fr paediatric endopyelotomy stent for postoperative stenting is not suitable for such a procedure. However, the number of paediatric cases was not given in their paper.

Bogaert et al.[19] demonstrated the efficacy of retrograde endopyelotomy in children. However, they recognized that this technique, at present, is recommended only for children over 4 years. The principal limiting factor for the retrograde procedure appears to be the size of the ureter, demanding from the manufacturers smaller catheters that will make the procedure possible in small children. As the frequently recommended stent after adult endopyelotomy (14–7 Fr taper)[7] is inappropriate for children, they used standard double-J catheters with good results. This approach was supported by the experimental study of Moon et al,[13] who demonstrated that there is no advantage in using a 14 Fr stent rather than a 7 Fr stent.

Conclusions

Summing up, although there is only a small series in the literature, and too brief a period of follow-up for firm conclusions to be drawn about the role of endopyelotomy in the management of UPJ obstruction in children, endoscopic endopyelotomy has proved its merits technically and effectively. The low morbidity and long-term success of open pyeloplasty in this age group are excellent, thus limiting the relative advantage of an endoscopic approach. With the availability of newer, smaller endoscopes, accessory instruments and smaller stents, endopyelotomy may become a more popular approach in small children with UPJ obstruction.

References

1. Gerber G S, Lyon E S. Endopyelotomy: patient selection, results and complications. Urology 1994; 43: 2–10

2. Bolton D M, Bogaert G A, Mevorach R A et al. Pediatric ureteropelvic junction obstruction treated with retrograde endopyelotomy. Urology 1994; 44: 609–613

3. Saing H, Chan F L, Yeung C K et al. Pediatric pyeloplasty: 50 patients with 59 hydronephrotic kidneys. J Pediatr Surg 1989; 24: 346–349

4. Motola J A, Badlani G H, Smith A D. Results of 212 consecutive endopyelotomies: an 8-year followup. J Urol 1993; 149: 453–456

5. Davis D M. Intubated ureterotomy: a new operation of ureteral and ureteropelvic stricture. Surg Gynecol Obstet 1943; 76: 513

6. Thomas R. Endopyelotomy for ureteropelvic junction obstruction and ureteral stricture disease: comparison of antegrade and retrograde techniques. Curr Opin Urol 1994; 4: 174–179

7. Siegel J F, Smith A D. The ideal ureteral stent for antegrade and retrograde endopyelotomy: what would it be like? J Endourol 1993; 7: 151–154

8. Smith A D. Percutaneous ureteral surgery and stenting. Urology 1984; 23: 37

9. Mardis K K, Kroeger R M. Ureteral stents: materials. Urol Clin North Am 1988; 15: 471

10. Macaluso J N Jr. Evaluation of the J-Maxx ureteral stent. J Endourol 1990; 4: 114

11. Saltzman B. Ureteral stents: indications, variations and complications. Urol Clin North Am 1988; 15: 481

12. Oppenheimer R, Hinman F Jr. Ureteral regenaration: contracture versus hyperplasia of smooth muscle. J Urol 1955; 74: 476

13. Moon Y T, Kerbl K, Pearle MS et al. Evaluation of optimal stent size after endourologic incision of ureteral strictures. J Endourol 1995; 9: 15–22

14. Smith J M, Butler M R: Splinting in pyeloplasty. Urology 1976; 8: 218–221

15. Meretyk I, Meretyk S, Clayman R V. Endopyelotomy: comparison of ureteroscopic retrograde and antegrade percutaneous techniques. J Urol 1992; 148: 775–782

16. Eshghi M: Endoscopic incisions of the ureter 1–3. AUA Update Series, 9 (37–39), 1989

17. Clayman R V, Basler J W, Kavoussi L et al. Ureteronephroscopic endopyelotomy. J Urol 1990; 144: 246–252

18. Badlani G H, Smith A D. Stent for endopyelotomy. Urol Clin North Am 1988; 15: 433

19. Bogaert G A, Kogan B A, Mevorach R A et al. Efficacy of retrograde endopyelotomy in children. J Urol 1996; 156: 734–737

20. Netto Jr. N R, Ikari O, Esteves S C et al. Antegrade endopyelotomy for pelvi-ureteric junction obstruction in children. Br J Urol 1996; 78: 607–612

21. King L R, Coughlin P W, Ford K K, et al. Initial experiences with percutaneous and transurethral ablation of post-operative ureteral stricture in children. J Urol 1984; 131: 1167–1169

22. Kavoussi L R, Meretyk S, Dierks S M, Shapiro E et al. Endopyelotomy for secondary ureteropelvic junction obstruction in children. J Urol 1991; 145: 346–349

23. Towbin R B, Wacksman J, Ball W S. Percutaneous pyeloplasty in children: experience in three patients. Radiology 1987; 163: 381

24. Tan H L, Najmaldin A, Webb D R. Endopyelotomy for pelviureteric junction in children. Eur Urol 1993; 24: 84–88

25. Faerber G J, Ritchey M L, Bloom D A. Percutaneous endopyelotomy in infants and young children after failed open pyeloplasty. J Urol 1995; 154: 1495–1497

32

ESWL: to stent or not to stent?
F. A. G. Bloem and J. J. M. C. H. de la Rosette

Introduction

The first ureteral stents were utilized during incisional surgery to facilitate upper tract drainage or to align the ureter. The initial report was by Gustav Simon in the 19th century, who placed a tube in the ureter while performing an open cystostomy. The first catheter purposely created for use in the ureter was made in the early 1900s by Joaquim Alobarrano.[1] A long period of hiatus, when little work was directed toward refining ureteral stents, ended in 1967, when a report by Zimskind and associates touched off an explosion in research on the development of ureteral stents.[2] Following this work, design modifications were directed at preventing antegrade or retrograde migration. The proximal and distal ends of a silicone tube were coiled in the shape of a J. Such tips were malleable and could be straightened and strengthened by an internal guidewire that was utilized for stent passage. Once the wire was removed, the J memory would prevent stent migration. In 1978, Finney[3] and Hepperlen and associates[4] described the double-J stent, which since has been adapted for passage cystoscopically or percutaneously. Since then, great efforts in research and development have been made to create a stent that would alleviate upper urinary tract obstruction while being painless and safe and would permit maximal indwelling time.

The daily use of ureteral stents has increased enormously because of the important roles of ureteropyeloscopy, percutaneous renal surgery and extracorporeal shock-wave lithotripsy (ESWL) in modern urology. Today, most stones are treated with ESWL, which is highly effective in pulverizing stones. Elimination of the stone fragment can be more difficult and the primary complication of ESWL is ureteral obstruction by fragments and the associated morbidity.[5] The use of double-J stents is considered to contribute to successful stone passage[6] and to reduce post-treatment morbidity,[5] but there also have been reports of complications that might have been caused by indwelling ureteral stents.[7] Therefore, the question may be raised whether to stent or not to stent following ESWL treatment. In this chapter this point is discussed, and the authors' current approach and recommendations in the use of double-J stents following ESWL is presented.

Rationale and indications for stent placement

Urologists perform internal ureteral stenting as a therapeutic or prophylactic procedure prior to ESWL. A stent normally drains through its lumen; however, drainage around the stents is frequent. It is often observed that, in the presence of a stent, urine increasingly flows around the stent and causes a gradual dilatation of the ureter. Moreover, when ureteroscopy is performed on a ureter that has been stented for some time, the orifice rarely requires dilatation for insertion of the instrument. These two observations — the intraluminal and extraluminal drainage and the ureteral dilatation — provide the rationale for the use of stents to facilitate elimination of stone debris after ESWL. On the other hand, not every patient needs to be stented prior to treatment and the decision whether to stent depends on several considerations.

Indications for immediate stenting are as follows: (1) obstructive pyelonephritis secondary to a renal pelvic, ureteropelvic or ureteral stone; (2) renal colic or pain refractory to analgesia and hydration; (3) renal failure secondary to bilateral renal obstruction or an obstructing stone in a solitary kidney; (4) prevention of more distal ureteral migration of a stone, precluding easy access to lithotripsy; and (5) establishment of secure outflow from the kidney.

Patients who need prophylactic stenting are those with minimum or manageable symptoms whose stent is placed to minimize post-procedural morbidity during particle passage. Not only stone size (burden), but stone composition, renal anatomy, the patient's age and body habitus, associated disease, and compliance must be judged in selecting patients for stenting. Indications for stenting also include the presence of ureteropelvic junction oedema, ureterovesical angulation secondary to benign prostatic hyperplasia (BPH), long-standing hydronephrosis, or urinary tract infection prior to treatment (Table 32.1).

As mentioned before, the number of ESWL patients receiving pretreatment stents has increased rapidly, yet controversy continues over which patients receive the maximum benefit from stenting.

Table 32.1. *Patients who may benefit from stenting prior to ESWL*

Compliant patient (balance of pros and cons)
Anatomical arguments: stone burden with UPJ* oedema
UVJ† angulation secondary to BPH
Long-standing hydronephrosis
Struvite stones or known urinary tract infections
Health status: advanced age
immobility
poor medical condition

* UPJ, ureteropelvic junction.
† UVJ, ureterovesical junction.

Results of ureteral stenting with ESWL

Multiple studies have been performed to determine the benefit of stenting, compared with ESWL in situ for renal pelvis and ureteral stones.

Shabsigh et al.[8] included 820 patients with renal pelvic stones in a retrospective study. None of the patients had ureteral stones or ureteral obstruction. The study population was divided into two groups: group 1 comprised patients with ureteral stents; group 2 comprised those who did not have stents. The incidence of multiple ESWL treatments increased with stone burden, but was unaffected by the use of stents. Auxilliary procedures, such as percutaneous nephrostomy, percutaneous lithotripsy or ureteroscopy, were necessary in 6.5% of patients. Where the stone burden was 15–29 mm, there was almost no difference between groups; however, when the stone burden exceeded 30 mm, significantly more procedures were performed in the group treated with ESWL in situ. The incidence of

complications (haemorrhage, obstruction; urinary infection) was lower when ureteral stents were used, regardless of stone size and number of stones although, overall, patients with larger stones had a higher complication rate than those with smaller stones.

In an analysis of complications after ESWL by Libby et al.,[5,9] comparing stented patients and patients treated in situ, it was shown that the rate was significantly less in the internally stented group. In more recent studies, the advantage in stenting patients with a large stone burden prior to ESWL treatment, as advocated above seems to decline. In a retrospective study by Kirkali et al.[10] 351 patients with renal stones larger than 30 mm were reviewed to determine the effectiveness and the complications of double-J stents. Stents were inserted prior to ESWL in 85 patients, and 266 patients were treated without stents. The stone-free rate in the stented group did not differ significantly from that in the non-stented group (31% and 30%, respectively). The auxiliary treatment rate for the *steinstrasse* was 15% in the stented group and 18% in the non-stented group. Additionally, four of the stented patients (5%) were treated endoscopically because of encrustation or migration of the stent. Half of the patients in the stented group complained of mild bladder discomfort and disturbances, which were relieved after removal of the stent (Table 32.2).

Cass[11] reviewed the results of the ureteral stent used with ESWL in 3096 patients with renal calculi less than 3 cm in diameter. With an 80% follow-up rate at 3 months, indwelling ureteral stents were associated with a higher stone-free rate in patients with a single stone, but a lower stone-free rate in patients with multiple stones, compared with those treated without a stent. An indwelling ureteral stent, however, resulted in symptoms of urinary frequency and bladder discomfort in most patients.

Another study by Cass[12] determined whether a stent is an advantage in treating patients with ESWL for ureteral stones. The outcome of ESWL treatment of 1712 single ureteral stones was reviewed retrospectively; in 1425 cases an indwelling stent was used and the other 287 stones were treated in situ. The stone site, size and treatment parameters were similar in both groups. The treatment rate, post-ESWL secondary procedure rate and stone-free rate were 5, 5 and 79%, respectively, with a stent and 6, 9 and 79% without a stent, respectively.

Table 32.2. *Results of ESWL with and without stenting prior to treatment, in different studies*

Study	Stone size/location	Stent (n)	In situ (n)	Stone-free rate (%) < 30 months		Stent complications (%)		
				Stent	In situ	Migration	Encrustation	Discomfort
Kirkali et al.[10]	> 30 mm / renal	85	266	31	30	5	5	50
Nakada et al.[13]	— / mid-ureteral	14	8	71	63	—	—	—
Cass[12]	— / ureter	1,425	287	79	79	—	—	—
Bierkens et al.[15]	> 200 mm² / renal	41	23	44	35	24	15	42

Cass concluded, therefore, that a stent is not necessary in treating ureteral stones with ESWL.

Other authors have also investigated the use of stents in patients with ureteral stones treated with ESWL. Nakada et al.[13] concluded, in their retrospective study of 26 patients with mid-ureteral stones, that stenting before treatment confers no advantage over ESWL treatment in situ.

The use of auxiliary procedures (including stenting) prior to ESWL treatment for calculi in a solitary kidney was investigated by Heimbach et al.[14] In their study, 54 patients were reviewed. In 52% of cases the stones measured more than 1 cm, in 43% between 0.4 and 1 cm and in 5% less than 0.4 cm in diameter. A single ESWL treatment was successful in 73% of cases. In eight patients, ureteric stents were placed prior to ESWL treatment, because of obstruction of the upper urinary tract. Following ESWL, percutaneous nephrostomy was performed in four patients and a ureteric stent was placed in two patients because of urinary obstruction. It was concluded that, if there is no ureteric obstruction present prior to ESWL, the majority of patients with a solitary kidney do not present extraordinary problems and do not need auxiliary procedures.

In the authors' own department, Bierkens et al.[15] randomized 64 patients with large renal calculi (stone burden more than 200 mm²) for treatment in situ or treatment with a prophylactically inserted stent. A round 6 Fr stent with single-coiled ends or a triangular stent with double-coiled ends was used. After 3 months the results of treatment and post-ESWL morbidity was evaluated. In the in situ group (23 patients), treatment complications consisted of fever in three, pyelonephritis in one and *steinstrasse* in three patients. After 3 months,

eight patients (35%) were free of stones. In the stented population (41 patients), treatment complications consisted of fever in seven, pyelonephritis in one, *steinstrasse* in six and bladder discomfort in almost half of the patients. Stent calcification and stent migration were also seen in seven and ten patients, respectively. Calcified stents had been in situ longer than non-calcified stents. The round stents migrated and calcified more often than the more rigid triangular stents. After 3 months, 18 of the stented patients were stone free (44%). Bierkens et al.[15] concluded that ureteral stents do not reduce post-ESWL complications, are clearly associated with morbidity and do not markedly improve stone passage.

Discussion

Today, most renal stones are treated with ESWL, which is highly effective in pulverizing stones. As endo-urologists gain experience with ESWL, progressively larger stones are being treated. However, the larger the stone, the greater the number of fragments generated and the greater the incidence of colic and obstruction and the longer the time necessary for complete stone passage. For stones larger than 3 cm in diameter, percutaneous debulking before ESWL treatment or ESWL with prophylactic ureteral stenting is advocated.[16] For complete staghorn calculi, good results with ESWL monotherapy combined with prophylactic ureteral stenting have been reported.[17] The use of double-J stents has been shown to contribute to successful stone passage[4] and to reduce post-ESWL morbidity,[5] but there have also been reports of complications that might have been caused by indwelling ureteral stents.[7]

Elimination of the fragments can be difficult, depending on the location of the stone, the initial stone burden, the anatomy of the individual patient and the size of the fragments after ESWL treatment. To prevent urinary obstruction, ureteral stents were employed in the outpatient setting on the basis of the following assumptions. Indwelling ureteral catheters allow continued passage of urine through and around the stent, while allowing some spontaneous passage of particles (some up to 5 mm in diameter).[18] the ureter responds to the insertion of a catheter by constriction around the foreign object and hyperperistalsis, followed by fatigue and dilatation; thus, on removal of a ureteral stent several days later, larger particles may pass through a relaxed ureterovesical junction. Larger fragments will be held in the kidney by an indwelling stent, preventing their passage through the ureteropelvic junction, necessitating re-treatment. Finally, renal function is preserved on the treated side.[19]

Thus, when should we stent and which type of stent should be used? Major indications for stenting are as follows: obstructive pyelonephritis secondary to a stone; renal colic or pain refractory to analgesics; renal failure secondary to bilateral obstruction or obstruction by a stone in a solitary kidney; prevention of a distal migration of a stone and establishment of secure outflow from the kidney. More or less minor indications for stenting are the stone size (burden) itself, the stone composition, renal anatomy, the patient's age and body habitus, associated diseases and compliance of the patient. In the retrospective study of Shabsigh et al.,[8] with 802 consecutive patients, none of whom had ureteral stones or ureteral obstruction, the decision to stent depended on the clinical judgement of the individual urologist[8] (Table 32.3).

Although an impressive variety of stents have been developed, an ideal stent does not exist. Stents differ in texture (from soft to stiff), size, shape (from round to square) and composition. Silicone stents are non-irritant, more or less resistant to encrustation and ideal for long-term use. Unfortunately the flexibility of silicone makes these stents difficult to insert and it is also necessary to create thicker-walled tubes with correspondingly smaller lumina to prevent kinks or collapse of the stent. Stents made of polyurethane (Soft-Flex) are more stiff than silicone, but are more elastomeric than polyethylene, which becomes brittle

Table 32.3. *Advantages and disadvantages of the use of stents prior to ESWL treatment*

Advantages	Renal function is preserved
	Large particles will be held in kidney by indwelling stent to facilitate re-treatment
	Incidence of colic, *steinstrasse* and urinary tract infection can be reduced, especially in patients with large stones or large aggregate stone burden
Disadvantages	Complaints due to stents: urgency and frequency
	Migration of stents
	Stent encrustation
	Invasive procedure in combination with ESWL

after some time. Polyurethane stents have good flow rates, which suggest reliable drainage over a longer period of time. C-Flex is a material softer than polyurethane but less likely to develop encrustation, despite long periods of contact with urine. The memory of C-Flex, however, is inferior to that of stents made of polyurethane and therefore the migration rate is somewhat higher.[20] Because stent migration is a well-recognized phenomenon,[21] several types of stents have been designed. The tip of a stent should prevent migration.[22] Soft silicone stents have the highest incidence of migration, compared with polyurethane stents, which have a good memory. Libby et al.,[5] using silicone stents, reported an expulsion incidence of 10%. In the study by Bierkens et al.,[15] polyurethane stents were used, which migrated in about 25% of cases and resulted in premature cystoscopic stent removal.[15] Stents that have migrated downwards can be removed without problems, but those that have migrated upwards should be removed either ureterorenoscopically or by an open surgical procedure.

Stone formation has been reported as a complication of indwelling ureteral stents. Spirnac and Resnick[23] recommended that ureteral stents should be used with caution in any person with a history of stone formation (!).[23] Pyelonephritis resulting from severe encrustations on ureteral stents have also been reported.[24] In the authors' opinion, therefore, stents in patients with stones should be removed within 8 weeks or as soon as possible after ESWL treatment. Fragments are sometimes prevented from passing until stent removal.

If, however, significant obstructive stone fragments persist, the stent should be replaced.

Irritative voiding symptoms with bladder discomfort is another morbid factor associated with indwelling ureteral stents. Patients can have alarming symptoms of bladder spasms, reflux, haematuria, incontinence and cystitis.[18] Riehle et al.[19] interviewed 50 patients treated with ESWL after the internal stent had been removed from each. Of these patients, 30% reported episodic or constant discomfort in the flank during the post-treatment period, 26% reported bladder urgency, spasm or incontinence, and 42% reported at least one episode of gross haematuria after leaving the hospital. In an attempt to quantify the subjective symptoms, patients were asked to rate the experience of having the stent in situ: 22 patients (44%) experienced moderate to severe or intolerable discomfort, which was relieved dramatically after removal of the stent. The polymer composition, and thus the stiffness of the stent, did not appear to relate directly to the degree of discomfort.

Conclusions

Internal ureteral stents may be helpful in minimizing the morbidity of ESWL for large renal stones. In view of the morbidity caused by stents, and the minimal advantage over not stenting, the indications are limited. Only in selected patients is stenting advocated. The choice of type of stent seems to have no major bearing on the results of ESWL and its morbidity.

References

1. Herman J R. Urology: a view through the retrospectroscope. New York: Harper and Row, 1973
2. Zimskind P D, Fetter T R, Wilkerson J L. Clinical use of long-term indwelling silicone rubber ureteral splints injected cystoscopically. J Urol 1967; 97: 840
3. Finney R P. Experience with new double-J ureteral stent. J Urol 1978; 120: 678
4. Hepperlen T W, Mardis H K, Kammandel H. Self-retained internal ureteral stents: a new approach. J Urol 1978; 119: 731
5. Libby J M, Meacham R B, Griffith D P. The role of silicone ureteral stents in extracorporeal shock-wave lithotripsy (ESWL) of large renal calculi. J urol 1988; 139: 15
6. Littleton R H, Goodman N. Extracorporeal shock-wave lithotripsy — use of double-J stent. J Urol 1987; 137(2): 143A (abstr 158)
7. Pollard S G, Macfarlane R. Symptoms arising from double-J ureteral stents. J Urol 1988; 139: 37
8. Shabsigh R, Gleeson M J, Griffith D P. The benefits of stenting on a more-or-less routine basis prior to extracorporeal shock-wave lithotripsy. Urol Clin North Am 1988; 15(3): 493
9. Libby J, Griffith D. Large calculi and ESWL: is morbidity minimized by ureteral stents? J Urol 1986; 135: 182A (abstr)
10. Kirkali Z, Esen A A, Akan G. Place of double-J stents in extracorporeal shock-wave lithotripsy. Eur Urol 1993; 23(4): 460
11. Cass A S. Ureteral stenting with extracorporeal shock-wave lithotripsy. Urology 1992; 39(5): 446.
12. Cass A S. Nonstent or noncatheter extracorporeal shock-wave lithotripsy for ureteral stones. Urology 1994; 43(2): 178
13. Nakada S Y, Pearle M S, Soble J J et al. Extracorporeal shock-wave lithotripsy of middle ureteral stones: are ureteral stents necessary? Urology 1995; 46(5): 649
14. Heimbach D, Wirth M, Hofmockel G, Frohmuller H. Are auxiliary methods necessary prior to ESWL in patients with a solitary kidney? Urol Int 1994; 52(3): 131
15. Bierkens A F, Hendrikx A J, Lemmens W A, Debruyne F M. Extracorporeal shock-wave lithotripsy for large renal calculi: the role of ureteral stents. A randomized trial. J Urol 1991; 145(4): 699
16. Anderson P A, Norman R W, Awad S A. Extracorporeal shock wave lithotripsy experience with large renal calculi. J Endourol 1989; 3(1): 31
17. Pode D, Verstandig A, Shapiro A et al. Treatment of complete staghorn calculi by extracorporeal shock wave lithotripsy monotherapy with special reference to internal stenting. J Urol 1988; 140: 260
18. Riehle R A Jr, Naslund E. Patient management after shock wave lithotripsy. In: Principles of extracorporeal shock wave lithotripsy. New York: Churchill Livingstone, 1987
19. Riehle R A Jr. Selective use of ureteral stents before extracorporeal shock-wave lithotripsy. Urol Clin North Am 1988; 15(3): 499
20. Salzman B. Ureteral stents, indications, variations and complications. Urol Clin North Am 1988; 15(3): 481
21. Oswald G C, Buechsen A J, Lloyd L K. Upward migration of indwelling ureteral stents. J Urol 1979; 122: 249
22. Hofmann R, Hartung R. Ureteral stents — materials and new forms. World J Urol 1989; 7: 154
23. Spirnac J P, Resnick M. Stone formation as a complication of indwelling ureteral stents: a report of 5 cases. J Urol 1985; 134: 349
24. Abber J C, Kahn R I. Pyelonephritis from severe encrustations on silicone ureteral stents: management. J Urol 1983; 130: 763

33

Uretero-intestinal stricture stenting
Z. Markovic and S. Perovic

Introduction

Reconstruction, involving uretero-intestinal anastomosis, may be indicated following severe trauma or radical pelvic surgery for malignant disease. Sometimes these procedures also necessitate the construction of an ileostomy or colostomy which may be permanent or temporary. These are complicated operations with an unpredictable outcome. One of the long term complications can be stricture at the anastomosis between ureter and bowel.

Earlier, in the 'pre-nephrostomic' era, uretero-intestinal anastomoses were used much more frequently than today. The increasing use of interventional uroradiological methods has brought a new clinical quality to the treatment of ureteral strictures. If percutaneous balloon catheter recanalization is used as the sole method for the management of uretero-intestinal strictures, permanent recanalization is not obtained in over 50% of cases.[1,2] However, in recent years, the use of metal stents as adjuncts to balloon recanalization has established the clinical role of this procedure in this group of indications.

Causes of stricture

Stricture aetiology at the site of anastomosis may vary. Postoperative fibrosis at the site of anastomosis due to insufficiency of the microcirculation occurs from several weeks to a year after the surgery (Fig. 33.1a). Post inflammatory strictures cannot be predicted and they may occur early in the postoperative course (Fig. 33.2a) or several years later. The strictures may develop as long as 20 years after the operation and their cause may remain obscure.[2] During differential diagnosis in uretero-intestinal anastomosis patients with ileostomy or colostomy, stenosis of the outflow from the intestinal stoma should be ruled out. Knowing the primary disease, rapid deterioration of renal function raises the suspicion of uretero-intestinal anastomosis obstruction. This can

be visualized by echotomography and antegrade ureterography, while additional diagnostic information may be obtained with retrograde contrast exploration of the intestinal segment. Uretero-intestinal strictures may be intermittent (incomplete) or permanent (complete). In cases of bilateral obstruction, bilateral antegrade ureterography is performed in one procedure for most precise morphological grading.

Indications for the use of metal stents

Indications for the application of a metal endoprosthesis in cases of uretero-intestinal anastomosis include stricture relapse after repeated percutaneous balloon catheter recanalization and contraindications for repeated surgical reconstruction. Contraindications for stent use include irreversible renal deterioration, severe urinary infection (pyonephrosis), poor general condition and bleeding disorders.

Procedure

Technically, the percutaneous insertion of a metal stent to the site of anastomosis calls for knowledge of, and skill in, modern methods of interventional uroradiology (percutaneous nephrostomy, balloon catheter dilatation, catheter stents).[3] Percutaneous nephrostomy is the first step in the management of this type of urinary obstruction. Nephrostomy, in addition to urine deviation and renal function preservation (Fig. 33.2a), has a diagnostic significance for subsequent imaging of the anastomosis with contrast media and helps in the recovery of ureteral peristalsis. As the distal end of the stent-carrying catheter is rigid, the incision for the nephrostomy should be through the mid or upper calyx. This eases the subsequent passage of the balloon catheter and stent-carrying catheter from the renal pelvis into the ureter.

Selection of anaesthesia for this procedure is determined by the general condition of each patient.

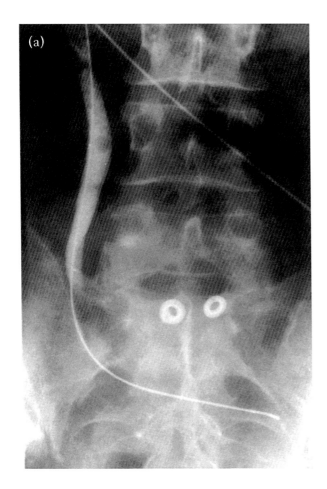

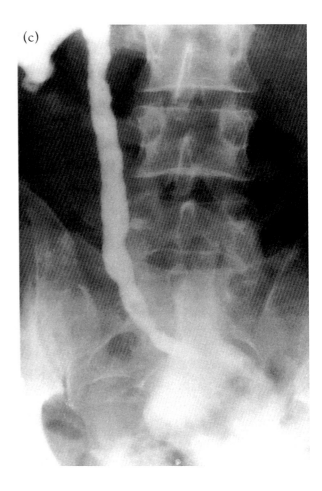

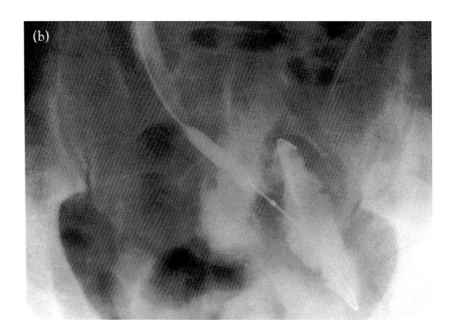

Figure 33.1. *(a) Stricture of ureterointestinal anastomosis — nephrostomal wire percutaneously placed via the stricture into the intestine; (b) balloon catheter recanalization of a stricture at the site of anastomosis; (c) Strecker stent insertion — complete recanalization.*

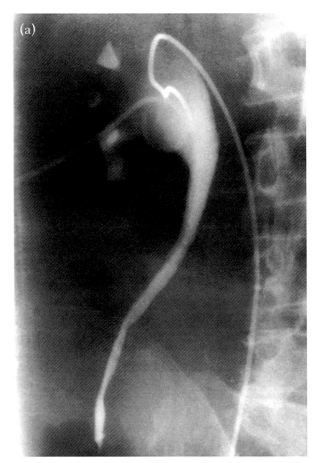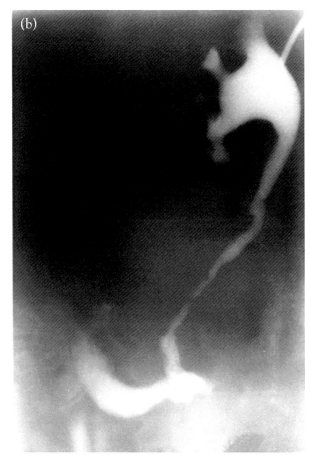

Figure 33.2. *(a) Complete obstruction of uretero-intestinal anastomosis — visualization via percutaneous nephrostomy; (b) recanalization using a Strecker stent (4 cm long and 7 mm wide).*

Most commonly, spinal anaesthesia is used, but local anaesthesia may also be used with the addition of systemic analgesia and sedation.

Balloon or self-expandable stents 4–8 cm long and 5–11 mm wide are used for recanalization of strictures of uretero-intestinal anastomosis (Figs. 33.1c, 33.2b). Placement of a balloon-expandable Strecker stent requires dilatation of the access tract up to 14 Fr and placement of a temporary angiographic sheath through which the stent-carrying catheter is passed. Not using this sheath may cause stripping of the stent from the catheter at the level of the renal fascia or perirenal tissues. Narrowing of the ureter at the site of anastomosis (angulation of the ureter, stricture of the ureteropelvic junction, high ureteral insertion, etc.) may also hinder the passage or cause displacement of the balloon-expandable stent from the catheter. Before stent insertion, 'preliminary dilatation' with a balloon catheter (Fig. 33.1b) is performed by fractionated

balloons with increasing calibre (2 mm, 4 mm, 6 mm).[4] The balloon catheters have a distention strength of 16 – 22 atm (≈1.62–2.22 MPa). The aim of recanalization and dilatation is to prepare the space for stent insertion. The degree of dilatation is checked by contrast injection through the visceral opening of the balloon catheter. This is important, as the balloon catheter may only push aside the walls of the stricture, which bounce back immediately after deflation of the balloon. In such a case the tip of the catheter with the stent can be placed only to the cranial end of the stricture. The whole procedure is performed over a nephrostomic guidewire of minimum length 125 cm, which is passed into the intestine with at least 10 cm of the guidewire in the intestine. Precise insertion of the stent is radiographically guided. Stent positioning is an important part of the procedure. Irrespective of the type of anastomosis, the distal part of the stent should enter the intestinal lumen as little as possible to prevent possible displacement and its expulsion with the intestinal contents.

In cases of recanalization of a uretero-sigmoidal anastomosis, a percutaneous and colonoscopic approach may be combined for percutaneous placement of the nephrostomic guidewire and other catheters, and their retrieval through the colonoscope. After stent insertion, the percutaneous nephrostomy is left in place for 2 weeks.[5,6] Percutaneous nephrostomy acts as a 'safety valve' to prevent stent obstruction with clots and also enables effective management of a possible infection.[7]

Clinical experience

In the authors' institution over a 3-year period, recanalization of strictures of uretero-intestinal anastomosis using a metal stent has been performed in 13 patients, using balloon-expandable Strecker stents 4–8 cm long and 7 mm wide. The patients were followed-up initially by echotomography, and 3 months after the procedure by urography and renal function tests. In nine cases an ileostomy or colostomy was present simultaneously. In four cases (31%), displacement and spontaneous expulsion of the stent occurred. In five cases intermittent urostasis occurred at

the stent level due to tissue proliferation into the lumen. Permanent stricture recanalization after stent insertion was obtained in six cases (46%) over an 18-month follow-up after insertion. Neither irritative symptoms nor other post-procedureal complications were observed.

In addition to the use of metal stents, strictures of uretero-intestinal anastomoses can be managed by other interventional uroradiological methods, such as balloon catheter dilatation followed by catheter prosthesis (8–10 Fr) insertion with prolonged percutaneous nephrostomy. However, utilization of these methods for creating a granulation/fibrous lumen around the catheter prosthesis failed to improve the final outcome in comparison to cases in which only balloon dilatation was used.[8,9] Moreover, in other distal ureteral strictures of different aetiologies, starting with balloon dilatation has been shown to reduce urethral and periurethral tissue reactions.[10,11]

A special aetiological group (which is classified) within that of ureter-intestinal anastomosis strictures is that of strictures developing at the site of anastomosis between the ureters and the orthotopic bladder (Fig. 33.3a). These anastomoses are characterized by a high percentage of postoperative strictures. Until the advent of interventional uroradiology (balloon catheter

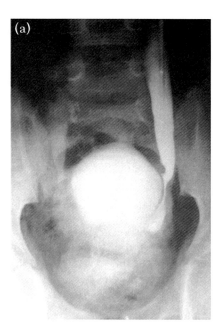 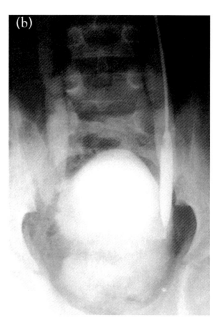 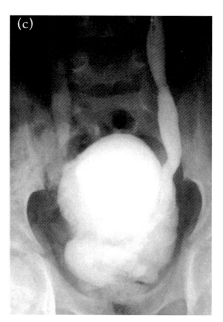

Figure 33.3. (a) Anterograde urography: postoperative stricture at the site of ureter with orthotopic bladder; (b) percutaneous balloon catheter 'preliminary dilatation' with a balloon 5 mm wide and 6 cm long; (c) insertion of balloon-expandable Nitinol Strecker stent (4 cm/7 mm): complete recanalization was visualized by application of contrast medium through a percutaneous nephrostomy.

dilatation and stent insertion), these strictures were managed by repeated surgery, which unavoidably led to further shortening of the ureter. In the authors' institution in the last 2 years, metal stents for recanalization of strictures at the site of ureteral anastomoses with an orthotopic bladder have been mostly used in paediatric urology. In eight patients (average age 5.5 years), Strecker stents 5–7 mm wide and 4–8 cm long were applied. Post-procedureal recanalization was established in all eight cases (Fig. 33.3b,c). In six cases (75%), 12 months after the insertion good upper-tract urodynamics were established, with normal pyelocalyceal morphology. In two cases the stent was obliterated by proliferative tissue 6–9 weeks after the insertion.

Conclusions

Recanalization of uretero-intestinal strictures by metal stent insertion is used only in very extreme cases. A high percentage of tissue proliferation into the stent lumen, the probability of stent displacement and the fact that the implanted stent cannot be extracorporeally controlled make the method imperfect. Nevertheless, it is the therapeutic method of choice in selected indications. Future application of new generations of coated and biodegradable stents will yield a better therapeutic outcome in this group of indications also.

References

1. Cornud F, Cheretin Y, Bonnel D et al. Long-term result of angioplasty balloon dilatation of uretero-digestive anastomoses. Effect of prolonged pattern with large caliber prosthesis. J Urol 1991; 97: 11–13
2. Markovic Z, Masulovic D. Recanalization of the postoperative strictures of the uretero-digestive anastomoses using percutaneous approach. Radiol Arch Serbia 1993; 4: 325–329
3. Lang E K. Interventional radiology of the lower urinary tract. In: Mueller P R (ed) A categorial course in diagnostic radiology — interventional radiology. Chicago: RSNA, 1991: 49–55
4. Masulovic D, Markovic Z, Goldner B, Tulic C. The postoperative uretero-intestinal strictures dilatation using percutaneous approach. J Endourol 1995; 9: 95
5. Gort H B, Mail W P, van Waees P F. Metallic self-expandable stenting of ureteroileal strictures. AJR 1990; 152: 422
6. Dardenne A N, Van Cange P J. Endoscopic and percutaneous management of ureteral strictures and fistulas. In: Dondelinger R, Rossi P (eds) Interventional radiology. New York: Thieme, 1990; 246–255
7. Reinberg Y, Ferral H, Gonsales R et al. Intraureteral metallic self-expanding endoprosthesis (Wallstent) in the treatment of difficult ureteral strictures. J Urol 1994; 151: 1619–1622
8. Castaneda-Zuniga W R, Tadavarthy S M, Hunter D W et al. Recanalization in nonvascular interventional radiology. In: Castaneda-Zuniga W R, Tadavathy S M (eds) Interventional radiology, 2nd edn. Baltimore: Williams and Wilkins, 1992: 777–989
9. Shapiro M J, Banner M P, Amendole M A et al. Balloon catheter dilatation of ureteroenteric strictures: long-term results. Radiology 1988; 168: 385–387
10. Markovic Z. Algorithm of interventional radiological methods in treatment of distal ureteral strictures. Radiol Arch Serbia 1994; 5: 407–412
11. Lugmayr H, Pauer W. Selbstexpandierende Metall-Stents bei malignen Ureterstenosen. Dtsch Med Wochenschr 1991; 116: 573

34

Metallic stents in the management of ureteric obstruction

R. Kulkarni

Introduction

Insertion of a stent in the ureter has truly altered the practice of urology. The possibility of relieving upper tract obstruction with an internally placed tube would be attractive to any patient especially when it can avoid the need of a painful open operation.

The first use of a ureteric stent dates back to Gustav Simon in the 19th century.[1] Despite the obvious logic behind the concept, it did not flourish. Joaquin Albarrano made the first purpose built ureteric catheter in 1900.[1] Yet another period of 67 years went by until Gibbon described a silicone stent for use in the ureter. Finney and Hepperlen first introduced the present version of the pigtail stent in 1978.[1]

The advantages of such a device became obvious and the application of the technique began to proliferate. This brought to light the difficulties and problems associated with stents. They encrust, migrate, fragment, and irritate the urothelium and cause pain.[1,2] Biofilm formation on the stent surface and its microbial colonization is universal. Flow of urine through and around the stents has been studied extensively.[3,4] Ureteric dilatation is induced by the presence of a stent. However, stents are also known to cause obstruction – both by dampening the peristalsis of the ureteric muscle as well as by its very presence in the lumen of the ureter.[3] Extra-anatomic placement of stents also has been attempted.[5] However, they need regular replacement. Long-term use of a pigtail stent is therefore fraught with problems.

The quest for an improved stent has led to many alterations in design and material during the past two decades. In addition to the reduction (and increase) of stent diameter, the design has seen many other changes. Single-J, tail and spiral stents are examples of important shape modifications, aimed at reducing symptoms.[6] While the latter also aimed to improve the flow of urine, simultaneous insertion of multiple stents has also been used to achieve this.[7]

The undesirable side-effects of stents stem not only from the reaction between the stent material and the host but also the mechanical effect of the stent itself. This has intuitively led to the development of stents that would only occupy the obstructing segment of the ureter.

The development of the Wallstent in the management of ureteric obstruction caused by malignancy introduced a new concept of stenting only the obstructing part of the ureter.[8,9] It also ushered in the era of metallic stents into the armamentarium of the endourologist.

History of metallic ureteric stents

The introduction of metallic stents in surgery dates back many years.[10] These devices had already been successfully used in the biliary tract and coronary as well as peripheral arteries. But perhaps the obvious fear of encrustation, when metal came in contact with urine, discouraged urologists.

Milroy and colleagues reported the use of metal stents in the management of urethral strictures.[11] These and similar metallic stents have been reported by other authors.[12]

The first publication of Wallstent on the management of malignant ureteric obstruction was made by Pauer and Lugmayer.[8,9] The results were mixed. There was good relief of upper tract obstruction. However, this was not sustained due to the ingrowth of tumour tissue through the mesh of the stent. Endoscopic removal of these stents is extremely difficult.

The unique property of an alloy made from nickel and titanium was discovered over 40 years ago – it has a thermal memory for shape. A device made from a specially manufactured version of this alloy maintains its shape above 55°C. A particular thermoreactive combination of nickel and titanium gives the alloy another unique property – it becomes soft below 10°C, and regains its shape when rewarmed to 55°C. A device made from this alloy can be delivered at the site of obstruction in its unexpanded form and heated to 55°C to induce expansion to a predetermined shape. This has led to the concept of Nitinol urological stents.

In 1991, Danish engineers and medical practitioners developed a prostatic stent made from Nitinol for the relief of symptomatic benign prostatic hyperplasia. It was a tightly coiled wire of 0.7 mm diameter which had a wide end aimed at the verumontanum. This was called the Memokath stent. A ureteric stent made with the same concept in mind was introduced in 1995. It had a similar design but the wire was much thinner – 0.4 mm diameter and the wide fluted end faced towards the renal pelvis. Its shaft had an external diameter of 9 Fr (3 mm) and the wide end expanded to 14 Fr (4.6 mm).

The Memokath ureteric stent

We performed the first insertion of this stent (Memokath 051 to differentiate it from the prostatic version Memokath 028) in November 1996 in a patient with extraluminal ureteric obstruction due to metastatic lymph nodes from transitional cell carcinoma of the bladder. A total of 49 stent insertions have been carried out in 39 patients to date. Our interim results encouraged us to explore the use of this stent in more complex strictures.[13,14] Initially, this study included patients with malignant ureteric obstruction. Patients with refractory benign strictures were later included. As this was a pilot study, patients were included consecutively and were not randomized. The details of the indications and location of strictures is outlined in Tables 34.1 and 34.2.

After the first few insertions, the stent design was changed. The new, wider version now has an external diameter of 10.5 Fr (3.5 mm) and its wide fluted end expands to 20 Fr (6.6 mm). The original Memokath 051 stent was available in a fixed length of 100 mm. The current version is available in 30, 60, 100, 150 and 200 mm lengths. It is available for retrograde insertion (Memokath 051 CW) as well as antegrade insertion down a nephrostomy tract (Memokath 051 USDW).

Memokath stent design

The stent is packed in its unexpanded form. The metallic stent is mounted on a black catheter. A pair of plastic lugs traverses through the stent and emerges at its far (yet unexpanded) end. The lugs are kept apart by a guidewire, which runs through the entire assembly. These lugs and the catheter secure the two ends of the stent until it is ready for expansion and deployment. The stent is protected by a pair of plastic 'shells'. These shells are removed prior to insertion by cutting the plastic retainers with the blade provided (Fig. 34.1).

The stent is introduced into the ureter through a 14 Fr diameter introducer sheath provided with the stent assembly. The latter is mounted over a dilator. The dilator sheath, its core and the stent assembly can be firmly connected to each other by a locking mechanism.

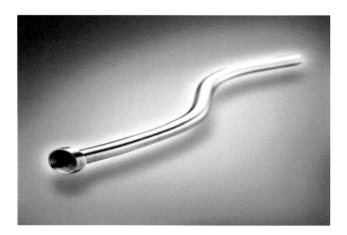

Figure 34.1. *The Memokath 051 ureteric stent.*

Table 34.1. *Indications for Memokath stenting malignant ureteric obstruction*

Aetiology	Patients
Colorectal carcinoma	8
Gynaecological cancers	8
Carcinoma of prostate	2
Transitional cell carcinoma bladder	3
Carcinoma of breast	2
Carcinoma of pancreas	1
Lymphoma	1
Total	**25**

Table 34.2. *Indications for Memokath stenting benign strictures*

Aetiology	Patients
Iatrogenic	4
Ischaemia of ureteroileal anastomosis	3
Post radiotherapy	1
UPJ obstruction	2
Retroperitoneal fibrosis	2
Endometriosis	1
Post transplant	1
Total	**14**

UPJ, uteropelvic junction.

Memokath insertion technique

The procedure is carried out under general or regional anaesthesia. It is essential to have the necessary endourological equipment as well as fluoroscopy (C-arm) in the operating theatre.

The first step of the stent insertion involves defining the stricture limits by a retrograde ureterogram. It may be useful (indeed vital in some cases) to use an antegrade study in combination with the retrograde injection of contrast to clearly identify the upper and the lower limits of the ureteric stricture. These are marked externally on the skin with metallic markers. This step is important in the accurate placement of the stent. A guidewire is passed across the stricture into the renal pelvis. It is advisable to insert two parallel guidewires in patients with long and tight strictures. One of these acts as a 'safety' guidewire.

The length of the stricture is measured in several ways. The distance between the metallic markers measured over the skin frequently underestimates the true length. It is best assessed by inserting a ureteric catheter over the guidewire. Measurement is taken while the catheter is withdrawn between the proximal and the distal ends of the stricture.

This measurement is important, as it is used to select the appropriate length of the Memokath 051 stent for that patient. It is advisable to use a slightly longer stent than the length of the stricture to avoid residual obstruction especially in dealing with malignant strictures.

The stricture is dilated to 14 Fr with the dilator provided. The blue core of the dilator assembly can be removed once the dilator sheath has passed the superior limit of the stricture. (This step would be reversed in an antegrade insertion of the stent.) The hollow dilator sheath is radiopaque. A contrast study through the dilator sheath ensures complete dilatation.

The stent is now exposed by removing its protective shells. It is introduced into the dilator sheath under fluoroscopic guidance. When the stent has entered the upper limit of the dilator sheath, the latter is withdrawn under fluoroscopic control. The stent is fully exposed when the dilator sheath and stent assembly are locked.

Although the stent and its dilator are packed separately, they are tailor-made for each other. When fully locked, the stent will be completely exposed at the working end of the dilator sheath.

The assembly is manoeuvred in the appropriate direction so that it lies across the stricture. The external makers are invaluable during this procedure. The guidewire inside the stent assembly is removed. Any additional (safety) guidewires introduced in the ureter are removed. About 20 ml of sterile water preheated at 55°C is injected through the port of the dilator sheath to induce expansion of the stent. The position of the stent assembly is accurately maintained under fluoroscopy during this step. The expansion of the stent is virtually instantaneous.

The white lugs are now removed. The supporting black catheter is removed. The internal end of the dilator sheath would be at the lower end of the Memokath stent. A contrast study can be performed at this stage to ensure free flow through the stent as well as successful decompression of the obstructed system. The dilator sheath is now removed. Ureteroscopy may be performed up to the lower end of the stent if felt necessary.

It is important to avoid excessive pressure while injecting contrast for a retrograde study or ureteroscopy immediately after the insertion of the stent. The stent is liable to migrate proximally before it is 'gripped' by the surrounding tissue.

The author has used a urethral catheter overnight especially in males. This is removed the next day. A plain X-ray, renal function tests and urine culture is taken the following day. The patient is allowed home a day after stent insertion on oral antibiotics for 5 days.

The protocol of follow-up consists of intravenous urography, renal function tests and urine culture at 6 weeks. These are repeated at 3 months. DTPA renography is undertaken if necessary. Subsequent assessment of the upper tracts can be safely undertaken with ultrasonography combined with plain X-ray, renal function tests and urine culture at 3 monthly intervals.

Memokath removal technique

The unique property of the alloy permits the removal of this stent. The metal needs to be cooled below 10°C. The pre-cooled irrigant is passed through the stent for a few minutes. The irrigant can be cooled by keeping the bag of irrigating fluid in a refrigerator overnight prior to use. Once the stent had been cooled, its lower end is held in a suitable forceps and the stent is removed by pulling the metal wire. The stent unfurls easily as long as the metal is kept below 10°C (Fig. 34.2).

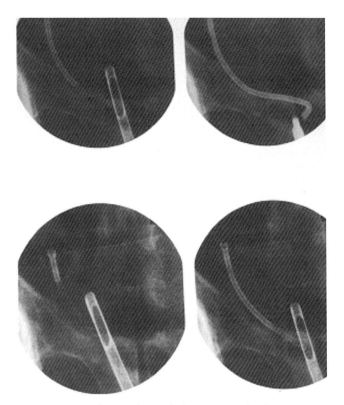

Figure 34.2. *Technique of Memokath stent removal. The stent is softened with cold irrigant (<10°C) and removed by suitable forceps.*

Results

The author has performed a total of 49 stent insertions in 39 patients to date (1996–2002). The first 13 patients were treated with the previous narrow version of the stent. The remaining 26 were treated with the new wide design stent. The initial application of the stent was restricted to the patients suffering upper tract obstruction due to malignancy. The study included patients with very refractory strictures referred from other institutions and hence was not randomized.

The indications for using the Memokath stent are outlined in Tables 34.1 and 34.2. A total of 26 patients had obstruction caused by malignancy. The remaining 13 had recurrent benign strictures. The benign strictures treated in this study have had several attempts with open as well as endourological surgery prior to referral.

The vast majority of the strictures (22 patients) were located in the lower third of the ureter. In 2 patients it was in the upper third, in 3 in the middle third, in 6 it was across the middle and the lower third of the ureter. In four patients, the entire ureter was obstructed whereas two patients had a pelviureteric obstruction.

Bilateral ureteric obstruction was treated with this stent in two patients by simultaneous insertion on both sides while in one patient, the stents were inserted three months apart.

The author has observed no major complications following the insertion of these stents. The mean length of stay has been 1.5 days (1–3 days). There was no operative mortality. No patient has been readmitted with stent-related complications.

Migration was observed in three patients who had the previous narrow version of stent. Upper tract decompression was maintained in these patients. However, the lower end of the stent entered the bladder and caused irritative symptoms requiring reinsertion of a short stent, with good results. Stent migration was seen in four patients with the wide version. Three of these patients do not have residual ureteric obstruction and have not needed a stent. The fourth patient has been treated with a specially designed stent for a recurrent ureteroileal stricture (Fig. 34.3).

Progression of disease (carcinoma of the prostate) caused obstruction at a different level in one patient requiring insertion of a longer stent two years after original insertion.

Fifteen patients have died with functioning stents. These patients benefited from the stent insertion for a period ranging from 2 months to 4 years. Eighteen patients are alive with functional stents for a mean period of 12 months (2 months to 4 years).

Ureteroscopy was performed 4 months after stent insertion in the first few patients. As no visible encrustation or urothelial ingrowth was observed, endoscopy is no longer felt to be necessary.

Cine intravenous urography was undertaken in the first two patients. Return of peristalsis was observed in the ureter above and below the stent.

Discussion

The Memokath stent offers many benefits over the conventional Double-J stents. It harnesses the possibility of selective decompression of the obstructed segment of a ureter. There are several advantages in stenting only the obstructed segment of a ureter. The lack of bladder component to a stent offers two important benefits. In addition to the lack of irritative symptoms, reflux is avoided.

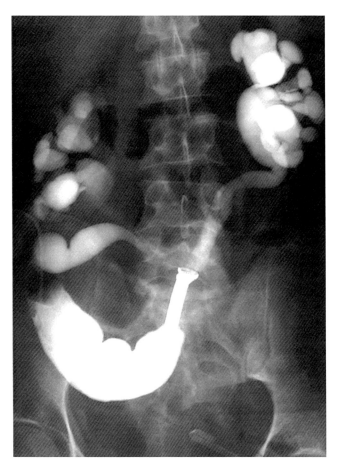

Figure 34.3. *A recurrent ureteroileal stricture managed by insertion of a modified Memokath stent.*

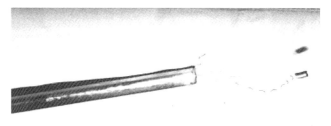

Figure 34.4. *A removed stent that has been partly remodelled by warming to demonstrate the property of the metal.*

Milroy et al. first reported the use of metallic stents in the management of urethral strictures.[11]

Pauer and Lugmayr[8,9] reported the benefits of the Wallstent in the management of ureteric strictures. The problems they encountered with these stents included ingrowth of the urothelium or tumour tissue and difficulty of stent removal.

The alloy of nickel and titanium has a unique shape memory. Depending on the manufacturing process, the alloy can be designed to soften below 10°C and regain its predetermined shape when rewarmed to 55°C (Fig. 34.4). The first reported use of the ureteric stents made from a similar alloy was in 1997.[15] The Memotherm stents Pandian et al. reported in this study could be deployed endoscopically but they cannot be softened by cooling and hence endoscopic removal was not possible.

The author undertook the first insertion of the Memokath 051 ureteric stent in November 1996. The intermediate results encouraged us to use this stent in difficult and recurrent strictures.[13] A total of 49 stents have been inserted in 39 patients. Improvements in the stent design and the delivery system have been made to improve the ease of introduction and reduce migration. The initial use of the stent was restricted to patients with malignancy. Patients with complex strictures due to benign disease were included later. Most patients were referred from tertiary centres for management with this stent as a last resort (having failed conventional endourological as well as open procedures). Hence, the study was not randomized.

This device has some important advantages:

Quality of life. A significant number of patients in this study had malignant disease. They needed regular hospital admissions for stent changes and stent-related complications. These significantly lowered their quality of life. One of the patients in this series had a solitary functioning kidney which was repeatedly obstructed by encrustation of the Double-J stent. This required frequent insertions of a nephrostomy tube. The quality of her life in the terminal months was enormously improved after the introduction of this stent (Fig. 34.5).

Cost. The use of long-term Double-J stents is sometimes necessary. This would invariably lead to regular stent changes. The cost-benefit of this stent becomes evident if more than two stent changes are necessary in a patient (based on UK hospital costs).

Bilateral ureteric obstruction. The introduction of bilateral Double-J stents can cause a significant increase in morbidity. This can be reduced enormously by the insertion of Memokath stents because the 'crowding' effect of the two lower ends of the Double-J stents in the bladder is avoided.

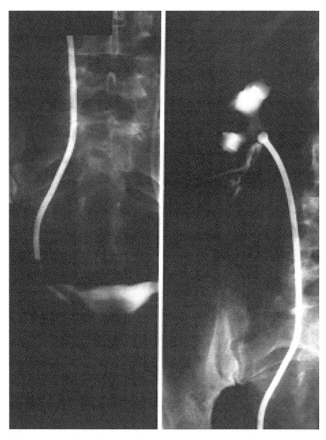

Figure 34.5. *Long Memokath stent insertion for a total ureteric obstruction in a solitary kidney caused by retroperitoneal lymph nodes from carcinoma of the breast.*

Points of technique. A few points of technique deserve special mention. Prior Double-J stent is helpful but not essential. Accurate placement of external markers and selection of appropriate stent length cannot be overemphasized. Although it may be possible to insert two or more stents in one ureter, multiple strictures at different levels are best treated with a single long stent. Benign strictures are often more difficult to dilate. Balloon dilatation (if used) must not exceed 14 Fr. The author feels the stent should not protrude into the bladder as the risk of encrustation may increase. Although there are no data to support this concept, encrustation has been observed in prostatic stents that have migrated into the bladder (Ellis, personal communication). The authors also feel that the stent should be placed with caution if the obstructed kidney has poor function, as stasis may lead to encrustation (Philp, personal communication).

Conclusions

The Memokath stent has several useful features. It combines the probability of selective decompression of an obstructed segment of a ureter, which prevents the unwanted side-effects associated with conventional stents. The unique property of its metal alloy allows removal when necessary in contrast to other stents. The alloy seems less prone to encrustation and so may be left in situ longer. This is a major advantage to the patients with malignancy.

The developments in stent design and indeed this metal alloy continue and will surely bring to the endourologist newer versions for use in the most awkward of strictures.

References

1.   Saltzman B. Ureteral stents. Indications, variations and complications. Urol Clin North Am 1988; 15: 481
2.   Ringel A, Richter S, Shalev M et al. Late complications of ureteral stents. Eur Urol 2000; 38: 41
3.   Dolcimo S G, Dewolf W. High failure rate of indwelling ureteral stents in patients with extrinsic obstruction: experience at 2 centres. J Urol 1989; 142: 277–179
4.   Cormio L, Koivusalo A, Makisalo H, Wolff H, Ruutu M. The effects of various indwelling JJ stents on renal pelvic pressure and renal parenchymal thickness in the pig. Br J Urol 1994; 74: 440–443
5.   Minhas S, Irving H C, Lloyd S N et al. Extra-anatomic stents in ureteric obstruction: experience and complications. Br J Urol 1999; 84: 762
6.   Dunn M D, Portis A J, Kahn S A et al. Clinical effectiveness of new stent design: Randomised single-blind comparison of tail and double pigtail stents. J Endourol 2000; 14: 195
7.   Gross A J, Plothe K D. The use of 2 ipsilateral ureteral stents for relief of ureteral obstruction from extrinsic compression. J Urol 1998; 160: 505
8.   Lugmayr H F, Pauer W. Wallstents for the treatment of extrinsic malignant ureteral obstruction: Mid term results. Radiology 1996; 198: 105
9.   Paue W, Lugmayr H. Metallic Wallstents: a new therapy for extrinsic ureteral obstruction. J Urol 1992; 148: 281
10. Gillams A, Dick R, Dooley J et al. Self expandable stainless steel braided endoprosthesis for biliary strictures. Radiology 1990; 174: 137–140
11. Milroy E J, Chapple C R, Cooper J E et al. A new treatment for urethral strictures. Lancet 1988; 1: 1424
12. Machan l, Rolf J, Adam A et al. Benign prostatic hypertrophy: treatment with a metallic stent. Am J Radiol 1989; 153: 779–181
13. Kulkarni R, Bellamy E. A new thermo-expandable shape memory Nickel-Titanium alloy stent (Memokath 051) for the management of ureteric strictures. Br J Urol 1999; 83: 755–759
14. Kulkarni R, Bellamy E. Nickel-Titanium shape memory alloy Memokath 051 ureteral stent for managing long-term ureteral obstruction: 4 year experience. J Urol 2001; 166: 1750–1754
15. Pandian S S, Hussey J K, McClinton S. Metal ureteral stents – an early experience. J Endourol 1997; 11: S92

35

A stent/nephrostome for the management of post-renal transplantation complications

M. F. Trapeznikova and S. B. Urenkov

Introduction

Ureteral complications, associated with stricture of ureter and ureteral fistula with urinoma, are the most frequent urological complications seen in renal transplantation. From 1 to 12% of kidney recipients suffer from ureteral complications[1-4] and, of these, an average of 30% lose the transplanted kidney, and up to 20% die because of these complications.[1,2,5]

Traditionally, such ureteral complications in renal transplant recipients have been managed by open reconstructive plastic surgery. Recently, better results have been achieved using various percutaneous techniques such as percutaneous nephrostomy, bougienage or balloon dilatation of the ureter followed by antegrade stenting.[4,6-17] In many cases these procedures have obviated traumatic secondary open surgery.

As a rule, obstructive complications and ureteral leakages, that develop during the first weeks after transplantation are caused by technical errors such as narrow, submucosal tunnel kinking of the ureter or narrow submucosal tunnel. One of the most frequent causes of late ureteral stenosis is wall ischaemia, as well as fibrosis of the area around the transplant. In the majority of cases the stricture is situated in the distal part of ureter and progresses within a period from 1 month to 5 years.[1,2,6]

Materials and methods

From January 1990 to December 1995, 561 renal transplantations were performed at the authors' institute. Ureteral complications were registered in 20 cases (3.6%), 14 of which were stricture of the ureter and six patients had ureteral fistula with urinoma in our study.

In patients after renal transplantation the clinical manifestations of ureteral complications are non-specific, and are often misinterpreted as chronic or acute rejection of the transplant. The results of treatment of ureteral complications depends directly on when they are detected.

Ultrasonography is the main method used for diagnosing ureteral complications after renal transplantation: in almost all cases, stricture of the ureter and ureteral fistula with urinoma can be diagnosed by this means (Fig. 35.1a).

Antegrade pyeloureterography is the most informative method for determining the localization of a stenosis or fistula, as well as the calibre of the lumen, length of the stricture and size of the urinoma. However, to reduce the risk of infection and decrease trauma to the transplant, this diagnostic method should be performed only during percutaneous nephrostomy (Fig. 35.1b), which will be followed by a choice of treatment options.

All 20 recipients were initially managed with this percutaneous approach. At the first stage of treatment percutaneous nephrostomy was performed using the standard technique under ultrasonographic guidance. Two patients of the six with ureteral fistula had large urinoma which were also drained percutaneously. In all cases the procedure was performed under local anaesthesia.

After percutaneous nephrostomy, the subsequent treatment stragegy was decided. In five cases open surgical correction was necessary because of complete obstruction of ureteral fistula (two patients) and when the stricture was more than 2–3 cm in length (three patients). During these operations the ureter was stented with a double-pigtail stent to prevent recurrence of the stricture.

In the remaining 15 cases of stricture of the ureter, percutaneous procedures such as bougienage (Fig. 35.2) and/or balloon dilatation (Fig. 35.3) of the narrow part of ureter with further antegrade stenting were performed. In those cases in which it was difficult to pass the guidewire through the stenosis under X-ray control, it was negotiated under endoscopic control using a flexible ureteroscope. The balloon dilatation was preceded by endoscopic incision of the stricture.

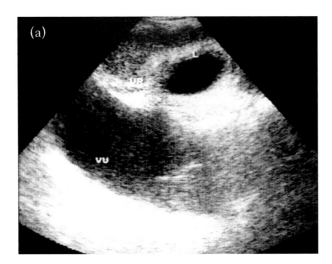

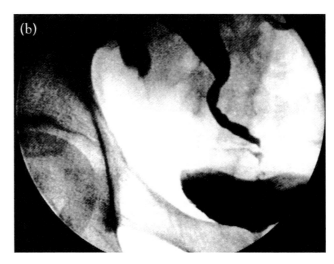

Figure 35.1. *Stricture of ureter after renal transplantation: (a) ultrasound image; (b) antegrade pyeloureterography showing the stricture. VU, bladder; UR, ureter; L, dilated renal pelvis.*

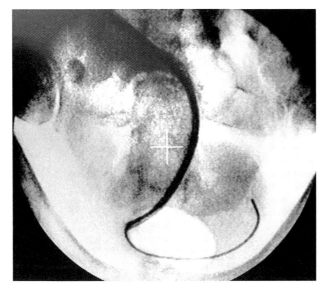

Figure 35.2. *Bougienage of ureteral stricture of renal transplant.*

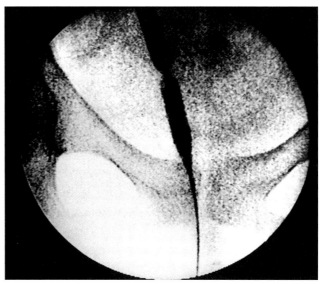

Figure 35.3. *Balloon dilatation of ureteral stricture of renal transplant.*

Results

In all cases of antegrade stenting special stent-nephrostomies, developed in the authors' department, was used (Fig. 35.4). The stent-nephrostomy represents a drainage device, combining a nephrostome and a ureteral stent. A special 'coupling' is fixed on the stent at the level of stricture of the ureter as seen during antegrade X-ray; this 'coupling' helps to prevent recurrence of the stricture. A 6 or 8 Fr (rarely 10 Fr) stent-nephrostomies was normally used. The stent-

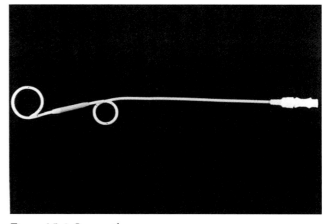

Figure 35.4. *Stent-nephrostomy.*

nephrostomies were adjusted for every patient individually, according to the ureteral length and localization of the stricture. The length of the ureter was determined either by ultrasound or X-ray. Experimental prototypes of the stent-nephrostomy were produced by the Moscow region-based firm "Meditcina, Informatciya, Technologiya" (MIT Ltd) in cooperation with the Department of Urology, Moscow Regional Research Clinical Institute (MONIKI).

Use of this stent-nephrostomy (Fig. 35.5), with its further transformation into the ureteral stent, has some distinct advantages over ordinary stents, as follows:

1. This stent simultaneously acts as a nephrostomy;
2. It enables the position of the stent's coils in the pelvis of the transplanted kidney and in the bladder to be regulated;
3. If the stent becomes obstructed during the early postoperative period, the patency of the lumen can be restored or the stent can be replaced.

Usually 3–5 days after the procedure the stent-nephrostomy is transformed to a ureteral stent by removal of the nephrostomy part (Fig. 35.6). The stent is finally removed 12–16 weeks after the operation. All percutaneous antegrade stentings were performed under epidural anaesthesia. No complications with regard to placement of the stent-nephrostomy were noted during these percutaneous operations.

Four patients with ureteral fistulas treated by percutaneous technique, despite the fact that the fistula healed within 5–7 days after percutaneous nephrostomy, underwent antegrade stenting by stent-nephrostomy to prevent stenosis of the ureter in the site of the fistula.

It should be noted that eight of the 11 patients with ureteral strictures treated by percutaneous technique underwent antegrade stenting by stent-nephrostomy performed simultaneously with percutaneous nephrostomy, bougienage and/or balloon dilatation of the stenosis. In cases of ureteral fistula, in order to avoid damaging the ureter in the segment of the fistula, antegrade stenting was always delayed. Stenting was performed 10–14 days after percutaneous nephrostomy when radiography showed the resolution of the fistula. As a rule, necrosis of the ureteral wall is accompanied by dense periureteral fibrosis. In turn, this leads to narrowing of the ureter at that particular site. Before

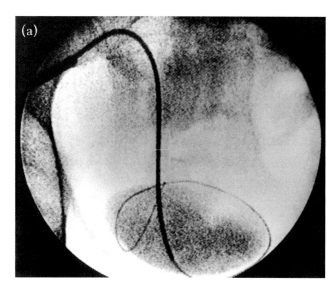

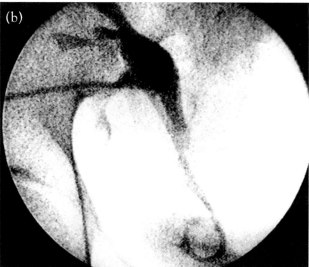

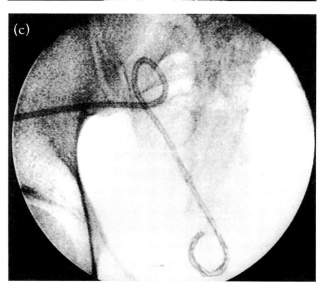

Figure 35.5. *Antegrade stenting of renal transplant ureter by stent-nephrostomy: (a) antegrade placing of stent-nephrostomy along the guidewire; (b,c) removal of the guidewire from stent-nephrostomy.*

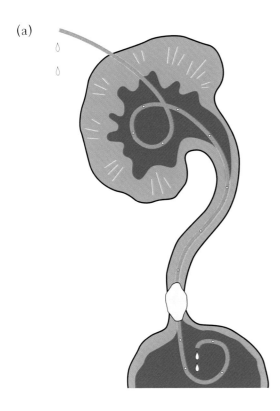

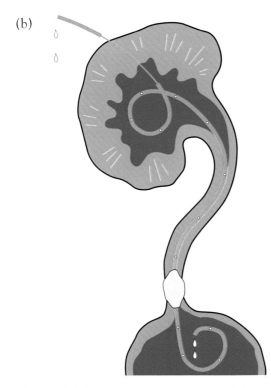

Figure 35.6. *Diagrammatic representation of the use of a stent-nephrostomy during treatment of ureteral complications after renal transplantation: (a) immediately after operation; (b) 3–5 days after operation (the nephrostomy component has been removed.)*

antegrade stenting, balloon dilatation of the ureter was performed at the site of the closed fistula. In the 15 cases of ureteral stricture, after antegrade stenting with the stent-nephrostomy during early postoperative period, ultrasound monitoring was performed every day (Fig. 35.7). This enabled the position of the stent-nephrostomy, as well as any obstruction of the stent, to be determined. After discharge, patients were recommended to attend for weekly ultrasound examinations.

The complications attendant on the long-term use of ureteral stents in patients with renal transplants are fragmentation of the stent, proximal and distal stent

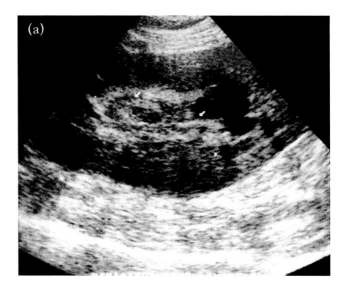

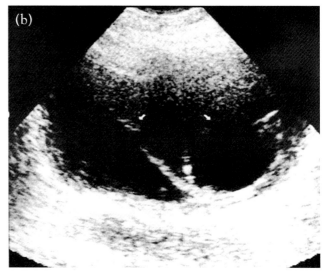

Figure 35.7. *Ultrasound monitoring after antegrade stenting: (a) proximal part of stent in pelvis of transplant; no dilatation of collecting system of transplant and no obstruction of stent; (b) distal part of stent in bladder.*

Table 35.1. *Stent-related complications*

Complications	Number of cases	Time since stent placement	Management
Stone formation	1	3 months	Extracorporeal shock-wave lithotripsy and stent removal
Proximal migration	1	5 days	Stent replacement
Distal migration	2	6 and 10 weeks	Not required

migration, stone formation on the stent and its obliteration, urinary tract infection and haematuria.[17] Complications related to placement of the stent-nephrostome were noted in four cases. All these complications were resolved without open surgical operations and the grafts were saved (Table 35.1).

In one patient 3 months after stent placement, a stone formed on its distal end (Fig. 35.8). This caused stent obstruction, distension of the collecting system and malfunction of the transplant, necessitating immediate intervention. Because of the relatively large size of the stone (2.0 × 0.9 cm), to achieve its complete fragmentation extracorporeal shock-wave lithotripsy was performed twice before removal of the stent. However, in this particular case the nephrostomy part was not removed because of the high risk of obstruction of the transplant with stone fragments. After removal of the stent in due course, encrustation of the stent without concomitant obstruction was observed in three patients. In one case proximal migration of the stent occurred, disrupting urine outflow (Fig. 35.9). This complication took place on day 5 after antegrade stenting and before removal of the nephrostomy part.

Replacement of the same stent in correct position with the help of a guidewire under X-ray control was performed.

If such a complication occurs after removal of the nephrostomy part of the stent, an additional percutaneous intervention to remove the migrated stent and to replace it with a new stent is necessary. This case confirms the advantage of using the stent-nephrostomy in the management of ureteral complications in patients after renal transplantation.

In two cases, distal migration 6 and 10 weeks after stent placement did not cause any disturbance of urine outflow and transplant function remained stable. All patients reported some dysuria. Ultrasonography revealed slight and insignificant distension of the transplant pelvicalycal system. As the dysuria and microhaematuria after placing the stent in the transplant were not considered to be serious complications, early removal of stents was not necessary and all stents were removed in due course.

Figure 35.8. *Stone formation at the bladder end of the stent.*

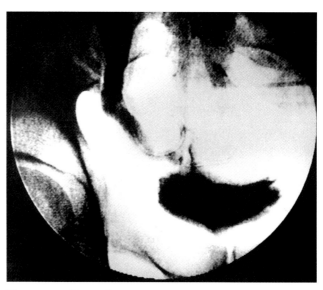

Figure 35.9. *Proximal stent migration.*

Urinary infection was noted to some extent in all patients. Percutaneous intervention, indwelling stent placement, as well as immunosuppression, are risk factors for the development of transplant pyelonephritis, which may lead to urosepsis and loss of the renal graft. However, adequate antibacterial therapy helps to avoid this complication. In this study no patients developed transplant pyelonephritis, either during stenting or after stent removal.

During the follow-up period (12–48 months), recurrence of stricture was observed in two cases, 5 and 18 months after stent removal. When the obstruction caused malfunctioning of the transplants, secondary percutaneous manipulation, such as percutaneous nephrostomy, endoscopic incision of the stricture in combination with balloon dilatation and antegrade stenting with the stent-nephrostomy were necessary. Stenting of ureter in these cases continued for longer periods, and the stents were removed 6 and 8 months after their placement. No serious complications were observed during secondary stenting.

Conclusions

This experience has shown that the use of antegrade stenting with the stent-nephrostomy in the management of ureteral complications in patients with a kidney transplant enables these complications to be resolved effectively and in a minimally invasive manner for the recipients.

In patients who develop stricture of the ureter after percutaneous nephrostomy, if the patient's condition allows further operative intervention, the authors recommend immediate dilatation of the stricture percutaneously, followed by antegrade stenting. In those cases in which the patient's condition requires time to prepare him for further treatment, the intervention is divided into two stages: during the first stage, only percutaneous nephrostomy is performed; as a subsequent second stage the ureteral obstruction is treated and antegrade stenting is carried out. A similar tactic is recommended in patients with ureteral fistula, because an attempt to place a stent immediately after percutaneous drainage of the transplant creates a high probability of further damage of the ureteral wall at the site of the fistula.

The use of a stent-nephrostomy significantly facilitates the management of patients with ureteral complications after renal transplantation during the early postoperative period; it drains the graft well and helps to prevent such complications as obstruction and migration that are encountered with regular stents.

References

1. Loughlin K L, Tilney N L, Richie J P. Urological complications in 718 renal transplant patients. Surgery 1984; 95: 297–302
2. Mundy A R, Podesta M L, Hartley L C J et al. The urological complications of 1000 renal transplants. Br J Urol 1981; 53: 397–402
3. Meech P R, Hardie I R, Hartley L C J et al. Further experience with an external ureterovesical anastomosis in renal transplantation. Aust N Z J Surg 1979; 49: 629–635
4. Kinnaert P, Hall M, Janssen F et al. Ureteral stenosis after kidney transplantation: true incidence and long-term follow after surgical correction. J Urol 1985; 133: 17–20
5. Sagalowsky A I, Ransler C W, Peters P C et al. Urological complications in 505 renal transplants with early catheter removal. J Urol 1983; 129: 929–932
6. Trapeznikova M F, Filiptsev P Y, Urenkov S B et al. Ureteral stricture: treatment in kidney recipients. Urol Nefrol (Mosk) 1994; 3: 42–45
7. Swierzewski S J, Konnak J W, Ellis J H. Treatment of renal ureteral complications by percutaneous techniques. J Urol 1993; 149: 986–987
8. Warner J J, Matalon T A, Rabin D N et al. Percutaneous interventional radiologic procedures for diagnosis and treatment of urological complications in renal transplant patients. Transplant Proc 1987; 19: 2203–2207
9. Bennett L N, Voegeli D R, Grummy A B et al. Urological complications following renal transplantations: role of interventional radiological procedures. Radiology 1986; 160: 531–551
10. Streem S B, Novick A C, Steinmuller D R et al. Long-term efficacy of ureteral dilation for transplant ureteral stenosis. J Urol 1988; 140: 32–35
11. Lamballe A K, Winfield M E, Brun M E et al. Percutaneous nephrostomy in renal transplant patients. Transplant Proc 1985; 17: 2143–2144
12. Glanz S, Rotter M R, Gordon D H et al. Interventional radiologic procedures in the management of the renal transplant patient. Urol Radiol 1985; 7: 97–101
13. Voegeli D R, Grummy A B, Mc.Dermott J C, Jensen S R. Percutaneous dilation of ureteral stricture in renal transplant patients. Radiology 1988; 169: 185–189
14. Leiberman R P, Glass N R, Grumm A B et al. Nonoperative percutaneous management of urinary fistulas and strictures in renal transplantation. Surg Gynecol Obstet 1982; 155: 667–672
15. Nicholson M L, Vietch P S, Donnelly P K, Bell P R F. Urological complications of renal transplantation: the impact of double J ureteric stents. Ann R Coll Surg Engl 1991; 73: 316–321
16. Thomalla J V, Leapman S B, Fil R S. The use of internalised ureteric stents in renal transplant patients. Br J Urol 1990; 66: 363–368
17. Nicol D L, P'ng K, Hardie D R et al. Routine use of indwelling ureteral stents in renal transplantation. J Urol 1993; 150: 1375–1379

Recanalization of metal ureteral stents obliterated by proliferative tissue

Z. Markovic

36

Introduction

Extensive advances in modern endoscopy, new surgical techniques and interventional radiology have contributed significantly to better surgical therapy of urinary tract obstruction. However, the high incidence of recurrent ureteral strictures remains one of the basic urological preoccupations. This particularly applies to patients who have contraindications for anaesthesia, repeated reconstructive operations with poor outcome, postirradiation retroperitoneal fibrosis and congenital malformations of the collecting system.

Metal stents are used for recanalization of ureters in an attempt to provide permanent patency to chronic strictures and to overcome imperfections of the previous methods used in interventional radiology (e.g. balloon catheter dilatation, various types of catheter prostheses and endoprostheses). Initial caution was induced by the fact that the first experimental and clinical results were unsatisfactory, that the implanted stent was not extracorporeally controlled and that the percentage of obliterations with tissue was high.[1] In the course of recent years, the new generation of stents, showing excellent results in recanalization of occlusive lesions of the blood vessels, reaffirmed their use in the management of ureteral strictures, as well.

Tissue proliferation into the stent lumen cannot be predicted according to mere duration, as it may occur 3–4 weeks or 4–6 months after stent insertion. In almost all cases, the stent becomes embodied in the ureteral wall, to some degree. This process is not related to the possible subsequent proliferation of tissue into the lumen, and should not be confused with tissue proliferation.

Localization of obstruction in relation to stent insertion depends on the site of predominant proliferation. Tissue proliferation may obstruct the stent partially or along the entire lumen. Stent ends are the most usual sites for the development of tissue obstruction: either lower (Fig. 36.1) or upper (Fig. 36.2) ends may be affected. Localization of the stent

obstruction should always be discussed in relation to the underlying disease and contrast image of the whole ureter. The stent may be patent, with obstruction occurring proximally (Fig. 36.3a) or distally (Fig. 36.3b) to the stent.

The obliterated stent is easy to diagnose by history, renal echotomography and blood analysis. The definite diagnosis is established by antegrade urography. Exact morphological gradation of the urodynamic disorder is an important prerequisite for planning the stent recanalization procedure.

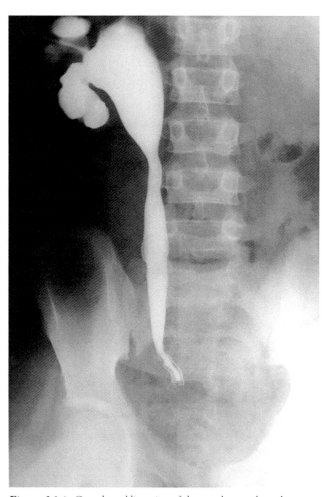

Figure 36.1. *Complete obliteration of the metal stent along the entire lumen of the distal end of the stent (filling through percutaneous nephrostomy).*

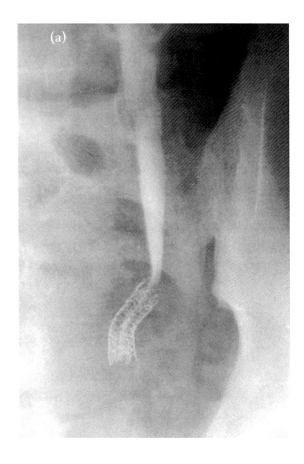

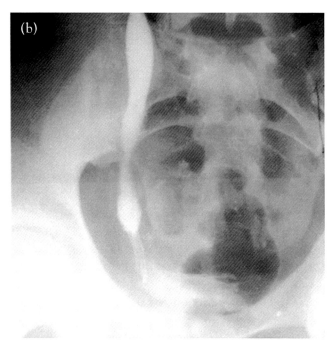

Figure 36.2. *Complete (a) and subtotal (b) obliteration of the stent by proliferative tissue on the proximal end of the stent.*

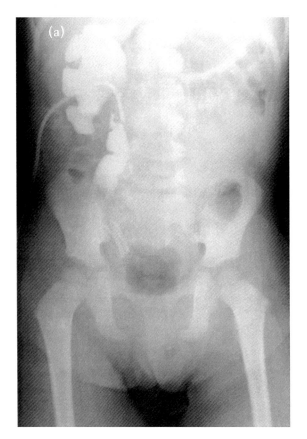

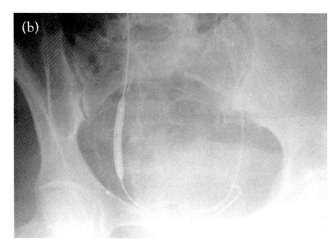

Figure 36.3. *(a) Contrast image through percutaneous nephrostomy: ureterohydronephrosis due to urostasis at the level of the ureteral mid-third. (b) Percutaneous balloon catheter recanalization of ureteral stricture localized distally from the metal stent.*

Recanalization methods

Recanalization of an obliterated stent usually implies the combination of several interventional uroradiological and/or endoscopic therapeutic methods. Management of urostasis caused by tissue proliferation into the stent lumen necessitates skilful application of modern methods of interventional uroradiology (percutaneous nephrostomy, balloon catheter dilatation and transurethral catheter stent placement).[2–4] Technically, recanalization of an obliterated stent lumen implies a return to the original therapy — percutaneous nephrostomy. Several approaches to recanalization of an obliterated stent are possible, and all have proved effective in indicated situations.

Mechanical ablation of proliferated tissues

Percutaneous placement of the broad end of a nephrostomic metal guide through the stent lumen is achieved through a percutaneous nephrostomy with the tip placed 1–3 cm proximally to the stent (Fig. 36.4). The metal guide is passed several times distally through the lumen of the obliterated stent, enabling recanalization to be achieved by mechanical ablation.

A more radical form of mechanical recanalization of the stent lumen implies use of manual or electric rotating metal baskets with a catheter of less than 5 Fr and fragmentation basket 5–7 mm in diameter (Arrow-Trerotola PTD 3000-R). Other systems, for percutaneous blood vessel recanalization and thrombectomy, can also be used in a modified form. This type of mechanical ablation usually results in minimal recanalization to form a tract through the stent to enable other recanalization methods, since it alone is insufficient for longer-lasting prevention of progression of tissue proliferation into the lumen.[5]

A special form of mechanical recanalization of the obliterated stent is compressive ablation of proliferated tissue. It implies balloon catheter dilatation with hyperextension of the obliterated stent. The procedure is preceded by placement of a nephrostomic guide through the obliterated stent, which is used as a dilatation tract.

Greatly distended pressure balloons (>16 atm ≈ 1.62 MPa) which are 6–8 mm wide and 5–10 cm long, are used in accordance with the length and lumen of the obliterated stent. The balloon is distended to its full width (Fig. 36.5). The inflated balloon is kept in place for about 10 minutes. Repeated dilatation during the same procedure has proved beneficial. Patency of the recanalized stent is monitored simply by the application of contrast medium through the same catheter. Uncontrolled dilatation (without manometric control) may result in balloon rupture. Pieces of the balloon

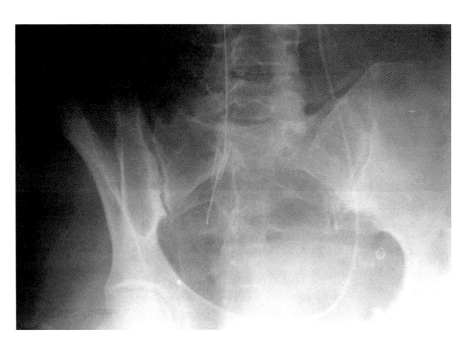

Figure 36.4. *Percutaneous recanalization of obliterated stent by metal wire (0.038 inch).*

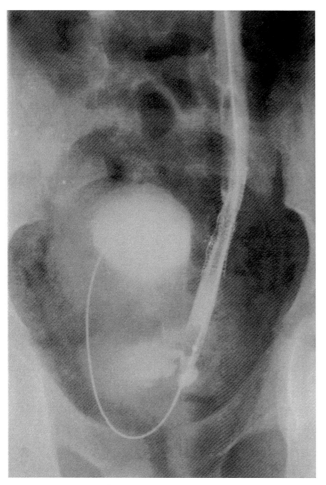

Figure 36.5. *Recanalization along the whole length of an obliterated Strecker stent (size 8 cm x 7 mm) by percutaneous balloon catheter dilatation.*

walls entering between the stent wires may result in catheter obstruction during pullout. A retrograde approach may be used as a alternative method to percutaneous placement of the balloon catheter. The site of stent obstruction determines the choice of approach: a retrograde approach is preferred in cases of predominant obliteration of the proximal end of the stent; with all other localizations, a percutaneous approach is preferred. After percutaneous recanalization the percutaneous nephrostomy is left in place for 2 weeks. Thus, control of stent patency is possible, as well as repetition of the procedure, if required. If a retrograde approach is used, a double-J catheter is left in place after the procedure. It is pulled out transurethrally, as it has the same purpose as the percutaneous nephrostomy in the antegrade approach. This type of recanalization is associated with a primary success rate of more than

75%. In the subsequent 9 months, proliferation and lumen obstruction ensue in about one-third of cases.[6,7]

Stent-in-stent recanalization technique

Overlapping stents provide the most effective method for recanalization of an obliterated system. The method is based on the encouraging experience in recanalization of obliterated urethral self-expandable stents.[8,9] This overlapping may be either partial or complete. The new stent to be inserted has to cover part ($\approx$5 mm) of the ureteral lumen beyond the primary stent. This applies to the proximal, distal or both ends of the obliterated stent. The stent used for recanalization should be the same width as (or somewhat wider than) the primary one. It is placed without preliminary dilatation, as this has been shown to increase firmness of the placement (Fig. 36.6). The stent-in-stent technique is associated with the most favourable permanent results: success is achieved in 85% of cases. Good permanent results with this type of recanalization have directly influenced the construction of a new generation of overlapping stents (Cook-Z stents, Covert Ultraflex stents) that are currently used as the stents of choice for recanalization of malignant oesophageal strictures.[9,10]

Recanalization by haemolysis (necrosis) of proliferated tissue

This is a new method that is, in fact, an imitation of the clot fibrinolysis used in atherosclerosis of the blood vessels. The primary aim of this type of recanalization is not to achieve permanent postprocedural patency, but to retard or terminate proliferation of tissues into the stent lumen, thereby providing conditions suitable for other, mechanical, types of recanalization. The method implies percutaneous placement of an occlusive balloon immediately caudally to the stent and jet-lysis perfusion of the fibro-necrotic substance. Special jet-lysis catheters of 5–7 Fr (Angiomed, Medi-tech) are used. Necrosis of proliferative tissue can be achieved by substances based on free radicals, such as glutathione peroxidase, glutathione-S-transferase, superoxide dismutase (LIP-SOD), C-vitamin solution, urokinase, streptokinase and other fibronecrotic factors.[10] Combinations of these substances may also be used: for example, 300–700 mg glutathione peroxidase is dissolved in about 500 ml fluid, and the obliterated

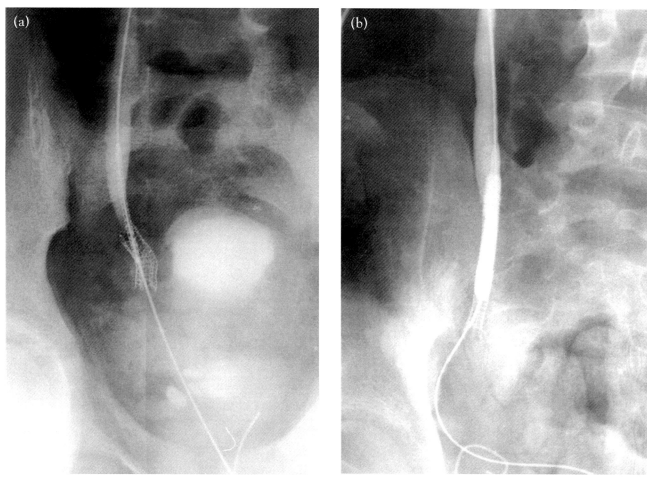

Figure 36.6. *Recanalization of obliterated stent by stent-over-stent technique. (a) Guidewire placed through obliterated stent to the urinary bladder. (b) Recanalization of the stent by a second metal stent insertion (size 4 cm/7 mm).*

lumen is perfused. An occlusive balloon prevents leakage of fluid distally, while jet-lysis enables postprocedural aspiration. A percutaneous nephrostomy is kept in place for 2–3 weeks as a tract for reperfusion. The perfusion is repeated daily for 1–2 weeks. In addition to local application, systemic therapy may be prescribed according to a special protocol implying initial determination of the basal oxidative status. In 12 of 20 cases (60%) the method successfully established primary recanalization of the stent lumen.[10] However, in about 45% of cases, obstruction recurred within 3 months. Use of this technique may stop tissue proliferation into the stent lumen. In addition to jet-lysis perfusion, the concept of application of fibronecrotic substances, in indications such as postirradiation fibrosis of the distal ureter, holds promise. For such applications, biodegradable stents containing fibronecrotic substances can be used.

Recanalization by retrogradely placed double-J catheter

Long-term (3–9 months) placement of an internal derivation system with double-J probe has proved to be a simple and relatively effective method of recanalization of obliterated stents. This particularly applies to the application of metal stents in paediatric urology (Fig. 36.7). Symptoms of urinary obstruction occur before the onset of stent encrustation. Therefore, tissue obliterated by a metal stent is never so thick that it will prevent application of a retrograde catheter of less than 5 Fr. In cases when catheter placement is impossible, previous introduction of a guide and minimal balloon dilatation with 3–5 Fr catheters has been found useful. Recanalization starts with 5 Fr, ending with 10–12 Fr. This type of recanalization prevents urinary stasis and infection proximally to the stent.

With regard to other recanalization techniques, laser recanalization of an obliterated stent has been used experimentally.[10] The method is equivalent to laser angioplasty. Initial results on the animal model have shown that the method is ineffective, and that it is difficult to control the reaction of a stent stricture on heating or disintegration, which results in necrosis or urethral rupture.

Selection of the recanalization method depends on the overall evaluation, implying the cause of primary insertion of the stent, time of obliteration, duration of urostasis due to the obstructed stent, and kidney function. Recanalization of the obliterated stent implies consistent utilization of all available alternatives. Therapy may last for several weeks. The methods available may be combined in various sequences, and the last in the algorithm is the stent-in-stent procedure.

When all the available alternatives are used to eliminate obstruction, primary recanalization of occluded stent is usually successful. However, recurrence of obliteration remains a threat. Postprocedural obliteration cannot be prevented in cases where the indications were incorrect. If a stent is inserted in inflammatory stricture, in postoperative strictures in the early postoperative course, and in strictures of other aetiologies where substantial fibroproliferative reaction of the urothelium is to be expected, such obliteration cannot be prevented. The best permanent results are achieved in patients with postoperative ureteral fibrosis characterized by avascularity and urothelial tissue reduction. The use of metal stents is not recommended in cases of stricture of unknown aetiology. Metal stents are not indicated if the more well established methods of interventional radiology and endoscopy have not been used in an attempt to recanalize the stricture.

The application of metal stents in the recanalization of ureteral strictures is a method that holds clinical promise. This will be determined by further technical improvements in stent design and manufacture. With the introduction of covered stents, tissue proliferation into the stent lumen among the thin wires of the stent will be greatly reduced.

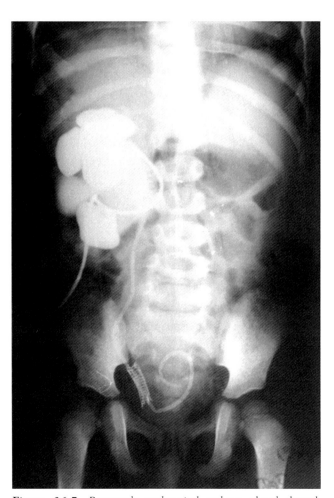

Figure 36.7. *Retrograde pyelovesical catheter placed through obliterated metal stent.*

References

1. Charnsangavej C, Carrasco C H, Wright S et al. Expandable Stents. In: Dondelinger F, Rossi P, Wallace S (eds) Interventional Radiology. New York, Thieme Medical, 1989: 686–706
2. Bettmann M A, Perlmutt L, Finkelsten J et al. Percutaneous placement of soft, indwelling ureteral stent. Radiology 1985; 157: 817–818
3. Bigongiari L R. Transluminal dilatation of ureteral strictures. In: Lang E K (ed) Percutaneous and interventional urology and radiology. Berlin: Springer, 1986: 113–118
4. Fritzsche P J. Antegrade and retrograde ureteral stenting. In: Lang E K (ed) Percutaneous and interventional urology and radiology. Berlin: Springer, 1986: 91–111
5. Markovic Z, Goldner B, Masulovic D, Bozovic Z. Recanalization of postoperative ureteral strictures with metal stent. Cardiovasc Intervent Radiol 1996; 19 (suppl 2): 203–204
6. Markovic Z, Masulovic D, Bozovic Z et al. Recanalization of postirradiation strictures of distal ureter with systemic and local therapy with free oxygen radicals: initial experience. Cardiovasc Intervent Radiol 1996; 19 (suppl 2): 139–140
7. Wright K C, Dobben R L, Magal C et al. Occlusive effects of metallic stents on canine ureters. Cardiovasc Intervent Radiol 1993; 16: 230–234
8. Mitty H A. Ureteral stenting facilitated by antegrade transuretral passage of guide wire. AJR 1984; 142: 831–832
9. Ell C, May A, Hahn EG, Gianturco-Z. Stents in the palliative treatment of malignant esophageal obstruction and esophagotracheal fistulas. Endoscopy 1995; 27: 495–500
10. Markovic Z. Recanalization of ureteral strictures with metal stents. In: Markovic Z (ed) Interventional radiology of uroobstruction. Belgrade: Srbostampa, 1996: 142–161

Ureteric stents: side-effects and health-related quality of life (HRQOL)

H. B. Joshi, F. X. Keeley Jr. and A. G. Timoney

37

Following an initial description of a long-term indwelling ureteric silicone stent by Zimskind in 1967, there has been considerable expansion in this field.[1] Over time, indications for stent insertion and their use have continued to expand. Since the development of stents, it has been realized that all types of stents are associated with side-effects and their use, in this respect, remains far from satisfactory. A number of side-effects, such as local discomfort or pain (loin and bladder region), lower urinary tract[2–8] and possible sexual dysfunction, have been observed following insertion of ureteric stents, which can distress patients both physically and psychosocially.

The history of the development of stents highlights some of the side-effects and morbidity associated with the stents. The ureteric catheters used in the early days were made of fabric coated with varnish and caused significant irritation to the bladder epithelium and urinary tract resulting in rapid development of encrustations. This limited ureteric catheterization to a few days because of patient discomfort and poor drainage. Similarly, the silicone rubber tubing, used subsequently, caused patient irritation as it impinged on the bladder.[9] In fact, the side-effects associated with stents have remained important stimuli to bring improvements in stent design and in the search for an ideal stent.

Indwelling ureteric stents: a source of problems

The literature on the subject of side-effects of stents and their impact on the patient is scant. The incidence of various symptoms associated with ureteric stents noted from the few studies in the literature is shown in Table 37A.1. Overall, the results from these studies highlight an array of side-effects associated with the stents. These studies indicate that the increase of lower urinary tract symptoms vary between 30% and 70%, while that of stent-related pain is 18–50%. In addition, some studies have identified additional problems, such as experiencing symptoms of urinary tract infection (UTI) and the need to take antibiotics. In addition, a study by Dunn et al. compared side-effects associated with two different stent designs (double-pigtail and tail).[8] Although they did not specify the incidence of the individual symptom assessed, the results revealed that both designs were associated with significant urinary tract symptoms and additional problems, such as fever, UTI, emergency room visits and the need for painkillers.

It is expected that these side-effects would have a negative influence on patients' health-related quality of life (HRQOL). Many factors, related to the stent (e.g. diameter, length, composition) and the patient (e.g. reflux renal pain, level of physical activities) may influence the incidence of side-effects. However, their cause-effect relationship has been difficult to establish. There were many shortcomings in these studies in terms of the methodology and the contents of the assessment. These studies did not use validated QOL measures. This has made the results of these studies weak.

It is interesting to note that despite improvements in stent design and composition, which have the important aim of achieving improved patient comfort and little or no morbidity, structured in-depth assessment of symptoms due to stents and their impact on patients' daily life has not been performed until recently.[10] Health-related quality of life (HRQOL) has become a relevant measure of efficacy and outcome in clinical trials. Its assessment is generally best performed using patient self-report techniques that measure subjective quality of life objectively, and forms an important valid outcome measure, as long as the tool is appropriate, well developed and reliable.[11–12]

Table 37A.1. *Ureteric stents and reported incidence of side-effects*

Side-effects Authors	Cadela et al.[4]	Bregg et al.[5]	Preminger et al.[6]	Lennon et al.[14]		Irani et al.[15]		Pollard et al.[16]
				Firm stent	Soft stent	1 week	Before removal	
	(n=60)	(n=50)	(n=70)	(n=78)	(n=77)	(n=20)	(n=39)	(n=20)
Method of Assessment	Q	Q	T	Q		Q		Q
Urinary symptoms								
Frequency (day)	62%		51%	65%	55%	85%	74%	50%
Urgency	67%		43%	58%	43%	59%	45%	
Nocturia	47%			50%	35%	56%	53%	55%
Haematuria	85%	42%	40%	54%	40%	64%	34%	40%
Dysuria	72%		34%	40%	22%	31%	13%	40%
Incontinence	20%		30%					
Debris in urine		0%						0%
Pain								
Loin/flank pain	18%	50%	43%	58%	38%	54%	40%	50%
Reflux pain				36%			51%	
Suprapubic pain		26%		46%	26%	49%	53%	
Bladder pain		38%	36%					
Lower abdominal pain								50%
Other								
Fever or chills		20%	13%					
Need for painkillers			41%			41%	21%	
Taking antibiotics		66%						
Migration		10%						
Infection			16%					
Pyelonephritis		8%						

Q, questionnaire; T, telephone.

Ureteric Stent Symptoms Questionnaire (USSQ): a valid approach for the assessment of the impact of stents

Lack of a reliable measure that could assess quality of life issues in patients undergoing ureteric stent insertion hampered understanding of stent-related symptoms and their true impact on patients' HRQOL. To deal with this problem, the Ureteric Stent Symptoms Questionnaire (USSQ), a new intervention-specific, comprehensive, reliable, and psychometrically valid multi-dimensional measure has been developed.[10] The development of the USSQ involved considerable input from clinicians and patients. The USSQ was developed using a multi-step, multi-disciplinary approach and adhered to the standard methods and rigorous guidelines of instrument development used in the field of measurement psychology.

A total of 309 patients were asked to participate during different phases. In Phase I, a structured literature search, patient interviews (n = 9) and studies using existing instruments (n = 90) formed the foundation for the initial draft of a new questionnaire (USSQ). In Phase II, the USSQ was pilot tested, reviewed by experts and field tested (n = 40) to produce a final 38-item draft. This addressed various domains of health (6 sections and 38 items) affected by stents covering urinary symptoms, pain, general health, work performance, sexual matters and additional problems (Appendix 1).

In Phase III, formal validation studies were performed to assess validity, reliability and sensitivity to change (n = 55). These studies showed it to be internally consistent (Cronbach's alpha >0.7) with good test-retest reliability (Pearson's coefficient >0.84). The questionnaire demonstrated good construct validity and sensitivity to change shown by significant changes in the score with and after removal of stents. The USSQ discriminated patients with stents from healthy controls ($P<0.001$) and patients with urinary calculi without stents and lower urinary tract symptoms.

Ureteric stents: symptoms and quality of life

The validation studies of the new USSQ described the incidence of stent-related side-effects and their impact on patients' HRQOL in detail for the first time.[13] A large proportion of patients undergoing stent insertion is in employment and the stents are found to have a significant impact on patients' work performance. Assessment of this aspect of stents as well as utility evaluation has clearly demonstrated the negative impact of stents.

Evaluation of 85 patients with unilateral indwelling ureteric stents who participated during the validation phases of the USSQ revealed a variety of side-effects due to stents. Urinary symptoms and pain that affected work performance and general health were important stent-related problems: 78% of patients reported bothersome urinary symptoms that included storage symptoms, incontinence and haematuria; over 80% of patients experienced stent-related pain affecting daily activities; 32% of patients reported sexual dysfunction; 58% of patients reported reduced work capacity and negative economic impact. The mean EuroQOL utility values (based on the results of the EuroQOL questionnaire survey), used commonly by health economists and indicate patients' satisfaction with the treatment, were significantly reduced following stent insertion.

Conclusions

In conclusion, it is evident that ureteric stents have a significant impact on patients' HRQOL. Urinary symptoms and pain associated with indwelling ureteric stents interfere with daily activities and result in reduced QOL in up to 80% of patients. Stents are associated with negative functional capacity and reduced utility values. The new Ureteric Stent Symptoms Questionnaire (USSQ) is a valid and reliable instrument that is expected to become a standard outcome measure. The USSQ has undergone linguistic validation for use in languages other than English and continues to undergo international evaluation within clinical trials. Future studies using the USSQ will help us to understand the mechanisms underlying stent-related symptoms and the therapies used in their treatment. It will also be possible to compare current and future stent types. The results may help to identify and establish a stent with minimum side-effects and maximum benefits ('gold standard' stent). This will be helpful in all future stent studies as the results and comparisons can be standardized.

References

1   Saltzman B. Ureteral stents, indications, variations and complications: Urol Clin North Am 1988; 5(3): 481–491
2. Tolley D. Ureteric stents, far from ideal. Lancet 2000; 356: 872–873
3. Thomas R. Indwelling ureteral stents: Impact of material and shape on patient comfort. J Endourol 1993; 7(2): 137–140
4. Candella J, Bellman G. Ureteral stents – impact of diameter and composition on patient symptoms. J Endourol 1997; 11(1): 45–47
5. Bregg K, Riehle R. Morbidity associated with indwelling internal ureteral stents after shock wave lithotripsy. J Urol 1989; 1141: 510–512
6. Preminger G, Kettlehurst M, Elkins S, Seger J, Fetner C. Ureteral stenting during extracorporeal shock wave lithotripsy: help or hindrance? J Urol 1989; 142: 32–36
7. Pryor J, Jenkins A. Use of double pigtail stents in extracorporeal shock wave lithotripsy. J Urol 1990; 143: 475–478
8. Dunn M D, Portis A J, Kahn S A et al. Clinical effectiveness of new stent design: Randomized single-blind comparison of tail and double-pigtail stents. J Endourol 2000; 14(2): 195–202
9. Mattelaer J J. History of ureteral and urethral stenting. In: Yachia D (ed) Stenting the urinary system (1st edn). Oxford: ISIS Medical Media, 1998: 18–26
10. Joshi H B, Newns N, Stainthorpe A, Keeley F X, MacDonagh R P, Timoney A G. Ureteric stent symptoms questionnaire: Development and validation of a new outcome measure. J Urol 2003; 169(3): 1060–1064
11. Fallowfield L. Quality of quality-of-life data. Lancet 1996; 348: 421
12. Streiner D L, Norman G R. Health measurement scales: A practical guide to their development and use. In: Streiner D L, Norman G R (eds), 2nd edn. Oxford University Press 1995: 1–3
13. Joshi H B, Stainthorpe A, Keeley F X Jr, MacDonagh R P, Timoney A G. Ureteric stent symptoms questionnaire: Evaluation of symptoms, Quality of Life and utility in patients with indwelling ureteric stents. J Urol 2003; 169(3): 1065–1069
14. Lennon G M, Thornhill J A, Sweeney P A, Grainger R, McDermott T E D, Butler M R. Firm versus soft double pigtail ureteric stents: A randomised Blind Comparative Trial. Eur Urol 1995; 28: 1–5
15. Irani J, Siquier J, Pires C, Lefebvre O, Dore B, Aubert J. Symptom characteristics and the development of tolerance with time in patients with indwelling double-pigtail ureteric stents. BJU Int 1999; 84: 276–279
16. Pollard S G, MacFarlane R. Symptoms arising from double J ureteral stents. J Urol 1988; 139: 37–38

APPENDIX 1

URETERIC

STENT SYMPTOMS QUESTIONNAIRE

Questionnaire 1 (*Stent in situ*)

We are interested to know about various aspects of your health, following insertion of the stent and the effect stent has had on your health.

Please complete the following questionnaire, which has different sections. Please answer all questions in each section.

(We would be grateful if you could complete and post the questionnaire within seven days)

Please complete:

Today's Date: /   /

Date of Birth: /   /

Please return to:

Post Code:

Hospital Number:
(for office use)

You will see that some questions ask if you have a symptom occasionally, sometimes or most of the time.

Occasionally	=	less than one third of the time
Sometimes	=	between one and two thirds of the time
Most of the time	=	more than two thirds of the time

URINARY SYMPTOMS

Please answer the questions thinking about the urinary symptoms you have experienced following insertion of the stent.

Please put a tick in one box for each question. ✔

Please think about your experience since insertion of the stent.

U1. During the day, how often do you pass urine, on average?

Less than hourly ₅

Hourly ₄

Every 2 hourly ₃

Every 3 hourly ₂

Every 4 hours or more ₁

U2. During the night, how many times do you have to get up to pass urine, on average?

None ₁

1 ₂

2 ₃

3 ₄

4 or more ₅

U3. Do you have to rush to the toilet to urinate?

Never ₁

Occasionally (less than one third of the time) ₂

Sometimes (between one and two thirds of the time) ₃

Most of the time (more than two thirds of the time) ₄

All of the time ₅

U4. Does urine leak before you can get to the toilet?

Never ₁

Occasionally ₂

Sometimes ₃

Most of the time ₄

All the time ₅

U5. Do you leak urine without feeling the need to go to the toilet?

Never ₁

Occasionally (less that one third of the time) ₂

Sometimes (between one and two thirds of the time) ₃

Most of the time (more than two thirds of the time) ₄

All of the time ₅

U6. How often do you feel that your bladder has not emptied properly after you have passed urine?

Never ₁

Occasionally ₂

Sometimes ₃

Most of the time ₄

All of the time ₅

U7. Do you have a burning feeling when you pass urine?

Never ₁

Occasionally ₂

Sometimes ₃

Most of the time ₄

All of the time ₅

U8. How often do you see blood in your urine?

Never ₁

Occasionally ₂

Sometimes ₃

Most of the time ₄

All of the time ₅

U9. How much blood do you see in your urine?

Do not see any blood ₁

Urine is slightly blood stained ₂

Urine is heavily blood stained ₃

Urine is heavily blood stained and has clot(s) ₄

U10. Overall, how much of a problem are your urinary symptoms to you?

Not at all ₁

A little bit ₂

Moderate ₃

Quite a bit ₄

Extreme ₅

U11. If you were to spend the rest of your life with the urinary symptoms, if any, associated with the stent just the way they are, how would you feel about it?

Delighted ₁

Pleased ₂

Mostly satisfied ₃

Mixed feelings (about equally satisfied and dissatisfied) ₄

Mostly dissatisfied ₅

Unhappy ₆

Terrible ₇

BODY PAIN:

This section asks about the **body pain or discomfort, which you associate with the stent.**

Please think about your experience **following insertion of the stent.**

P1. Do you experience body pain or discomfort in association with the stent?
YES ₁, **please go to question P2**
NO ₂, **please go to next section on General Health**

P2 (for women): Think of the drawings below as the drawings of your body. Please **mark (X) or shade the site(s)** **where you experience pain or discomfort in association with the stent typically (e.g. during the day to day** **activities, whenever you pass urine)**
   If you get pain at more that one site, please use a separate mark for each site.

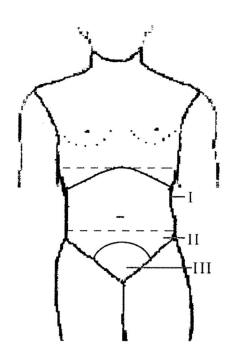

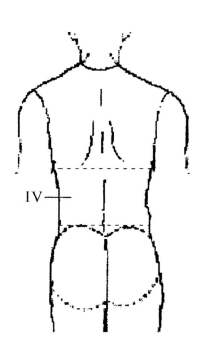

Front View   Back View

The numbers I – IV represent following areas for the right and left sides
   I – Kidney front/side area   **III** – Bladder area
      II – Groin area   **IV** – Kidney back (loin) area
Please use O for any other marked area and write the name of the site

P2 (for men): Thinking the drawings below as the drawings of your body, **mark (X) or shade the site(s) where you experience pain or discomfort in association with the stent typically (e.g. during the day to day activities, whenever you pass urine)**

If you get pain at more than one site, please use a seperate mark for each site.

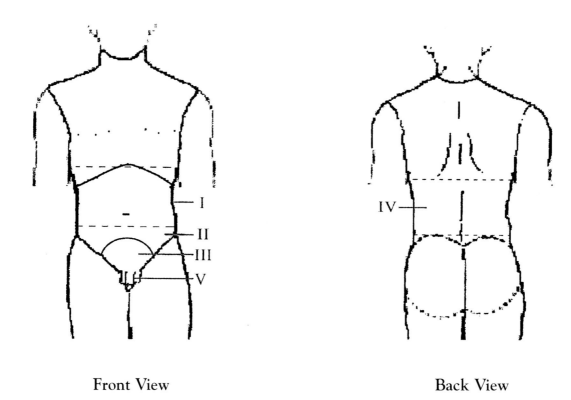

Front View   Back View

The numbers I –V represent following areas for the right and left side.

    I – Kidney front/side area   IV – Kidney back (loin) area

     II – Groin area   V – Penis

     III – Bladder area

Please use **O** for any other marked site and name that site.

P3. Please place a mark (X) to a point on the line below that indicates your pain or discomfort in association with the stent. **Please put a separate mark for each site** if the pain or discomfort is different in severity and write the corresponding number of each site used in the drawing above.

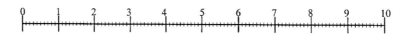

          No Pain or discomfort   **Worst Possible**

          Pain

P4. Which of the following statements best describe your experience regarding <u>physical activities</u> and the pain or discomfort in association with the stent?

I **do not experience any pain** or discomfort during physical activities ₁

I experience pain or discomfort only when I perform **vigorous activities** ₂
(e.g. strenuous sports, lifting heavy objects)

I experience pain when I perform **activities of moderate severity** but not with basic activities ₃
(e.g. walking few hundred yards, driving a car)

I experience pain even when I perform **basic activities** of daily living ₄
(e.g. walking indoors, dressing)

I experience pain while also **being at rest** ₅

P5. Does the pain or discomfort, in association with the stent, interrupt your sleep?

Never ₁   Most of the time ₄

Occasionally ₂   All of the time ₅

Sometimes ₃

P6. Do you experience pain or discomfort, in association with the stent, while passing urine?

Never ₁   Most of the time ₄

Occasionally ₂   All of the time ₅

Sometimes ₃

P7. Do you experience pain or discomfort, in the <u>kidney area</u>, while passing urine?

No ₁

Yes ₂

P8. How frequently have you required painkillers to control the pain or discomfort associated with the stent?

Never ₁   Most of the time ₄

Occasionally ₂   All of the time ₅

Sometimes ₃

P9. Overall, how much does the pain or discomfort, in association with the stent (as distinct from other symptoms) interfere with your life?

Not at all ₁   Quite a bit ₄

A little bit ₂   Extremely ₅

Moderately ₃

GENERAL HEALTH:

Following insertion of the stent:

G1. Have you had difficulty in performing light physical activities (e.g. walking short distances, driving a car)?

Usually with no difficulty ₁   Usually did not do because of the stent ₄

Usually with some difficulty ₂   Usually did not do for other reasons ₀

Usually with much difficulty ₃

G2. Have you had difficulty in performing heavy physical activities (e.g. strenuous sports, lifting heavy objects)?

Usually with no difficulty ₁   Usually did not do because of the stent ₄

Usually with some difficulty ₂   Usually did not do for other reasons ₀

Usually with much difficulty ₃

G3. Have you felt tired and worn out?

Never ₁   Most of the time (more than one third of the time) ₄

Occasionally (less than one third of the time) ₂   All of the time ₅

Sometimes (between one and two thirds of the time) ₃

G4. Have you felt calm and peaceful?

All of the time ₁   Occasionally (less than one third of the time) ₄

Most of the time (more than two thirds of the time) ₂   Never ₅

Sometimes (between one and two thirds of the time) ₃

G5. Have you enjoyed your social life (going out, meeting friends and so no)?

All of the time ₁   Occasionally ₄

Most of the time ₂   Never ₅

Sometimes ₃

G6. Have you needed extra help from your family members or friends?

Never ₁   Most of the time ₄

Occasionally ₂   All of the time ₅

Sometimes ₃

WORK PERFORMANCE:

W1. Regarding your employment status, are you

In full time employment	1	Student	4
In part time employment	2	Unemployed, looking for work	5
Retired on health ground	3	Retired for other reason (including age)	6
Not working for other reason (please specify)	7	_____	

W2. Following insertion of the stent, how many days did the symptoms associated with the stent keep you in bed all or most of the day?

Day(s)

W3. Following insertion of the stent, for how many half days or more did you cut down your routine activities because of the symptoms associated with the stent?

Half day(s)

Please answer the questions below (W4 – W7) only if you are in active work.

(Otherwise ignore questions W4 – W7).

W4. a) Job title or description of your role:_____

b) Are you an: Employee $_1$ Employer $_2$ Self employed $_3$

Please answer following questions if you have worked after insertion of the stent,

---

W5. Have you worked for short periods of time or taken frequent rests because of the symptoms associated with the stent?

Never	1	Most of the time	4
Occasionally	2	All of the time	5
Sometimes	3		

W6. Have you worked at your usual job, but with some changes because of the symptoms associated with the stent?

Never	1	Most of the time	4
Occasionally	2	All of the time	5
Sometimes	3		

W7. Have you worked your regular number of hours?

All of the time	1	Occasionally	4
Most of the time	2	Never	5
Sometimes	3		

SEXUAL MATTERS:

Please tick one box for each question by thinking about **your experience following insertion of the stent**.

S1. Currently, do you have an active sex life?

No   ₁, Please answer question S2 and go to next section (Ignore questions S3 and S4).

Yes   ₂, Please go to question S3 (Ignore question S2).

S2. (i) If NO sex life, how long ago did this stop?

After insertion of the stent   ₁   Before insertion of the stent   ₀
(ii) AND, why did this stop?

Because of the problems associated with the stent   ₁₀

Did not attempt any sexual activity   ₀

Some other reason – not to do with the symptoms of the stent   ₀

(Ignore questions S3–S4)

Please answer questions S3 and S4, only if you have answered 'yes' to question S1.
Please think about your experience following insertion of the stent.

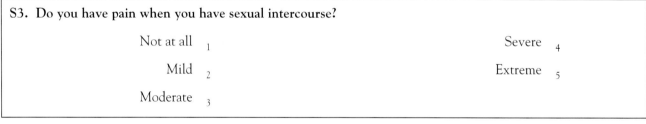

S3. Do you have pain when you have sexual intercourse?

Not at all   ₁   Severe   ₄

Mild   ₂   Extreme   ₅

Moderate   ₃

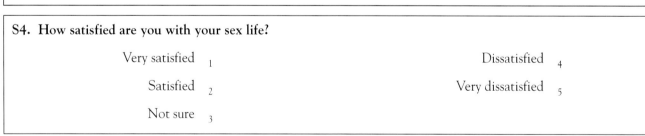

S4. How satisfied are you with your sex life?

Very satisfied   ₁   Dissatisfied   ₄

Satisfied   ₂   Very dissatisfied   ₅

Not sure   ₃

ADDITIONAL PROBLEMS:

The following questions ask about your experience following insertion of the stent. Please indicate your experience by ticking the appropriate box.

A1. How many times have you felt you may be suffering from a urinary tract infection (e.g. running temperature, feeling unwell and pain while passing urine)?

Never ₁   Most of the time ₄

Occasionally ₂   All of the time ₅

Sometimes ₃

A2. Have you needed to take antibiotics as a result of insertion of the stent? (Please ignore the course of antibiotics, which may have been given at the time of insertion of the stent.)

Not at all ₁   Two Courses ₃

One Course ₂   Three or more Courses ₄

A3. Have you needed to seek help of a health professional (such as GP, nurse) due to any problem associated with the stent?

Never ₁   Twice ₃

Once ₂   Three or more times ₄

A4. Have you needed to visit the hospital due to any problem associated with the stent?

Never ₁   Twice ₃

Once ₂   Three or more times ₄

GQ. In the future, if you were advised to have another stent inserted, how would you feel about it?

Delighted ₁   Mostly dissatisfied ₅

Pleased ₂   Unhappy ₆

Mostly satisfied ₃   Terrible ₇

Mixed feelings (about equally satisfied and dissatisfied) ₄

AQ. If there are any comments you would like to make about the questionnaire or any of your symptoms, please use the space below.

THANK YOU VERY MUCH FOR YOUR HELP

All information will remain confidential

QUESTIONNAIRE SCORING

Calculation of the scores for each section:

1. <u>Urinary Index Score</u>: Addition of the scores for the questions U1–U11

2. <u>Pain Index Score</u>: Addition of the scores for the questions P3–P9
   - Responses to the question P2 help to calculate the percentage of people reporting pain at individual sites (e.g. loin/bladder/groin)
   - P3 is the sum of the VAS scores for all sites of the pain

3. <u>General Health Index Score</u>: Addition of the scores for the questions G1–G6

4. <u>Work Performance Score</u>:
   - Days in bed
   - Loss of activity for half day or more
   - Quality of work: Addition of scores for the questions W5 – W7

(The answers to the individual question W5 – W7 can be additionally mentioned as % of people reporting problems for that attribute.)

5. <u>Sexual Matters Score</u>:
   - Percentage of patients unable to have sex due to stents
   - Quality of sex: total of S3 and S4

6. <u>Additional Problems with the stent in situ</u>: Responses to questions A1 to A4:
   Percentage of people reporting the problem and /or the number of times that problem has been reported. There is no single summated score.

7. <u>Global Quality of life with the stent in situ</u>: Response to the question GQ

37

Ureteric stents: development of a validated booklet for patients
H. B. Joshi, F. X. Keeley Jr. and A. G. Timoney

Due to the expansion in endourological techniques, both the diversity of ureteric stents available, and the indications for their use have increased significantly.[1] However, the side-effects of stents are a source of concern to patients.[2] The quality of information provided can greatly influence the way patients cope with stents. The provision of adequate patient information, as a part of shared decision making, contributes to good clinical practice and a satisfactory outcome.

Health information designed for patients serves to promote health awareness, encourages self-care, reduces inappropriate service use and improves the effectiveness of clinical care. Commonly, provision of patient information remains a one-sided affair and there is sufficient evidence that patients do not receive the information they want and need,[3,4] regarding their medical conditions, treatments and the outcome.[5] Explaining and understanding patient concerns, even when they cannot be resolved, results in a significant fall in anxiety.[6] These aspects are very important in patients undergoing placement of an indwelling ureteric stent.

There has been no validated and widely accepted patient information about ureteric stents available in the literature or clinical practice. The authors assessed the way patients are informed about stents, their expectations and satisfaction about such information. By using the results of these observations, and applying qualitative research methodology, the authors developed a scientific approach that incorporates patients' views and preferences, towards the development of a reliable and validated patient information booklet about ureteric stents. This booklet can be incorporated in daily clinical practice.

Methodology

Phase I: assessment of quality of current information and patient expectations
This involved qualitative research methodologies that include a survey of patients with indwelling ureteric stents. Semi-structured interviews of four patients (2 male and 2 female) were conducted to identify various issues related to the prior information they received about ureteric stents. The interviews focused on patients' understanding and knowledge of stents, their side-effects and how they managed while the stent was in place. The interviews explored the way in which patients received communication about the stents and their expectations and satisfaction with such communication. The interviews were audiotaped and transcribed to analyse emerging themes.

Using the themes generated in the interviews, a questionnaire was devised to further explore these themes across a wider cross section of patients with ureteric stents. The questionnaire asked about the presence of side-effects associated with the stents, the method used to inform patients about stents (e.g. verbal, written information), the adequacy of the information provided and the need for more details. Patients were also asked about the appropriate time for providing such information, the preferred format for its provision, and based on their experience of the stent, what information should be provided when a stent is placed. The questionnaires were sent to patients with different stent indwelling times, age groups, occupational status and to both sexes.

A structured search of the literature using all electronic databases and cross-references was performed to review the scientific literature concerning ureteric stents. Further opinions were sought from urologists about the use of ureteric stents and how patients were informed about them. In addition, currently available patient information material about kidney diseases and urological conditions were examined. The information thus compiled was used in the proposed material about ureteric stents.

The results of the questionnaire were analysed and, together with the information collected from the literature review and urologists' opinions, a preliminary draft of an information booklet (16 pages, size A5) entitled *Having a Ureteric Stent: What to Expect and How* to *Manage* was prepared. The booklet was divided into two sections. Part 1 entitled 'Urinary system and ureteric stents', covered information about the urinary system, details of the stents and indications for their use. Part 2 of the booklet, entitled 'Living with a ureteric stent', covered possible side-effects and the impact of the stents on daily life, the care that needs to be taken while a stent is in place and when to call for help. The booklet covered the important criteria set out by the King's Fund's work on patient information booklets.[6] The booklet is available on *http://www.blackwell-science.com/products/journals/suppmat/BJU/BJU2356/hrishi.pdf*

Phase II: validation of the booklet
The first draft of the information booklet was pilot tested by face-to-face interviews with five patients and was also reviewed by three urologists. This was aimed at assessing understanding, acceptability and content adequacy, and to clear any ambiguities in the booklet. Following pilot testing, necessary changes were made to finalize the contents of the booklet.

Formal validation studies were then conducted. Based on the work carried out by the King's Fund group, a questionnaire was designed to evaluate the new booklet.[7] The questionnaire asked for opinions on the six core attributes. These were:

- Content adequacy
- Relavance
- Matching of information with the individuals' experience
- Understanding
- Balanced view
- Visual appeal

The questionnaire asked readers to rate each attribute on a 6-point rating scale (poor) 1–6 (excellent) and an overall score out of 10.

The booklet, along with the questionnaire, was sent to a panel of clinicians, comprising 10 urologists and 10 general practitioners, and 30 patients with ureteric stents for evaluation. The booklet was also sent to five stent manufacturers for their opinions.

Results and discussion
The patient interviews highlighted a lack of communication between patients and the clinicians regarding the use of stents and the symptoms to expect while the stent was in place. A total of 26 (84%, 19 men and 11 women, mean age 49) patients completed the questionnaire in Phase I. The indwelling time for the stent at the time the patients were surveyed was 2–7 weeks. The interviews revealed widespread dissatisfaction about the content of the information and the way it was provided. The patients felt that the information did not match their experiences. They experienced various problems while the stent was in situ and struggled to get the necessary, basic information and the reassurance that, in their opinion, could have been provided before the intervention. Overall, it was apparent that patients were interested in getting more information that was scientific and realistic.

The analysis of the data collected is shown in Table 37B.1. The patients wished to know more about why stents are used, how they are placed and how they stay in. They were keen to know all possible side-effects, such as various urinary symptoms and associated pain, even though not everyone experienced these side-effects. One 2 of the 30 patients expressed the view that they did not wish to have detailed information about stents.

The patients did not receive information about the possible impact of an indwelling stent on work

Table 37B.1. *Survey of patients' views regarding provision of information about ureteric stents*

Questions	Patients (%) (n=30)
Experience of side-effects of stents	86
Did not receive adequate information	80
Information provided	
• Oral	53.3
• Written	6.7
• None	40
Patients requesting more information	85
Appropriate time to provide information: prior to stent placement	100
Modes (format) of information requested	
• Written with drawings	84
• To see an actual stent	40
• To see a model	30
• Computer based	0

performance, general health and daily life. This information, in the patients' opinion, would have been very helpful for them to prepare for stent-related problems and to cope with them more easily while the stent was in place. There was agreement among the patients about the importance of receiving this information prior to the placement of stent. As explained by a patient during the interviews:

> Getting the information about stents would not have stopped me having the stent put in but I would have liked to have known for my own personal benefit what the experiences were going to be. It would have made no difference to me saying yes to have the stent put in. The advice was that I would be better off with the stent and I was prepared to take the advice.

This fact was in contradiction to the urologists' view that information about the stent, especially the side-effects, should be given only after the stent was in place. Finally, all patients expected the stent to be much smaller than its true length. No patient showed preference towards computer-based information as this was perceived to be less easily accessible for frequent use.

The results of this study clearly indicated that patients were not receiving satisfactory information about ureteric stents. The information provided was inadequate, in a form that was not the preferred mode and did not take into account patients' needs and expectations. This lack of adequate patient information may also have contributed to patient dissatisfaction about the stents and the difficulties encountered in coping with them. The reasons for this may be multiple. The information involved is, in part, complex and includes technical details. There are limitations on the consultation time and constraints within the clinical situation (e.g. patients presenting in an acute situation requiring urgent or semi-urgent stent insertion). Importantly, there is no effective written information available that could be given to the patients. The common question faced in a day-to-day clinical practice is: What is the best way to provide information that is adequate, valid, evidence-based and incorporates patients' expectations? The need for more information was highlighted in this study where patients wanted more information about stents in addition to seeking a better understanding of their disease and the treatment offered. They were even interested to see a real stent and/or the models to show how a stent is located in the body.

Patients preferred written details along with illustrative drawings as the preferred method of receiving information about the stents. It has been shown that an average of 75% of patients wanted written information with their medication and such information is read by the vast majority (80%) of patients. The same is applicable to a medical investigation, treatment or hospital admission.[8,9] Hence, the authors decided to provide this information in a booklet form. In the booklet illustrative diagrams and photographs were included that would satisfy the patients' need to observe a model or an actual stent. The little support for the provision of the information on computer demonstrated the importance of the booklet in the paper form as this was considered to be easily accessible. Such leaflets can play an important part in supplementing and reinforcing information as long as they conform to the highest standards of scientific accuracy, comprehensibility and relevance.[10]

Various checklists have been proposed to enhance the quality of the health information.[11] The main way to improve patient understanding and to incorporate it in patient communications is by seeking their active participation in the preparation of such information.[7] In Phase I, the principles of social survey and qualitative research methods followed, as this is the most relevant method to explore and incorporate patients' perspectives.[12] Once important issues were identified after interviewing four patients with ureteric stents, these themes were further explored using a questionnaire survey, which was relatively easy to conduct.

It has been shown that written information, prior to surgery, can result in better post-surgical adjustment and sometimes in faster recovery.[13] The findings of this study match these views as all patients in the study expressed the view that information about stents should be given prior to stent placement, as this would have helped them to cope better. The clinicians appeared to disagree with this view. It may be that patients need be given a choice on this issue and the timing of provision of the information may be decided on an individual basis so that it would fit with their methods of coping and information needs.

In Phase II, the results of the pilot testing showed the booklet to be acceptable and adequate in content. Some sentences required alteration to improve patient understanding. The diagrams were felt to be appropriate and easy to understand. Of the 30 patients and 20 clinicians, 23 (77%) and 10 (50%), respectively, returned the booklet evaluation questionnaires. Four of five stent manufacturers reviewed the booklet. The mean patient booklet rating score was 9.2 (range 8–10) while the mean score given by the clinicians' was 8.1 (range 7–9.5) out of 10. Analysis of each of the six attributes revealed that the mean score for all the attributes was in the range between 4 and 5 (Fig. 37B.2). The highest scores were given to adequacy and relevance of the content.

There was no important areas that were omitted or required to be added. The only major point raised by the clinicians was the timing of provision of this information. The clinicians thought that giving this information prior to stent insertion might make patients feel very anxious and worried. Hence, such information should best be provided only after insertion of the stent. All the stent manufacturers who reviewed the booklet found it to be satisfactory and only minor amendments were suggested.

The results of the validation study showed satisfactory acceptance of the booklet by the patients, clinicians and the stent manufacturers although it is difficult to satisfy every reviewer on all the attributes. In this regard it is essential to incorporate a multidisciplinary approach so that important aspects of the information can be covered. During Phase II, involvement of the consultant urologists and the manufacturers has been on a national basis while patients involvement was on a regional basis. Patients involvement on a national basis may help to take into account cultural differences related to such information, if any, so that the booklet can be validated in a wider context.

Conclusions

There is a lack of provision of enough patient information about ureteric stents that would satisfy their needs. Using an approach that included qualitative research methodologies the authors developed a validated information booklet on ureteric stents that

Category	Clinicians	Patients
Content adequacy	4.5	5.1
Relevance	4.4	5.2
Matching of information with the individual's experience	4.3	4.9
Understanding	4.0	4.9
Balanced view	4.4	4.8
Visual appeal	4.0	4.7

Figure 37B.2. *The mean rating scores for the booklet given by patients and clinicians for each category (0–6, poor–excellent).*

incorporated patients' expectations and views. This approach can be used to develop various other patient information materials. The new booklet is expected to be an effective tool for patient communication that should enable patients to cope better with problems associated with ureteric stents.

References

1. Saltzman B. Ureteral stents: Indications, variations and complication. Urol Clin North Am 1988; 15(3): 481–491
2. Joshi H B, Stainthorpe A, Keeley F X Jr, MacDonagh R, Timoney A G. Indwelling ureteric stents: evaluation of patient's quality of life to aid outcome analysis. J Endourol 2001; 15(2): 151–154
3. Korsch B M, Negrate V F. Doctor patient communication. Sci Am 1972; 227: 66–72
4. What seems to be the matter; communication between hospitals and patients: Audit Commission. London: HMSO, 1993
5. Ley P. Giving information to patients. In: Eiser J R (ed) Social psychology and behavioural medicine. New York: Wiley, 1982
6. Coulter A, Entwistle V, Gilbert D. Sharing decisions with patients: is the information good enough? BMJ 1999; 318: 318–322
7. Coulter A, Entwistle V, Gilbert D. Informing patients: an assessment of the quality of patient information material. London: King's Fund, 1998
8. Morris L A, Groft S. Patient package insertion: a research perspective. In: Melmon K (ed) Drug therapeutics: concepts for clinicians. New York: Elsevier, 1982
9. Visser A P. Effects of an information booklet on the well being of hospital patients: Pat Couns Health Educ 1980; 2: 51–64
10. Coulter A. Evidence based patient information: is important, so there needs to be a national strategy to ensure it. BMJ 1998; 317: 225–226
11. Entwistle V A, Watt I S, Davis H, Dickson R, Pickard D, Rosser J. Developing information materials to present the findings of technology assessments to consumers. Int J Technol Assess Health Care 1996; 8: 425–437
12. Pope C, Mays N. Reaching the parts other methods cannot reach: an introduction to qualitative methods in health and health services research. BMJ 1995; 311: 42–45
13. Matthews A, Ridgeway V. Health care and human behaviour. In: Steptoe A, Matthews A (eds) London: Academic Press, 1984

HAVING A URETERIC STENT

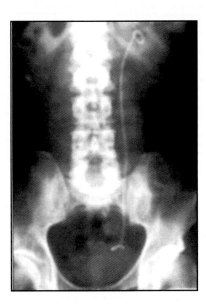

WHAT TO EXPECT AND
HOW TO MANAGE

INTRODUCTION

In patients who have, or might have, an obstruction (blockage) of the kidney, an internal drainage tube called a 'stent' is commonly placed in the ureter, the tube between the kidney and the bladder. This is placed there in order to prevent or temporarily relieve the obstruction.

The booklet contains general information about ureteric stents, explains the benefits to be derived from them and mentions some of the drawbacks that patients might experience.

Your urologist is planning to use such a stent for you.

The booklet is divided into two parts.

- The first part explains about the urinary system, obstruction of the kidneys and treatment of this obstruction using ureteric stents.
- The second part describes what to expect while the stent is in place and any possible side-effects.

Your urologist will explain the specific details applicable to you.

The booklet is designed for use by patients who are going to have a stent inserted. It will also be of help to health care professionals involved in your care or anyone who wishes to know more about ureteric stents. At the end there is information about your kidney condition and stent.

The information provided in the booklet is also available on the Bristol Urological Institute's web site. The web address is **http://www.bui.ac.uk**

INDEX TO THE CONTENTS

Page

Part I: THE URINARY SYSTEM AND URETERIC STENTS

The Urinary System and the Ureter

The kidneys produce urine. Normally there are two kidneys situated in the upper part of the abdomen, towards the back. The urine formed in the kidney is carried to the bladder by a fine muscular tube called a ureter. The urinary bladder acts as a reservoir for the urine and when it is full it is emptied via the urethra (water passage).

Figure 1: The Urinary System

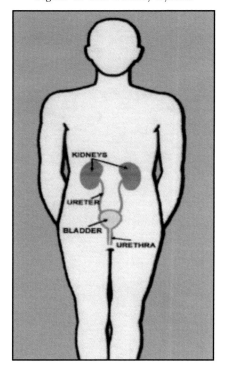

How does a kidney become obstructed?

Common causes of obstruction of the kidneys and ureter are:

- a kidney stone or its fragment moving into the ureter, either spontaneously, or occasionally following such treatment as shock wave therapy.
- narrowing (stricture) of the ureter anywhere along its path. This can be due to various causes e.g. scarring of wall of the ureter, narrowing of the area where ureter leaves from the kidney (pelvi-ureteric junction).
- temporarily, following an operation or after an instrument has been inserted into the ureter and kidneys.

Occasionally, obstruction can occur because of diseases of the prostate or tumours of the urinary system.
Your urologist will provide further details applicable to you.

What are the effects of obstruction?

Whenever there is an obstruction, pressure builds up behind the kidney. Due to high pressure, the function of the kidneys starts to suffer over a period of weeks.

The obstruction can also cause stagnation of the urine, which can lead to infection and further damage to the kidneys. It is, therefore, important to relieve or prevent obstruction of the kidneys.

Temporary relief of the obstruction

It is not always possible to identify what has caused an obstruction and to treat this immediately. It is therefore essential to relieve the obstruction on a temporary basis before treatment is carried out.

Also, following an operation on the ureters, it takes time for the ureters to heal and a temporary measure to prevent obstruction becomes essential. This is commonly achieved by inserting a ureteric stent to make a channel for the urine to pass and allow the kidneys to drain.

What is a Ureteric Stent?

A ureteric stent is a specially designed hollow tube, made of a flexible plastic material that is placed in the ureter. The length of the stents used in adult patients varies between 24 to 30 cm. Although there are different types of stents, all of them serve the same purpose (see Figure 2).

Figure 2: A type of a ureteric stent

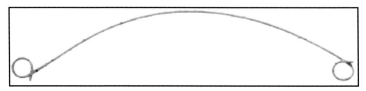

How does a stent stay in place?

The stents are designed to stay in the urinary system by having both the ends coiled. The top end coils in the kidney and the lower end coils inside the bladder to prevent its displacement. The stents are flexible enough to withstand various body movements.

How is a ureteric stent put in place?

Usually a stent is placed under a general anaesthetic using a special telescope (cystoscope) which is passed through the urethra into the bladder. The stents are then placed in the ureter and kidney via the opening of the ureter in the bladder. The stent may be inserted as an additional part of an operation on the ureter and kidney (e.g. ureteroscopy). Occasionally they are placed from the kidney down to the bladder using special x-ray techniques. The correct position of a stent is checked by taking an x-ray.

How long will the stent stay in the body?

There is no hard and fast rule about this. The stent has to be kept in place as long as necessary, i.e. until the obstruction is relieved. This depends on the cause of obstruction and the nature of its treatment.

In the majority of patients, the stents are required for only a short duration, from a few weeks to a few months. However, a stent in the right position can stay in for up to three months without the need to replace it. When the underlying problem is not a kidney stone, the stent can stay even longer. There are special stents, which may be left in for much longer time.

Your urologist will tell you how long he expects your stent to remain in place.

How is a stent removed?

This is a short procedure and consists of removal of the stent using a flexible cystoscope, usually under local anaesthesia. Sometimes a stent can be left with a thread attached to its lower end that stays outside the body through the urethra. Doctors can remove such stents by just pulling this thread.

Figure 3: A stent placed inside the urinary system

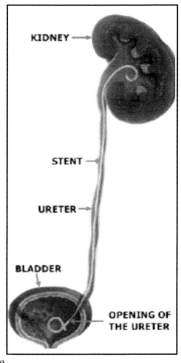

Is there an alternative option to the use of a stent?

There is no simple alternative option. In some patients, a tube draining the urine to the outside called a 'nephrostomy tube' may be placed in the kidney. However, this involves carrying a urine collection bag attached to your back, which requires proper care.

If you need this treatment your urologist will explain in detail what is involved.

Part 2: LIVING WITH A URETERIC STENT

Introduction

Ureteric stents are designed to allow people to lead as normal a life as possible. However, they may not be without side-effects. In placing a stent, there is a balance between its advantages in relieving the obstruction and any possible side-effects. Most side-effects are not a danger to your health or your kidneys although they can be a nuisance. Below, we have described all the possible side-effects associated with a ureteric stent.

What are the possible side-effects associated with a stent?

Many patients do not experience problems with the stents. In the majority of the patients experiencing side-effects they are minor and tolerable. However, sometimes they can be moderate to severe in nature.

Commonly noted side-effects are:

- The majority of patients with a stent in place will be aware of its presence most of the time.

- *Urinary symptoms*
  There might be:
  – an increased frequency of passing urine

- the need to rush to pass urine (urgency)
- a small amount of blood in the urine. This is quite common and the situation can improve with a greater fluid intake.
- the stents can also result in a sensation of incomplete emptying of the bladder.
- very occasionally, especially in women, there is a slight risk of episodes of incontinence.

These effects are possibly due to the presence of the stent inside the bladder causing mechanical irritation. These effects should disappear when the stent is removed.

- **Discomfort or pain**

Stents can cause discomfort or pain, commonly in the bladder and kidney (loin) area, but sometimes in other areas such as the groin, urethra and genitals. The discomfort or pain may be more noticeable after physical activities and after passing urine.

Complete understanding of these side-effects and their causes is not clear at present. It has also not been possible to predict, before placement of a stent, which patients are likely to experience side-effects and what they will be.

Duration of side-effects associated with a stent – can they improve?

There is some evidence that some of the symptoms, such as pain while passing urine and blood in the urine, may improve with time. However, this remains unpredictable. It has been reported that around 20–70% of patients with stents experience one or more of these side-effects.

Medical science and the stent manufacturers are working to develop a stent that will cause the least possible side-effects.

Can the side-effects interfere with my day to day life?

The stents are not expected to cause much disruption to your normal daily life. However, you may experience some side-effects that can cause some problems, either directly or indirectly.

Let us look at this in relation to various daily activities:

- **Physical activities and sports:**
  You can carry on with various physical activities while the stent is in place provided the underlying kidney condition and your health allows you to do it. However, you may experience some discomfort in the kidney area and passing of blood in your urine, especially if sports and strenuous physical activities are involved. Sometimes side-effects associated with a stent can make you feel more tired than normal.

- **Work activities:**
  You can continue to work normally with the stent inside your body. However, if the work involves lot of physical activities, you may experience more discomfort. Occasionally side-effects, such as urinary symptoms and pain associated with the stent, may make you feel tired. If the stent causes significant problems, you can discuss it with your manager and colleagues so that possible temporary adjustments can be made at your work place.

- **Social life and interactions:**
  The presence of a stent should not affect this in a significant way. In case you get urinary symptoms such as increased frequency and urgency, you may need to use public toilets more frequently while taking part in outdoor activities. Occasionally you may need a little more help from family members or colleagues, because of any pain or tiredness you may feel.

- **Travel and holidays:**
  It is possible to travel with a stent in place, provided the underlying kidney condition and your general health allows this. However, presence of significant side-effects associated with the stent may make travel and holidays less enjoyable. Also there is a small possibility that you may require additional medical help while the stent is in place.

- **Sex:**
  There are no restrictions on your sex life due to the presence of a stent. Few patients experience discomfort during sexual activities. Occasionally the side-effects associated with the stent may have an effect on the sexual desire.

  If you have a stent with a thread coming outside the body through the urethra, sexual activities may be difficult. Care will be required so as not to dislodge the thread, which could then in turn displace the stent.

Can a stent get displaced? What other complications are possible?

Occasionally a stent may develop a crystal coating on its surface although this is not a significant problem. Very occasionally a stent may get displaced, usually slipping towards the bladder, and it may even fall out.
If this happens, you should contact the hospital or your GP.

Is there a possibility of a urinary tract infection?

The presence of a stent, along with the underlying kidney problem, makes it more likely that you could get a urinary tract infection. Some of the symptoms that you may experience if you get a urinary tract infection are raised temperature, increased pain or discomfort in the kidney or bladder area, a burning sensation while passing urine and feeling unwell. This usually requires treatment with antibiotics.

What care do I need to take?

- **It is essential that you drink at least 1½ to 2 litres (approximately four pints) of fluids, mainly water, a day.** This will help to cut down the risk of getting an infection and will reduce the amount of blood in the urine. It will also help in the treatment of stones.
- If you experience bothersome pain you can take painkillers for relief, on the advice of a doctor.
- If you have got a stent with a thread coming down from the urethra outside the body, then more care will be needed so as not to dislodge the thread.
  If in any doubt please seek medical help (contact your GP/Local Hospital).

When should I call for help?

You should contact a doctor or a hospital:-
- if you experience a constant and unbearable pain associated with the stent.
- if you have symptoms of urinary tract infection as mentioned above (e.g. a raised temperature, pain during passing urine and feeling unwell).
- the stent gets dislodged or falls out.
- if you notice a significant change in the amount of blood in your urine.

Authors: MR. H. B. Joshi (Clinical Research Fellow in Urology), N Newns (Staff Nurse), Mr. F. X Keeley JR. (Consultant Urologist), Mr. A.G. Timoney (Consultant Urologist) – Southmead Hospital, Westbury-on-trym, Bristol BS10 5NB.

Publication Month: February 2000.

Sponsorship (in part): Southmead Hospital Research Foundation

If you have any questions to ask about the stent or your kidney problem, please write them down below so that you can ask your doctor at the next meeting.

_____

_____

_____

_____

_____

Further Reading:

If you would like to know more about ureteric stents here are the details of some relevant articles for further reading:

1. Ureteral stents – Materials; Endourology update: Mardis HK, Kroeger RM: Urological Clinics of North America, 1988, Vol. 15, No. 3, 471–479.
2. Ureteral stents – indications, variations and complications: Saltzman B: Endourology update: Urological Clinics of North America, 1988, Vol. 15, No. 3, 481–491.
3. Self retained internal stents: Use and complications: Mardis HK: AUA update series, 1997, Lesson 29, Volume XVI.

USEFUL INFORMATION

This patient has a ureteric stent, a temporary internal drainage tube, placed between the kidney and bladder.

Patient Name:	_____
Patient Address:	_____
Date of Birth:	_____
Unit Number:	_____
G.P. Name:	_____
G.P. Surgery Address:	_____
Diagnosis:	_____

URETERIC STENT

Side of the stent: Right   Left

Date of stent insertion:	_____
Date of stent removal:	_____
Type of stent:	_____
Consultant:	_____
Hospital:	_____

> ✪ **If you need urgent medical help please contact the GP or local Hospital on following numbers:**
>
> Telephone Number: (Working hours)
> Telephone Number   (Out of hours)

Ureteral stents: non-urological diseases

VI

Temporary ureteral stenting for the management of symptomatic hydronephrosis during pregnancy

T. D. Zwergel, B. Wullich, M. Uder and U. Zwergel

38

Introduction

Pregnant women with dilatation of the upper urinary tract, and especially those with renal colic, present a challenge to urologists and gynaecologists. Renal colic may precipitate premature delivery, and X-ray exposure, medication, anaesthesia and invasive diagnostic and therapeutic procedures may be potentially harmful to the foetus.[1–3] Physicians therefore fear to endanger the pregnancy by insufficient or excessive interventions.[4] Primarily, they have difficulty in distinguishing between those symptoms due to dilatation of the upper urinary tract and/or ureteric obstruction and those related to pregnancy, but not to dilatation of the upper urinary tract.[5–7]

In this chapter, the aetiology, diagnosis and management of ureteric dilatation or obstruction in pregnancy are discussed, and the use of ureteric stents in pregnant women is described.

Incidence and causes of upper urinary tract dilatation and hydronephrosis during pregnancy

Dilatation of the upper urinary tract in pregnancy is a normal phenomenon, to be found in up to 90% of pregnancies.[8–10] It is well known that only few cases result from intrinsic blockage (i.e. calculi).[11] There have been several reports that the total incidence of stone disease is unchanged and low in pregnancy (0.03–0.53%),[12–16] despite many abnormal anatomical and metabolic changes in the urinary tract that would be expected to enhance nephrolithiasis.[8,17] On the other hand, in reports published after 1980, a trend towards increasing incidence of renal calculi has been suggested, which may be associated with the more frequent use of calcium supplements during pregnancy.[2]

Debate continues as to the probable cause of the urinary tract dilatation. It appears that both anatomical and hormonal mechanisms make a contribution[9,18] (Table 38.1). As primary mechanisms, partial ureteric compression is caused by the gravid growing uterus and by dilated ovarian veins.[11,19] The smooth muscle relaxant properties of progesterone, in addition, produce a degree of hormonal ureteric dilatation.[18] The preponderance of affected right kidneys may be due to the gravid uterus being particularly deflected to the right side and to the lack of intestinal stuffing, again on the right side.

Dilatation of the upper urinary tract should, especially, be more readily suspected in women with pregnancies complicated by an overdistended uterus — for instance in cases of multiple pregnancy or polyhydramnios.[11] The preponderance of primigravid patients in several other series (confirmed by the authors' own data) has been discussed, but is not yet well understood.[11]

Forced diuresis, small stones or other unrecognized factors (oedema, blood clots)[3] may cause decompensation of ureteral function, which may progress from physiological dilatation of the upper urinary tract to symptomatic acute hydronephrosis during pregnancy. Regardless of the exact aetiology of the acute ureteric obstruction (with consequent hydronephrosis), severe pain and serious complications such as renal infection, or even sepsis or premature delivery may then result.

Table 38.1. *Causes of physiological dilatation of the upper urinary tract during pregnancy*

Anatomical changes:	Preponderance of the right kidney:
Gravid growing uterus	Uterus deflection to the right side
Dilated ovarian veins	Lack of intestinal stuff on the right side
Hormonal changes:	
Progesterone elevation	

Symptoms of upper urinary tract dilatation during pregnancy

Upper urinary tract dilatation during pregnancy is usually painless, asymptomatic and without renal damage.[7,20–22] However, some pregnant women describe various symptoms, the most common (more than 80%), *with* or *without* urinary tract dilatation and *with or without stone* confirmation being flank pain (ref. 2 and authors' own data). Many women also complain of dysuria, haematuria and/or fever due to urinary tract infection (pyelonephritis, cystitis). It may be very difficult to distinguish between those symptoms due to urological changes and those related to pregnancy; many of the presenting signs and symptoms may be masked by the pregnancy.

Overall, the variability of symptoms emphasizes the difficulty of clinical diagnosis, particularly because the symptomatology for both groups — pregnant women with and without urolithiasis — is very similar.

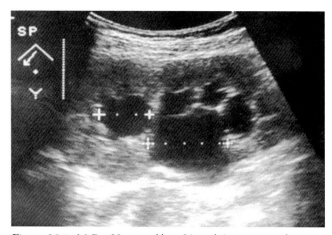

Figure 38.1. M.B., *28 years old, at 31 weeks' gestation with pain in the right loin during the last trimester of her pregnancy; ultrasound of the dilated calyces (29 mm) and the dilated renal pelvis (45 mm) (grade III).*

Diagnosis of upper urinary tract dilatation during pregnancy

Nowadays, a dilated ureter can easily be diagnosed by real-time ultrasound examination.[5–7] Abdominal ultrasound is performed to determine renal pelvic and *calyceal* diameters. The grading system is based on maximal calyceal and not on renal pelvic diameter, since the latter shows a number of physiological variations.[7] Figure 38.1 shows the ultrasound image of severe dilatation of the right kidney in a 28-year-old pregnant woman (at 31 weeks' gestation).

Careful interpretation of ultrasonic diameter size and comparison with the unaffected side, as well as meticulous ultrasonic searching for calculi, is necessary to discover and to distinguish physiological urinary dilatation in contrast to pathological hydronephrosis during pregnancy. Ultrasonic studies have confirmed the existence of physiological dilatation, with the right side affected more than the left,[7] but sometimes also found on both sides (as shown by the authors' own data).

Urine microscopic analysis, monitoring of blood pressure and gynaecological examination are routine assessments in the follow-up of symptomatic pregnant women and should be repeated within intervals of at least 2 weeks in cases of upper urinary tract dilatation.

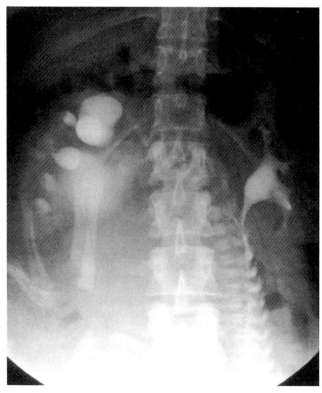

Figure 38.2. S.B., *24 years old, at 30 weeks' gestation; intravenous pyelogram with dilatation of the right upper urinary tract.*

If conservative therapy does not reduce the main symptoms and urinary dilatation is reconfirmed by ultrasound examination, a single-shot intravenous pyelogram may be performed, or a retrograde pyelogram is immediately done (under local anaesthesia) to look for intrinsic blockage (for instance ureteric stone), to confirm the site of the obstruction and to prevent renal infection, should there be stone formation or ureteric stenosis. Figure 38.2 shows the intravenous pyelogram of a 24-year-old woman with right renal pelvic dilatation at 30 weeks' gestation; Figure 38.3 shows the retrograde pyelogram of a 24-year-old pregnant patient with a ureteric stone on the right side.

Rapidly dividing cells are more sensitive to X-rays, so the potential for teratogenesis is greatest within the first

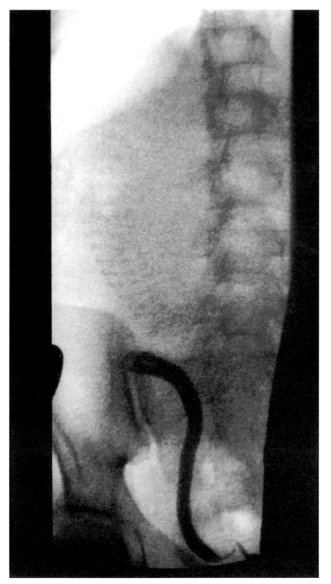

Figure 38.3. *F.M., 24 years old, at 30 weeks' gestation, having a ureteric stone with consequent massive dilatation of the right upper urinary tract: retrograde pyelogram before application of a ureteric stent.*

trimester, when radiation exposure should be particularly avoided.[2,12] In the second and third trimesters of pregnancy, X-rays can be used more safely, with careful attention to restricting the foetal dose of radiation by limiting the number of films, using new digital X-ray-monitoring systems and shielding the foetus as much as possible.[1,9]

Conservative therapy of symptomatic upper urinary tract dilatation during pregnancy

Initially, conservative treatment in pregnant women with symptomatic upper urinary tract dilatation consists of (a) positioning the patient on the left side in case of right hydronephrosis (as often as possible),[6,19] (b) analgesia and (c) antibiotics. The authors recommend that drugs suitable for the pregnant women and her foetus, with minimal risks of negative side effects and teratogenesis, are selected.

Acute symptomatic dilatation of the upper urinary tract during pregnancy that fails to respond to tried and tested conservative measures may also be managed by beta-1-adrenoceptor blockers.[23–25] These drugs may stimulate the contractile activity of the renal pelvis and ureter, in order to improve upper urinary tract urodynamics. However, to date, no precise experience with beta-1-adrenoceptor-blockers has been obtained by the authors and no wider experience or controlled studies exist to confirm the efficacy of this medication.

Interventional therapy for symptomatic upper urinary tract dilatation during pregnancy

Suitable therapy of upper urinary tract dilatation in symptomatic pregnancy is controversial, particularly because of the difficulty of differentiation between truly pathological ureteric obstruction and physiological dilatation of the upper urinary tract. The management also depends on the personal experience of the urologist in handling ureteric stents, percutaneous nephrostomies and/or ureteroscopy.

Up to the mid 1980s, management of an obstructed ureter in pregnant women depended on the gestational age of the foetus. Pregnancies in the early phase were treated conservatively or, in selected cases, by temporary nephrostomy tube. When the foetus was considered to be mature, delivery was induced.[11]

In recent years, the use of ureteric stents has been described in the management of all types of obstructive uropathies, and also during pregnancy.[9,17,20–22] Other authors still prefer the use of percutaneous nephrostomy tubes.[27,28,30,31] Recently, ureteric endoscopy and, if necessary, stone fragmentation and extraction, has also been suggested as a means of management of ureteric dilatation or obstruction during pregnancy.[3,16,32,33]

Ureteral stenting: indications and management during pregnancy

Since Finney[34] initiated the application of double-pigtail stents in 1978, improvements in materials and design have made the use of stents routine in urological practice.[35,36]

Apart from the fact that X-ray exposure should be minimized during pregnancy, stent application in pregnant women does not differ from that in the normal population, but the indications for ureteral stenting during pregnancy are particularly debated.[1,9,17,21,37]

Overall, in each woman the course of disease must be discussed and decided individually. Symptomatic hydronephrosis in pregnancy is rare and only a few patients really show intrinsic ureteric blockage (the total incidence of calculus is up to 0.53%).[12–16] Therefore, only a few pregnant women with flank pain really need ureteral stenting; the others, with unobstructed but only dilated ureters and renal pelves do not require invasive procedures, since physiological dilatation of the upper urinary tract does not harm the kidneys.[20–22]

As the rate of spontaneous stone passage during pregnancy has been documented as 74–86%, most patients need only conservative management to pass their calculi either before, during or after delivery.[2,6,38] In summary, ureteral stents during pregnancy are rarely indicated.

Whenever the application of a ureteric catheter is deemed necessary, a double-pigtail ureteric stent may be passed transurethrally under local anaesthesia. Nowadays, the authors prefer, for instance, Urosoft® stents (7 or 8 Fr) (Bard Angiomed, Karlsruhe, Germany) or silicone as material (Porgès, Le Plessis Robinson, France).

After manipulation, patients are required to complete a course of a suitable antibiotic.[11] In the authors' experience, the stents are usually removed 4–6 weeks post partum under local anaesthesia, when physiological renal tract changes of pregnancy are considered to have resolved.[29]

The placement of a double-pigtail stent allows pregnancy to continue without the need for external drainage and its risks of infection.[39] If urinary obstruction occurs in the presence of ureteric obstruction by calculi or because of a pre-existing abnormality such as primary pelvic hydronephrosis (for instance, due to pyelo-ureteral stenosis), it allows definitive treatment (lithotripsy or surgery) to be performed electively postpartum if necessary.[40,41]

Clinical experience with pregnant women with symptomatic dilatation of the upper urinary tract

The outcome in 124 pregnant women with symptomatic urinary dilatation and, in particular, the authors' experience with ureteric stents in 39 patients with urinary symptoms (e.g. flank pain) in pregnancy has been described.[29] At first sight the data (39 stents and two nephrostomies in 124 pregnant women) suggest that acute symptomatic dilatation of the upper urinary tract or hydronephrosis is not infrequent, but it should be stressed that this is a highly selected group.

Over a 6-year period, from 1990 to 1995, the pregnant women initially presented to obstetrical departments and thereafter to the urological clinic in Homburg/Saar (Germany) because of symptomatic dilatation of the upper urinary tract (for instance with dysuria, persistent loin pain, urinary infection and/or fever). All were in the second half of pregnancy; 99 patients were in their first, 18 in their second and seven in their third pregnancy. The mean duration of gestation at presentation was 32 weeks. A total of 96 women complained of unilateral loin pain, 21 of pain on both sides, and 97 complained of voiding symptoms and nausea with or without vomiting.

In 104 patients, urine microscopy showed significant pyuria and these patients were treated with antibiotics (irrespective of stent application).

Table 38.2. *Ultrasonic grading system in 124 pregnant women with upper urinary tract dilatation*

Grade	Dilatation	Calyceal diameter (mm)	Affected kidney (no. of women)		
			Right	Left	Both
I	Mild	5–10	65	4	13
II	Moderate	10–15	26	3	4
III	Severe	> 15	7	1	1

The ultrasound results are summarized in Table 38.2. In most cases the women showed mild or moderate urinary dilatation on the right side.

Table 38.3 summarizes the treatment in 124 consecutive patients with symptomatic ureteric dilatation. Double-pigtail ureteric stents were placed in 39 patients: 26 of these patients experienced only moderate relief, at least initially for 2 days; 17 of them continued to have problems post-therapeutically, namely frequency, nocturia and strangury (for a maximum of 10 days) (Table 38.4).

All patients completed a course of a suitable antibiotic after manipulation. As microscopic analysis of the urine was repeated at short intervals, especially during the stenting period, re-infections (n = 8) could be treated immediately (Table 38.5).

All but three women received benefit from anticholinergic, antibiotic and analgesic agents. Three women complained of persistent loin pain: two catheters were obstructed by encrustation and one woman developed a small stone in the renal pelvis; it was necessary to replace these three stents once (Table 38.3 and 38.5). In 26 patients, urinary tract dilatation was reduced but not erradicated (Table 38.6); nevertheless, these patients did not need stent replacement.

In two cases, percutaneous nephrostomy tubes were placed, one because of pyelo-ureteral stenosis and the

Table 38.3. *Treatment of 124 pregnant women with symptomatic dilatation of the upper urinary tract*

Treatment	No. of women
Antibiotics	104
Ureteric stent	39
Stent replacement	3
Percutaneous nephrostomy	2

Table 38.4. *Symptoms (for max. 10 days) after stenting symptomatic dilatation of the upper urinary tract in pregnancy (n = 17, including n = 14 with more than one symptom)*

Symptom	No. of women[*]
Frequency < 3 h	13
Stranguria	10
Haematuria	4
Loin pain	4

[*]Total no. of women = 17 (14 had more than one symptom).

Table 38.5. *Follow-up after stenting symptomatic dilatation of the upper urinary tract in pregnancy*

Finding	No. of women[*]
Stent replacement	3
Re-infection	8
Persistent dilatation[†]	22

[*]Total no. = 30.
[†]Median stenting duration 8.6 weeks (range 12 days – 22.5 weeks), with one exception of 14 months.

Table 38.6. *Ultrasonic follow-up of 26 patients with persistent urinary tract dilatation during pregnancy*

	Dilatation before stenting			Dilatation after stenting		
Grade	R. kidney	L. kidney	Both	R. kidney	L. kidney	Both
I	–	–	–	13	3	3
II	11	2	3	6	–	1
III	8	1	1	–	–	–

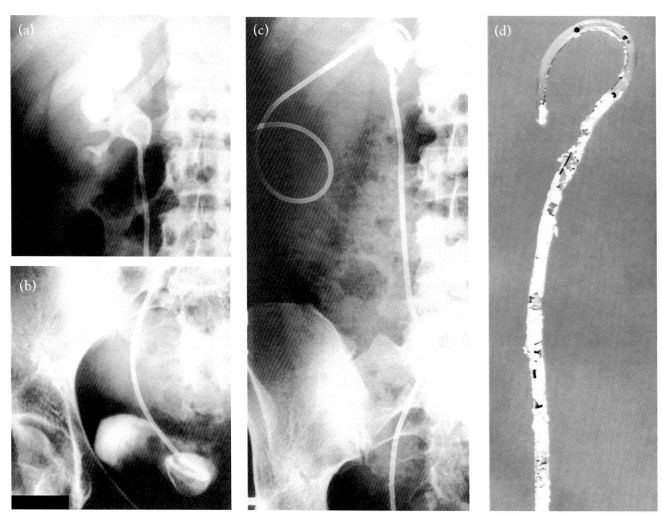

Figure 38.4. G.D., *27 years old, post partum, 14 months after stent application: (a,b) intravenous pyelogram with stone formation along the stent, especially in the renal pelvis and in the bladder; (c) plain film after additional application of a percutaneous nephrostomy tube; stone reduction after extracorporeal piezoelectric lithotripsy; (d) the ureteral catheter after removal, with extensive encrustation.*

other because of an impacted ureteric stone. Ureteric stents could not be placed correctly. Neither patient experienced major problems with the nephrostomy tube.

All pregnancies progressed uneventfully and all women were delivered after a mean of 38 weeks' gestation.

After delivery, urological diagnostic procedures and treatment were initiated. In four cases calculi were passed spontaneously. Seven patients were successfully treated by extracorporeal lithotripsy.[41] One patient had stone removal by ureteroscopic lithotripsy, but only post partum. Finally, all but one woman had their stents removed uneventfully under local anaesthesia, and none showed persistent infection on further follow-up.

In one special case, stones were found, attached to the full length of the stent. This woman had neither history of stone formation nor concomitant hypercalciuria, and did not return to the authors' clinic for more than a year after stent application (after delivery of her child). Extracorporeal piezoelectric lithotripsy[41] enabled the stent to be removed without further problems (Fig. 38.4).

Morbidity and complications after ureteral stenting during pregnancy

Symptoms after stenting

The use of ureteral stents may bring about several symptoms and complications: discomfort, voiding problems, pyelonephritis, encrustation and clinically significant stone formation with renal colic have been reported.[8,26,39,42]

Minor problems (dysuria, pollakiuria) after stenting may persist (in up to 45% of the authors' patients), but these are insignificant and the patients usually do not need stent replacement or other interventional therapy.

Difficulties with stent application

Usually, stents can be placed easily in the correct position and their application does not differ from that in the normal population.[40] In rare cases, not seen in the authors' own series, catheters may have migrated up the ureter and require removal by ureteroscopy under anaesthesia[11] Since the ureter in pregnant women may be elongated, the length of the catheter should be adapted to the changed situation.

Urinary infection and stent encrustation

Enhanced stent encrustation in pregnancy is the subject of debate.[6,8,26,39] Increased encrustation rates might seem to depend on frequent concomitant urinary infections. There is a consensus of opinion that infection undoubtedly enhances detritus accumulation, urinary stasis and/or the rate of stone growth, probably by alteration of the urinary epithelium, and thus encourages earlier stent obstruction. However, stasis and infection are not the only factors: endocrine changes also play a significant role. The presence of hypercalciuria during pregnancy (presumbly secondary to enhanced placental formation of 1,25-dihydroxycholecalciferol) is not generally accepted.[6] Calcium excretion may even be somewhat reduced, owing to augmented foetal needs. Furthermore, stone inhibitors seem to be elevated in the urine of pregnant women,[13] in order to reduce stone formation.

To sum up, pregnancy does not seem to exert a major and constant effect on stone development. The number of stone episodes during pregnancy is close to that predicted from the average rate of stone occurrence observed in unselected, non-pregnant patients. On the other hand, there is a possible trend towards increasing incidence of renal calculi, which may be associated with external factors, such as the frequent use of calcium supplements during pregnancy.[2] Of 39 cases of stenting, only one patient suffered severe problems with extensive encrustation. The one case report of major stone formation and stent encrustation is distinct, since stone formation and stent encrustation were not caused by changed circumstances during pregnancy, such as hypercalciuria, but by long-term stenting (> 1 year).

Persistent dilatation after stenting

Ureteric stenting does not guarantee that dilatation will disappear. In 26 of the authors' patients, urinary tract dilatation was only reduced after stenting. This is not surprising since dilatation depends on different anatomical and hormonal changes of the upper urinary tract in pregnancy.[7,8,10,18,20–22] Since the dilatation may persist, indications for stenting must be especially well evaluated during pregnancy. On the other hand, the authors did not note any major complications after stenting (except in one special case). According to their experience, the exceptional case of 'overtreatment' (stenting because of dilatation without stone) may be better than lack of interventional procedures, which are essentially needed in cases of acute ureteric obstruction.

Stent breakage

Complications with long-term indwelling stents are mainly due to stent encrustation or stone formation. Breakage of long-term stents (especially without encrustation) is uncommon, especially if catheters are left in situ for less than 6 months and if, for instance, silicone is used. Mardis and Kroeger[35] studied stent material and found that silicone stents did not lose tensile strength after an indwelling period of 20 months; only elasticity diminished somewhat. Witjes[36] reported a case in which the silicone catheter had broken into several pieces after 29 months.

Stent versus nephrostomy

Ureteric stents also increase the risk of ascending pyelonephritis by causing vesico-ureteral reflux; some authors therefore, prefer to use percutaneous nephrostomies.[27,28,30] The nephrostomy tubes can be easily placed under local analgesia and ultrasound guidance, thus minimizing (or even avoiding) radiation exposure during pregnancy. Maintenance of nephrostomy also allows the uneventful continuation of pregnancy to full term and effectively preserves and helps the recovery of renal function (as demonstrated in the authors' two cases). However, nephrostomies also have disadvantages, most problems with nephrostomy tubes being mechanical: the tubes become dislodged or drainage is blocked by formation of sediment with its risks of ensuing infection. The two patients in question did not have any difficulty with external drainage. In summary, the authors' positive, but limited, experience with nephrostomies during pregnancy does not encourage them to recommend these tubes; they preserve them for very special circumstances.

Stent versus ureteroscopy

Since Kolligian[32] found that his patients experienced severe morbidity after stenting during pregnancy (contrary to the present authors' experience), he proposed the use of (rigid) ureteroscopy. He and other authors[2,16,33] reported that pregnant women with suspected ureteral obstruction and stable pregnancy well tolerated endoscopy without major adverse reactions. However, Ulvik[2] had one patient who suffered a ureteric perforation during ureteroscopy; both Ulvik[2] and Scarpa[16] therefore concluded that this procedure should be performed with the greatest possible care. Both authors also mention that some of the ureteroscopic procedures could have been avoided, since the interval between medication and intervention had, perhaps, been too short, and since only about one-half of the pregnant women (13 of 24)[3] were proved to have ureteric stones, and 50–80% of calculi pass spontaneously. Therefore, the authors' do not consider ureteroscopy during pregnancy as a useful option, even though it combines diagnostic procedure (stone confirmation) with definitive treatment (stone extraction). It is also advisable to refrain from using ultrasound for ureteric stone fragmentation in pregnant women,[3] as it is possible that the high-pitched audible sound produced by the sonotrode during stone disintegration may be harmful to the foetus and may cause hearing injury. The authors opt to postpone definitive diagnosis and treatment until after delivery of the child. In their series, only one patient needed stone removal post partum by ureteroscopic lithotripsy.

Conclusions

Dilatation of the upper urinary tract in pregnancy should initially be treated by well-known conservative measures. If acute urinary tract dilatation or even hydronephrosis fails to respond to such conservative treatment, it can be managed by interventional methods (for instance ureteral stenting or, in special cases, by percutaneous nephrostomy).

Since double-pigtail stents are usually placed without any major problems and are tolerated with only minor

and short post-therapeutic discomfort, the authors prefer ureteral stenting as a simple, safe and effective method of internal upper tract drainage in cases of symptomatic ureteric dilatation and/or obstruction during pregnancy. They recommend this form of therapy, even when urinary obstruction is only suspected and conservative treatment has been ineffective. The final diagnosis and treatment are postponed until after delivery.[2,6,14,20,21]

Overall, each course of pregnancy and disease has to be individually evaluated. In cases where symptoms persist because of acute urinary tract dilatation or hydronephrosis, ureteral stenting is usually preferred, according to the experience of the urologist.[9,17,20–22] Percutaneous nephrostomy tubes and/or ureteric endoscopy during pregnancy may be reserved for very special cases of ureteric dilatation and obstruction.

References

1. Duncan P G, Pope W D, Cohen M M et al. Fetal risk of anesthesia and surgery during pregnancy. Anesthesiology 1986; 64: 790–794
2. Stothers L, Lee L M. Renal colic in pregnancy. J Urol 1992; 148: 1383–1387
3. Ulvik N M, Bakke A, Hoisaeter P A. Ureteroscopy in pregnancy. J Urol 1995; 154: 1660–1663
4. Kroovand R L. Stones in pregnancy and in children. J Urol 1992; 148: 1076–1078
5. Cietak K A, Newton J R. Serial qualitative maternal nephrosonography in pregnancy. Br J Radiol 1985; 58: 399–404
6. Denstedt J D, Razvi H. Management of urinary calculi during pregnancy. J Urol 1992; 148: 1072–1075
7. Lentsch P, Schretzenmaier M, Dierkopf W et al. Die Dilatation der oberen Harnwege in der Schwangerschaft — Inzidenz, Schweregrad und Verlaufsbeobachtungen. Urologe A 1987; 26: 122–128
8. Goldfarb R A, Neerhut G J, Lederer E. Management of acute hydronephrosis of pregnancy by ureteral stenting: risk of stone formation. J Urol 1989; 141: 921–922
9. Lipsky H. Dilatation of the urinary tract during pregnancy and its management. Eur J Urol 1984; 10: 372–376
10. Waltzer W C. The urinary tract in pregnancy. J Urol 1981; 125: 271–276
11. Eckford S D, Gingell J C. Ureteric obstruction in pregnancy — diagnosis and management. Br J Gynaecol Obstet 1991; 98: 1137–1140
12. Cass A S, Smith C S, Gleich P. Management of urinary calculi in pregnancy. Urology 1986; 28: 370–373
13. Coe F L, Parks J H, Lindheimer M D. Nephrolithiasis during pregnancy. New Engl J Med 1978; 298: 324–327
14. Hendricks S K, Ross S O, Krieger J N. An algorithm for diagnosis and therapy of management and complications of urolithiasis during pregnancy. Surg Gynec Obst 1991; 172: 49–54
15. Horowitz E, Schmidt J D. Renal calculi in pregnancy. Clin J Gynec Obst 1985; 28: 324–326
16. Scarpa R M, De Lisa A, Usai E. Diagnosis and treatment of ureteral calculi during pregnancy with rigid ureteroscopy. J Urol 1996; 155: 875–877

17. Jarrard D J, Gerber G S, Lyon E S. Management of acute ureteral obstruction in pregnancy utilizing ultrasound-guided placement of ureteral stents. J Urol 1993; 42: 263–268

18. Clayton J D, Roberts J A. The effect of progesterone on ureteral physiology in a primate model. J Urol 1972; 107: 945–948

19. Rubi R A, Sala N L. Ureteral function in pregnant women: Effect of different positions and of fetal delivery upon ureteral tonus. Am J Obstet Gynecol 1968; 101: 230–237

20. Loughlin K R, Bailey R B. Internal ureteral stents for conservative management of ureteral calculi during pregnancy. N Engl J Med 1986; 315: 1647–1651

21. Loughlin K R. Management of urological problems during pregnancy. Urology 1994; 44: 159–164

22. Lowes J J, Mackenzie J C, Abrams P H et al. Acute renal failure and acute hydronephrosis in pregnancy: use of double-J stent. J Soc Med 1987; 80: 524–525

23. Hettenbach A, Tschada R, Hiltmann W D et al. Untersuchungen zum Einfluß von β-Stimulation und β-1-Blockade auf die Motilität des oberen Harntraktes. Z Geburtshilfe Perinatol 1988; 192: 273–277

24. Tschada R, Mickisch G, Rassweiler J et al. Succès et échecs avec la sonde double J. Analyse de 107 cas. J Urol (Paris) 1991; 97: 93–97

25. Tschada R, Mickisch G, Hettenbach A et al. Untersuchungen zur internen Urinableitung bei komplizierter schwangerschaftsbedingter Harnstauung. Z Geburtshilfe Perinatol 1992; 196: 123–128

26. Docimo S G, Dewolf W C. High failure rate of indwelling ureteral stents in patients with extrinsic obstruction: experience at 2 institutions. J Urol 1989; 142: 277–279

27. Mandal A K, Sharma S K, Goswami A K et al. The use of percutaneous diversion during pregnancy. Int J Gynecol Obstet 1990; 32: 67–70

28. Quinn A D, Kusuda L, Amar A D et al. Percutaneous nephrostomy for treatment of hydronephrosis of pregnancy. J Urol 1988; 139: 1037–1040

29. Zwergel T, Lindenmeir T, Wullich B. Management of acute hydronephrosis in pregnancy by ureteral stenting. Eur J Urol 1996; 29: 292–297

30. Kavoussi L R, Albala D M, Basle J W et al. Percutaneous management of urolithiasis during pregnancy. J Urol 1992; 148: 1069–1071

31. Holman E, Toth C S, Khan M A. Percutaneous nephrolithotomy in late pregnancy. J Endourol 1992; 6: 421–425

32. Kolligian M, Eshgi M. Management of upper urinary tract obstruction and ureteroscopy during pregnancy. J Urol 1996; 155: 672A

33. Vest J M, Warden S S. Ureteroscopic stone manipulation during pregnancy. Urology 1990; 35: 250–251

34. Finney R P. Experience with new Double J catheter stent. J Urol 1978; 120: 678–681

35. Mardis H K, Kroeger R M. Ureteral stents: materials. Urol Clin North Am 1988; 15: 471–474

36. Witjes J A. Breakage of a silicone double pigtail ureteral stent as a long-term complication. J Urol 1993; 150: 1898–1899

37. Harvey E B, Boice J D, Honeyman M et al. Prenatal x-ray exposure and childhood cancer in twins. N Engl J Med 1985; 312: 541–543

38. Jones W A, Correa R J, Ansell J S. Urolithiasis associated with pregnancy. J Urol 1979; 122: 333–335

39. Spirnak J P, Resnick M I. Stone formation as a complication of indwelling ureteral stents: a report of 5 cases. J Urol 1985; 134: 349–351

40. Sibley G N, Graham M D, Smith M L et al. Improving splinting techniques in pyeloplasty. Br J Urol 1987; 60: 489–491

41. Zwergel U, Neisius D, Zwergel T et al. Results and clinical management of extracorporeal piezoelectric lithotripsy (EPL) in 1321 consecutive treatments. World J Urol 1987; 5: 213–217

42. Pollard S G, Macfarlane R. Symptoms arising from double-J ureteral stents. J Urol 1988; 139: 37–38

39

Stenting in benign gynaecology and gynaecological oncology
M. M. Altaras, S. Richter and A. Fishman

Introduction

Since the introduction, 30 years ago of cystoscopically inserted long-term indwelling ureteral stents as a new treatment modality, new horizons have been opened in research and development in this field and in stenting procedures, including their potential implementation in gynaecology in general, and in gynaecological oncology in particular. In addition, the development of 'interventional radiology' as a new subspecialty, as well as the marked advances in this discipline relating to diagnosis and management of urological problems, have expanded the indications and the development of new procedures as a result of collaboration between the two disciplines of urology and interventional radiology during the past two decades. All these advances have provided the possibility of offering curative therapy to some patients, with the ability to perform several interventions almost at the bedside, by eliminating the need for general anaesthesia, avoiding extensive surgery with its attendant morbidity and allowing surgery in critically ill patients to be deferred until their general condition has been optimized.

The purpose of this chapter is twofold. First, it is intended to provide an update in stenting methods and to emphasize the importance of follow-up of stented patients with their management problems; to outline the potential use of stenting in benign gynaecology and gynaecological oncology and, to evaluate the results of such treatment in various fields where the use of stenting is becoming more frequent. Secondly, although many papers have been published describing clinical studies and case reports on this subject, such data have not been included in gynaecology textbooks or in books on gynaecological oncology published in recent years. In the authors' opinion, this chapter will be of use to obstetrics and gynaecology residents, specialists and all gynaecological oncologists with various degrees of experience. Attending gynaecologists practising in regional clinics may also benefit from recognition of problems encountered in the follow-up of their patients carrying stents.

The most common and least invasive technique for stent insertion is retrogradely through cystoscopy. In the event of problems with one-step retrograde stent insertion, it is advisable to introduce an open-ended ureteral catheter over a guide wire. After a couple of days, it is usually quite easy to exchange the ureteral catheter for an internal ureteral stent.

In emergency cases with severe hydronephrosis or pyonephrosis, or when every attempt at retrograde insertion fails, the nephro-ureteric unit should be approached without delay, through the insertion of a nephrostomy tube. After the affected kidney has properly recovered its function, an attempt can be made to introduce a stent in an antegrade fashion. Whenever a ureteral stent is inserted, either retrogradely or antegradely, it is recommended that this should be done under fluoroscopic guidance in order to have on-line information available at every step. Some cases have been reported in the literature in which a combined antegrade/retrograde approach has been used to overcome a problem in stent insertion.[1,2]

Ureteral stents are intended to remain in place for periods of 3, 6 or 12 months, depending on the material from which they are made (Fig. 39.1). The better their biocharacteristics, the longer the time they can remain indwelling. Nevertheless, there are inherent risks attached to the use of indwelling ureteral stents. A stent placed blindly without fluoroscopic guidance or control is predisposed to inappropriate positioning and to migration either upwards (distal and above the ureteral meatus) or downwards (proximal and below the ureteropelvic junction). As previously stated, vesico-ureteral reflux can occur in up to 61% of cases.[3] It is important to note that a patient bearing a ureteral stent and nephrostomy tube on the same side may have no bladder voided urine at all, since urine from the contralateral kidney may flow up through the stent and out through the nephrostomy tube. This is not a

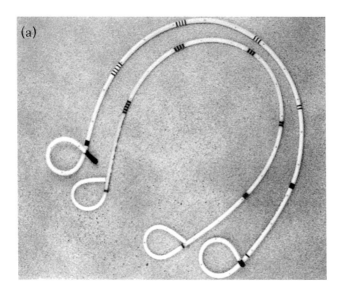

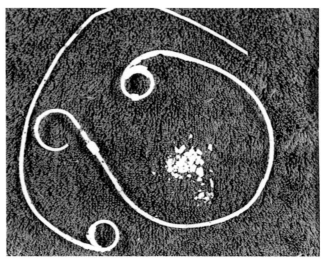

Figure 39.2. *Encrustation causing obstruction of the stent.*

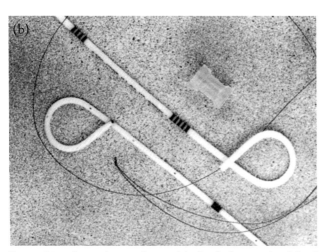

Figure 39.1. *Internal ureteral stents (a); detail of proximal and distal pigtail tip for self-retaining (b).*

pathological condition but the consequence of reflux. Urinary infection as a consequence of an uncomplicated indwelling stent has been rarely reported. Although it is advisable to administer some antibiotic during the perioperative period, there is no consensus on whether to continue with permanent antimicrobial therapy. There is an important difference between infection and colonization when stents are present. In the latter event, urine culture may be positive but the patient is asymptomatic and it is not necessary to institute any treatment. None the less, colonization may accelerate stent encrustation, stone forming and potential obstruction (Fig. 39.2). An occluded stent is consequently an infected one, and should be removed

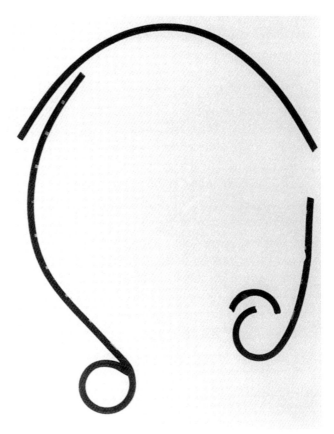

Figure 39.3. *A broken Double-J stent after its removal.*

and replaced immediately. Stent encrustation may be so severe as to hinder stent retrieval and to cause its fragmentation. Stents may break in situ without any symptomatology. This complication is usally discovered by a routine X-ray film before exchange is due, and hinders removal of the fragments, necessitating concomitant procedures such as cystoscopy, ureteroscopy and nephroscopy (Fig. 39.3). It has been proved that silicone stents are the best for long-term use, presenting the lowest incidence of complications.[4] Figures 39.4–39.8 show displacement of a ureteral stent that was diagnosed 4 months after its insertion.

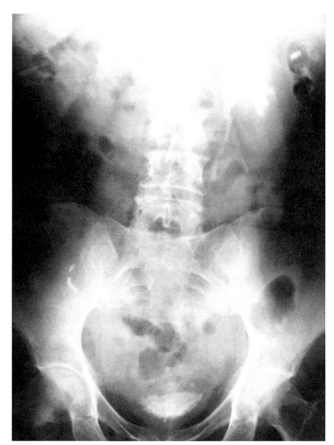

Figure 39.4. *Malignant obstruction of the left ureter causing hydronephrosis in a 62-year-old woman after cytotoxic therapy for adenocarcinoma of the right Batholin's gland.*

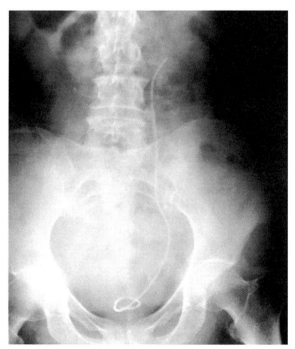

Figure 39.5. *Functional pigtail stent in normal position.*

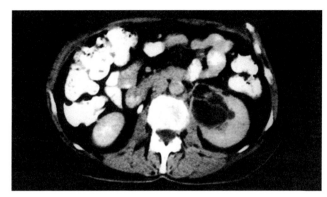

Figure 39.6. *CT scan of persistent left hydronephrosis and functional right ureter 4 months after placement of a pigtail-stent.*

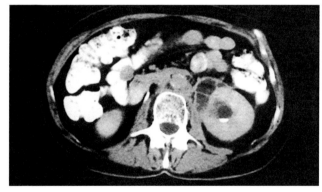

Figure 39.7. *Delay in appearance of radiopaque material in left hydronephrotic kidney.*

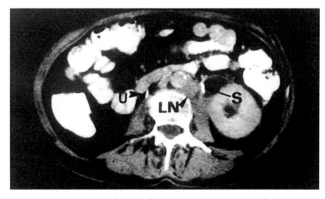

Figure 39.8. *Proximal tip of the stent in presence of hydronephrotic kidney indicating downward stent displacement. Note the pressure of the enlarged para-aortic lymph nodes on the stented non-functional ureter. Arrows indicate (U) right functional ureter, (S) tip of the pigtail stent, (LN) left para-aortic enlarged lymph nodes.*

Indications for stent placement in gynaecology

An important adjunct to open surgery encompassing the urinary tract is the correct employment of ureteral stents in general and in benign and gynaecological oncology in particular.

Uretero-ureterostomy, ureteroneocystostomy and external diversions of the ureter all depend on the accurate placement of a stent to protect and defend the anastomosis from vascular compromise, urinary leakage with subsequent periureteral fibrosis, infection or kinking.[5]

Women with a history of abdominal and gynaecological surgery should be considered to be at risk for various kinds of ureteral injuries when they undergo further pelvic surgery. In this respect Daly and Higgins[6] reported 16 ureteral injuries occurring during 1093 (1.5%) extensive procedures: of these 16, eight occurred in women who had undergone hysterectomy. The injuries involved were transection (nine patients), ligation (six patients) and fulguration in one patient. Daly and Higgins stated that previous open surgical procedures in the pelvis, endometriosis, ovarian neoplasms, pelvic adhesions, and distorted anatomical features of the pelvis should be considered as risk factors for surgical ureteral injuries.[6] In patients at risk for ureteral injury, preoperative evaluation of the ureters by an intravenous pyelogram (IVP) or contrast-enhanced computerized tomography (CT) scan are useful to anticipate the course of the ureter. The best method of preventing ureteral injuries is stent placement, compared with other methods such as IVP and/or insertion of a ureteral catheter. However, it should be borne in mind that stent placement may cause ureteral oedema, which may lead to temporary ureteral obstruction following stent removal shortly after surgery. Another disadvantage of retrograde manipulations is that they may add to the operative time and carry inherent risks of ureteral injury and upper urinary tract infection.[7]

Precise specification of the most appropriate time to use a stent constitutes part of the clinical judgement that the surgeon can gain only with experience. In this section the indications and potential use of stents in benign gynaecology and in gynaecological oncology patients are discussed.

Prevention

It is well established that preoperative placement of unilateral or bilateral ureteral stents is extremely helpful for intra-operative identification of the ureters. The indication for the use of such stents may be related partly to the experience of the surgeon and partly to the various clinical characteristics of the pathological entity treated surgically in patients with no such previous surgery. However, the indications for surgery in relation to the pathological entity warrant careful evaluation in some patients. Those who have previously undergone pelvi-ureteric or ureteric surgery, patients who have previously been treated surgically for endometriosis, those with non-malignant ureteric obstruction diagnosed prior to surgery, before planning the operation and especially when it is clear that ureteral dissection will be difficult, should be evaluated carefully. Proven retroperitonal fibrosis is also an indication for placement of ureteral stents for further surgery when required. In some circumstances the decision for the placement of preventive stents may be taken after open surgery, in the light of the problems encountered, such as traumatic dissection of the ureter(s) resulting in abrasion(s) in their wall(s) or when their devascularization occurs. Pocock et al.[8] reported on stent insertion prior to surgery in six patients with non-malignant ureteric obstructions yielding a 100% success rate of insertion. The same authors also performed stent insertion in seven patients with idiopathic retroperitoneal fibrosis with a good success rate. High rates (6–9%) of ureteric fistula have been reported in patients treated by a combination of pelvic radiation and radical hysterectomy.[9] Such patients, or any women with previous pelvic irradiation subjected to pelvic or urological surgery, should be considered candidates for preventive stent placement.

Stent placement at the time of surgery

During the course of surgery ureteral injuries may be caused by crush, avulsion, partial or complete transection, ligation, or devascularization. Such injuries evidently result in fistula or stricture formation if missed or left untreated.[10] Excision of a portion of the ureter has also been reported as a possible ureteral injury.[11]

When the ureter is injured it may become obstructed, creating hydronephrosis, or a fistula may occur leading to urinary extravasation (urinoma) into the retroperitoneum or the peritoneal cavity. The same complication can occur when the injury results in complete transection of the ureter. If injury to an adjacent structure occurs at the time of ureteral injury, a fistula may develop between them. Most fistulas are to the vagina, skin or bowel. Extravasated urine can induce an intense inflammatory reaction, resulting in secondary periureteral fibrosis and ureteral obstruction. If the urine is infected, an abscess and possibly life-threatening sepsis may develop, requiring emergency surgical intervention.[10]

Surgical ureteral injuries occur in 0.5–1% of all pelvic operations.[12] It is estimated that about 50% of these, or even more, are related to gynaecological surgical procedures.[7,13] Their aetiology in relation to benign gynaecological or gynaecological oncology surgery, is reported to be related to radical or simple abdominal and vaginal hysterectomies, salpingo-oöphorectomy, vesicovaginal fistula repair, dilatation and curettage, excision of cervical stump, cystocoele repair, colpocleisis, laparoscopy and the Marshall–Marchetti–Krantz operation for vesico-urethral suspension.[10] Zinman et al.[14] reported that only 20–30% of all ureteral injuries can be recognized at the time of surgery. When a ureteral injury is suspected during surgery, an indigo carmine injection test may indicate the possibility of an extravasation. However, there is not an ideal method for precisely diagnosing a ureter that was injured at the time of surgery but which looks normal; this is true also for the recognition of ureteral devascularization.

Ureteral laceration, transection and avulsion

Once the injury has been fully delineated and assessed, treatment can be selected. If a partial laceration is present and the ureter that is still in continuity is viable, placement of an indwelling Double-J stent and closure of the wound is the most established procedure, yielding good results. The insertion of a stent provides minimal extravasation from the anastomosis site.[10] Some authors advocate a somewhat different approach for the management of a partially transected or damaged ureter beyond repair, based on the level of damage. If the ureteral damage is above the brim, a simple reanastomosis is done. One end of a Double-J stent is inserted into the bladder through the distal ureter, with the proximal part in the upper segment of the ureter,

and both ends are anastomosed.[15] This should be followed by a contrast study 6–8 weeks after injury to determine the need for further intervention.[12] Several options for successful open ureteral repair at the time of surgery can be considered.[7] In circumstances when the ureter has been injured partially, or transected completely during surgery distal to the pelvic brim, the preferred repair procedure is ureteroneocystotomy requiring also a Double-J stent to protect the ureteral anastomosis to the bladder. The use of stents is also necessary in very selected candidates for transuretero-ureterostomy to protect the anastomotic site. The protective stent in both procedures described above should be left in place for at least 14 days.[15]

Barone et al.[12] reported on a simple technique for intra-operative stenting of a transected ureter requiring neither cystoscopy nor a separate incision in the bladder or skin. They stressed that some controversy may exist in the use of ureteral stents during ureteral repair, and added that most physicians would agree that stenting is warranted for distal ureteral injuries and injuries occurring in a radiated field. The advantages of ureteral stenting include a reduced risk of angulation or obstruction in the event of adhesions forming at the site of the ureteral anastomosis, and reduced extravasation through the anastomosis, as described by Sieben et al.[16] Thus, the optimal management of a totally or partially transected ureter at the time of benign gynaecological or gynaecological oncology surgery is intra-operative insertion of a fenestrated ureteral Double-J stent and anastomosis of the ureter over the stent. The most important advantage of this approach as described by Barone et al., is that the stent is completely internal and operative time is not prolonged.[12,17] Transurethral retrograde placement of a stent prolongs the operative time and may not be possible in some patients with previous ureteral injury or stricture. In addition to internal stenting it is recommended that a tube drain be placed to the site of the anastomosis.

Crush injury

At the time of operation, the surgeon may crush the ureter by placing a clamp on it, or may ligate the ureter and then remove the ligature. Since there is no accurate test to use at the time of surgery to diagnose whether the clamping or ligation may lead to necrosis or fistula creation, in these circumstances the surgeon has to decide whether to perform a segmental resection of the ureter followed by insertion of ureteral stents and reanastomosis, or only to insert an indwelling ureteral stent. Such a complication associated with clamping of the ureter is, in the authors' experience, thought to be caused by the presence of the ovarian artery above the brim, which was managed successfully by the insertion of a Double-J stent to prevent unpredictable complications and removed uneventfully 3 weeks later.

Stent placement for urinary tract injuries diagnosed in the postoperative period

Ureteral injuries are reported to occur in 10–30% of all radical hysterectomies and 1.5–2.5% of all gynaecological procedures, as described by Dowling et al.[13] An early series reported ureteral fistula rates in radical hysterectomies as being 8–20%.[9] However, during the last two decades, the use of techniques that avoid ureteral devascularization, vacuum suction of retroperitonal spaces and permanent bladder drainage, plus the availability of potent antibiotics, has resulted in ureterovaginal fistula rates of 1–2% and vesicovaginal fistula rates of less than 1%.[18]

For the majority of patients with delayed diagnosis of ureteral injuries, an initial endo-urological procedure is an excellent approach. Percutaneous nephrostomy (PCN), with or without antegrade stent placement, can stabilize the septic or unstable patient with a ureteral obstruction. Occasionally PCN or stent placement will allow resolution of the injury without further intervention. However, stents and PCN are also useful as a temporary measure until more definitive therapy can be performed.[7]

Ligation injuries

Injury of the ureter may also occur inadvertently by its ligation, or from the placement of surgical clips during abdominal or vaginal procedures or in vesico-urethropexy. The approach in this kind of complication may not be universal, except where a vesico-urethropexy is the source of the injury. Following the diagnosis, placement of a percutaneous tube in the kidney, followed by an antegrade stent insertion as a sole and definitive treatment, can be attempted. If the procedure succeeds, the stent is to be left in place until the resorption of the suture material, which takes 3–4 weeks for catgut or 6–8 weeks for polyglycollic

acid.[13,19,20] De-ligation of the ureter by open surgery and insertion of a preventive Double-J stent is also an accepted approch. According to Corriere, at the time of vesico-urethropexy large amounts of tissue are caught in the suture, so devascularization is less of a problem than is the mechanical obstruction of the ureter from angulation. Thus, if the ureter has been ligated loosely, a stent can be placed through the narrowed lumen.[10] Harshmann et al.[19] reported on three patients with ureteral obstruction secondary to suture entrapment which occurred in two patients during the Marshall–Marchetti–Krantz operation and in the third during vaginal hysterectomy with anteroposterior colporhaphy. All were managed by PCN in all, and also by stent placement in two until the resorption of suture material.

Ureteral fistulae

Ureteral fistulae are one of the major areas in which ureteral stents are commonly used as described above. As a result of various types of ureteral lacerations and injuries, and after their repair, if necrosis occurs, ureteral fistulae may develop. According to Lang,[20] ureteral fistulae can be classified into five groups; reflecting their location: these are (1) ureterovaginal, (2) ureterocutaneous, (3) uretero-enteric, (4) lymphatico-ureteric and (5) ureteroretroperitoneal (urinoma). The most common symptoms of ureteral fistulae diagnosed after surgery in a female patient following benign gynaecology or gynaecological oncological surgery are (a) flank pain, (b) fever above 100°F, (c) anuria and (d) vaginal urine leak.[10]

Since the introduction of newer stenting methods, a revolution has occurred in the management of fistulae of all aetiologies. Goldin[21] was the first to use percutaneous ureteral stents successfully, when he treated four cases of urinary fistula and one patient with uretero-ileal anastomosis stricture.

Lang[20] reported on the diagnosis and management of ureteral fistulae by PCN and antegrade stent catheter in 15 patients. Of these, 33% (5/15) developed ureteral fistulas as complications occurring during the treatment of cervical carcinomas (four patients) and subsequent total abdominal hysterectomy in one. One of the four patients with advanced stage IV cervical carcinoma developed a ureterocolic fistula following radiation therapy. All were treated by placement of an antegrade stent, despite an apparent discontinuity of ureteral segments or sequestration of the ureter from the bladder in some cases. None of the 15 study patients responded to surgery, and endoscopic introduction of a retrograde indwelling catheter proved impossible prior to utilization of PCN and stent insertion.[20]

Andriole et al.[22] described their experience with 87 patients treated with indwelling Double-J ureteral stents for temporary and permanent urinary drainage. In this patient series, upper urinary tract fistula was the third major indication for stent placement in 10 of 87 patients (11.5%). Three of the ten had ureterovaginal fistulae following a total abdominal hysterectomy, whereas one had received palliation by pelvic irradiation for cancer. Five of the ten fistulae healed within 2–4 months. Andriole et al.[22] concluded that the Double-J ureteral stent was reliable and useful as an internal diversion for upper urinary tract fistulae.

The results obtained after using Double-J stents among 100 patients for various indications have been reviewed by Pocock et al.[8] Fifteen patients with complications of urological surgery and an additional four patients following benign gynaecological surgery were treated for persistent leakage of urine. Seven of the 15 had initially undergone ureteral surgery for various indications. In all seven patients, and in four others undergoing gynaecological surgery for benign conditions, the fistulae were closed within a few days of inserting the stent, and any patients with pain due to obstruction became asymptomatic.

Dowling et al.[13] achieved a success rate of 73% (11/15) by using the antegrade method of stent placement for ureteral obstructions, or for the management of ureteral fistulae.[13]

Chang et al.[23] managed 12 cases of fistula using PCN and placement of stent, resulting in a success rate of 85%. The major reason for failure in the management of ureteral fistula by placement of stent was when the fistula was present for more than 4 months, owing to epithelialization of the tract preventing the spontaneous closure of old fistulae.[19]

Barton et al.[24] documented five patients with ureteral fistulae out of 40 women who were all treated by stents for various types of gynaecological malignancy or their complications. As far as the authors are aware, this is the largest gynaecological oncology patient series ever to be reported for treatment for various indications using ureteral stents. In two of the five, ureterovaginal and ureterocutaneous fistulae had developed after radical hysterectomy. An additional two patients had previously undergone total pelvic exenteration and had developed uretero-ileal and ureteroperineal fistulae. Thus, four of the five patients with fistulae were managed by ureteral stents alone and four fistulae were closed.[24]

Ureteral strictures

The accepted treatment for urodynamically significant strictures of the ureter in the ureteropelvic junction has, in general, been surgical. However, since the late 1970s and early 1980s, less-aggressive management procedures have been reported.[17,21,25,26] Although chronic ureteral stenting provides effective palliation for ureters that are obstructed by malignant disease, it is not ideal for benign post-surgical ureteral strictures. The introduction of self-retaining Double-J stents has also paved the way for the development of alternative, less-aggressive management modalities in the treatment of this complication resulting from various types of surgical procedure and ureteral damage.

Bigongiari et al.[17] published data obtained with the conservative management of non-malignant ureteral strictures diagnosed in 14 renal units among nine patients. Of 14 strictures, eight (57%) were successfully stented and three were converted to indwelling ureteral stents, yielding a 78% success rate using only ureteral stenting, without significant complications.[17]

Catheter dilatation of benign ureteral strictures followed by stenting was reported by Banner et al.,[25] who treated 27 ureteral strictures in 23 patients followed by stent placement in 22. Of the 23 patients treated, eight (35%) had undergone benign gynaecological and gynaecological oncological surgery, including radical hysterectomy (two), radical hysterectomy with ureterovaginal fistula (three) and other benign gynaecological surgery (three). Using the method described, they reported that, of 27 strictures, 13 (48%) were successfully dilated and 26 of 27 renal units (96%) were stented. In 11 of the 23 patients (48%), urinary conduits had been placed and dilatation was successful in seven of these cases (64%). In addition, ten of these 11 patients (90%) were stented. Although all patients that had undergone gynaecological surgery were stented, dilatation was successful in the only two patients who only underwent benign gynaecological surgical procedures.[25]

One year later, Banner et al.[26] reported their accumulated experience from 44 patients, who initially had been reported for dilatation of ureteral stenosis. Gynaecological surgical procedures such as radical hysterectomy with ureterovaginal fistula (five), radical hysterectomy (one), gynaecological surgery for benign conditions (five) made up 25% of all patients treated. In this study they achieved successful results identical (48%) to those in their previous report.[25,26] One of the important conclusions of the authors was that strictures that follow radical hysterectomies, particularly those associated with urine leakage, usually are not responsive to treatment by dilatation. However, stenting of an ureteral fistula that develops after radical hysterectomy, followed shortly by prophylactic dilatation of the ureter at the former fistula site, may prevent stricture formation, whereas a single indwelling stent probably will not. An additional conclusion of this study is that uretero-enteric strictures can be effectively treated percutaneously in about 40% of cases. Analysis of 20 uretero-ileostomy stricture dilatations after pelvic exenteration for recurrent cervical carcinoma suggests that, usually, dilatation cannot be achieved in these patients. This is probably due to ureteral ischaemia associated with radical hysterectomy and, in some patients, high-dose radiotherapy to pelvic parts of the ureter. This is in contrast to strictures that follow ureteral ileostomy for benign or malignant bladder disease, which may be amenable to catheter dilatation.[26] In a very important study, Cormio et al.[27] analysed the results of treatment of 23 patients with bilateral ureteral injuries diagnosed between 1971 and 1991 after benign gynaecological (four) and gynaecological oncology (19) surgical procedures, comprising radical hysterectomy (three), radical hysterectomy combined with radiotherapy (16) and simple hysterectomy in (four). Of 46 ureters, 43 were compromised with strictures and three with vaginal fistulae. Four of 19 patients were not treated because they were not symptomatic, whereas 19 women were treated with various kinds of treatment modalities: ureteral stents alone were used in four patients; in nine subjects, treatment was by reconstructive procedures; internal diversion was used in two and external diversion in four. Treatment results in 14 of 19 patients (74%) were considered to be good. The success rate was markedly higher (85%) in those treated with stents and/or reconstructive procedures than in those treated with diversions (50%). The authors concluded that ureteral stenting and bilateral reconstructive procedures, when feasible, constitute the simplest and safest way to repair most ureteric injuries. In the management of extensive injuries, nephrostomy represents a safe and valid alternative to open surgical diversions, which do not improve the quality of life and may even be life threatening.[27]

Radiation injury of the ureter

This type of injury is an extremely rare condition that may develop after a considerable period following radiation therapy and which is mostly associated with ureteral stricture.

Buchler et al.[28] and Underwood et al.[29] described an occurrence rate of 0.04–4% non-symptomatic ureteral stricture with no demonstrable disease. However, the occurrence of ureteral stricture or obstruction, in patients treated previously by irradiation or surgery combined with irradiation for cervical carcinoma, is caused in as many as 95% of cases by reactivation of the disease. For symptomatic patients with unproven active disease treated previously by surgery and combination of irradiation alone, catheter dilatation of the stricture by placement of an internal stent may be considered, as discussed in the preceding section.[17,25,26]

In patients with previous recurrent disease, initially an indwelling ureteral stent should be inserted, in order to gain time and allow evaluation for pelvic exenteration, with the aim of achieving a cure. If the patient is not found to be eligible for exenteration, palliation by re-irradiation or cytotoxic therapy can also be attempted. The important role of unilateral or bilateral stenting in such conditions is to preserve renal function in these patients. Surgical correction of strictures with no evidence of recurrent disease may also be attempted, considering the surgery that will have to be done in irradiated areas, with a radiation effect existing in the bladder and in the pelvic part of the ureter that has been exposed to irradiation. These local conditions may be worse than the irradiation effect if the patient has previously undergone a radical hysterectomy as well.[9,10]

Malignant ureteral obstruction

Reversible ureteral obstruction is a not infrequent complication of gynaecological malignancy or its treatment. Diagnosis of an obstructed ureter comprises a urologic emergency warranting surgical intervention. In the past, open nephrostomy has been a standard method of management in such patients. However, non-operative urinary diversion techniques in the management of malignant ureteral obstruction (MUO) have undergone major changes due to the availability of percutaneous drainage techniques and endoscopically inserted ureteral stents.[30] Mann et al.[31] were the first to report on the use of ureteral stents in gynaecological malignancies. Ureteral obstruction due to malignant conditions can be detected at the time of tumour diagnosis, following completion of the treatment or in instances where the disease has progressed while treatment is being administered (Figs 39.9–39.10). Zadra et al.[32] reported on 98 patients (57 women and 41 men), who were referred with bilateral malignant ureteral obstruction. The most common origin of the disease was the cervix (28%), followed by the prostate (17%), bladder (16%) and ovary (10%). The remaining sites of origin were gastrointestinal (9%), breast (8%), lymph (5%), testis (4%), lung (2%) and uterus (1%). In this patient series, gynaecological origin comprised the highest rate of 39% among the 98 patients studied. Malignant bilateral ureteral obstruction (BUO) was caused in 73.4% of patients by tumours arising from pelvic organs.[32] Gasparini et al.[34] also reported similar rates. The following figures were from 22 patients with MUO caused by malignancies of gynaecological organ origin in 35% (8/22) of patients evaluated, and in 65% arising from non-gynaecological organs. Nevertheless, in relation to pelvic organ origin, the rate of MUO was found to be 65.6%,[2,22,33] which is very similar to that in the series of Zadra et al.[32] However, in the series reported by Fallon et al.,[35] composed of 100 patients (35 female and 65 male), the aetiology of MUO was related to pelvic organs in 86%, with most (37%) being in the prostate, followed by the bladder (29%), cervix (15%), ovary (4%) and vulva (1%).

Prior to the use of stents in MUO, the classic mode of management was an open nephrostomy when the obstruction was bilateral, causing uraemia, or in symptomatic patients when it was unilateral. This approach has resulted in a median survival rate of less

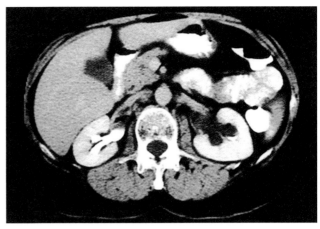

Figure 39.9. *CT scan of right normal and left hydronephrotic kidney in a 64-year-old patient treated by surgery and pelvic irradiation for stage IIIB endometrial carcinoma 18 months previously.*

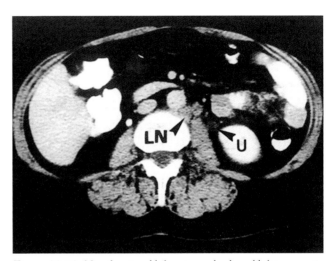

Figure 39.10. *Non-functional left ureter and enlarged left para-aortic lymph nodes. Arrows indicate (LN) enlarged (left) para-aortic lymph nodes, (U) non-functional (left) ureter.*

than 6.3 months. The rate of complications was 40–50% whereas only 31% of patients recovered uneventfully. Mortality rates in relation to surgery in such patients was reported to vary from 3 to 8%.[32]

The advances that have occurred in the last two decades in endo-urologic instrumentation and its concomitant use with fluoroscopy, the use of transureteral manipulation and the experience gained in this field, have enabled the urologist to divert the majority of renal obstructions of benign and malignant aetiology in either a retrograde or an antegrade fashion.[36]

In suitable patients, most diversions can be performed in an antegrade fashion, providing a cure, considerable patient comfort, short hospital stay, and longer survival with a marked increase in the number of days at home. Furthermore, a marked reduction has occurred in the incidence of serious direct complications and a decrease in the use of external appliances [32,34,36]. In this respect, Zadra et al.[32] reported their experience of treating 135 patients between 1978 and 1984 with unilateral (37) or bilateral (98) MUO using stenting methods. They showed that, during the study period, open nephrostomy was hardly ever necessary. Initial retrograde ureteral stenting was successful under local anaesthesia in 41% of patients. Percutaneous nephrostomy was performed in 47 patients. A total of 21 patients underwent miscellaneous open procedures, mostly in the earlier years, with a 57% morbidity rate compared with minimal morbidity associated with the newer techniques. The overall mean survival after diversion was 9.9 months, which was significantly longer than that reported after open procedures. This is one of the largest studies in which the beginning of the study period concurs with the period of initial insertion of self-retaining J stents, and represents the results obtained in a transitional period from open urinary diversion procedures to the current use of newer techniques.[32]

Experience gained in the use of indwelling double-J ureteral stents for temporary and permanent urinary drainage in 87 patients was described by Andriole et al.[22] The study period was between 1980 and 1982 (30 months), and this was one of the first and largest patient series, in which the indication for stent placement was ureteral obstruction in 57 subjects, 36 of whom had MUO. Although the rates of female patients and of those with gynaecological cancer have not been reported for the 36 patients treated, the results from the point of view of ease of stent insertion and a low rate of complications were excellent. No patient, of the 36 with MUO, was hospitalized for urologic obstruction for more than 4 days, and all were able to return home without significant morbidity. Although 12 of the 36 patients died of cancer, kidney function in all of them was almost normal (creatinine < 2.2). Mean survival was 4 months from the time of insertion of the stent (range 2–10 months). In 12 patients, eight stents were changed cystoscopically under local anaesthesia in the outpatient clinic. Overall, complications occurred in 28% of patients (24/87). Obstruction rate of stents was 15%,

severe irritation requiring medical treatment was 7% and stent site problems were diagnosed in 6% of patients.[22]

Of 100 patients who underwent a double-J stent placement between 1982 and 1986 with various indications and who were reviewed by Pocock et al.,[8] 17 were referred initially with MUO and the number of gynaecological oncology patients were not recorded. A total of 32 attempts at placement were made, and endoscopic insertion was successful in only 50% of 20 attempts. After insertion failure, four patients subsequently underwent successful antegrade placement. The authors concluded that their results were disappointing in patients with malignant obstructions.[8]

Much-improved results in the use of stenting methods in the management of MUO have been reported.[37] Gasparini et al.[34] managed 22 patients with MUO between 1986 and 1989. This study period started 3 years after that of Zadra et al.[32] Of the 22 patients, eight were male. All evaluated patients had advanced stages of disease. Of the 14 women, eight (57%) had gynaecological malignancies. The mean survival period between diversion and the analysis of results was 75 weeks (17 months; range 1–144 weeks). Three of the 22 patients (14%) had survived for 52, 56 and 244 weeks, respectively, at the end of the study period. The majority of patients (77%) were discharged from the hospital and this group spent 86% of their survival time at home. Mean survival at home was 64.7 weeks (range 0–98 weeks). After completion of the study, mean survival after diversion was 140 weeks in seven stented patients and in 15 (11 with failed stent placement) with PCN was 44.4 weeks.[34] Complications were infrequent and did not greatly affect survival or quality of life. Figures 39.11–39.12 depict malignant ureteral obstruction diagnosed by CT and treated by stent placement.

In a recent study, Barton et al.[24] described 40 women with gynaecological cancer who were treated with PCN and stents between 1986 and 1991. The indications were as follows. On initial presentation, nine had ureteral stenosis, 18 had persistent or recurrent cancer, nine had no evidence of disease (seven with ileal conduit) and four had operative ureteral damage. Thirty-five patients had ureteral stenosis (bilateral 24 and unilateral 11) and five had ureteral fistulae. Unilateral stents were inserted in 17 patients and 12 received bilateral stents. Renal function was initially

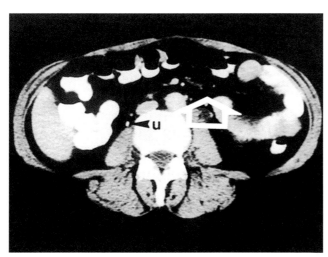

Figure 39.11. *Entrapment of left non-functional ureter by enlarged left para-aortic lymph nodes. Entrapped ureter appears inside the large arrow. U, functional right ureter.*

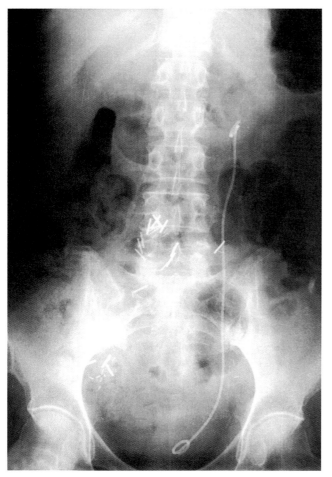

Figure 39.12. *Double-J stent in normal position inserted retrogradely.*

abnormal in 26 patients (65%); among these, improvement or normalization of renal function was

achieved in 62% (16/26) and in 23% (6/26) respectively. The overall median time of 5.5 months from the insertion of stents till death, was achieved in 22 cases of recurrent cancer, whereas it was 12 months in primary patients. By the end of the study period, 18 patients were alive: 12 of these were without clinical evidence of the disease with a median of 38 months, one was lost during follow-up and five were alive with clinically detectable disease with a median of 16 months.[24] No serious complications had occurred, haematuria being the most common complication. Failed first attempts at stent insertion occurred in 34% of 41 cases (12 bilateral and 17 unilateral) of renal units stented. Migration or dislodgement of the stents occurred in 17% (7/41) of the units stented, either during placement of the stent or 3 days later. Infection or sepsis was diagnosed in 44.8% of 29 patients stented, five of whom had a history of urinary tract infection prior to stent insertion. Curative or palliative treatment by irradiation and/or cytotoxic therapy in the presence of stents was carried out in 18 women. The authors concluded as follows: (1) the techniques used were safe and often improved renal function; (2) the general improvement and survival differs in women with primary and recurrent gynaecological cancer, in those without evidence of disease, and in women with ileal conduit. Figure 39.13 shows bilateral ureteral stents inserted in a 68-year-old woman with BUO. This study is an excellent example of the management of gynaecological patients using PCN and stents.

Mata et al.[36] reported their experience in the management of 105 obstructed renal units between 1983 and 1986, 30 (28%) of which were MUO. The majority of these were secondary to carcinoma of the cervix, many after previous radiation therapy and most before planned nephrotoxic chemotherapy. Of 30 obstructed ureters, 24 (80%) were successfully stented internally — a very high rate of success in relation to the insertibility procedure and the impact on patient management. On the other hand, data concerning survival time after stent placement, survival rate at home, comprehensive rates of stent displacement or dislodgement, and rates of infection or haematuria rates and other complications were not recorded. One of the aims of this study was to present an endo-urological algorithm that has been developed by the authors for bypassing and stenting ureteral obstructions, and that

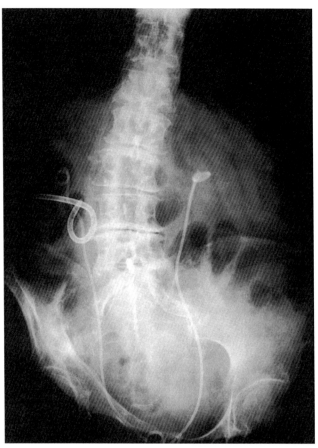

Figure 39.13. *Bilateral ureteral stents placed because of cervical carcinoma stage III B in stump, causing BUO associated with grade II cervical prolapse before removal of left nephrostome. Right stent was placed antegradely and left retrogradely.*

encompasses alternative techniques for the insertion of ureteral stents.[36]

Feuer et al.,[37] reviewing nine retrospective studies of PCN and surgical nephrostomy and adding their own experience, noted five independent prognostic factors that were consistently identified as absolute contraindications for PCN placement and were used for patient selection. These factors were (1) progressive disease during or immediately after optimal therapy, (2) lack of available therapy that has a reasonable possibility of being effective, (3) Zubrod performance status of more than 2, (4) the presence of tumour-related medical problems threatening the patient's life and (5) uncontrollable pain while on optimal medication. Using the same criteria, Feuer et al. showed clearly the efficacy of their selection method, in that no patient survived more than 160 days in the group in which treatment was contraindicated, whereas 20% of

patients survived more than 700 days among those who fulfilled the treatment criteria. Similar significant results were also obtained regarding number of 'days at home': in the group in which treatment was contraindicated this was a maximum of 25 days (approximately) compared with the more than 600 days at home that was achieved in 20% of patients who fulfilled the treatment criteria suggested by the authors.[37]

Conclusions

Despite the advances that have occurred in the development of stenting technology, as yet no stent exists that is ideal with regard to its material and its useful characteristics. On the other hand, during the last two decades, new developments and experience gained in the use of modern endo-urological methods have opened up new avenues in patient management, particularly for those needing temporary or prolonged periods of urinary diversion. It has been proved that stent placement, in conjunction with current endo-urological methods, is safe, effective and associated with low morbidity rates.

One of the major fields in which the newer stenting methods have provided higher treatment success rates, is the management of unilateral or bilateral MUO, yielding a stent placement rate of over 80% in relation to gynaecological oncological conditions. This has resulted in a significantly improved rate of survival, or even a cure in some previously untreated patients, as well as in those with recurrences, by providing preservation or often improvement of their renal function, compared with old methods involving open surgery. Furthermore, substantially higher treatment success rates have been achieved in the definitive treatment of most patients who have developed fistulae or symptomatic ureteral strictures, as well as in the treatment of surgical injury of the ureters, diagnosed mostly during the postoperative period, with no need for repeat surgery. In addition, the contribution of stents in the development of ultraradical surgery, particularly in the field of gynaecological oncology for urinary diversion, with the aim of achieving a cure, cannot be over-emphasized.

Finally, the literature shows clearly that more than 50% of ureteral injuries, and their possible early or late complications occurring in pelvic operations, are related to benign and malignant gynaecological oncological surgical procedures, compared with other specialities. It is also true that the main cause of MUO in general is related to gynaecological organ sites. Therefore gynaecological surgeons, as well as attending gynaecologists practising in regional clinics, should be familiar with the potential use of stenting methods. In addition, their use in the prevention of ureteral injury, as well as in all issues pertaining to follow-up strategies in stented patients, should be considered.

Acknowledgement

The authors thank Mrs S. Newman for her editorial assistance and typing of the manuscript.

References

1. D'Souza R, Tait P, Thomson R W, Trewhello M. An alternative approach to stenting the obstructed ureter. Case Report. Br J Radiol 1993; 66: 460–461
2. Edwards R D, Cockburn J F. Antegrade ureteric stenting using a 'pull-through' technique. Case Report. Br J Urol 1994; 73: 593–594
3. Culkin D J, Zitman R, Bundrick W S et al. Anatomic, functional and pathologic changes from internal ureteral stent placement. Urology 1992; 40: 385–390
4. Arsdalen K N, Pollack H M, Wein A J. Ureteral stenting. Semin Urol 1984; 11: 53
5. Saltzman B. Ureteral stents. Indications, variations and complications. In: Smith A D (ed) Endourology update. Urol Clin North Am 1988; 15(3): 481–491
6. Daly J W, Higgins K A. Injury of the ureter during gynecologic surgical procedures. Surg Gynecol Obstet 1988; 167: 19–22
7. St Lezin M A, Stoller M L. Surgical ureteral injuries. Urology 1991; 38: 497–506
8. Pocock R D, Stower M J, Ferro M A et al. Double-J stents. A review of 100 patients. Br J Urol 1986; 58: 629–633
9. Smith E B. Gynecology for the urologist. In: Gillenwater J Y, Grayhack J T, Howards S S, Dockett J M (eds) Adult and Pediatric Urology. Chicago: Year Book Medical, 1987; 2: 1328–1342
10. Corriere J N Jr. Ureteral injuries. In: Gillenwater J Y, Grayhack J T, Howards S S, Ducket J M (eds) Adult and Pediatric Urology. Chicago: Year Book Medical, 1987; 1: 436–443
11. Tarkington M A, Dejter S W Jr, Bresette J F. Early surgical management of extensive gynecologic ureteral injuries. Surg Gynecol Obstet 1991; 173: 17–21
12. Barone J G, Vates T S, Vasseli A J. A simple technique for intraoperatively stenting a transected ureter. J Urol 1993; 149: 535–536
13. Dowling R A, Corriere J N Jr, Sandler C M. Iatrogenic ureteral injury. J Urol 1986; 135: 912–915
14. Zinman R M, Libertino J A, Roth R A. Management of operative ureteral injury. Urology 1978; 12: 641–644
15. Berek J S. Surgical techniques. In: Berek J S, Hacker N F (eds) Practical gynecologic oncology, 2nd edn. Williams and Wilkins: Baltimore, 1994: 544–551
16. Sieben D M, Homerton L, Amin M et al. The role of ureteral stenting in the management of surgical injury of the ureter. J Urol 1978; 119: 330–331
17. Bigongiari L R, Lee K R, Moffatt R E et al. Percutaneous ureteral stent placement for stricture management and internal urinary drainage. AJR 1984; 143: 789–793
18. Boyce I, Fruchter R, Nicastri A. Prognostic factors in stage I carcinoma of the cervix. Gynecol Oncol 1981; 12: 154–165
19. Harshmann M V, Pollack H M, Banner M P, Wein A J. Conservative management of ureteral obstruction secondary to suture entrapment. J Urol 1982; 127: 121–123
20. Lang E K. Diagnosis and management of ureteral fistulas by percutaneous nephrostomy and antegrade stent catheter. Radiology 1981; 138: 311–317
21. Goldin A R. Percutaneous ureteral splinting. Urology 1977; 10: 165–168
22. Andriole G L, Bettmann M A, Garmie M B, Richie J P. Indwelling double-J ureteral stents for temporary and permanent urinary drainage: experience with 87 patients. J Urol 1984; 131: 239–241
23. Chang R, Marshall F F, Mitchell S. Percutaneous management of benign ureteral strictures and fistulas. J Urol 1987; 137: 1–26
24. Barton D P J, Morse S S, Fiorica J V et al. Percutaneous nephrostomy and ureteral stenting in gynecologic malignancies. Obstet Gynecol 1992; 80: 805–811
25. Banner M P, Pollack H M, Ring E J, Wein A J. Catheter dilatation of benign ureteral strictures. Radiology 1983; 147: 427–433
26. Banner M P, Pollack H M. Dilatation of ureteral stents: techniques and experience in 44 patients. AJR 1984; 143: 789–793
27. Cormio L, Ruutu M, Trabicante A et al. Management of bilateral ureteric injuries after gynecological and obstetric procedures. Int Urol Nephr 1993; 25: 551–555
28. Buchler D A, Kline J C, Peckham B M et al. Radiation reactions in cervical cancer therapy. Am J Obst Gynecol 1971; 111: 745–750
29. Underwood P B Jr, Lutz M H, Smack D L. Ureteral injury following irradiation therapy for carcinoma of the cervix. Obstet Gynecol 1977; 149: 663–669
30. Coddington C C, Thomas J R, Hoskins W J. Percuteneous nephrostomy for ureteral obstructions in patients with gynecologic malignancy. Gynecol Oncol 1984; 18: 339–348
31. Mann W J Jr, Peter Jander H, Orr J W Jr et al. The use of percutaneous nephrostomy in gynecologic oncology. Gynecol Oncol 1980; 10: 343–349
32. Zadra J A, Jewett M A S, Keresteci A G et al. Non operative urinary diversion for malignant ureteral obstruction. Cancer 1987; 60: 1353–1357
33. Finney R P. Experience with double-J ureteral catheter stent. J Urol 1978; 120: 678–681
34. Gasparini M, Caroll P, Stoller M. Palliative percutaneous and endoscopic urinary diversion for malignant ureteral obstruction. Urology 1991; 38: 408–412
35. Fallon B, Olney L, Culp D A. Nephrostomy in cancer patients: to do or not to do? Br J Urol 1980; 152: 237–242
36. Mata J A, Culkin D J, Venable D D. Techniques for bypassing and stenting ureteral obstructions. J Urol 1994; 152: 917–919
37. Feuer G A, Fruchter R, Seruri E et al. Selection for percutaneous nephrostomy in gynecologic cancer patients. Gynecol Oncol 1991; 42: 60–63

40

Endo-urological management of iatrogenic ureteral injuries
D. M. Lask and N. Erlich

Introduction

Since the introduction of modern upper urinary tract endo-urology and minimal invasive surgical techniques, both the aetiology of, and the ability to treat, iatrogenic ureteral injuries have, dramatically altered. Up to 20 years ago a wide variety of major open abdominal surgical techniques (end-to-end ureteral anastomosis, ureteroneocystostomy, psoas hitch, Boari flap, transuretero-ureterostomy, intestinal interposition, urinary diversion, renal autotransplantation and nephrectomy) were used. The concurrent morbidity and prolonged hospitalization associated with these procedures is well documented.[1,2] However, improved instrumentation and endo-urological techniques have provided less invasive means of managing iatrogenic ureteral injuries, with a concomitant decrease in morbidity and cost.[3]

Endo-urological methods consist of ureteral repair without removal of the injured portion of the ureter, which is made possible by the phenomenon of spontaneous ureteric regeneration. Since the classic clinical report by Davis,[4] many experimental studies have demonstrated the sequelae of ureteral regeneration,[5] indicating complete restoration within 3–6 weeks and a possibility of continued ureteral peristalsis, even after transmural incision.[6,7] Although ureteric regeneration occurs whether or not a stent is present, the use of stents is preferable as it provides a framework for epithelization and avoids early urine flow through the defect.[8–10]

Since Zimskind's pioneer straight silicone stent and the multiple-barb silicone stents developed by Gibbons and colleagues, which were prone to migration and caused placement difficulties, the silicone double-J stent has been developed.[11–14] Such stents can be straightened for insertion by an internal guidewire and then return to their original shape when the guidewire is removed. Double-J ureteric stents, however, are not free from problems, including catheter migration, encrustation and breakage, bacterial adhesion,

alteration of renal pelvic dynamics, vesico-ureteric reflux with reduction of ureteric peristaltic activity, ureteral epithelial ulceration, hyperplasia and metaplasia of the mucosa, and wall thickening.[15–21]

Nowadays, endo-urologic techniques provide the means of repairing iatrogenic ureteral injuries. However, the indications, effectiveness and long-term results, as well as the safety of the prosthetic materials, remain to be defined.[22]

Aetiology of iatrogenic ureteral injuries

Iatrogenic ureteral injuries may occur during surgical or laparoscopic procedures performed in the retroperitoneal space or pelvis (urological, general, gynaecological and vascular surgery), as well as during ureteroscopic procedures.[23,24]

Urological procedures

Ureteroscopy accounts for most ureteral injuries, occurring in 9% (range 0–28%) of all procedures, including perforation (7%), avulsion (0.4%) and postoperative strictures (1.4–11%).[24–26] Although the upper ureter has a thinner mucosal lining and less muscle support than the lower part, most injuries occur in the distal third, where the majority of procedures are performed. Perforations occur when forcing against resistance, and avulsion, when the ureter wall is captured within basket wires. Strictures are due to relative ischaemia (large instruments used for prolonged periods), and extravasation of urine due to mechanical or thermal injury. The rate of complications following ureteroscopic manipulation appears to be related directly to the experience of the individual operator.[27,28] The ureter may be injured during transurethral resection of the prostate or bladder tumours, bladder diverticulectomy, or radical — and even retropubic — prostatectomy.[29] Recently, extracorporeal shock-wave lithotripsy has been reported to cause ureteral stricture.[30]

General surgical procedures

Abdominal perineal resection is the colorectal surgical procedure most frequently associated with ureteral injury (0.3–5.7%), with predominance of the left ureter due to its close proximity to the mesocolon.[31,32]

Gynaecological procedures

The overall rate of ureteral injuries due to gynaecological procedures is 0.5%–1.5%.[33,34] Two-thirds occur during abdominal procedures and one-third during vaginal surgery.[35] The incidence of ureteral injury following radical hysterectomy may vary from 5 to 30%, 2.5% after hysterectomy for benign disease and 0.1% after caesarean section.[36–38] Rare cases of ureteral injury have also been reported after bladder neck suspension, laparoscopic procedures (sterilization, fulguration of endometriosis and assisted vaginal hysterectomy) and oocyte harvesting for in vitro fertilization.

The three most common sites of ureteral injury during gynaecological surgery are (a) at the pelvic brim (the ureter is close to the ovarian vessels); (b) at the level of the infundibulopelvic ligament (the ureter is under the uterine artery), and (c) at the ureterovesical junction.[39]

Vascular surgery

Injury to the ureter may occur following aortoiliac or aortofemoral bypass, but its incidence has not been established. Goldenberg et al.[40] have demonstrated, in a prospective study in 1988 on 181 kidneys of 93 patients who underwent aortofemoral bypass, that mild to moderate hydronephrosis can be noted in 15 kidneys 1 week after surgery, but in only 1 kidney at 1-year follow-up. Thus, hydronephrosis is not uncommon, but rarely has clinical significance.[40] The incidence of urinary fistula following aortofemoral bypass is quite rare, but always of clinical significance. Blasco and Saladie,[41] reviewing 154 patients with ureteral obstruction following vascular surgery, observed that ureteric fistula occurred in 19 patients (12%).

Other procedures

Ureteral injuries have also been known to be caused by lumbar disc surgery,[42] lumbar surgical and computed tomography (CT)-guided chemical sympathectomy,[43,44] arthrodesis of the hip joint[45] and total hip replacement.[46]

Diagnosis and symptomatology

More than 80% of ureterical injuries are diagnosed in the late postoperative period.[47] The non-specific nature of complaints, such as abdominal or flank pain, nausea or vomiting, are usually attributed to the patient's postoperative condition rather than to ureteral injury. On the other hand, postoperative anuria, after elimination of causes of acute renal failure, may suggest bilateral ureteral ligation, or unilateral ligation in cases where only one kidney is functioning. In some patients, urinary leakage through the surgical incision (abdominal or vaginal) is noted days or weeks after partial or complete ureteral transection.[48] The watery discharge can be identified as urine by its creatinine content, or by intravenous injection of indigo-carmine, which will stain the discharge dark blue.[49] When the urine is trapped in the retroperitoneum, urinoma formation will occur, manifested by malaise, fever and vague gastrointestinal symptoms.

Intravenous urography (IVU) is essential to determine the diagnosis and to provide information about the contralateral kidney. Lask et al.[50] noted various degrees of hydronephrosis in all their patients with ureteral injuries. Apart from hydronephrosis, other abnormalities, such as complete obstruction, retroperitoneal extravasation, and ureterovaginal or ureterosigmoid fistula, can be diagnosed.[50,51] IVU may determine the site and length of iatrogenic ureteral strictures, but when complete obstruction is diagnosed, it is essential to perform retrograde pyelography to visualize the distal part of the ureter.[52] Renal ultrasonography, with its moderate degree of specificity, may reveal the presence of hydronephrosis in up to 80% of patients.[50] Ultrasonography, as well as CT and magnetic resonance imaging (MRI), are useful in diagnosing urine extravasation and urinoma formation.[52]

Treatment

Until the 1980s, ureteral injuries always required open reconstructive surgery. Nowadays, minimal invasive and endo-urological techniques have provided new approaches to overcome such lesions.

Ureteral stenting

Turner et al.[53] proposed that retrograde endoscopic placement of an indwelling double-J stent to bridge the damaged area should be attempted whenever possible. In case of failure, decompression of the obstructed kidney by percutaneous nephrostomy tube insertion is mandatory in order to preserve renal function, relieve flank pain, overcome urinary tract infection and to divert urine from the injured site of the ureter.

In 1984, Andriole et al.[54] reported a 50% success rate in the treatment of ureteric fistulas using an indwelling double-J ureteral stent. An even higher success rate of 83–90% was observed by Chang et al.[55] and Turner et al.[53] Stenting the ureter is possible, either by a retrograde approach or by percutaneous antegrade stent placement.[56,57]

Percutaneous nephrostomy drainage alone

Harshman et al.[58] suggested that ureteral obstruction following gynaecological procedures is due to entrapment of the ureter by a suture, which is eventually absorbed and may be best treated by proximal drainage alone. They treated three patients with ureteral injury, in whom insertion of a percutaneous nephrostomy tube resulted in complete recovery.[58] Lang et al.[59] reported on five patients with ureteral injuries, including four with ureterovaginal fistula, who were successfully treated by percutaneous nephrostomy alone. Dowling et al.[60] reported good results in 11 of 15 patients managed with percutaneous drainage alone or with antegrade ureteric stenting. In the authors' personal series, complete spontaneous recovery of the injured ureter occurred in 16 of 20 patients with good long-term results. Only one patient needed additional treatment by balloon ureteral dilatation.[50]

Although primary management of ureteral injuries by insertion of a percutaneous nephrostomy tube results in significantly decreased reoperation and morbidity rates, and has enabled spontaneous recovery of the injured ureter in a significant number of patients, it seems that the need for prolonged external drainage is not well accepted by patients. With the availability of other techniques, this method should only be used in selected cases.

Ureteral dilatation

Since the invention of the percutaneous trochar nephrostomy by Goodwin et al.[61] and the balloon catheter by Gruntzig et al.,[62] the technology of instrumentation and the development of refined biocompatible well-tolerated stents with reliable internal drainage have been described. The availability of such tools, and the fact that most narrowed ureteral segments can be negotiated, dilated and stented, suggests that catheter or balloon ureteral dilatation, followed by stent insertion, should be the initial method of ureteral stricture management. From accumulated data on 181 patients, with follow-up ranging from 1 to 60 months, the success rate was 57% to 76%.[29,63–65] This success rate depends on several factors. The best results were achieved in 11 of 13 patients with strictures after ureteroscopy or ureteral ligation (85%), but successful outcome was seen in only five of 10 patients with anastomotic stricture (50%).[63] In addition, the success rate is much lower if the duration of the stricture is more than 3 months.[63,64] The length of the stricture also influences the outcome: Chang et al.[64] reported a 100% success rate in strictures less than 1.5 cm. and a failure rate of 86% with longer or multiple strictures. Similar results are reported by Netto et al.,[65] who noted better outcome in strictures shorter than 2 cm. Smith[29] observed that distal ureteral strictures managed by balloon dilatation responded far better than those of the middle or upper ureter.[29]

As no consensus exists about several technical points regarding balloon dilatation of the ureter (route of access — antegrade or retrograde — balloon size, duration of inflation, single versus multiple dilatation and the use of stents following the procedure), it is impossible to define the best method of dilating ureteral strictures.[3]

In conclusion, ureteral dilatation and stenting should be recommended as the initial treatment in most patients with ureteral strictures. A high success rate is predicted in short, non-anastomotic strictures of less than 3 months' duration. In addition, late reconstructive surgery of recurrent strictures is not compromised by the endoscopic procedure.[66]

Endoscopic ureterotomy

Recurrent ureteral strictures following balloon dilatation will not usually benefit from a repeated procedure.[67] Endoscopic incision (endo-ureterotomy) should be recommended and is likely to be more successful than open reconstructive surgery. The advantages of endo-ureterotomy compared with open surgical repair include a low rate of morbidity and minimal interference to the ureteral blood supply.

This technique includes full-thickness incision until the periureteral fat is exposed. The incision should be extended 1–2 cm above and below the stenotic area and, in cases of dense periureteral fibrosis, even balloon dilatation of the incised open ureter is recommended.[68–70] Care should be taken, regarding the direction of the incision, to avoid injury to major periureteral vessels. In general, strictures between the ureteropelvic junction and iliac vessels should be incised in a posterolateral direction, whereas those below the vessels are incised anteromedially or even by direct anterior incision.[68,69] Meretyk et al.[68] suggest that extreme proximal strictures can be marsupialized to the renal pelvis, and distal strictures to the bladder. The incision can be performed with a cold-knife which may result in less periureteral scarring, or by electrocautery (3 Fr Greenwald electrode), which allows a more precise incision of the proper depth with simultaneous cauterizing of small vessels.[68,70–72] Following the incision, the ureter is usually stented for 6 weeks, the time required for full regeneration of its wall.[68] However, successful results with endopyelotomy have been observed within 4 days of splinting.[71] The most common stent used is a tapered (14/7 Fr) double-pigtail catheter.[68]

From cumulative data on 262 patients from nine series, the success rate with endo-ureterotomy is 57–100%,[68,72–79] with few major complications, such as urinoma formation and severe haemorrhage, requiring emergency laparotomy.[68,73] The success rate with endo-ureterotomy is higher when managing strictures shorter than 1.5 cm and the results are poor in patients after irradiation therapy.[74]

Lingeman et al.[77] reported their experience in nine patients with total ureteral occlusion. This technique consists of a combined retrograde and antegrade approach using a 'cut-to-the-light' with a fascial incising needle and balloon dilatation. The success rate was 100% with a mean follow-up of 22 months. A combined approach to treat complete obstruction at the level of the ureterovesical junction was reported by Strup and Bagley,[78] with successful results in six of seven patients.

Acucise® endo-ureterotomy

The Acucise (Applied Medical Technologies, Laguna Hills, CA, USA) cutting balloon catheter provides an alternative method for performing endo-ureterotomy. Although there has been extensive experience regarding the treatment of ureteropelvic junction stenosis, this technique has been used in only a small number of patients with ureteral stricture.[80,81] With this technique, proper orientation of the cutting wire is achieved by fluoroscopic guidance and there is no need for upper tract access but it is essential that the stricture be wide enough to allow passage of the device.

Other techniques

Finally, several additional endo-urological techniques have been reported in the last few years, including the use of free urothelial grafts (harvested from the bladder and placed endoscopically),[82] the use of metallic stents (expandable and non-expandable)[83–85] and the use of laparoscopy in the repair of ureteral strictures (reanastomosis using fibrin glue).[86] A reliable assessment of the efficacy of these techniques in patients with ureteral strictures requires further study.

Conclusions

At present, endo-urology provides new opportunities to repair ureteric injuries which, until the 1980s, always required open reconstructive surgery.

These new techniques reduce hospital stay, co-morbidity and also costs. Endoscopic placement of an indwelling double-J catheter in the damaged ureter should be attempted whenever possible. Balloon dilatation is most effective for short non-anastomotic strictures of the distal ureter of less than 3 months' duration. Recurrent obstruction will benefit from endo-ureterotomy techniques, although there is a risk of significant haemorrhage, due to the alteration of the normal anatomical relationship of the iliac vessels and the ureter. Surgery should be reserved for patients in whom endo-urological techniques have failed.

References

1. Fry D E, Milholen L, Harbrecht P J. Iatrogenic ureteral injury. Arch Surg 1983; 118: 454–457

2. Silverstein J L, Libby C, Smith A D. Management of ureteroscopic ureteral injuries. Urol Clin North Am 1988; 15: 515–524

3. Goldfischer E R, Gerber G S. Endoscopic management of ureteral strictures. J Urol 1997; 157: 770–775

4. Davis D M. Intubated ureterotomy: new operation for ureteral and ureteropelvic stricture. Surg Gynecol Obstet 1943; 76: 513–523

5. Hinman F Jr. Ureteral reconstruction. In: Bergman H (ed) The Ureter. New York: Springer-Verlag, 1981: 179–185

6. Openheimer R, Hinman F Jr. Ureteral regeneration: contracture vs. hyperplasia of smooth muscle. J Urol 1955; 74: 476–484

7. Hanna M K, Jeffs R D, Sturgess J M, Barkin M et al. Ureteral structure and ultrastructure: part 1. The normal human ureter. J Urol 1976; 116: 718–724

8. McDonald J H, Calams J A. Experimental ureteral stricture: ureteral regrowth following ureterotomy with or without intubation. J Urol 1960; 84: 52–59

9. Oppenheimer R, Hinman F Jr. The effect of urinary flow upon ureteral regeneration in the absence of splint. Surg Obstet Gynecol 1956; 103: 416–422

10. Witherington R. Ureteral splints. Urology 1974; 3: 257–263

11. Zimskind P D, Fetter T R, Wilkerson J R. Clinical use of long-term indwelling silicone rubber ureteral splints inserted cystoscopically. J Urol 1967; 97: 840–843

12. Gibbons R P, Correa R J Jr, Cummings K B, Mason J T. Experience with indwelling ureteral stent catheters. J Urol 1976; 115: 22–26

13. Finney R P. Experience with new double-J ureteral catheter stent. J Urol 1978; 120: 678–681

14. Hepperlen T W, Mardis H K, Kammandel H. Self-retained internal ureteral stents: a new approach. J Urol 1978; 119: 731–734

15. Bagley D J, Huffman J L. Ureteroscopic retrieval of proximally located ureteral stent. Urology 1991; 37: 446–448

16. Holmes S A V, Cheng C, Whitfield H N. The development of synthetic polymers that resist encrustation on exposure to urine. Br J Urol 1992; 69: 651–655

17. Reid G, Denstedt J D, Kang Y S et al. Microbial adhesion and biofilm formation on ureteral stents in vitro and in vivo. J Urol 1992; 148: 1592–1594

18. Payne S R, Ramsay J W A. The effects of double J stents on renal pelvic dynamics in the pig. J Urol 1988; 140: 637–641

19. Mosli H A, Farsi H M A, Fawzi Al-Zimaity M et al. Vesicoureteral reflux in patients with double pigtail stents. J Urol 1991; 146: 966–969

20. Marx M, Bettman M A, Bridge S et al. The effects of various indwelling ureteral catheter materials on the normal canine ureter. J Urol 1988; 139: 180–185

21. Ramsay J W A, Crocker R P, Ball A J et al. Urothelial reaction to ureteric intubation. A clinical study. Br J Urol 1987; 60: 504–505

22. Cormio L. Ureteric injuries — clinical and experimental studies. Scand J Urol 1995 (suppl 171): 20

23. Selzman A A, Spirnak J P. Iatrogenic ureteral injuries: A 20-year experience in treating 165 injuries. J Urol 1996; 155: 878–881

24. Huffman J R. Ureteroscopic injuries to the upper urinary tract. Urol Clin North Am 1989; 16: 249–254

25. Weinberg J J, Ansong K, Smith A D. Complications of ureteroscopy in relation to experience: report of survey and author experience. J Urol 1987; 137: 384–385

26. Lytton B, Weiss R M, Green D F. Complications of ureteral endoscopy. J Urol 1987; 137: 649–653

27. Motola J A, Smith A D. Complications of ureteroscopy: prevention and treatment. AUA Update Series, 1992; 11: 162 (lesson 21).

28. Assimos D G, Patterson L C, Taylor C L. Changing incidence and etiology of iatrogenic ureteral injuries. J Urol 1994; 152: 2240–2246

29. Smith A D. Management of iatrogenic ureteral strictures after urological procedures. J Urol 1988; 140: 1372–1374

30. Dogra P M, Jadeia N A. Urosepsis and ureteric strictures following extracorporeal shock wave lithotripsy. Eur Urol 1994; 52: 109–112

31. Hughes E S R, McDermott F T, Polglase A L, Johnson W R et al. Ureteric damage in surgery for cancer of large bowel. Dis Colon Rectum 1984; 27: 293–295

32. Anderson A, Bergdahl L. Urological complications following abdominoperineal resection of the rectum. Arch Surg 1976; 111: 969–971

33. Mann W J, Arato M, Patsner B, Stone M L. Ureteral injuries in an obstetrics and gynecology training program: etiology and management. Obstet Gynecol 1988; 72: 82–85

34. Daly J W, Higgins K A. Injury to the ureter during gynecological surgical procedures. Surg Gynecol Obstet 1988; 167: 19–22

35. Tarkington M A, Dejter S W, Bresette J F. Early surgical management of extensive gynecological ureteral injuries. Surg Gynecol Obstet 1991; 173: 17–21

36. Gangi M P, Agee R E, Spence C R. Surgical injury to the ureter. Urology 1976; 8: 22–27

37. Solomons E, Levin E J, Bauman, J, Baron J. A pyelographic study of ureteric injuries sustained during hysterectomy for benign conditions. Surg Gynecol Obstet 1960; 111: 41–48

38. Eisenkop S M, Richman P, Platt L D, Paul R H. Urinary tract injury during cesarean section. Obstet Gynecol 1982; 60: 591–596

39. Boyd M E. Care of the ureter in pelvic surgery. Can J Surg 1987; 30: 234–236

40. Goldenberg S L, Gordon P B, Cooperberg P L, McLoughlin M G. Early hydronephrosis following aortic bifurcation graft surgery: a prospective study. J Urol 1988; 140: 1367–1369

41. Blasco F J, Saladie J M. Ureteral obstruction and ureteral fistulas after aortofemoral or aortoiliac bypass surgery. J Urol 1991; 145: 237–242

42. Flam T A, Spitzenpfeil E et al. Complete ureteral transection associated with percutaneous lumbar disk nucleotomy. J Urol 1992; 148: 1249–1250

43. Kuzmarov I W, MacIsaac S G, Sioufi J, De Domenico I. Ureteral injury secondary to sympathetic ganglion blockade. Urology 1980; 16: 617–619

44. Trigaux J P, Decoene B, van Beers B et al. Focal necrosis of the ureter following CT-guided chemical sympathectomy. Cardiovasc Intervent Radiol 1992; 15(3): 180–182

45. Egawa S, Shiokawa H, Uchida T et al. Delayed presentation of ureteric injury following arthrodesis of the hip joint. Br J Urol 1994; 73: 212–213

46. Carrieri G, Callea A, Gala F et al. Avulsione dell'uretere pelvico in corso di artroprotesi dell'anca. Atti Soc Urol Il Centro-Mer Isole 1986; 22: 269–273

47. Witters S, Cornelissen M, Vereecken R. Iatrogenic ureteral injury: aggressive or conservative treatment. Am J Obstet Gynecol 1986; 155: 582–584

48. Gerber G S, Schoenberg H W. Female urinary tract fistulas. J Urol 1993; 149: 229–236

49. McAninch J W. Injuries to the genitourinary tract. In: Tanagho E A, McAninch J W (eds) Connecticut: Appleton and Lange, 1988: 302–318

50. Lask D, Abarbanel J, Luttwak Z et al. Changing trends in the management of iatrogenic ureteral injuries. J Urol 1995; 154: 1693–1695

51. Bayer I, Kyzer S, Chaimoff C. Iatrogenic ureterosigmoid fistula — a rare complication of sigmoidectomy. Colo-proctology 1989; 9: 370–373

52. Lezin M A, Stoller M L. Surgical ureteral injuries. Urology 1991; 38: 498–506

53. Turner W H, Cranston D W, Davies A H et al. Double-J stents in the treatment of gynaecological injury to the ureter. J R Soc Med 1990; 83: 623–624

54. Andriole G L, Bettman M A, Garnick M B, Richie J B. Indwelling double-J ureteral stents for temporary and permanent urinary drainage: experience with 87 patients. J Urol 1984; 131: 239–241

55. Chang R, Marshall F F, Mitchell S S. Percutaneous management of benign ureteral strictures and fistulas. J Urol 1987; 137: 1126–1131

56. Bigongiari L R, Lee K R, Moffat R E et al. Percutaneous ureteral stent placement for stricture management and internal urinary drainage. Am J Radiol 1979; 133: 865–868

57. Pingoud E G, Bagley D H, Zeman R K et al. Percutaneous antegrade bilateral dilation and stent placement for internal drainage. Radiology 1980; 134: 780

58. Harshman M W, Pollack H M, Banner M P, Wein A J. Conservative management of ureteral obstruction secondary to suture entrapment. J Urol 1982; 127: 121–123

59. Lang E K, Lanasa J A, Garrett J et al. The management of urinary fistulas and strictures with percutaneous ureteral stent catheters. J Urol 1979; 122: 736–740

60. Dowling R A, Corriere J N, Sandler C M. Iatrogenic ureteral injury. J Urol 1986; 135: 912–915

61. Goodwin W E, Caset W C, Woolf W. Percutaneous trochar (needle) nephrostomy in hydronephrosis. JAMA 1955; 157: 891–894

62. Gruntzig A R, Senning A, Siegenthaler W E. Nonoperative dilatation of coronary artery stenosis: percutaneous transluminal coronary angioplasty. New Engl J Med 1979; 301: 61–68

63. Beckman C F, Roth R A, Bihrle W III. Dilatation of benign ureteral strictures. Radiology 1989; 172: 437–441

64. Chang R, Marshall F F, Mitchell S. Percutaneous management of benign ureteral strictures and fistulas. J Urol 1987; 137: 1126–1131

65. Netto N R Jr, Ferreira U, Lemos G C, Claro J F A et al. Endourological management of ureteral strictures. J Urol 1990; 144: 631–634

66. Kramolowsky E V, Tucker R D, Nelson C M K. Management of benign ureteral strictures: open surgical repair or endoscopic dilation? J Urol 1989; 141: 285–286

67. Kwak S, Leef J A, Rosenblum J D. Percutaneous balloon catheter dilatation of benign ureteral strictures: effect of multiple dilatation procedures on long-term patency. AJR 1995; 165: 97–100

68. Meretyk S, Albala D M, Clayman R V et al. Endoureterotomy for treatment of ureteral strictures. J Urol 1992; 147: 1502–1506

69. Eshghi M. Endoscopic incisions of the urinary tract. Part I & II. AUA Update Ser 1989; 8: lessons 37,38

70. Conlin M J, Bagley D H. Incisional treatment of ureteral strictures. In: Smith A D (ed). Smith's Textbook of Endourology 1996: 497–505

71. Abdel-Hakim A M. Endopyelotomy for ureteropelvic junction obstruction: is long term stenting mandatory? J Endourol 1987; 1: 265

72. Schneider A W, Conrad S, Busch R, Otto U et al. The cold-knife technique for endourological management of stenoses in the upper urinary tract. J Urol 1991; 146: 961–965

73. Yamada S, Ono Y, Ohshima S, Miyake K et al. Transurethral ureteroscopic ureterotomy assisted by a prior balloon dilation for relieving ureteral strictures. J Urol 1995; 153: 1418–1421

74. Thomas R. Choosing the ideal candidate for ureteroscopic endoureterotomy. J Urol 1993; 149(part 2): 314A (abstr 404)

75. Eshghi M, Franco I, Hernandez-Gravlav J, Schwalb D. Cold knife endoureterotomy of 79 strictures: technique and 5-years follow-up. J Urol 1992; 147(part 2): 471A (abstr 1036)

76. Selikowitz S M. New coaxial ureteral stricture knife. Urol Clin North Am 1990; 17: 83–89

77. Lingeman J E, Wong M Y, Newmark J R. Endoscopic management of total ureteral occlusion and ureterovaginal fistula. J Endourol 1995; 9: 391–396

78. Strup S E, Bagley D H. Endoscopic ureteroneocystostomy for complete obstruction at the ureterovesical junction. J Urol 1996; 156: 360–362

79. Cornud F, Lefebvre J F, Chretieny et al. Percutaneous transrenal electro-incision of uretero-intestinal anastomotic strictures: long-term results and comparison of fluoroscopic and endoscopic guidance. J Urol 1996; 155: 1575–1578

80. Chandhoke P S, Clayman R V, Stone A M et al. Endopyelotomy and endoureterotomy with the Acucise ureteral cutting balloon device: preliminary experience. J Endourol 1993; 7: 45–51

81. Cohen T D, Gross M B, Preminger G M. Long term follow-up of Acucise incision of ureteropelvic junction obstruction and ureteral strictures. Urology 1996; 47: 317–323

82. Urban D A, Kerbl K, Clayman R V, McDougall E. Endo-ureteroplasty with a free urothelial graft. J Urol 1994; 152: 910–915

83. Reinberg Y, Ferral H, Gonzales R et al. Intraureteral metallic self-expanding endoprosthesis (Wallstent) in the treatment of difficult ureteral strictures. J Urol 1994; 151: 1619–1622

84. Pauer W, Lugmayer H. Metallic Wallstents: a new therapy for extrinsic ureteral obstruction. J Urol 1992; 148: 281–284

85. Cussenot O, Bassi S, Desgrandchamps F et al. Outcomes of non-self-expandable metal prostheses in structured human ureter: suggestions for future developments. J Endourol 1993; 7: 205–209

86. McKay T C, Albala D M, Gehrin B E, Casttell M. Laparoscopic ureteral reanastomosis using fibrin glue. J Urol 1994; 152: 1637–1640

Reinforced endo-ureteral stent in tumour-induced hydronephrosis

R. W. Schlick and K. Planz

41

Introduction

The management of patients with ureteral obstruction in advanced cancer can be difficult. Metastases from primary malignancies anywhere can spread to the retroperitoneum and lead to ureteral obstruction. Secondary involvement of the retroperitoneum by malignant tumours occurs either by direct extension of the adjacent malignancy or by metastasis to the retroperitoneal lymph nodes. Tumours that spread to the retroperitoneum by direct extension usually involve the pelvic part of the ureter. The tumours may simply compress the ureteral wall, but they can also invade the entire ureter. Metastatic tumours involving the retroperitoneum and the periureteral lymphatic nodes tend to produce obstruction, which may be limited or quite extensive in area.[1] Tumours of varying origin can progress in this way; they include metastases from carcinomas of the breast, stomach, lung, pancreas, lymphoma and colon.[2,3] Tumours arising from pelvic structures can be similarly involved; typically, these include tumours of the bladder or prostate, the cervix, sigmoid colon and rectum. Theoretically, any secondary tumour mass spreading to the retroperitoneum can advance upon the ureter with subsequent obstruction and hydro- or pyonephrosis.[4,5] Ureteral obstruction may occur within 2 years of the primary diagnosis in 60–70% of patients, but it may occur up to 20 years later,[6] or may be the first sign in gynaecological cancer.[3] Sometimes the decrease in urine output is not suspected until the patient develops signs of uraemia due to obstruction of both ureters or anuria becomes manifest.[2,3] The obstruction usually can be seen in the distal or pelvic part of the ureter, although it can occur anywhere and may be located at multiple sites.

Urinary diversion can be accomplished with internal ureteral stents, percutaneous nephrostomies, or cutaneous ureterostomy. Some unusual means such as subcutaneous urinary diversion have also been suggested.[7] Nowadays, nephrostomy is widely used because of the easy percutaneous approach, but nephrostomies appear to have a significant incidence of associated infections and stone formation.[8] Double-J ureteral catheters, introduced in 1978 by Finney, have become the preferred long-term option because of their relative ease of insertion, but it is important to be aware that even well-placed indwelling ureteral stents may not ensure sufficient urinary drainage,[9] particularly in the presence of extrinsic ureteral obstruction: it has been noted that 46% of silicone stents and 41% of polyurethane stents, both with side-ports, failed in the presence of extrinsic ureteral compression. Furthermore, the comment has been made that silicone ureteral stents may be appropriate for long-term stenting in patients where a flow around the stent can be expected, but not for urinary drainage.[10]

In the belief that this high failure rate reflects the existence of high extrinsic pressures against the stents and is not attributable to potential aperistaltic ureteral segments in such cases, the authors have attempted to develop a new indwelling ureteral stent in the well-known double-J configuration. This new design should resist high extrinsic pressures, should be placed easily, guaranteeing adequate drainage of urine and should be comfortable for the patient.

The first Bard-angiomed tumour stent™, with an external diameter of about 14 Fr and an internal diameter comparable to that of a normal 6 Fr stent, did not gain sufficient acceptance owing to its extremely large external diameter. However, the idea was correct, to develop a ureteral stent that could resist external pressure and could provide sufficient drainage of the collecting system, but without having a larger external diameter than normal stents in use.

Materials and methods

The aim was to develop a ureteral stent for use in tumour patients with pelvic or retroperitoneal masses causing obstructive renal failure, or just to relieve pain. This 'tumour stent' (Bard-Angiomed, Karlsruhe,

Germany), is currently in use in Europe (and has been submitted for FDA approval), is available in diameters from 6 to 8 Fr and in lengths of 24–32 cm. The body of the stent consists of a high-stability combination of plastic (polyurethane–polyamide) with adequate elasticity (Fig. 41.1). Both ends of the stent consist of extremely elastic and smooth J-parts for fixation, and are marked for easy radiological identification (Fig. 41.2). To conform to common Double-J stents of the same external diameter, the new stent has a sufficiently large interior diameter to allow antegrade urine drainage (Tables 41.1–3).

The management of this stent does not differ from that of commonly used stents; there is, therefore, no need of special instrumentation and no learning curve is

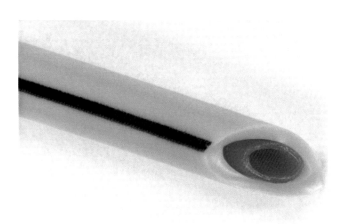

Figure 41.1. *Body of the tumour stent (cross-section) constructed from a highly stable combination of polyurethane and polyamide.*

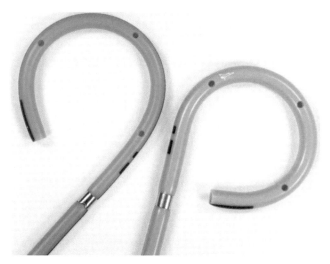

Figure 41.2. *Flexible ends of stents with platinum markers.*

Table 41.1. *Characteristics of new endo-ureteral 'tumour stent'*

Outside diameter	6–8 Fr
Inside diameter	0.98–1.3 mm
Length available	24–32 cm
Material	Combination of polyurethane/ polymide
Max. indwelling time (manufacturer's recommendation)	6 months
Marked as tumour stent	Platinum markers make the special stent immediately obvious as a 'tumour stent' on X-ray

Table 41.2. *Internal diameter of 'tumour-stent' vs the Bard stent*

	Internal diameter (mm)	
Calibre (Fr)	Tumour stent	Bard stent
6	0.98	1.24
7	1.00	1.32
8	1.30	1.60

Table 41.3. *Drainage parameters of 'tumour-stent'*

External diameter, tumour stent (Fr)	Renal pelvic drainage (ml) (physiological expectation > 20 ml) tested parameters	Drainage time (min)
6	40	1.50
7	40	1.39
8	40	1.16

required. The high internal stability of the body results in a high degree of pressure resistance (Table 41.4).

From April 1995 to October 1996, in 29 patients suffering from retroperitoneal metastatic masses or pelvic tumour progression, in one patient with distal ureteral stenosis due to tuberculosis and in two patients with retroperitoneal fibrosis, 42 'tumour stents' were placed at the Department of Urology and Paediatric Urology at Fulda Medical School, University of Marburg, Fulda, Germany. The 29 tumour patients included 17 in whom the urinary diversion was changed from nephrostomies to internal stenting with 'tumour stents', because conventional endo-ureteral stents had

Table 41.4. *Maximum resistance of 'tumour-stent' against external pressure*

Tumour stent (external diameter; Fr)	Maximum resistance against extrinsic pressure (N)
6	30
7	50
8	70

provided insufficient urine drainage. No intra-operative problems were encountered.

In the short term (0–3 months) the 'tumour stents' had to be removed because of obstruction in the one patient suffering from tuberculosis, who developed bilateral pyonephrosis. The urinary diversion had to be changed to nephrostomies, which in turn had to be changed eight times owing to recurrent obstruction; the patient died 6 months after the initial treatment.

In the long term (more than 3 months), four tumour stents had to be replaced owing to external encrustation, but none of those patients had a recurrence of hydronephrosis, which showed that the internal (stent) drainage was adequate. Tumour-induced compression of the stent or a higher rate of encrustation than that normally encountered with Double-J stents were not noted.

The average indwelling time was 7 (range 1–15) months. All patients tolerated these stents well, and none required an alternative palliative urinary diversion. A survey of 18 patients (of 22 patients still living), including those who previously had carried nephrostomies, indicated a clear improvement of their quality of life after insertion of the tumour stent. Five patients suffered from slight urgency incontinence after insertion of the tumour stent, which could be treated conservatively by medication in three cases; none suffered from severe incontinence.

Summary and discussion

Frequently, urologists are called upon to perform palliative urinary diversions in patients with advanced cancer. Pressure to perform such a diversion may be exerted by the patient himself or his family. Physicians, chemotherapists or radiotherapists often try to gain additional time for adjuvant therapies to be used. However, often following palliative urinary diversion the patients have a downhill course and die weeks or months later without, or shortly after, leaving hospital. Unfortunately, the fate of such patients has received little attention in the literature. In Grabstald and McPhee's, series in 1973, reviewing the survival of 170 cancer patients undergoing nephrostomy, 43% did not leave hospital after the procedure and 70% of the procedures performed to relieve ureteral obstruction resulted in a poorer survival rate than those performed for other indications. These and other data show the poor length of survival and quality of life after urinary diversion for ureteral obstruction. The occurrence of severe ureteral obstruction, with some exceptions, therefore appears to be a sign of an extremely late stage of the malignant disease. The difficult decision in cancer patients, whether to stent, may perhaps depend on the estimated rate of survival, in that further treatment may be more feasible in patients with a better prognosis than in those with cancer diseases in which the survival rate is known to be poor.

In Bordinazzo's series,[11] reviewing the outcome of 28 patients with prostate cancer and associated ureteral obstruction, and who had undergone percutaneous nephrostomy, the overall survival rate was 60% at one year and 32% at 2 years. Those patients previously receiving hormonal treatment prior to nephrostomy had a poor survival rate of 46% at 1 year and only 17% at 2 years. However, of ten patients with severe renal failure (serum creatinine > 7 mg%), eight achieved an adequate return of renal function (serum creatinine < 3 mg%) and 55% survived more than 1 year.[11]

In a study by Paul et al.,[12] of upper urinary tract decompression in patients with prostate cancer and with renal failure due to ureteral compression, those patients with hormonal therapy after decompression had a mean survival rate of 646 days. Among these patients, decompression improved survival and reduced the amount of time that they spent in hospital. In those patients undergoing androgen depletion before decompression, survival was very poor (80 days). In all patients, percutaneous nephrostomy was the commonest method of palliative urinary diversion.[12]

In a study by Lee,[13] of patients with ureteral obstruction due to advanced cervical cancer, no significant difference in survival rates could be noted between those patients with unilateral or bilateral ureteral obstruction and those without obstruction.

In a review of patients with advanced squamous cell cancer of the cervix, in a retrospective analysis (1970–1985), all patients with renal failure died within 16 months; the mean survival of patients undergoing percutaneous nephrostomy was 8 months and 66% died of the disease within 1 year.[14] In the age of better oncological and/or radiotherapeutic options these circumstances may have changed, and possibly the survival rates may have improved. However the fact remains that currently about 40% of patients suffering from advanced tumour disease and who undergo a palliative urinary diversion for ureteral obstruction, die within 6 months.[15]

Regarding the benefit to the patient with respect to quality of life, even if adjuvant procedures with major effects may have altered the rate of mortality and length of life, they have to be extremely beneficial to be preferred to palliative urinary diversion. The difficulties in selection of patients with advanced tumour disease for intervention remain and only few guidelines exist. Thus, the urologist's responsibility lies in deciding whether a palliative urinary diversion may be helpful and what kind of diversion should be selected. In most of the investigations discussed above — and in most of those that have not been referred to percutaneous nephrostomy has been chosen as the initial or long-term means of palliative upper urinary tract diversion, which may thoroughly compromise the quality of life of the patients.

As previously stated, since their introduction double-J ureteral catheters have become the preferred long-term option because of their relative ease of insertion, but they do not guarantee adequate drainage of urine in the presence of extrinsic ureteral obstruction. The disadvantage of highly flexible endo-ureteral stents (Double-J) in cases of tumour-induced extrinsic compression of the ureter is insufficient radial stability of the stents, leading to stent compression and subsequent hydro- or pyonephrosis. The failure rate with the commonly used perforated silicone stents or polyurethane stents with side-ports has been described as about 40%. In the series described here, using the newly developed 'tumour stent', the overall complication rate was 14%, comprising stent

obstruction in a patient with tuberculosis, and external stent encrustation; however, recurrent hydronephrosis occurred only in the patient with distal ureteral stenosis due to tuberculosis. No serious complications were noted during stent placement or while it was in situ. All patients tolerated the stent well; some suffered from mild urgency, which could be treated conservatively.

In conclusion, the new stabilized endo-ureteral stent can be seen as a better solution than percutaneous nephrostomy or frequent stent changing in patients with tumour-induced extrinsic ureteral compression, and one which leads to a better quality of life in patients with cancer.

References

1. Megibow A J, Mitnick J S, Bosniak M A. The contribution of computed tomography to the evaluation of the obstructed ureter. Urol Radiol 1982; 4: 95
2. Thomas M H, Chisholm G D. Retroperitoneal fibrosis associated with malignant disease. Br J Cancer 1973; 28: 453
3. Kuhn W, Loos W, Graeff H. Hydronephrosis as the first manifestation of primary metastatic breast cancer. Geburtshilfe Frauenheilk 1994; 54(5): 308–310
4. Abrams H C, Spiro R, Goldstein N. Metastases in carcinoma; analysis of 1000 autopsied cases. Cancer 1950; 3: 75
5. Kaufman R, Grabstald H. Hydronephrosis secondary to ureteral obstruction by metastatic breast cancer. J Urol 1969; 102: 569
6. Brin E, Schiff M, Weiss R. Palliative urinary diversion for pelvic malignancy. J Urol 1975; 113: 619–622
7. Lingam K, Paterson P J, Lingman M K et al. Subcutaneous urinary diversion: an alternative to percutaneous nephrostomy. J Urol 1994; 152(1): 70–72
8. Resnick M I, Kursh E D. Extrinsic obstruction of the ureter. In: Walsh P C, Retik A B, Stamey T A, Vaughn E D Jr (eds) Campbell's Urology, 6th edn. Philadelphia: Saunders, 1992: 533–569
9. Docimo S G, DeWolf W. High failure rate of indwelling ureteral stents in patients with extrinsic obstruction: experiences at 2 institutions. J Urol 1989; 142: 277–279
10. Khori K, Yamate T, Amasaki N et al. Characteristics and usage of different ureteral stent catheters. Urol Int 1991; 47(3): 131–137
11. Bordinazzo R, Benecchi L, Cazzaniga A et al. Ureteral obstruction associated with prostate cancer: the outcome after ultrasonographic percutaneous nephrostomy. Arch Ital Urol Nefrol Androl 1994; 66(4 suppl): 101–106
12. Paul A B, Love C, Chisholm G D. The management of bilateral ureteric obstruction and renal failure in advanced prostate cancer. Br J Urol 1994; 74(5): 642–645
13. Lee S K, Jones H W III. Prognostic significance of ureteral compression in primary cervical cancer. Int J Gynaecol Obstet 1994; 44(1): 59–65
14. Hopkins M P, Morley G W. Prognostic factors in advanced squamous cell cancer of the cervix. Cancer 1993; 72(8): 2389–2393
15. Esk P C, Seidl E, Schindler E. Durchzugsnephrostomie — Indikation und Bedeutung für die Lebensqualität des Patienten. Therapiewoche 1983; 3: 23–26

42

Double-pigtail stent with radiopaque adjustable collar
A. G. Martov, S. S. Zenkov and Y. G. Andreev

Introduction

Significant advances and growing experience in urologic endoscopic procedures, together with progress in balloon catheter technology (Acucise™), have generated clinical data in reported series in which percutaneous (antegrade) and transurethral (retrograde) endo-ureteropyelotomy have been utilized for the management of ureteropelvic junction (UPJ) and ureteral obstruction.[1–8] Although the efficacy, reproducibility, and overall decreased morbidity of endo-urological procedures have been clearly demonstrated, several issues are still debated, one of which is the optimal type of stenting after endo-ureteropyelotomy.

The introduction of the tapered 14/7 Fr and 10/5 Fr internal endopyelotomy stent (Retromax endo-pyelotomy stent, Microvasive, Watertown, MA, USA) and 14/7 Fr and 10/6 Fr endo-ureterotomy stent with a wide proximal segment (Endoureterotomy stent, Cook Urological, Spencer, IN, USA) has been a substantial technical achievement. This type of stent promotes tissue regeneration around its widest segment at the UPJ and, because of its gradually tapered shape and small distal end diameter, diminishes bladder discomfort. These stents are ideal for retrograde[3,8] and also for antegrade endopyelotomy. However, some controversial questions concerning their application after endo-ureterotomy in the middle and distal part of the ureter (reverse-fashion stent placement) have arisen.

In this chapter, the authors describe their experience with a novel double-pigtail stent with a adjustable collar (MIT Ltd, Zheleznodorozny, Moscow, Russia) used for temporary internal drainage following retrograde endo-ureteropyelotomy. This stent is suitable for postoperative drainage in all cases of stricture at any location along the ureter, including the UPJ. The novel construction of the stent makes it possible to place and fix the sheath at any location along the stent.

Materials and methods

Description and characteristics of the stent

The double-pigtail stent with an adjustable collar is manufactured from radiopaque polyethylene with some materials added to improve its sliding ability and diminish salt encrustation on the stent. The stent diameter is 6 and 7 Fr, and its length varies from 12 to 30 cm. The adjustable radiopaque silicone collars are available in diameters of 12, 14 and 16 Fr and in lengths of 6 and 8 cm (Fig. 42.1).

The stent set consists of (a) an open-ended double-pigtail stent with a adjustable collar, (b) a stent positioner, (c) an open-ended 6 Fr ureteral catheter and (d) a super-stiff guidewire 145 cm long and 0.038 inch in diameter with 3 cm flexible tip. The stent is stiff enough to permit its advancement over the guidewire, even when force is required to pass through scarred tissue at the ureter or UPJ targeted for incision. Lateral flexibility of the stent is helpful during its placement in tortuous ureters. The stent has drainage side-holes located every 1.5 cm along its length. A strip marked in centimetres is printed along the side of the stent for visualization during endoscopic passage.

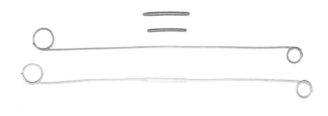

Figure 42.1. *Double-pigtail stent with adjustable collar.*

Coil strength of the stent has been evaluated according to the American Society for Testing and Materials (ASTM method D-1894, modified). The force (g) required to uncoil the proximal pigtail of a 6 Fr stent was 69 g, and that for a distal pigtail was 60 g; the force for a proximal pigtail of 7 Fr was 76 g and for a distal pigtail was 65 g.

Drainage efficiency was evaluated according to the experiments of Mardis et al.[9] At a pressure of 5 cmH$_2$O in the presence of a simulated mid-ureteral block (where the sleeve was located), the flow rate was 2.8 ml/s for a 6 Fr stent and 3.1 ml/s for a 7 Fr stent.

Biocompatibility was evaluated in three adult dogs (6 ureters). Specially designed 5 Fr polyethylene double-pigtail stents with silicone sheaths (9 Fr) 3 cm long (located in the middle of the stent in two ureters tested, near the distal coil in two and near the proximal coil in two) were placed retrogradely through an open transvesical approach using a small J-tipped super-stiff guidewire. Animals underwent urography at 6 weeks and then were killed. Mild hydronephrosis was noted in four instances, and was not related to the sheath localization. Mild epithelial erosion, hyperplasia, inflammatory infiltration and oedema of the lamina propria was noted in nine of 12 ureter specimens. These changes were detected both in the areas where the sheath contacted the ureteral wall and at the areas where the stent itself was adjacent to the mucosa. There were no cases of pyelonephritis and no renal pathological alterations were recorded.

Stent preparation

Stent preparation took place in the following steps:

1. To determine the correct stent length, the distance between the renal pelvis and the urinary bladder (ureteric orifice projection) was measured radiologically (the stent length is the distance between the proximal and the distal base of the pigtail).
2. The distance from the renal pelvis to the stricture and from the stricture to the urinary bladder (ureteric orifice projection), as well as the stricture length, were also estimated radiologically; this indicates the appropriate place for sheath placement.
3. With the stent held in one hand, the sheath is gently slid to the desired place with two fingers of the other hand, carefully pressing the sheath end nearest to the handling hand (Fig. 42.2).
4. Complete sheath fixation on the stent is achieved by pressing the sheath between the thumb and index finger of both hands, from its middle part towards the stent end (Fig. 42.3).
5. If the sheath is shifted on the stent, steps 3 and 4 are repeated. During positioning and fixation of the sleeve, forceful movements should be avoided, because they may damage the stent.

Patients

Over a 4-year period, 31 patients (19 male, 12 female, age range 4–70 years) with UPJ stricture (19 cases) and ureteral stricture (12 cases) were treated by retrograde endoureteropyelotomy. The stricture lengths varied from 0.4–2.7 cm. In 17 patients, obstruction was primary (15 UPJ, two ureter), and 14 patients had a

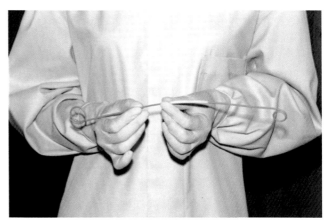

Figure 42.2. *Moving the sheath.*

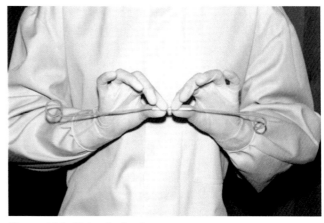

Figure 42.3. *Fixing the sheath.*

history of open urological, surgical and gynaecological operations. Over this period, nine further patients (six male, three female, age range 22–57 years) were treated with retrograde endopyelotomy (two patients) and endo-ureterotomy (seven patients) with simultaneous antegrade roentgen-endoscopic interventions because of impassable ureteral and UPJ obliteration. The length of the obliterated UPJ segment ranged from 0.3 to 1.7 cm. In five cases, obliteration followed various urological operations and in four cases it was a consequence of surgical or gynaecological intervention. All 40 patients had double-pigtail stents with adjustable collar inserted after endo-ureteropyelotomy.

Technique

With the patient in the lithotomy position under epidural anaesthesia, a small-calibre (7–8 Fr) Wolf or Storz rigid ureterorenoscope was used for the initial transurethral ureteropyeloscopy and endoscopic stricture evaluation. A super-stiff guidewire (0.038 inch, 145 cm long) was inserted into the working channel of the ureterorenoscope and passed through the stenotic segment under direct vision (Fig. 42.4). The ureterorenoscope was removed from the ureter leaving the guidewire in place, and then inserted again along the guidewire and advanced up to the stricture. An specially designed 3.5 Fr straight cold knife (MIT Ltd) was inserted into the working channel of the endoscope and the full thickness of the ureteral wall at the stricture level was completely incised (Fig. 42.5). The posterolateral or lateral wall was incised in the cases of the proximal ureteral and UPJ strictures. In the patients who had strictures localized in the distal and middle ureter, the incision was made at the anteriomedial section of the ureteral wall. In some cases, for retrograde endo-ureteropyelotomy a 3 Fr electrocautery cutting element was used through a small-calibre ureterorenoscope, and endoscissors and different cold knives were used through a regular 11.5 Fr Storz ureterorenoscope and 12 Fr Storz ureteroresectoscope. After the periureteral fatty tissue had been visualized through the incised ureteral wall, the ureterorenoscope was removed. The stricture area was dilated to approximately 16–20 Fr, using a standard balloon dilator (ureteral dilator set), which was passed over the super-stiff guidewire. Finally, the ureter was stented with a 6/12 (7/14) Fr double-pigtail stent equipped with

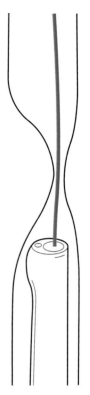

Figure 42.4. *Retrograde passage of the guidewire through the stricture.*

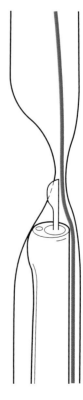

Figure 42.5. *Ureteroscopic cold-knife ureterotomy.*

adjustable collar (which was fixed beforehand at the estimated place of the incision). The stent was removed after 6 or more weeks.

In ureteral and UPJ obliterations that could not be negotiated by the guidewire before or at the beginning of the procedure, the approach was as follows (Figs. 42.6–42.11):

1. An angiographic catheter and guidewire or flexible ureteroscope (nephroscope) was antegradely introduced down to the stricture level for guiding the cold knife in the right direction (with simultaneous fluoroscopic control).
2. The obliteration was cut endoscopically through a retrograde approach with a small-caliber rigid ureterorenoscope (miniscope) and an originally designed 3.5 Fr cold knife.
3. A 0.038 inch super-stiff guidewire 145 cm long with 3 cm flexible tip was introduced into the renal pelvis through the miniscope after ureter (UPJ) recanalization.
4. Retrogradely inserted ureter dilators (balloon catheter, ureterorenoscope) were used to dilate further the treated area.
5. A double-pigtail stent with adjustable collar (6/12 or 7/14 Fr) was placed for at least 6 weeks.

Results

The average procedure time of the retrograde endo-ureteropyelotomy was 49 min. Clinical, radiological and functional success was achieved in 26 (84%) of the 31 patients (follow-up 6–48 months). One patient underwent nephrectromy for acute bleeding 30 days postoperatively; this was the only patient who received blood transfusions. One patient underwent ureteroneocystostomy for recurrent obstruction. In another three patients, who were asymptomatic, no evidence of positive radiological and functional changes were observed.

The 6/12 Fr stent was left indwelling for 6 weeks in nine patients, for 9 weeks in four and for 12 weeks in two patients. The 7/14 Fr stent was left indwelling for 6 weeks in 11 patients and for 9 weeks in five. No difficulties with stent insertion or removal were encountered in this group of patients.

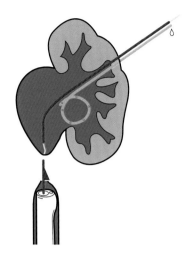

Figure 42.6. *Endoscopic endopyelotomy through a retrograde approach is guided by an angiographic catheter and guidewire antegradely introduced down to the stricture level.*

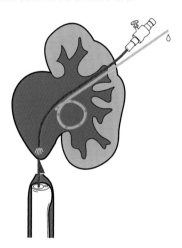

Figure 42.7. *Endoscopic endopyelotomy through a retrograde approach is guided by a flexible ureteroscope (nephroscope) antegradely introduced down to the stricture level.*

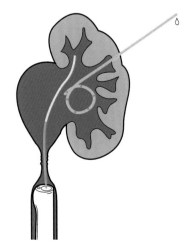

Figure 42.8. *Super-stiff guidewire with a flexible tip is introduced into the renal pelvis through a ureteropyeloscope after ureter/UPJ recanalization.*

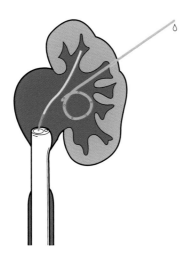

Figure 42.9. *Miniscope is advanced into the renal pelvis over the super-stiff guidewire after ureter/UPJ recanalization.*

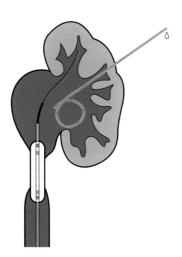

Figure 42.10. *Retrogradely inserted balloon catheter is used for further dilatation of the treated area.*

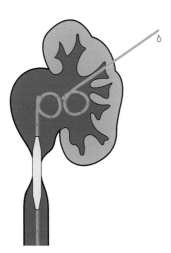

Figure 42.11. *Double-pigtail stent is placed with adjustable collar at the UPJ level.*

The average operative time of combined retrograde endo-ureteropyelotomy with antegrade intervention for the impassable obliterations was 72 min. Clinical, radiological and functional success was achieved in 8 (89%) of nine patients (follow-up 6–36 months). Figures 42.12–42.16 illustrate the clinical cases in such a patient, who underwent successful retrograde endopyelotomy of the obliterative UPJ. One patient had recurrent ureteral stricture and secondary endo-ureterotomy was performed successfully. In another patient, who developed recurrent ureteral obliteration, a ureteroneocystostomy was performed. Four (44%) of nine stents were considered difficult to insert and one (11%) was difficult to remove in this group of patients.

The 6/12 Fr stent was left indwelling for 6 weeks in three patients and for 9 weeks in two patients. The 7/12 Fr stent was left indwelling for 6 weeks in two patients, for 9 weeks in one patient, and for 12 weeks in one patient.

The incidence of symptoms related to the use of a double-pigtail stent with adjustable collar was evaluated in a total of 31 patients while the stent was in situ. Haematuria was noted in 15 (48%) patients, urinary frequency in 20 (65%), urgency in 16 (52%) and dysuria in 10 (32%) patients. Nine (29%) patients had renal and 14 (45%) suprapubic pain. There were two (6%) cases of distal stent migration with successful stent replacement.

No problem was encountered that could be attributed to the adjustable collar; all sheaths remained located in the places where they had been fixed before the insertion. No deterioration, spontaneous breakage or gross encrustation of the stents was noted. Polyethylene stents remained flexible, with a patent lumen in all patients during the indwelling time.

Discussion

Davis[10] popularized intubated ureterotomy in 1943, when he reported the open incision of strictures followed by splinting with a tube to guide the growth of the incised ureter around the tube. Davis et al.[11] believed that incision of the ureter followed by the placement of the ureteral splint promoted regeneration of, first, the mucosa and then of the muscular layer of the ureteral wall. Oppenheimer and Hinman[12] showed that smooth muscle regeneration was largely responsible for the re-establishment of the muscle layer during the

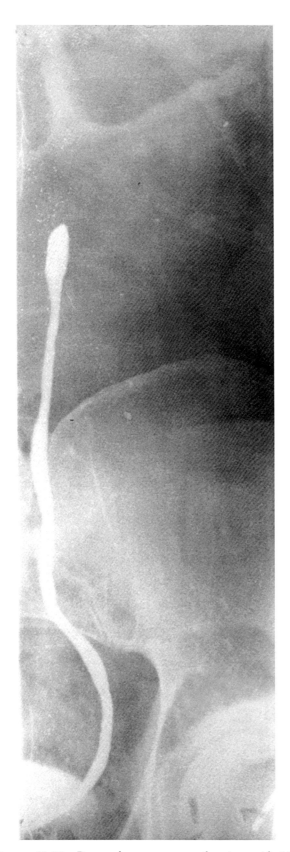

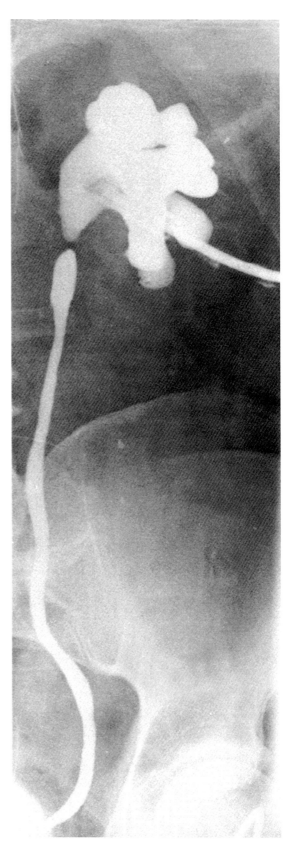

Figure 42.12. *Retrograde ureterogram of patient with UPJ obliteration.*

Figure 42.13. *Combined retrograde and antegrade pyelography demonstrating UPJ obliteration.*

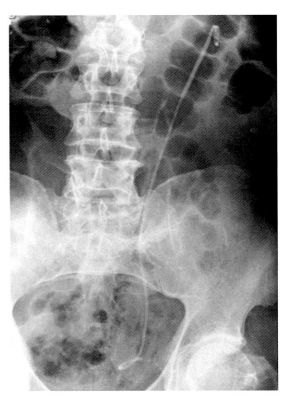

Figure 42.14. *Double-pigtail stent in place after retrograde UPJ recanalization.*

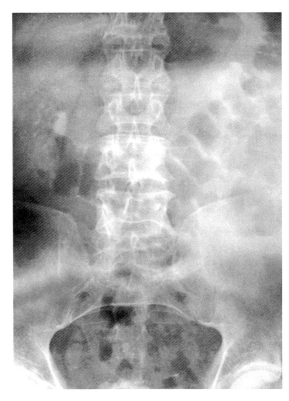

Figure 42.16. *IVP 2 years after retrograde endopyelotomy.*

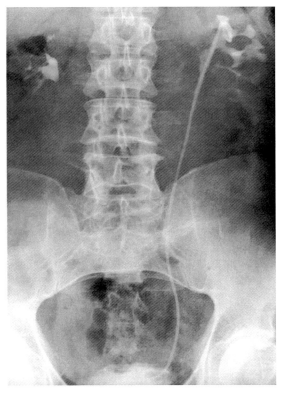

Figure 42.15. *Intravenous pyelogram (IVP) with double-pigtail stent and removable sleeve positioned at the UPJ level.*

healing process. In 1983, Wickham and Kellet[1] described the percutaneous version of this technique and, in 1986, Inglis and Tolley[2] described retrograde endopyelotomy. On the basis of this pioneering work, it is recommended that the indwelling stent is left in place for 6 weeks postoperatively because, after endoureteropyelotomy, the urothelium appeared to cover the incision site within 7 days, whereas muscle regeneration required longer (from 6 to 12 weeks).

Despite the widespread popularity of antegrade and retrograde endo-ureteropyelotomy, many aspects of this procedure remain controversial. Placement of a splinting tube is a vital component of the operation; however, there are many questions concerning such factors as the size, composition and construction of the stent. In the authors' opinion, an internal stent with a wide proximal segment is ideal for endoureteropyelotomy, and we recommend the double-pigtail stent, with a adjustable collar (6/12 Fr or 7/14 Fr) of radiopaque polyethylene, after retrograde endoureteropyelotomy.

Conclusions

Ease of insertion with low friction, a high flow rate with adaptable sheath localization for stricture splinting, plus a high rate of patient tolerance and efficacy, enable the double-pigtail polyethylene stent with a removable silicone sheath to be strongly recommended as a reliable and essential device for use after retrograde endo-ureteropyelotomy.

References

1. Wickham J E A , Kellet M J. Percutaneous pyelolysis. Eur Urol 1983; 9: 122–124
2. Inglis J A, Tolley D A. Ureteroscopic pyelolysis for pelvic ureteric junction obstruction. Br J Urol 1986; 58: 250
3. Clayman R V, Picus D D. Ureterorenoscopic endopyelotomy. Urol Clin North Am 1988; 15: 433–438
4. Van Congh P J, Jorion J L, Reese S X, Opsomer R J. Endoureteropyelotomy: percutaneous treatment of uretero-pelvic junction obstruction. J Urol 1989; 141: 1317
5. Motola J A, Badlani G H, Smith A D. Results of 212 consecutive endopyelotomies: an eight year follow-up. J Urol 1993; 149: 453
6. Eshghi M, Lifson B. Cold knife endoureterotomy. In: Smith A D (ed) Controversies in endourology. Philadelphia: Saunders, 1995: 302–309
7. Nakada S Y, Pearle M S, Clayman R V. Acucise endopyelotomy: evolution of a less-invasive technology. J Endourol 1996; 10(2): 133–139
8. Thomas R, Manga M, Klein E W. Ureteroscopic retrograde endopyelotomy for management of ureteropelvic junction obstruction. J Endourol 1996; 10(2): 141–145
9. Mardis H K, Kroeger R M, Hepperlen T W et al. Polyethylene double-pigtail ureteral stents. Urol Clin North Am 1982; 9(1): 95–101
10. Davis D M. Intubated ureterotomy: a new operation for ureteral and ureteropelvic stricture. Surg Gynecol Obstet 1943; 76: 513
11. Davis D M, Strong G H, Drake W M. Intubated ureterotomy: experimental work and clinical results. J Urol 1948; 59: 85
12. Oppenheimer R, Hinman F. Ureteral regeneration: contracture versus hyperplasia of smooth muscle. J Urol 1955; 74: 476

43

Use of self-expanding metal stents in ureteral obstruction due to malignant pelvic disease

E. F. Diaz-Lucas and J. L. Martinez-Torres

Introduction

The technique of ureteral stenting has been widely applied for many years to obtain adequate drainage of the obstructed upper urinary tract. Initially, the devices used consisted of single tubes of plastic material such as polyethylene, silicone or polyurethane, which underwent several modifications in their structure and composition in order to improve their stability and patency as well as to minimize urothelial damage.

Previously, these stents were placed during open surgery. Advances in endo-urological techniques allowed the retrograde insertion of ureteral stents through a cystoscope,[1] even with the aid of the Seldinger technique. Following the initial description of percutaneous nephrostomy by Goodwin and colleagues in 1955,[2] more than 15 years had to elapse before its value became recognized. Currently, this constitutes a way to approach the urinary tract in an antegrade manner for several purposes, including placement of stents.[3]

In the last few years, the development of metal stents has opened new perspectives for restoring the patency of any body conduit. These devices are metallic tubular structures, more or less flexible, with different-shaped walls (depending on the type), having a radial force higher than the pressure exerted by the surrounding tissues. Initially designed for arterial use, they are now used in the biliary tract, venous system, tracheobronchial tree, oesophagus, large bowel and urinary tract. The aim of this chapter is to report the authors' experience in the management of malignant ureteral obstruction by means of metal stents, as well as to highlight several features arising from the use of these devices in such particular indications.

Clinical considerations

A ureteral obstruction may occur in the course of several malignancies, either by direct infiltration of the ureter by the tumour (which may be a primary tumour of the urinary tract or from other nearby structures of the pelvis), or by extrinsic compression of enlarged retroperitoneal lymph nodes or masses, or by a combination of both mechanisms. A fourth situation can be iatrogenic as a result of development of fibrotic stenotic occlusion after transurethral resection (TUR) of bladder tumours or the prostate; or after ureterovesical or uretero-enteric anastomoses; or after iatrogenic accidents during major surgery for pelvic malignancy.

Theoretically, the ureteral blockage can be predicted because it is preceded by progressive impairment of renal function and by an increase in the degree of dilatation of the upper urinary tract detected by sonography, computed tomography (CT) or intravenous pyelography (IVP). In the management of this complication, surgical urinary diversion has been replaced by endo-urological procedures because of their low rate of complications and easier performance.[4] Several techniques have been used to provide adequate drainage of the upper urinary tract.

In the authors' opinion, percutaneous nephrostomy achieves drainage more rapidly (the authors' average time is 7–15 min), is performed under local anaesthesia and causes less discomfort to the patient. Nevertheless, this is an invasive procedure; in addition, the patient has to carry one or two drainage bags for long periods, thus impairing his quality of life.[5] Furthermore, the nephrostomy catheter needs changing periodically. There is also the possibility of accidental traction of the catheter, causing its dislocation.

Another option is the insertion of a plastic endoprosthesis. This can be carried out by either a retrograde or an antegrade approach. The retrograde approach, which is performed through a cystoscope, is uncomfortable for the patient unless it is performed under regional or general anaesthesia. Moreover, ureteral catheterization with this method can be difficult in the presence of a fistula or stricture,[6] and more difficult if this stricture becomes completely occluded or if intravesical masses hide the ureteral meatus. In these cases the percutaneous transrenal antegrade approach seems to have a higher rate of success, especially if complete occlusion or fistula exits,[7,8] or when attempted retrograde catheterization fails. This could be explained by the fact that the ureter, a long and relatively narrow conduit, constitutes a better support for the manipulation and torque control of the guidewire and the catheter, rather than the wide space offered by the vesical cavity. This is similar to what happens in the biliary tree.

Plastic stents may become obstructed after short periods because of encrustations,[5] debris or extrinsic compression by the tumour,[9] or because of tumour growth through the side-ports into the lumen. These conditions necessitate stent replacement at least every 6 months but in many cases this replacement is impossible.

Balloon dilatation is another alternative in the management of malignant or anastomotic strictures. The toughness or great elasticity (recoil) of the strictures is the cause of the immediate poor response after dilatation, or a high rate of late recurrence (up to 70% after 6 months).

Metal stents appear to possess some features that make them more attractive than the preceding plastic devices. One of these features is the easy placement of such stents in a single step; another is the fact that the delivery catheter of metal stents has a calibre similar to or smaller than that of conventional plastic stents, but delivers an endoprosthesis much larger in diameter, making them more useful. The self-expandable character of some types of the metal stents is important in cases of elastic lesions.

Materials and methods

Between April 1992 and August 1996, the authors reconstructed 12 ureters by implanting a total of 16 Wallstent® endoprostheses (Schneider, Bülach, Switzerland) (Fig. 43.1). To date, their experience has been limited to the antegrade approach.

The criteria for the selection of the patients were as follows:

1. Estimated survival of at least 6 months;
2. Progressive impairment of renal function assessed by increasing serum levels of creatinine and urea;

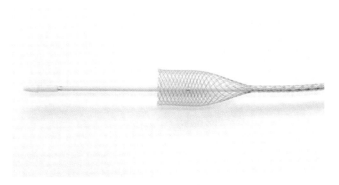

Figure 43.1. *Self-expanding Wallstent® endoprosthesis. The stent reaches its maximum diameter as the plastic cover (rolling membrane) is removed. Simultaneously, a shortening in length takes place.*

3. Presence of obstructive uropathy diagnosed by sonography, CT or IVP;
4. Acceptable urine quality and volume evaluated by progressive monitoring of selective samples obtained from the nephrostomy catheter or improvement of the parameters of renal function after drainage.

The initial number of candidates for metallic stent insertion was 12 (20 ureters), ranging in age from 40 to 76 (average 60.8) years; four were female and eight male. The primary malignant diseases affecting the patients were prostatic adenocarcinoma (three), transitional cell carcinoma of the bladder (five), uterine carcinoma (three) and ovarian cystic carcinoma (one). Each patient had previously undergone surgery. The period from the diagnosis of the disease to the development of the obstructive uropathy was between 1 month and 9.2 years (average 26.4 months).

All patients underwent unilateral or bilateral nephrostomy after an unsuccessful attempt at retrograde ureteral catheterization.

One patient (two ureters) was withdrawn from being a candidate after no improvement was observed in urine quality and volume or in the serum parameters of renal function.

Among the 18 ureters considered for stenting, 12 were completely obstructed, four presented tortuous stenosis and two had a wide extrinsic compression (Fig. 43.2). In all cases, the terminal segment of the ureters was affected, 16 at the ureterovesical junction and two (one patients) at the uretero-ileal anastomosis (Fig. 43.3).

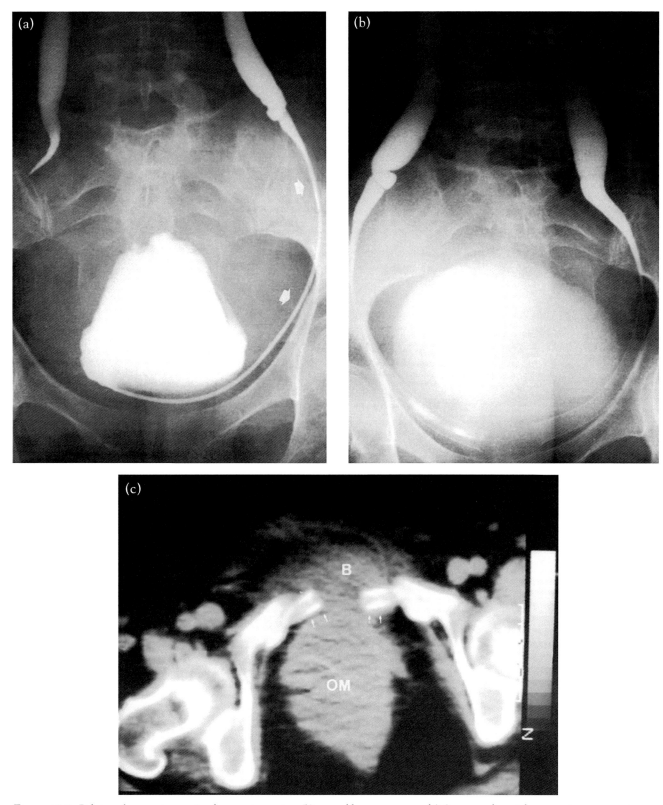

Figure 43.2. *Relapse of an ovarian cystic adenocarcinoma in a 58-year-old woman, resected 9.2 years earlier. A large ovarian mass compresses and obstructs both ureters. (a) Bilateral nephrostogram performed during the antegrade catheterization. The left ureteral obstruction has been initially passed by means of a 5 Fr Cobra; note its lateral displacement (arrows). (b) Bilateral nephrostogram performed 1 month after the implant of two 8 x 150 mm Wallstents, for the assessment of their patency in order to retrieve the nephrostomy catheters. Note the complete expansion of the stents. (c) CT scan obtained 18 months after stent implantation, showing the distal end of the stents in the bladder (B) and their relation to the caudal portion of the ovarian mass (OM). Loss of delimitation between these two structures, due to neoplastic infiltration, is also patent.*

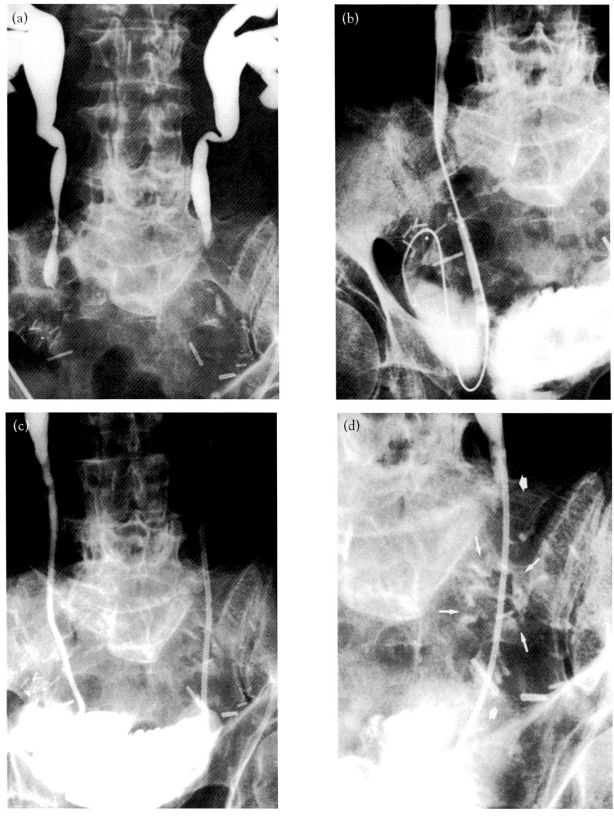

Figure 43.3. *Patient with ureteroileal anastomosis (Camey type II) and bilateral ureteral obstruction. (a) Initial IVP. (b) Placement of the right drainage catheter (8 Fr) necessitated previous dilatation with a 4 mm balloon. (c) X-ray with the internal–external catheters in place. Note urine drainage toward the ileal loop. (d) Irregular extravasation of contrast medium (thin arrows) around the middle portion of the infiltrated segment of the left ureter. The broad arrows indicate the extent of infiltration.*

Obviously the first step for stenting after nephrostomy was to negotiate the passage across the ureteral stricture or occlusion. This was performed at the time of nephrostomy in those cases where the condition of the patient permitted it. The time lag between the nephrostomy and the attempted antegrade ureteral catheterization enabled the percutaneous entry tract to mature and also the degree of dilatation and kinking of the ureter to diminish (Fig. 43.4a,b), which facilitated the manipulation.

Initially, the material employed to access the bladder was a SF-Cobra 2 Super-Torque® catheter (Cordis) and a 0.035-inch Standard or Stiff Micro-glide® steerable guide (Terumo) (Fig. 43.2a). In three patients (three ureters), in whom the lesion was very tight, the 5 Fr catheter could not be advanced through the obstruction after the guide was successfully placed in the bladder. The problem was solved by exchanging the 5 Fr catheter with a 4 Fr catheter of the same type; if this failed, the vesical end of the guidewire was extracted via the urethra by means of a snare. By tensing both ends of the guidewire, passage of the catheter could be accomplished. Occasionally, the authors have used this method for the insertion of plastic stents. The initial success rate in the antegrade catheterization was 15/18 ureters (83.3%); the three failures corresponded to completely obstructed ureters. In one of these cases — a patient with transitional cell carcinoma (TCC) — two successive attempts of bilateral ureteral catheterization had been unsuccessful because of the rigidity of the obstruction, probably due to the fibrotic component after transurethral resections (TUR). In the other patient, also with TCC, after antegrade catheterization failed, this became possible one week after a TUR. The definitive success rate in the antegrade catheterization, thus, was 16/18 ureters (888%).

After the tip of the 5 or 4 Fr catheter entered the bladder, a 0.035-inch guidewire of greater stiffness — the Rosen (Cook Europe, Bjaeverskov, Denmark) or the Amplatz Super-Stiff (Boston Scientific Corp., Watertown, Massachusetts, USA), which is coiled distally — was inserted. These guides are a good support for the introduction of an 8 Fr internal–external drainage catheter. Earlier, the authors used a Mueller biliary (Cook) and a customized Günter's pig-tail catheter (Cook); they are now using the biliary Temp-Tip catheter (Boston Scientific) (Fig. 43.5). This type of catheter seems to present some advantages with respect to the previous ones; its good rigidity during insertion is due to a plastic inner cannula that is subsequently retrieved, leaving a large lumen within the catheter; its tip dissolves after a few minutes of contact with urine, leaving an open end with an inner calibre of diameter equal to that of the catheter. In two patients (two ureters), the stricture needed dilatation with a 4 mm balloon (Fig. 43.3b) before the internal–external catheter could be advanced to the bladder.

This drainage system, with is proximal end closed, was left in place for approximately a week. As shown by the authors' previous experience with plastic stents, the residence in situ of the internal–external catheter for a few days provided a channel within the obstruction, larger than the 7 Fr calibre of the stent device, which enabled the stent to be positioned and delivered without difficulty in 100% of the implants. The presence of the catheter also indicated the tolerance of the ureter to a foreign body and to the distension. In two patients with uterine carcinoma (two more of the 18 ureters) the internal–external catheter was retrieved 2 and 3 days after insertion because of intractable pain in the hypogastrium and bladder. The nephrostograms did not reveal any abnormality to justify this event, apart from the presence of the catheter itself. A nephrostogram may also give warning of possible inadvertent lesions that could cause problems after the implant of a non-covered stent. Thus, in one patient with bladder carcinoma, uretero-ileal anastomosis and pyrexia of several days' duration immediately after bilateral catheterization the control nephrostogram showed a fistulous tract in the middle portion of the infiltrated segment of the left ureter (Fig. 43.3d). CT revealed a pelvic mass surrounding the ureter at this level, with a low-density necrotic centre.

In all the authors' cases, the Wallstent endoprosthesis (Schneider, Bülach, Switzerland) was used. Initially, one Wallstent of appropriate length and diameter was delivered. The diameter of the stent was chosen according to that of the ureter after it has been negotiated. In 12 stented ureters, the diameter of the stents used was as follows: 10 mm (in one larger ureter), 8 mm (in three); 7 mm (in ten); 6 mm (in two). The length of the stent was determined according to the extent of the lesion (Fig. 43.6a); too short a stent could cause the ureter to become L-shaped (Fig. 43.4c).

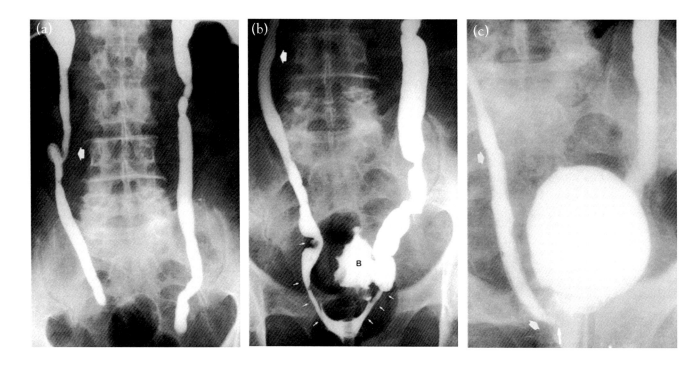

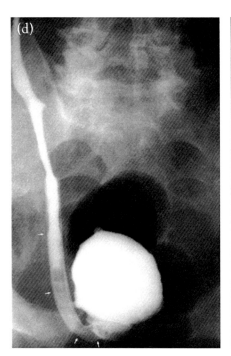

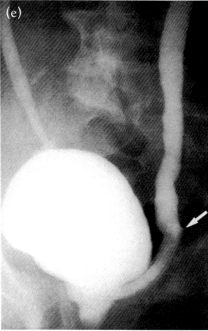

Figure 43.4. A 67-year-old male with a prostatic adenocarcinoma (Stage D2) (diagnosed 4.5 years earlier) causing anuria after 4.5 years of evolution. (a) Bilateral nephrostogram shows complete distal occlusion of the ureters. A ureteral loop is visible on the right side (arrow). (b) Monitoring nephrostogram 1 week after insertion of the 8 Fr internal–external catheters. Note the regression of the kinking in the right ureter (broad arrow) as well as better evaluation of the extent of the infiltrated segments of both ureters (small arrows) after the bladder has been opacified. Bladder (B) compressed by the prostatic growth. (c) After shortening, the right-side stent can be seen to have been deployed too proximally (broad arrows), leaving a residual distal stenotic segment uncovered (thin arrow). (d) X-ray after distal implantation of an additional stent (arrows). (e) Right oblique X-ray obtained one month after stent implantation. A slight tendency to formation of an L-shape can be seen at the proximal end of the stent on the left side (arrow).

Deployment was fluoroscopically controlled, leaving a sufficient length of stent in the bladder, preventing its further shortening. An externally closed 6 Fr nephrostomy (Günther; Cook) was left in the renal pelvis as a safety catheter (smaller in calibre than the initial one).

This catheter is clamped in place for one month approximately until the performance of the stent can be clearly assessed. It also permits further manipulations, such as additional implant, if required. 'Safety catheter' is an appropriate description since it provides

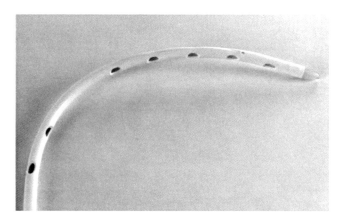

Figure 43.5. *Detail of the distal segment of an 8 Fr Temp-Tip® drainage catheter (Boston Scientific). The catheter is provided with 15 side-holes along its distal 21 cm. The tip, made of polyvinyl alcohol, dissolves after a few minutes of contact with fluids.*

alternative drainage of the urinary pathway if the stent fails during the observation period. This term has been employed by other authors, including van Sonnenberg.

Results and complications

Immediately after each implant, a nephrostogram was performed. This showed patency of the stent in 100% of cases, despite incomplete expansion (Fig. 43.6b). No complications related to the procedure itself were noted. During the days following the implant of the stent, some patients complained of bladder discomfort during micturition: their urine culture was negative. In only one patient, with uterine carcinoma, did the pain become intense; this was attributed to an excessive segment of stent protruding into the bladder.

Approximately 1 month later, the position and permeability of the stents were evaluated by antegrade pyelography through the safety nephrostomy catheter. In no case was displacement observed. The following findings were noteworthy:

1. Stenosis at the proximal end of the stent in five ureters (42%) perhaps caused by ureterospasm, oedema or even urothelial hyperplasia. These stenoses were not urodynamically significant, except in one ureter that needed insertion of an additional stent (Fig. 43.7a–d).

2. One residual proximal segment compressed by lymph nodes and not covered by the stent because of shortening of the stent after its full expansion. The patient in question also showed excessive tissue

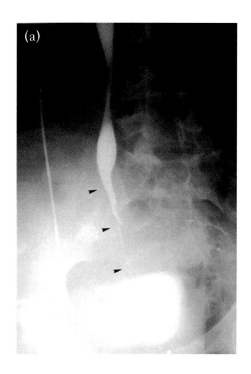

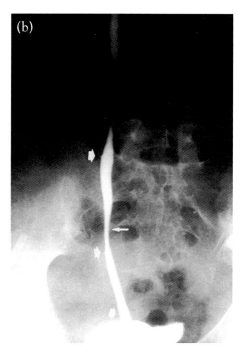

Figure 43.6. *A 40-year-old female with uterine cervical carcinoma detected in Stage IIIa–b, 10 months earlier. Obstructive anuria. The counterlateral nephrostomy was not considered because an atrophic hydronephrotic kidney of long evolution was observed at sonography. (a) Monitoring nephrostogram showing the right ureteral obstruction. The arrowheads mark the proximal extent of the infiltration which reaches 9 cm in length, approximately. (b) Repermeabilization of the ureter after insertion of 2 overlapping 6 and 7 mm stents (broad arrows). Immediately after their deployment, a good flow is obtained despite incomplete expansion of the proximal stent (thin arrow).*

protrusion through the mesh after 3 months, requiring an additional stent implant (patient 7, Fig. 43.8) (Fig. 43.9a–b).

3. In two ureters, owing to a change in posture of the patients during the deployment, in one patient the stent remained lodged too proximal (Fig. 43.4c–d) and in the second too distal to the lesion. Subsequently, an additional stent was inserted into these patients, one more distal to the previous stent in the first patient and another more proximal in the second patient. All patients who required an additional implant presented with urine leakage from the entry tract, around the nephrostomy catheter.

When drainage through the ureter was judged to be adequate the safety nephrostomy catheter was withdrawn.

For all the authors' patients, the follow-up period ranges from 3 months to 4.1 years (average 21.5 months). Follow-up examinations included periodical blood analysis, sonography (ultrasound), urography and occasionally CT. Both sonography and IVP almost always showed a mild degree of dilatation of the upper urinary tract (Fig. 43.7e). This did not necessarily imply malfunctioning of the stent, especially if the serum creatinine and urea values were normal. The presence of the stent at the level of the ureterovesical junction causes reflux from the bladder, especially when the patient is in the decubitus position; this reflux could be demonstrated during the performance of control antegrade pyelography after implanting a contralateral stent (Fig. 43.7d). External sonographic study of the stent to assess its permeability has not been conclusive, in most cases, because of interference by intestinal gas: only the segment closest to the bladder could be visualized. In one patient with signs of misfunction of the stent, increased echogenicity could be observed in its lumen (Fig. 43.9c,d).

The course of the patients depended on the extent of the malignant process. Three patients developed intestinal problems deriving from infiltration of the ileum or rectum. The patient with uterine carcinoma subsequently developed a rectovaginal fistula. One of the patients with prostatic carcinoma requiring urethral catheterization developed several episodes of urinary infection, probably due to difficulty in evacuating the bladder and to vesico-ureteral reflux. In two patients with upper urinary infection that was refractory to treatment, the infection disappeared after the implants. In one patient with TCC of the bladder, 19 months after stenting, a urothelial implant of the tumour was detected quite proximal to the endoprosthesis (Fig. 43.7e), and was resected by an antegrade approach through a new nephrostomy tract. This is a new urothelial neoplasm. The above is characteristic of this type of tumour which may appear in several locations along the urinary pathway.

In the authors' series, the first patients who had previously undergone combined chemotherapy died 3 months after stent insertion, as the result of renal failure caused by chronic parenchymatous damage. Successive sonographic studies revealed absence of obstructive uropathy until the death of the patient; for this reason, assessment of the functional renal recovery, particularly important in patients with bilateral drainage, was included as a fourth item among the selection criteria. To date, the longest recorded survival has been 4 and 4.1 years in two patients, the first patient having local recurrence of ovarian cystic adenocarcinoma and in whom the two stented ureters did not develop signs of obstruction until the last 3 months (patient 6, Fig. 43.8). In the second patient, with prostatic carcinoma and bilateral stents (patient 7, Fig. 43.8), infiltration of the right-side stent 2 years after implant, and 6 months later in the left-side stent, was noted. Nevertheless, the parameters of renal function continued to be within acceptable values. The patient died, 4 years and 1 month after stent implantation, after acute intestinal haemorrhage through the colostomy.

Discussion

It is well known that ureteral obstruction may appear in the course of several types of malignancy. The relative well-being of some patients encourages the adoption of a positive attitude to solve this problem in an attempt to extend the life expectancy, while causing as little 'bother' as possible. The middle- and long-term disadvantages of both internal plastic stents and the percutaneous nephrostomy are well known. The availability of metal ureteral stents gave a new perspective to the management of this condition. To the authors' knowledge, the first reference to the use of a metal stent in the ureter was by Gort et al.[10] in a case of uretero-ileal stricture. The present authors began to

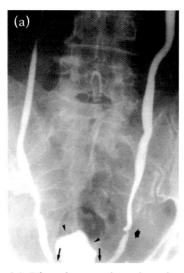

(a) Bilateral antegrade pyelography after nephrostomy. The thin arrows indicate the level of the obstructions. The right ureter, completely occluded, could not be catheterized until a TUR was performed. A second, more proximal, stenosis was observed in the left ureter (broad arrow). Through the left ureter, a small bladder with filling defects (arrowheads) is opacified.

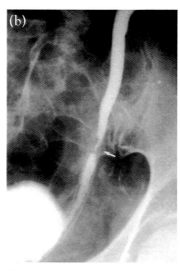

(b) One month after the implant, a monitoring nephrostogram shows the presence of severe proximal stenosis (arrow), which is irregular and asymmetric unlike that usually observed in the other ureters, attributable to spasm and/or oedema.

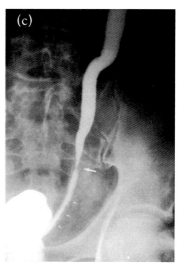

(c) Four months after the implant, the stenosis is apparently unchanged (large arrow) but the patient has started to leak urine around the nephrostomy catheter. Note the increase in the degree of dilatation of the upper urinary tract. The small arrows mark a higher protrusion of tissue through the mesh at the level of the initial proximal stricture.

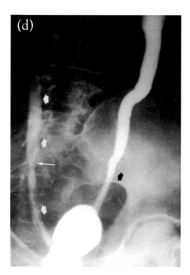

(d) An additional proximal implant at the left side (black arrow) solves the problem. On the right ureter, the reflux (white short arrows) as well as a mild ureterospasm (white long arrow) unmodified for 4 months can be observed.

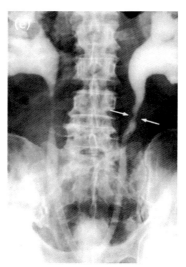

(e) Intravenous urography, 19 months after the implants, shows bilateral moderate dilatation of the renal pelvis and calyces. A filling defect (arrows) has been detected in the upper left ureter. At CT, a small mass corresponding to a new urothelial tumour was observed at this level, and was subsequently resected by a new antegrade approach.

Figure 43.7. (a–e) A 63-year-old male with a transitional cell carcinoma of the bladder. Urinary incontinence and marked volumetric decrease of the bladder probably related to several TURs and radiotherapy.

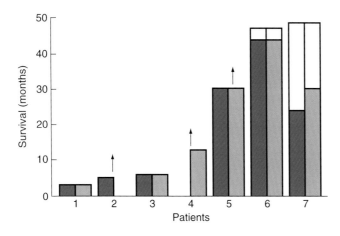

Figure 43.8. *Patient survival; arrows indicate those patients still alive. Dark bars represent the duration of good functioning of right ureteral stents; light bars represent the period of good functioning of left ureteral stents.*

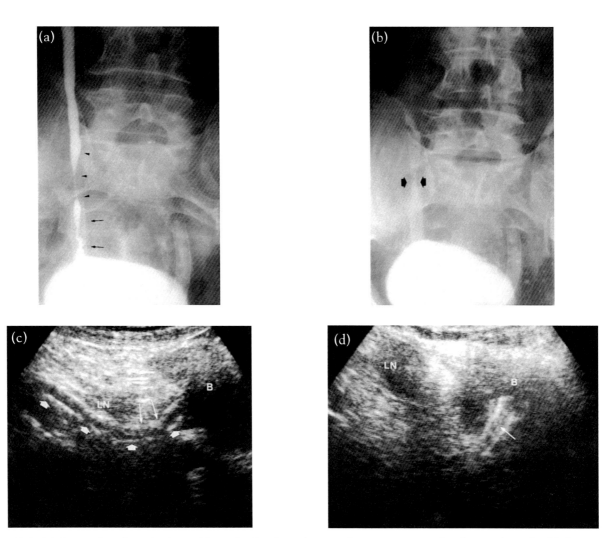

Figure 43.9. *(a) Antegrade pyelography obtained 3 months after the implant reveals a stenosis proximal to the stent (arrowheads) that was not covered by the first stent after shortening. In addition, excessive protrusion of tissue into the stent is observed. (b) After insertion of an additional implant, the X-ray shows narrowing of the stent at the level of the extrinsic compression; however, this obstruction resolved immediately. (c) Ultrasound examination 4 years after implants visualizes the two right-side stents (broad arrows), the bladder (B), and, adjacent to the ureter, a hypoechogenic mass corresponding to lymph node metastases (LN). An increase of echogenicity is apparent within the lumen of the stent at the same level where the protrusion of tissue took place within the first 3 months (thin arrows). The progressive dilatation of the ureter indicated malfunctioning of the stents. (d) Similar hyperechogenicity was also observed at the distal end of the stent (arrow).*

apply these devices in the ureter, as described by Lugmayr and Pauer,[11] as a logical extension of their applications on the basis of their principle of action. To date, reported experience of the use of metal stents in this situation is limited both in patient numbers and in the duration of the follow-up period, which may explain why a preference over the current methods has not been clearly defined. However, several benefits have now been noted while numerous questions have arisen, awaiting answers based on wider experience.

The main issue to evaluate is the patency of the stent, which appears to depend on several factors. A metal stent, like any other foreign body, exerts a stimulus on the ureter, which may respond by ureterospasm, oedema, urothelial hyperplasia or even fibrosis.[12,13] Theoretically, the speed and the intensity of the response would be proportional to that of the stimulus. Some authors have verified the early presence of oedema or urothelial hyperplasia, even causing obstruction in the days following the implant. For this reason, for a period of between 1 and 3 months they have added a double-J or pigtail stent to prevent this complication.[11,12] The urothelial reaction appears to stabilize when the stent has been urothelialized and subsequently incorporated into the ureteral wall.[12] The urothelialization has been macroscopically visualized at 8 weeks;[14] however, microscopic epithelialization may be observed within a few days. The extent of this reaction is limited to the length of the stent.[15] Other factors besides the presence of a foreign body should also be considered. What remains unknown is the influence of the type of metal or the alloy, structure of the stent, wire thickness, and their penetration into the ureteral wall. For the Wallstent, at the areas where the ends of the fine wires are lodged in the wall, a greater degree of urothelial activity has not been demonstrated.

One factor that probably affects the response and, perhaps, the patency of the lumen is overdistension of the ureteral wall.[15] This overdistension is attributable not only to the stent itself but also to the dilatations sometimes performed before or after stent implantation. The authors have avoided such dilatations, before and after the implant, as much as possible and they have opted for a progressive expansion of the ureter in order to minimize the stimulus and the subsequent inflammatory response. In the two cases where dilatation was required for the insertion of the drainage

catheter, this was performed with a balloon of minimal diameter (4 mm).

With respect to the stent, except in the first cases of the series, the authors tend to use those of smaller diameter (7 and 6 mm) in order to avoid overdistension of the ureteral wall. Therefore, progressive expansion is achieved firstly by the drainage catheter and then by the expansion of the stent itself. With regard to the self-expanding devices, the degree of dilatation should be closely related to their diameter. Although the authors have been unable to find any published report relating the diameter of the self-expanding stent to the magnitude of the oedema or urothelial hyperplasia, nevertheless a certain proportion should be expected. Pollack et al.[16] have noted their doubt about to what extent the use of relatively large Wallstents (10 mm diameter) in their series could contribute to poor patency. An excessive radial force pressing against the ureteral wall may facilitate the herniation of inflammatory or neoplastic tissue through the mesh of the stent. The present authors noted this protrusion of tissue partially obliterating the lumen from the first 24 hours after implant, both in the biliary tract and ureter, being more marked in the area of the constrictive lesion (Fig. 43.7c). Although the lumen can remain unchanged for many months without disrupting the flow of urine, this area of protrusion will be probably the site of recurrence of the obstruction.[16]

The fibrotic reaction found in some cases to compromise the stent lumen should not be attributed only to mechanical irritation, mesh penetration into the wall or radiation therapy: this reaction can have its basis in ischaemic changes secondary to overdistension.

Another issue that has arisen is interference of the stent with ureteral peristalsis. The Wallstent incorporated in the ureteral wall transforms this segment into a rigid tube. Although the remaining ureter retains its motility, peristalsis seems not to be essential for maintaining normal excretory function. Nevertheless, owing to the fact that, in all the authors' series of ureters, the stent was inserted into the ureterovesical junction, on several occasions reflux from the bladder has been verified fluoroscopically (Fig. 43.7d). This reflux may be favoured by a certain degree of residual ureteral hypotonicity and this may be responsible for the development of upper urinary tract infections under certain conditions, such as the addition of an intravesical obstacle. This could be responsible for the development of upper urinary tract infections under certain conditions.

A finding observed in 42% of the authors' series of stented ureters is the 'trumpetlike configuration' (as termed by Flueckiger et al.[12]) of the ureteral segments adjacent to the ends of the Wallstent (Fig. 43.10). Although in most cases this remains unchanged for a long period, in one ureter it became a severe stenosis 4 months after the first implant, requiring an additional overlapping stent (Fig. 43.7a–d). This development, as well as the decrease in ureteral calibre in the segment adjacent to the Wallstent (Fig. 43.10), suggested the possibility of an initial ureterospasm induced by the endwires that might lead to urothelial hyperplasia or even fibrosis.

Apart from these considerations, other factors may influence the permeability of the stent, such as tumoral ingrowth,[11] the formation of encrustations[17] and the presence of debris. The latter has been demonstrated, after implantation, by means of endoluminal sonography.[11] In selected cases, tumoral obliteration of the lumen can be managed by endoscopic resection or by adding a new stent to the first. Perhaps covered stents, used in a manner similar to that in other situations, may contribute to a longer patency of the ureter by delaying its infiltration.

With regard to the type of stent to use, the authors tend to use the Wallstent for several reasons: firstly, because it is self-expanding it exerts a constant pressure against the ureteral wall; secondly, the thinness of its wires give it great flexibility, enabling it to conform to the curves of the ureter; thirdly, because of its helical interwoven nature, constructed from continuous wires from end to end, if the Wallstent becomes kinked its surface remains smooth and its lumen unconstricted.

The disadvantages observed in the early devices were poor radiopacity and a certain imprecision in positioning because of an initial sudden slipping of the rolling membrane. ('Rolling membrane' is the term used by the manufacturer. This is the thin plastic invaginated membrane which covers the stent maintaining its constriction until the release.) The first problem has been corrected by the addition of tantalum to the mesh filaments; the second problem will probably be overcome by the new Placehit® (Schneider) releasing system. Anticipation of stent shortening after its

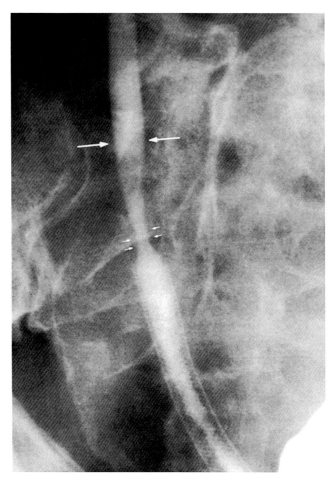

Figure 43.10. *'Trumpetlike configuration' of the ureteral segment adjacent to the stent. The diameter at this level (small arrows) is smaller than in the other parts of the ureter (large arrows), suggesting ureterospasm.*

complete expansion, in relation to the use of additional overlapping implants, is perhaps a matter of experience. The shortening basically depends on the diameter that the stent may attain, as well as on its length. Furthermore, the shortening at each end is different and varies according to the relative positions of the zone of greater stricture and the centre of the stent. The factors that may influence the speed of expansion are the disproportion between its diameter and that of the conduit that supports it, the elasticity of the surrounding tissue (which is not homogeneous along the segment) and, obviously, the performance of coadjuvant balloon dilatation. Generally, in the author's experience, if no additional dilatation is carried out, 48 hours later a slight narrowing at the level of the stricture is perceived;

this diameter becomes homogeneous after approximately 1 week.

Initially, use of the metal stent in the ureter was expected, by the authors, to give a patency similar to that of the biliary tract; however, better results were observed in the ureter. To date, apart from one case (4 years with stents and more than 6 years of malignant disease), the duration of permeability of the stent has not been less than the patient's length of survival. However, should obstruction occur, and if the patient's life expectancy and quality of life are good, the procedures described would be considered in order to rid the stent of obstruction.

To sum up, the implantation of a metal stent is a safe and easy procedure, particularly if the ureter is not completely obstructed. In this sense, it is important to chose the optimal time for the implant without delaying it until complete obstruction develops. The authors' experience, although limited, has enabled them to anticipate an acceptable rate of patency, thus avoiding long-term nephrostomy in their patients. The use of these stents has also reduced the necessity of cystoscopic manipulation to replace plastic stents in such patients, thus helping to decrease patient morbidity and discomfort and also reducing expenditure of time and money, in terms both of the procedure itself and of the anaesthesia required.

Acknowledgements

The authors would like to thank not only Mrs Márquez, Mrs Carrasco, Mrs Montes, Mrs Gijón and Mrs Velasco, who have probably spent a substantial part of their lives with X-rays, but also Mercedes Garcia Quesada for her special contribution to the translation of this manuscript.

References

1. Zimskind P D, Fetter T R, Wilkerson J L. Clinical use of long-term indwelling silicone rubber ureteral splints inserted cystoscopically. J Urol 1967; 97: 840–844

2. Goodwin W E, Casey W C, Woolf W. Percutaneous trocar (needle) nephrostomy in hydronephrosis. JAMA 1955; 157: 891–894

3. Günther R W, Alken P. Percutaneous nephropyelostomy: applications, technique and critical evaluation. In: Wilkins R A, Viamonte M Jr (eds) Interventional radiology. Oxford: Blackwell Scientific Publications, 1982: 333–355

4. Tadavarthy S M, Coleman C C, Hunter D W et al. Percutaneous uroradiologic techniques. In: Castañeda-Zuñiga WR, Tadavarthy SM (eds) Interventional radiology. Baltimore: Williams and Wilkins, 1988: 423–621

5. Hoe J W M, Tung K H, Tan E C. Re-evaluation of indications for percutaneous nephrostomy and interventional uroradiological procedures in pelvic malignancy. Br J Urol 1993; 71: 469–472

6. Evans P A M, Nisbet A P, Saxton H M. Antegrade ureteric stents in malignant disease. J Intervent Radiol 1988; 3(1): 9–13

7. Barton D P J, Morse S S, Fiorica J V et al. Percutaneous nephrostomy and ureteral stenting in gynecologic malignancies. Obstet Gynecol 1992; 80(5): 805–811

8. Fritzsche P J. Antegrade and retrograde ureteral stenting. In: Lang E K (ed) Percutaneous and interventional urology and radiology. Heidelberg: Springer-Verlag, 1986: 91–111

9. Docimo S G, Dewolf W C. High failure rate of indwelling ureteral stents in patients with extrinsic obstruction: experience at 2 institutions. J Urol 1989; 142: 277–279

10. Gort H B W, Mali W P, van Waes P F, Kloet A G. Metallic self-expandable stenting of a ureteroileal stricture. AJR 1990; 155: 422–423

11. Lugmayr H, Pauer W. Self-expanding metal stent for palliative treatment of malignant ureteral obstruction. AJR 1992; 159: 1091–1094

12. Flueckiger F, Lammer J, Klein G E et al. Malignant ureteral obstruction: preliminary results of treatment with metallic self-expandable stents. Radiology 1993; 186: 169–173

13. Reinberg Y, Ferral H, Gonzalez R et al. Intraureteral metallic self-expanding endoprosthesis (Wallstent) in the treatment of difficult ureteral strictures. J Urol 1994; 151: 1619–1622

14. Pauer W, Lugmayr H. Metallic Wallstents: a new therapy for extrinsic ureteral obstruction. J Urol 1992; 148: 281–284

15. Millward S F, Thijssen A M, Marriner J R et al. Effect of a metallic balloon-expanded stent on a normal rabbit ureter. JVIR 1991; 2: 557–560

16. Pollak J S, Rosenblatt M M, Egglin T K et al. Treatment of ureteral obstructions with the Wallstent endoprosthesis: Preliminary results. JVIR 1995; 6(3): 417–425

17. Lugmayr H, Pauer W. Selbstexpandierende metall-stents bei malignen ureterestenosen. Dtsch Med Wochenschr 1991; 116: 573–576

18. vanSonnenberg E, D'Agostino H B, O'Laoide R et al. Malignant ureteral obstruction: treatment with metal stents — technique, results and observations with percutaneous intraluminal US. Radiology 1994; 191: 765–768

Prostatic stents in benign prostatic hyperplasia

44

The Memokath thermoexpandable prostate stent
B. W. Ellis and J. Nordling

Introduction

Obstruction to the outlet of the bladder is one of the most frequent clinical scenarios that urological surgeons face. In the majority of cases, non-interventional therapy can be effective. However, there are many for whom the severity of symptoms is such that mechanical dis-obstruction of the prostatic urethra is essential. In addition are men who have developed acute or chronic urinary retention in whom attempts to remove the catheter have been unsuccessful or are undesirable.

Benign prostatic hyperplasia (BPH) is the most common underlying cause. The incidence of BPH rises with age. Thus, the number of patients requiring surgery is a function of the demographics of the population. The 2001 UK census has shown a notable increase in this elderly population (Fig. 44.1). For the first time there are more people over 60 than there are children (Fig. 44.2). The percentage of the population over 60 has risen from 16% to 21%. While the increase in under 50-year-olds is modest the over 70-year-olds have doubled, and the over 85-year-olds have increased more than fivefold. The increase in the absolute number of men over 70 is shown in Fig. 44.3. The rate of growth over this period is comparable with many European countries.

Transurethral resection of the prostate (TURP) is widely regarded as the 'gold standard' by which other techniques should be judged. Any urological surgeon who treats these elderly men will be faced with patients who ought to undergo TURP but whose comorbidity is such that the only options are a long-term catheter or risky surgery. Many of these patients will already have reached the stage of acute or chronic retention. Alternative techniques for dealing with advanced obstruction do exist but most rely on general or regional anaesthesia.

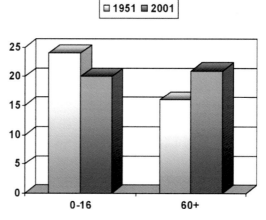

Figure 44.2. *For the first time there are more people in the UK over 60 compared to those under 16. Data from the UK population census.*

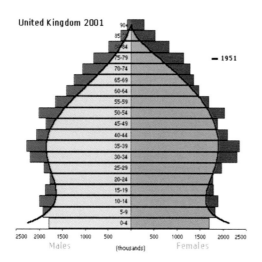

Figure 44.1. *Change in United Kingdom demography 1951–2001. In 50 years the over-70s have doubled and the over-80s have trebled. Data from the UK population census.*

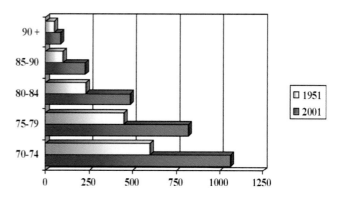

Figure 44.3. *Increase by decades of elderly men in the UK over 50 years.*

Most men faced with the prospect of lifelong catheterization would wish for a better option. Even with modern anaesthetic techniques not all men are fit for TURP. Brierly et al. investigated the morbidity of undertaking TURP on the over 80s; there was an early complication rate of 41% and a late complication rate of a further 22% in these elderly patients.[1] Recent stroke, myocardial infarction and significant cardiac dysrhythmias, often combined with severe respiratory problems, or the need for anticoagulants serve to compound the risks of age and frailty.

There is thus a need for a safe and effective alternative to TURP in this growing population of men.

Prostate stents

The first description of prostatic stenting involved a metallic spiral stent for temporary relief of obstruction.[2] In the cardiovascular system, metallic stents have been used for many years, commonly in association with materials such as woven Dacron. In this situation they have been used with great success. They were found to become colonized by endothelium and long-term patency was maintained. Stents have been used throughout the entire length of the gastrointestinal tract. Stents placed in the oesophagus have alleviated symptoms in patients with oesophageal carcinoma.[3-5] A Nitinol (nickel-titanium alloy) stent in the duodenum aided palliation of a high grade tumour.[6] Relief of obstructive jaundice due to unresectable malignancy has been reported with some success,[7,8] and in the colon in cases of malignant colorectal obstruction the use of stents is gaining wider acceptance.[9] Within the urinary tract Kulkarni has been instrumental in exploring the role of thermoexpandable metallic stents in the obstructed ureter.[10]

Depending on the characteristics of the stent the urothelium of the prostatic urethra will or will not grow over the stent so that it becomes incorporated in to urothelium. This feature used to be considered a positive attribute on the grounds that having the stent buried would reduce the risk of encrustation and infection; they were therefore termed 'permanent stents'. However, it was only rarely possible to ensure that the whole length of the stent would epithelialize and then, if problems did develop, the removal of these stents became little short of a nightmare and could never

realistically be contemplated under local anaesthesia. On the other hand, non-epithelializing stents are made of very inert materials and do not promote such urothelial reaction, they therefore do not get incorporated; they used to be termed 'temporary'. Thus, the distinction as permanent or temporary is really not helpful.

In developing the ideal stent, various characteristics are required. The stent must be easily placed under local anaesthesia. It should not cause any local side-effects, such as tissue hyperplasia or encrustation, and it should not migrate. The stents should be easily removable if necessary, and endoscopy through the stent should be feasible.

Epithelializing stents include the Urolume Wallstent® (American Medical Systems, Minnetonka, MN) and the Intraprostatic stent® (ASI Inc. San Clemente, CA). Initial responses to the use of these permanent stents were encouraging with good outcomes in select groups of patients.[11,12] However, longer-term follow-up showed that these devices were not without complications. These included epithelial ingrowth, encrustation, migration, recurrent urinary tract infection, and lower tract symptoms, such as dysuria and urgency.[13-15] These difficulties often necessitated stent removal, which required general anaesthesia, thereby negating the advantage of being able to avoid anaesthesia for the patient.[16]

Non-epithelializing stents, such as the Prostakath®, a rigid gold-plated spiral (Engineers & Doctors A/S Copenhagen, Denmark), were designed to be easy to insert and manipulate if necessary. Again, initial results were encouraging,[17] but longer-term data indicated success in a small percentage of patients,[18] with up to 50% needing to be removed within the first year.[19]

The Memokath® 028 intraprostatic stent (Engineers & Doctors A/S, Copenhagen, Denmark) is shown in Fig. 44.4. It is made of an alloy of nickel and titanium (NiTi) that exhibits a property known as 'shape memory'. The US Naval Ordinance Laboratory experimented with these alloys nearly 30 years ago but the shape memory effect was first discovered in gold and cadmium alloys over 65 years ago. In 1968, Bühler and Wang, while searching for non-magnetic, lightweight and corrosion-resistant material for submarines found the shape-memory behaviour in an alloy of nickel and titanium. However, it is only within the last few years

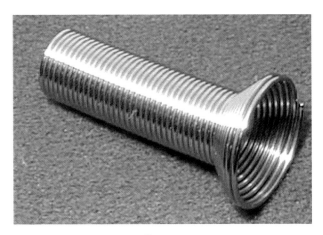

Figure 44.4. *The Memokath® 028 prostate stent.*

that more common applications have been developed for them.

A shape memory alloy (SMA) can 'remember' its shape and will return to that shape after it has been deformed if it is heated to a given temperature. The SMA of NiTi exists in two distinct crystalline forms, martensite and austenite. A martensite-type NiTi will, after a 'plastic' deformation within certain limits, return to its original shape when heated; it is the result of a specific type of phase-change known as martensitic transformation. Martensite is formed during a shear type process by cooling the high temperature phase (Austenite). In the absence of any outer stresses, several different directions of martensitic shear occur without any external macroscopic change. Applying a stress (e.g. a 'plastic' deformation), the martensite with many different orientations will be converted by a 'flipping-over' type of shear into a nearly single orientation. If the deformed martensite in this kind of nearly single orientation is now heated above a defined temperature, it transforms back to austenite with the initial original shape. The process is complex and the transition temperature depends on alloy mix, deformation and type and direction of applied stresses. Put more simply; the atomic structure of one crystalline lattice is floppy while that of the other is rigid.

Medical applications, such as orthopaedic implants (e.g. bone plates, rods, staples etc.), profit from the profound inertness of this alloy. Other applications take advantage of its super-elasticity feature in the austenitic configuration (e.g. guidewires and orthodontic wires).

Urological stents depend on both the inertness and the shape memory effect. The stent's memorized shape is

that of a tight coil opening into a funnel at one end. However, when unpacked it is a straight coil mounted on an introducing device. Only when it is correctly positioned in the prostate is it heated with water at 55°C; this then effects the transformation to its memorized shape and 'locks it into position'. When cooled using water at 10°C, it becomes soft and pliable and can be removed with relative ease under local urethral anaesthesia. The NiTi alloy is non-magnetic (and will therefore not bar the patient from having a magnetic resonance scan), it also has excellent biocompatibility properties. Its first use was described by Poulsen et al. in 1993.[20]

Patient selection

Patients for whom surgery is indicated but who are too frail or unfit and who would otherwise only be suitable for a long-term catheter or risky surgery should be considered for a stent rather than transurethral resection of the prostate (TURP). However, there are contraindications. Patients with bladder tumours should not be stented, because although a flexible cystoscope may be passed through a stent, a resectoscope cannot. Those with an existing bladder stone are best avoided in case they form a stone on their stent. Patients with urethral stricture (unless very distal) should not be stented as it is difficult to manage a stricture without jeopardizing the stent. On the other hand, it may be possible to stent both. Finally, patients with advanced detrusor failure will not respond to a stent any better than to TURP. Many stent failures are the result of attempting to treat these men with 'dead' bladders. If there is any doubt we would always consider simple urodynamic assessment by measuring the pressure volume profile during filling through the patient's catheter and also recording the volume at which there was a desire to void.

The majority of patients we stent have advanced cardiorespiratory and/or cerebrovascular disease. However, it is important that all chronic diseases should be stabilized. There is no contraindication to stent placement in a man who has had a recent stroke and has chronic obstructive pulmonary disease such that he is unable to lie flat. It is perfectly possible to place a prostatic stent without any sedation and with the patient semi-recumbent.

Preparation

Patients should understand why a stent is being suggested rather than 'conventional' surgery. They should know that the chances of success are not quite as high (approx. 75–80% satisfactory outcome vs approx. 90% for TURP). On the other hand, the technique is very safe and highly unlikely to aggravate any other disease state. We provide these men with a comprehensive instruction leaflet.*

It is important, where possible, to rid patients of active urinary infection. Of course this is not always easy, especially when there is an indwelling catheter. If infection does persist then the patient must have full cover with an antibiotic to which the infection has been shown to exhibit sensitivity.

Patients attend the day surgery unit for their stent placement. Premedication is with an oral antibiotic and rectal diclofenac 100 mg. Postoperative analgesia is not required but a five day course of an antibiotic is advisable.

Stent insertion

With the patient lying comfortably on the operating table the external genitalia are cleansed with a mild antiseptic and drapes applied. A flexible cystoscope is passed to the bladder to assess urethral patency and exclude the presence of bladder calculi and tumours. Next, the flexible cystoscope is held at the bladder neck and a marker is placed upon the cystoscope sheath at the tip of the penis (Fig. 44.5). The cystoscope is then

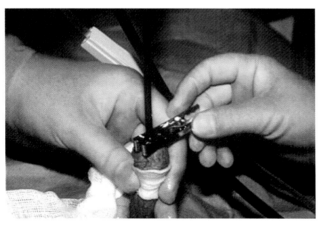

Figure 44.5. *A marker is placed while the tip of the cystoscope is held at the bladder neck.*

withdrawn to just below the apex of the verumontanum and a further marker is placed. The distance between the two markers gives an indication of the length of stent required. The stents are made in lengths from 30 mm to 70 mm in 10 mm steps. When selecting the stent, round up by at least 5 mm to the next size.

Further local urethral anaesthetic is applied prior to the passage of a 26/30 Ch sound to the bladder to ensure that the stent (24 Ch) will pass without hindrance. The stent, on its introducing sheath, is mounted onto the flexible cystoscope so that the tip of the cystoscope is proud of the stent by 2–3 mm. A check is made with the assistant nurse that the hot water is at the required temperature (57°C). The cystoscope is inserted into the urethra. It may be necessary to ask the assistant to hold the top of the cystoscope so that two hands can be used to get the stent through the urethral meatus. Next the cystoscope is advanced gently by pushing both on the introducing sheath and on the cystoscope. At the sphincter ensure that the tip of the cystoscope is accurately aligned, ask the patient to relax as best he can. Remember that the outside calibre is much greater than the cystoscope alone; sustained gentle pressure is occasionally required to open the sphincter. Once through the sphincter the assistant connects the hot water syringe and tubing to the input port on the introducing sheath. The cystoscope is further advanced until the tip just enters the bladder; often a slight give is felt at this point as the distal end, expanded very slightly by being mounted on the introducer thread, passes through the sphincter. After warning the patient, 50 ml hot water is flushed through the cystoscope, this expands the lower 4–6 mm into a cone shape (44 Ch) just proximal to the sphincter that 'locks' the stent into position. The cystoscope is then gently withdrawn through the stent. If there is any resistance, the introducing sheath can be rotated anticlockwise to ensure that the thread on to which the distal end of the stent was mounted is not catching on a coil of the stent. Just proximal to the thread at the end of the sheath are slits through which the hot water can get all around the stent to effect the expansion (Fig. 44.6). The final position is checked to ensure that the sphincter closes just below the distal end of the stent (Fig. 44.7) and the cystoscope and sheath are removed.

If the stent is too short it is much more likely to fail; the lower end will rotate posteriorly and impact on the

* Patient information sheets are available from: Department of Urology, Ashford Hospital, Ashford TW15 3AA, UK.

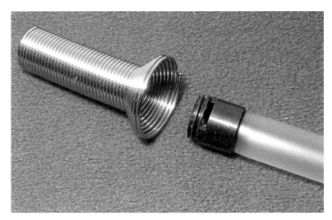

Figure 44.6. *The stent deployed from the sheath. The tip of the sheath has a short screw thread that holds the stent. When hot water is flushed through the sheath it comes out of the slits just behind the screw thread and the lower end of the stent expands off the sheath.*

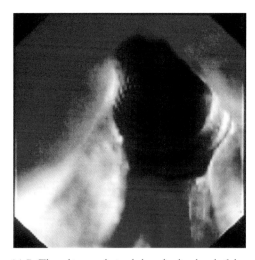

Figure 44.7. *The sphincter closing below the distal end of the stent.*

verumontanum (Fig. 44.8) or the upper end will lie below the bladder neck and occlude on the base of the middle lobe or bladder neck (Fig. 44.13). While it is wise to avoid too much stent lying free in the bladder a short amount is acceptable.

After insertion, the patient's bladder is usually full and they are able to urinate. About 10% of men will suffer temporary retention; for them a suprapubic catheter is placed until voiding is established.

Patients are asked to stay in the day unit until they have passed reasonable volumes of water twice and to their satisfaction. If there is doubt the bladder can be checked with a portable scanner. Prior to departure they are given a card indicating that they have a stent in the prostatic urethra and warning other medical personnel not to try and pass a catheter larger than 12 Fr.

Radiology

Stents are easily seen on plain radiographs (Fig. 44.9) and ultrasound (Fig. 44.10). The X-ray will not reveal the relationship of the stent to the prostate in the same way that ultrasound can. However, it will indicate the orientation of the stent, thus migration is simple to diagnose by X-ray as the stent will almost always lie horizontally (Fig. 44.11). Migration can also be appreciated on ultrasound (Fig. 44.12). An experienced ultrasonographer can usually determine the relationship between the bladder neck and the top of the stent to assess the possibility of a stent being placed too low (Fig. 44.13).

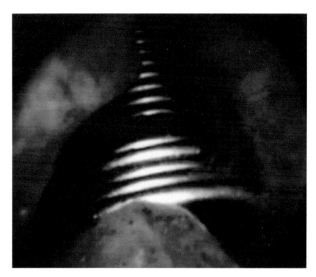

Figure 44.8. *The lower end of this stent is lying too high and has angulated posteriorly on to the verumontanum.*

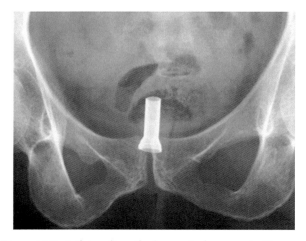

Figure 44.9. *A plain radiograph of a stent in the correct position.*

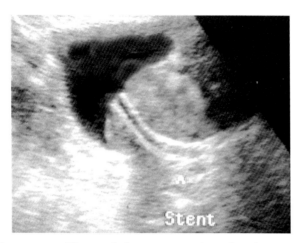

Figure 44.10. *Ultrasound of a prostate stent (sagittal view).*

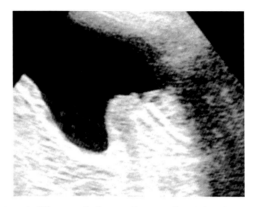

Figure 44.13. *Ultrasound of a stent lying too low. Note that proximal end of the stent clearly lies below the bladder neck.*

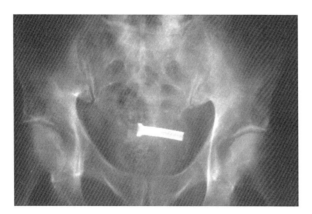

Figure 44.11. *Radiograph of a stent migrated to the bladder.*

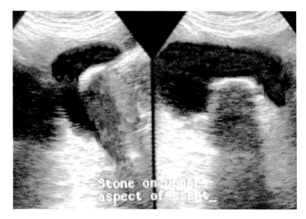

Figure 44.14. *Transverse and sagittal (longitudinal) ultrasound views of stone lying over the proximal end of the stent; note the acoustic shadow cast by the stone.*

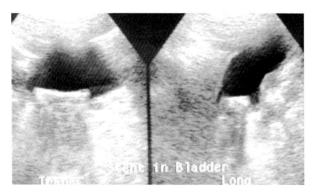

Figure 44.12. *Transverse and sagittal (longitudinal) ultrasound views of a stent migrated to the bladder.*

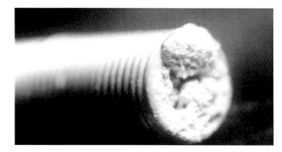

Figure 44.15. *Stent occlusion by stone. This was not visible on X-ray and ultrasound. Diagnosis was made by endoscopic inspection.*

Results

Ashford series[21]

Men were followed up every six months following their stent placement with assessment of their international prostate symptom score (IPSS) and satisfaction scores. Stent position was checked with a portable ultrasound scanner.

Stone formation is unusual (see below). It is almost always impossible to see on X-ray and is only visible on ultrasound in cases of gross encrustation (Fig. 44.14). Cystoscopy is necessary to diagnose significant stone occlusion (Fig. 44.15) or encrustation.

A total of 217 Memokath® stents was used in 211 men, all as a day case or outpatient procedure, unless the patient was already in hospital. The stents were placed under direct cystoscopic vision using urethral local anaesthesia; general anaesthesia was not used. In several patients with dementia mild sedation was necessary. The stents were placed with the expanded distal portion situated just proximal to or over the verumontanum. The stents used varied from 30 mm to 70 mm in length with the mode being 40 mm.

Over the same time period, 1511 transurethral resection of the prostate (TURP) operations were performed in our unit; therefore, 14% of interventions for prostatic bladder outflow obstruction involved the placement of an intraprostatic stent. The age differences of each cohort of patients are shown in Table 44.1 and Fig. 44.16. There is a decade difference in the mean age. The youngest patient stented was just 54. He suffered acute urinary retention during an episode of chronic rejection of a heart-lung transplant. A 62-year-old, the next youngest, developed retention after pneumonectomy, an ileofemoral bypass for critical lower limb ischaemia and a cardiovascular

accident while on anticoagulants. He had a successful TURP 15 months later.

The reasons for stent placement rather than TURP are listed in Table 44.2. The predominant reason was because of cardiovascular risk factors; general frailty was also a common cause. The listed factors are not mutually exclusive. A small number of men had a stent placed as a true temporary device, that is the stent was intended to be removed after a certain period of time (e.g. following coronary artery bypass grafting). Comorbidity as assessed by American Society of Anesthesiologists (ASA) grade was available in 158 of these patients (Table 44.3); there is clearly a notable difference between them and 792 of the 1511 patients undergoing TURP for whom ASA data was available.

Table 44.1. *Patients undergoing interventional treatment for bladder outflow obstruction secondary to prostatic enlargement: 1993–2001*

Treatment	No. of men	Mean age (range)
TURP	1511	70.2 (37–91)
Stent	211	80.2 (54–103)

TURP, transurethral resection of the prostate.

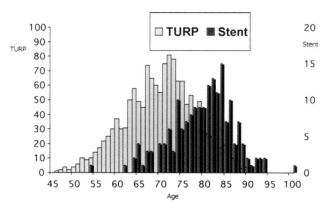

Figure 44.16. *Chart showing the comparative ages of men undergoing transurethral resection of the prostate (TURP) (blue) or stent insertion (red).*

Table 44.2. *Reason why a patient was unfit for surgery (not mutually exclusive)*

Reason	Number (%)
Severe cardiorespiratory disease (COPD/IHD/CVA)	95 (44)
Frail	117 (54)
Dementia	25 (12)
Anticoagulants/Clotting abnormalities	26 (12)
Temporarily unfit (e.g. prior to angioplasty, coronary artery bypass grafting)	12 (6)
Other (e.g. post-brachytherapy outflow obstruction)	11 (5)

COPD, chronic obstructive pulmonary disease; IHD, ischaemic heart disease; CVA, cerebrovascular accident.

Table 44.3. *ASA grades of 158 stent patients and 792 TURP patients*

ASA Grade	Description	Stent patients No. (%)	TURP patients No. (%)
1	Healthy	0 (0)	298 (38)
2	Mild systemic disease, no functional limitation	10 (6)	405 (51)
3	Severe systemic disease with functional limitation	74 (47)	81 (10)
4	Severe systemic disease, constant threat to life	74 (47)	8 (1)
5	Moribund	0	0

ASA, American Society of Anesthesiologists; TURP, transurethral resection of the prostate.

The IPSS were followed up in these men where possible. The mean score prior to stent insertion was 20.3 (N = 150, range 5–32, 95% confidence interval of the mean: 19.26–21.27). The scores pre- and post-insertion were both confirmed as having a normal distribution using the Kolmogorov-Smirnov test (P = 0.72 and 0.07, respectively). Following stent insertion the IPSS had fallen by 12.1 points to 8.2 (N = 151, range 0–25, 95% confidence interval of the mean: 7.25–9.08) a significant difference; P<0.0001 using a paired t-test. The 95% confidence interval for the pre- and post-insertion difference of paired samples was 10.03–12.79. The 'bother' score (0–6) fell by 59% from a mean of 4.1–1.7.

The post-insertion IPSS hardly changes over time. Figure 44.17 shows the IPSS before and after stent insertion and then annually for 7 years. The numbers of patients (i.e. sample size for each data point) for this symptom score analysis over time is also shown. Table 44.4 shows the change in IPSS by indication for intervention (symptoms, acute or chronic retention) cancer and dementia; these indications are not mutually exclusive. Patients treated for acute retention were asked to estimate their symptoms prior to the episode of retention.

Of the 217 stents placed, 52 (24%) were removed, however, eight of these men (4%) had their stents removed electively as they were no longer necessary (e.g. patients rendered fit again following coronary artery bypass grafting so that TURP could, once again, be considered). Removals occurred for many different reasons from worsening symptoms to migration. Several men had their stents removed because their prostates outgrew their stent; in these cases the middle lobe or bladder neck was then able to occlude the proximal

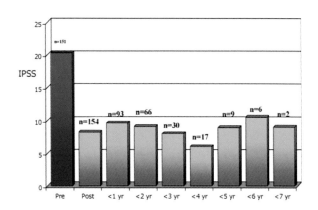

Figure 44.17. *The international prostate symptom score (IPSS) pre- and post-stent insertion over time. The number of men in each annual cohort is shown.*

aperture of the stent. In those men who had received benefit from their intraprostatic stent, a longer Memokath® stent was inserted (six patients).

Patients with high comorbidity have a risk of dying in the short term. Placement of a foreign body in the urinary tract also has a finite lifetime before failure. Although we have several patients whose stents are still in place after more than 6 years; it is nonetheless of importance, when considering the merits and demerits of a given treatment, to know whether the stent is likely to fail within the patient's expected lifespan. Figure 44.18 shows a Kaplan-Meier survival curve for those patients who either died or whose stents failed. The implication that can be drawn from these data is simple. Stents may well fail, but the patient is more likely to die first.

It is customary, when evaluating management for outflow obstruction from the bladder, to assess maximum and average flow rates before and after treatment. Although we started with this in mind it

Table 44.4. *Change in IPSS (pre- and post-insertion) by indication for intervention*

Indication	No.	IPSS			
		Pre	Post	Fall	Change (%)
Severe symptoms	105	20.6	8.7	11.9	58
Acute retention	77	19.6	7.9	11.7	60
Chronic retention	30	19.2	5.6	13.9	71
Cancer	17	23.4	9.5	13.9	59
Dementia	25	19.3	9.7	9.6	50

IPSS, international prostate symptom score.

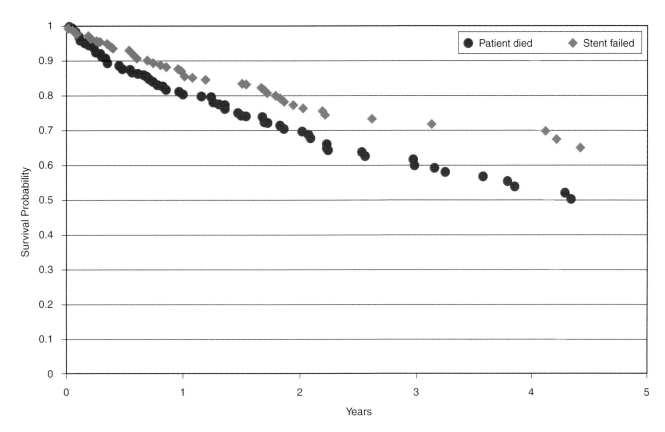

Figure 44.18. *Kaplan-Meier survival analysis of the stents in men living with intraprostatic stents in comparison to those men who died with their stents in situ (sample size 214).*

soon became clear that with men of this degree of comorbidity the logistics of obtaining flow rates were challenging for patients and staff alike. Furthermore, there seemed to be little correlation between those that were obtained and the patients' symptom scores. Because these stents are readily visible using ultrasound we find that, in practice, it is more helpful to check the patient using a portable scanner to establish that the stent remains in a satisfactory position and there is not a large residual volume and get an IPSS. After all, relief of symptoms is more important to the patient rather than the velocity of his stream.

Complications (Table 44.5)

We found a 10% rate of early acute urinary retention post procedure. A few days of suprapubic catheterization resolved the matter in almost all of these patients. We believe that some of these men suffer transient difficulty with sphincter relaxation as a result of the stent insertion; it might also be due to oedema or sphincter spasm induced by the insertion.

Stent migration occurred in 29 (13%). Migration did not always necessitate stent removal as methods of in situ repositioning were developed. Such a technique was carried out on 33 occasions, again under local anaesthetic as a day case or outpatient procedure.

Urinary tract infection was a problem in only 13 men (6%). Significant stent encrustation or stone formation was seen in five patients (2%) one of whom needed a general anaesthetic for stent/stone removal. Many stents, when examined after prolonged insertion, had a bronze appearance (when new they are a dull grey

Table 44.5. *Complications*

Migration	29 (13%)
Retention (post procedure)	21 (10%)
Incontinence	14 (6%)
Infection	13 (6%)
Pain	7 (3%)
Bleeding	6 (3%)
Stone formation	5 (2%)
Occlusion	3 (1%)

colour) (Fig. 44.19). When allowed to dry, in those stents removed, this bronze coating tended to come away from the stent as a fine powder. Its nature has not been established. Significant epithelial ingrowth has been seen in four patients. In later years, the stents were manufactured with a very much tighter coil so as to minimize this risk. It only became a problem in a single patient who had been fitted with an 'old' type of stent.

Impaired continence was a problem in 14 patients (6%). In many cases, it was probably as a result of unrestrained detrusor instability following prolonged obstruction; it often responded to anticholinergics. In two cases, the lower end of the coil became distracted and directly impaired sphincter function. Replacement of the stent was necessary in these men.

Discussion

The Memokath® 028 nickel titanium alloy intra-prostatic stent was placed in 211 men who were selected due to their unsuitability for transurethral surgery. The high proportion of stents inserted in our unit (14%) is a reflection of our interest in the technique, which has led to referrals from elsewhere.

The insertion of this stent is relatively easy to perform and they are normally placed as an outpatient procedure under local urethral anaesthesia. Placing the stent is no more uncomfortable than a flexible cystoscopic examination until the instillation of hot water into the urethra and bladder, which causes discomfort for 4–5 seconds. However, when men are forewarned of the 'hot flush' they tolerate it well. Having their hand held by a (female) nurse at this point usually engenders notable bravado! The whole procedure takes about 20 minutes. Most men void immediately after the procedure and the outcome of stent placement, as judged by the ability to void (and often with a stream that the patient finds extraordinary), is seen immediately.

Patient selection for any procedure aims to ensure that the planned procedure is appropriate to the patient's condition and circumstances so that there is the best possible chance of a satisfactory outcome. The men were chosen primarily for their willingness to have a surgical procedure but were of high surgical risk. This cohort of men obviously included many elderly men given an average age of 80.2 years. As noted earlier

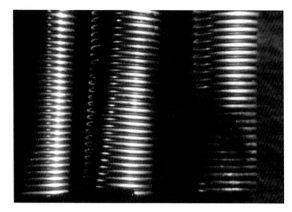

Figure 44.19. *Stent discoloration. The stent on the left is new. The middle one had been placed for 3 months; there is a very slight yellowing of the surface. The stent on the right had been in situ for 18 months.*

transurethral resection of the prostate (TURP) can benefit patients over 80 years of age, but they suffer high morbidity from age alone. The comorbid disease states present were those of old age, chronic obstructive pulmonary disease (COPD), ischaemic heart disease and dementia; these, of course, are not universal to this age but the prevalence is very much greater.

We have undertaken stent placement on 25 (12%) patients with dementia. In many of these cases the patients were deemed fit only for long-term catheterization, only to demonstrate their ability to remove their catheters! Their symptom scores were estimated by their carers, who were, for the most part, impressed that their charges instinctively knew when they had to find the toilet. Others did require regular toileting.

We placed stents in 17 patients with known prostatic carcinoma. Most of these patients had extensive local disease causing obstruction. Tissue ingrowth was not a problem in these cases. If patients need radiotherapy for prostatic cancer there should be uniform dosimetry to the gland assuming opposing ports are used. Studies have shown that there is an 18% reduction in dose to the far side of a stent and 20% enhancement on the near side.[22] Using conventional multi-port treatment protocols this is not likely to give any problems of uneven dosimetry. We have also used stents in patients following brachytherapy .

Patient sellection should not be based upon age and comorbidity alone. The failure rate of these stents is in part due to the fact that the bladder function in these elderly men may be poor. Urodynamic tests were performed in some men to assess detrusor activity prior to stent placement. In those men with a urinary catheter, the bladder was inflated with 500 ml of normal saline. If there was a sensory desire to micturate then it was considered that the bladder was suitable for this form of therapy. We believe that the number of stent failures has started to fall following this simple protocol.

The complication rate of these stents is low at this length of follow-up. Encrustation is rare, ingrowth uncommon and migration is relatively easy to rectify under local anaesthesia. The reason for the lack of encrustation on these stents is not known. It may be due to the exceptional smoothness of the surface of the stent, the inert property of the alloy or the gentle massaging action of subtle movement within the prostatic urethra. Increasing prostate growth causing stent obstruction has been managed by replacement with a longer stent. Bladder stone formation has not been seen and two bladder tumours, presenting with haematuria, have been diagnosed in patients with the Memokath® 028 stent. The stents allowed cystoscopic detection of these tumours but, once discovered, the management of these lesions has meant that the stents have had to be removed to allow the access of a resectoscope.

In our institution, patients who undergo transurethral surgery have a mean hospital stay of 2.2 days. They are followed up by telephone 8–10 weeks postoperatively by a nurse practitioner. The total cost of TURP is approximately £1050 per patient. That of the insertion of a prostatic stent is approximately £1200. Due to our special interest in these stents, their benefits and complications, we are undertaking long-term surveillance of the patients. The cost would be less if such protracted follow-up were not undertaken.

It is sometimes tempting to consider long-term catheterization as a simple and inexpensive option. However, Booth et al. have shown that the cost of care for a patient with an indwelling catheter is at least £700 per annum.[23] Most patients that we have stented who have had prolonged periods of catheterization remark on the liberation they feel in getting rid of the catheter. Furthermore, despite their comorbidity, a number of our patients have been able to enjoy some sexual activity that would otherwise have been difficult.

The reduction in the IPSS score is immediate and of a degree that comes close to that seen after TURP. In this series the mean fall was 12.1 points; that seen in the National Prostatectomy study of 5361 patients in 4 health regions in the UK was 12.9.[24] Furthermore, these patients are, on average, 10 years older than those undergoing TURP in our unit (Table 44.1). Their bladders cannot be expected to perform as well as they too are that much older!

The mean IPSS score remains at or below 10 during follow-up. It is possible that these long-term findings are favourably biased given that stent failures usually occur early so that, as time passes, those patients with a good outcome will predominate among those patients surviving beyond 1–2 years.

Patients sometimes report that they are aware of the presence of the stent for a week or two. Thereafter, they are usually quite unaware of it; in much the same way as we all get used to the feeling of a filling in a tooth.

The Kaplan-Meier survival graph (Fig. 44.18) shows a greater percentage of men who die with their stents than those who outlive the usefulness of the stent. This implies that generally the stents are well tolerated and have a reasonable life expectancy. They are less likely to produce severe side-effects compared to the benefit to the patient. They may be considered as 'permanent' stents in this elderly cohort of patients with significant comorbidity. Less than a quarter (23%) of stents were considered to have failed the patient either due to poor patient selection or where the stents caused unacceptable side-effects. During these eight years the important lessons that we have learnt include the need to:

- Slightly overestimate the length of the stent. A flexible cystoscope tends to run a more direct course from bladder neck to sphincter than the stent when in situ. Also, a slightly overlong stent is not a major problem whereas a slightly short one may obstruct.
- Try to clear urinary infection before stenting (not always easy).
- Ensure that there is some detrusor function.
- Ensure patient and/or carer has an information sheet on what is being done and why. In particular they must appreciate that if they ever need a urinary catheter it should be inserted suprapubically (only a 12 Ch catheter will pass through the stent).

Three of four patients stented can expect a satisfactory outcome. This is not as high as the satisfaction after

TURP (of an audited sample of 800 patients in our unit 92% declared that their outcome was as good as or better than their expectation). The difference is in part due to the fact that a foreign body lies within the prostatic urethra and in part due to the age of the patient's bladder. However, as a safe option for the patient with high comorbidity, we believe the thermoexpandable stent is a valuable addition to our therapeutic armoury. Three of every four of these men can expect a satisfactory solution to their clinical problem with minimal risk.

References

1. Brierley R, Mostafid A, Kontothanassis D, Thomas P, Fletcher M, Harrison N W. Is transurethral resection of the prostate safe and effective in the over 80 year old? Ann R Coll Surg Engl 2001; 83: 50–53

2. Fabian K M. [The intra-prostatic "partial catheter"; (urological spiral) (author's trans.)] (in German). Urologe A 1980; 19: 236–238

3. May A, Selmaier M, Hochberger J et al. Memory metal stents for palliation of malignant obstruction of the oesophagus and cardia. Gut 1995; 37: 309–313

4. Decker P, Jakschik J, Hirner A. [Self-expanding nitinol stent – use in esophageal carcinoma] (in German). Chirurg 1995; 66: 1258–1262

5. Singhvi R, Abbasakoor F, Manson J M. Insertion of self-expanding metal stents for malignant dysphagia: assessment of a simple endoscopic method. Ann R Coll Surg Engl 2000; 82: 243–248

6. Strecker E P, Boos I, Husfeldt K J. Malignant duodenal stenosis: palliation with peroral implantation of a self-expanding nitinol stent. Radiology 1995; 196: 349–351

7. Friedrich J M, Vogel J, Gorich J, Rieber A, Rilinger N, Brambs H J. [First clinical experience with a new nitinol stent in the biliary system] (in German). Rofo Fortschr Geb Rontgenstr Neuen Bildgeb Verfahr 1995; 162: 429–435

8. Smits M, Huibregtse K, Tytgat G. Results of the new nitinol self-expandable stents for distal biliary structures. Endoscopy 1995; 27: 505–508

9. Ahmad T, Mee A S. Expandable metal stents in malignant colorectal obstruction. Promising, but trials are needed on safety and cost effectiveness. BMJ 2000; 321: 584–585

10. Kulkarni R P, Bellamy E A. A new thermo-expandable shape-memory nickel-titanium alloy stent for the management of ureteric strictures. BJU Int 1999; 83: 755–759

11. Kirby R S, Heard S R, Miller P et al. Use of the ASI titanium stent in the management of bladder outflow obstruction due to benign prostatic hyperplasia. J Urol 1992; 148: 1195–1197

12. Oesterling J E. A permanent, epithelializing stent for the treatment of benign prostatic hyperplasia. Preliminary results. J Androl 1991; 12: 423–428

13. Anjum M I, Chari R, Shetty A, Keen M, Palmer J H. Long-term clinical results and quality of life after insertion of a self-expanding flexible endourethral prosthesis. Br J Urol 1997; 80: 885–888

14. Holmes S A, Kirby R S. Intraprostatic stents – a new complication. Br J Urol 1992; 69: 322–323

15. Chiou R K, Chen W S, Akbari A, Foley S, Lynch B, Taylor R J. Long-term outcome of prostatic stent treatment for benign prostatic hyperplasia. Urology 1996; 48: 589–593

16. Anjum M I, Palmer J H. A technique for removal of the Urolume endourethral wallstent prosthesis. Br J Urol 1995; 76: 655–656

17. Harrison N W, De S J. Prostatic stenting for outflow obstruction. Br J Urol 1990; 65: 192–196

18. Thomas P J, Britton J P, Harrison N W. The Prostakath stent: four years' experience. Br J Urol 1993; 71: 430–432

19. Nordling J, Ovesen H, Poulsen A L. The intraprostatic spiral: clinical results in 150 consecutive patients. J Urol 1992; 147: 645–647

20. Poulsen A L, Schou J, Ovesen H, Nordling J. Memokath: a second generation of intraprostatic spirals. Br J Urol 1993; 72: 331–334

21. Perry M J, Roodhouse A J, Gidlow A B, Ellis B W. Thermoexpandable intraprostatic stents in bladder outflow obstruction: an 8 year study. BJU Int 2002; 90(3): 216–223

22. Gez E, Cederbaum M, Yachia D, Bar D R, Kuten A. Dose perturbation due to the presence of a prostatic urethral stent in patients receiving pelvic radiotherapy: an in vitro study. Med Dosim 1997; 22: 117–120

23. Booth C M, Chaudry A A, Lyth D R. Alternative prostate treatments: stent or catheter for the frail? J Manag Care 1997; 1: 24–26.

24. Pickard R, Emberton M, Neal D E. The management of men with acute urinary retention. National Prostatectomy Audit Steering Group. Br J Urol 1998; 81: 712–720

45

Intra-urethral catheter (IUC) in the treatment of prostatic obstruction

I. Nissenkorn and S. Richter

Introduction

Transurethral resection of the prostate (TURP) is still the gold standard and most widely accepted treatment for clinically significant obstruction of urinary flow. Post-TURP mortality is low but morbidity is not insignificant. Common complications include urinary infection, epididymitis, impotence, incontinence and the need for transfusions. Furthermore, outcome studies reveal that about 20% of patients fail to achieve improvement in their voiding symptoms following prostatectomy and 15% of patients require reoperation for stricture, bladder neck contracture, recurrent 'prostatism' or other problems within 8 years of surgery.[1] These factors have fuelled the search for less-invasive and non-surgical treatments. The different treatment modalities may be temporary or become permanent, according to whether the patient will be viable or not fit for surgery. In the last decade the non-surgical armamentarium has grown tremendously with hyperthermia, balloon dilatation and pharmacological treatment, to mention just a few. Intra-urethral spirals or catheters, first described by Fabian[2,3] in the 1980s, have been modified by some[4] and innovated by others.[5,6] They have been put into clinical use mainly in Europe[2–4,7,8] and Israel.[5,6–9,10] These intra-urethral devices have enabled a new concept in the management of obstructed patients to be developed as, by remaining isolated from the extracorporeal surroundings, they have reduced to a minimum the danger of ascending urinary tract infection.

The main reason for leaving an indwelling catheter in place for a prolonged period is to relieve urinary retention. The risk of acquiring infection increases linearly with the number of days the catheter is left in place. Catheter-associated bacteriuria accounts for 40% of annual nosocomial infections.[11] The incidence of bacteriuria associated with indwelling urethral catheterization increases by about 5% per day. Thus, bacteriuria universally develops within 3–4 weeks, even when closed urinary drainage is strictly used.[11] It is estimated that 15–20% of all hospitalized patients undergo urinary tract catheterization.[11] The presence of an indwelling catheter is associated with nearly a threefold increase in mortality among hospitalized patients.[12–18] One of the authors' studies was designed to investigate the infectious complications caused by the intra-urethral catheter (IUC). The results of IUC insertion and the infection rate after IUC insertion are reported here.

In spite of the fact that an indwelling catheter is not an impediment for the appearance of penile erection, bearing one makes it extremely difficult to perform sexually. This can cause psychological problems, notably depression and loss of self-respect, in both the male and the female partner. As the authors have found in a pilot study of patients with an IUC, patients with such a device do not have any external appliances and may continue with their normal life, including sexual activity.[19]

Patients and methods

Patients

The indications for IUC insertion were either an indwelling catheter for prostatic obstruction or symptoms of prostatic enlargement and objective evidence of benign prostatic hyperplasia (BPH) as evaluated by digital rectal examination, transrectal ultrasound or a decreased peak urinary flow rate. All patients were considered to be at high risk for surgery, owing to severe concomitant diseases, or were men who refused to undergo surgery. Patients with previously known urethral stricture, spastic neurogenic bladder, or prostatic or bladder cancer were excluded.

Pretreatment evaluation included a complete physical examination, urine tests (urinalysis and culture) and abdominal ultrasonography to obtain an estimate of the residual volume and length of the prostatic urethra.

A total of 130 consecutive patients were enrolled in the study in whom the self-retaining IUC (Puroflex, Urosoft®, Angiomed, Karlsruhe, (Germany) was

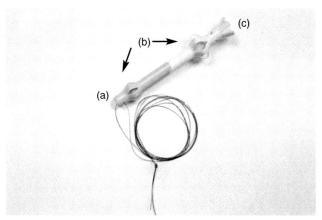

Figure 45.1. *Intraurethral catheter (IUC): (a) distal end with pull-back thread; (b) two self-retaining baskets; (c) crown-like intravesical proximal end.*

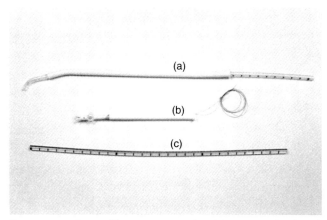

Figure 45.2. *Disposable IUC insertion kit: (a) insertion sheath with Tiemann catheter; (b) cartridge containing IUC; (c) pusher.*

inserted (Fig. 45.1). Of these 130 patients, 100 had an indwelling catheter before the current treatment.

Technique

The device is available in lengths of 35–70 mm to accommodate varying prostatic urethral lengths and is designed to be placed in the bladder neck and prostatic urethra through a specially designed disposable insertion kit (Fig. 45.2). The insertion technique of the device is simple and is performed under local anaesthesia with lignocaine (lidocaine) jelly, in the outpatient clinic. The length of each patient's prostatic urethra was known from ultrasonography. To ensure that the crown and proximal basket were located in the bladder neck, an IUC 10–15 mm longer than the prostatic urethra was chosen.

To facilitate the insertion of the IUC, 50–100 ml saline is infused through the indwelling catheter. The catheter is removed and the urethra lubricated with 10 ml lignocaine jelly. A penis clamp is attached for 10 minutes. The patient is placed in the lithotomy position and the insertion sheath with the Tiemann catheter in it is introduced into the bladder. The cartridge containing the IUC is approximated to the insertion sheath, and the IUC is advanced from the cartridge into the insertion sheath and further into the bladder, using the pusher (Fig. 45.3). The sheath is pulled back when the urologist senses (from low resistance within the sheath) that the crown and proximal basket of the IUC have left the insertion sheath. The pusher is kept in place until the IUC is expelled from the sheath. The sheath and pusher are removed from the urethra; the IUC is then partially in the bladder and partially in the urethra.

In order to position the IUC properly in the urethra, a urethroscopy is performed. The IUC is pulled back (using the thread connected to the end of the IUC), until its distal end is located 1–2 cm distal to the vermontanum. The suture is left outside the urethra for 24–48 h until the patient voids satisfactorily; it is then cut and removed. If necessary, the IUC can easily be removed by lubricating the urethra and pulling the suture out, or by using a biopsy forceps. The time of IUC insertion is essentially the same as the time necessary for cystoscopy.

There is also an additional possibility for IUC insertion through a 22 Fr cystoscope sheath, using a similar technique (Fig. 45.4). The IUC is pushed into the bladder through the cystoscope sheath with the help of the insertion sheath. Patients commonly experience discomfort and an urge to void for the first 2–3 days following IUC insertion. The reasons for that may be irritable bladder due to a long-standing (for weeks or months) indwelling catheter, the irritation caused by the IUC insertion and the commonly present urinary tract infection.

Monitoring

Antibiotic therapy was started 24–48 h before IUC insertion, and continued for 5–7 days. Patients were closely followed up after the procedure, for

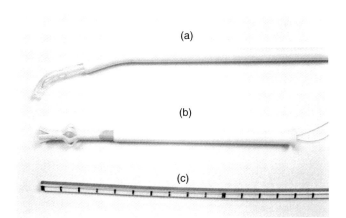

Figure 45.3. *Closer view of Figure 45.2.*

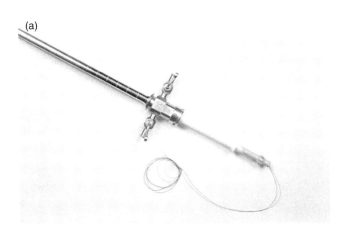

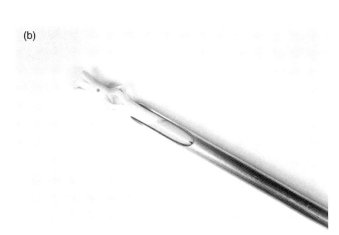

Figure 45.4. *(a) Pushing the IUC into the cystoscope sheath; (b) IUC exiting from the sheath towards the bladder neck.*

symptomatology, continence, residual urine volume and urinary infection. Urine cultures were taken weekly for the first 2 weeks, then monthly. Ultrasonography for measuring residual urine was also performed weekly for the first 2 weeks; subsequently the patients were seen monthly. Cystourethrograms were performed 10–14 days after insertion of the IUCs for the first six study patients. Urinary flow rates were assessed in the first 30 patients. Although all the patients were followed up for urinary infection, after the first 20 IUC insertions a special study was started to examine the infection rate after short- and long-term follow-up: short duration was defined as presence of the IUC for 1–4 weeks; long duration was defined as the IUC remaining in place for over 4 weeks. Only after completion of the study into the infection rate in the presence of IUC, did the follow-up involving urine cultures and ultrasound examinations become less intense.

A short study in a relatively younger group of patients, in whom the catheter was replaced by the IUC, was performed to evaluate the sexual behaviour of those men with the IUC. The patients and their female partners were either asked to answer a specific questionnaire or invited for a special interview to evaluate the patients's sexual activity while sustaining the IUC.

Results

A total of 130 IUCs were inserted in 112 patients (range 54–100 years), median 73.5 years). Of those patients, 100 had a catheter indwelling for from 1 week to over 3 years; 18 patients agreed to have their IUC changed after about 6 months, according to the authors' initial suggestion. In 105/130 cases the IUC remained in place successfully for an average period of 12 months (range 1–19 months). In almost 50% of cases the follow-up was of 6 months or more. Of the 130 insertions, 25 (19%) failed and the IUCs had to be removed earlier than anticipated. The reasons for early removal were incorrect placement (8), high residual urine and severe frequency (8), displacement of the IUC (5) and obstruction by clot (2), stone (1) or suture (1).

Six IUCs were removed at open prostatectomy, 6.5–8 months after successful insertion. One had a stone formed at the intravesical portion, which did not cause obstruction; of the other five, three had encrustations. No significant changes in the mucosa of the prostatic urethra were seen macroscopically during urethroscopy or on histological examination of the prostatectomy specimens. All the 105 patients were fully continent. Voiding was satisfactory, but 21% suffered some degree of frequency. In a subgroup of 30 patients with the device in place for over 3 months, the mean flow rates obtained were 8.2 ml/s. Residual urine was minimal and regarded as physiological in all cases.

A group of 65 patients were evaluated for urine infection rate in the presence of the IUC. Between October 1988 and October 1990, 83 IUC insertions were evaluated in this group of 65 patients, whose ages were 58—100 years, with a mean age of 74.4 years. Of these patients, 55 had an indwelling catheter for 1–153 weeks prior to the IUC insertion (mean duration 17.3 weeks). The underlying diseases contraindicating surgery in the group of patients are listed in Table 45.1.

Of 83 IUCs, 12 (14.5%) developed bacteriuria; only in three cases (3.6%) did clinical urinary tract infection (UTI) with high fever necessitate vigorous antibiotic therapy.

Short-term IUCs

In a group of patients with short-term IUCs, 12 devices remained in place for 1–3 months (mean duration of IUC 2.3 months). These patients were aged 60–93 years (mean age 75.5 years). All patients had a permanent indwelling catheter prior to IUC insertion, lasting from 2 to 108 weeks (mean 19.7 weeks). In this group bacteriuria was not observed in any of the urine cultures

Table 45.1. *Underlying diseases contraindicating surgery in patients with an IUC*

Contraindications	No. of patients
Recent MI or cardiac surgery*	8
Severe congestive heart failure	22
Recent cerebrovascular accident with residual hemiparesis	10
Severe chronic obstructive lung disease	7
Organic mental syndrome or mental retardation	4
Severe renal failure	3
Carcinoma of larynx or lung	3
S/A recent major abdominal surgery	3
General debilitation	5

* Under 8 weeks; MI = myocardial infarction.

obtained during the IUC period, from 1 week after insertion.

Long-term IUCs

The number of IUCs inserted for over 3 months was 78. The duration of the IUC ranged from 3.2 to 19 months (mean 13.8 months). Bacteriuria was observed in 12 of 78 cases (15.4%). On five occasions *Pseudomonas aeriginosa* was isolated; on six *Escherichia coli*, and on one occasion *Staphylococcus aureus* was isolated. In this group of 78 IUCs, only three were the cause of clinical UTI and were removed to enable control of infection.

Twenty-five couples, in whom the males were sustaining the IUC, were evaluated in order to find out if they were able to perform sexually; the age of these men ranged from 59 to 73 years. Among the 25 patients, 12 reported not having sexual activity since before onset of urinary retention. The reasons for abstinence were lack of sexual interest, fear of complications after myocardial infarction, and physical inability following cerebrovascular accident. The other 13 men had adequate sexual activity until the onset of complete urinary retention, had no sexual activity while they had a catheter, and renewed their sexual function after the catheter was replaced by the IUC.

Discussion

The damage caused by a permanent indwelling urinary catheter, as well as the discomfort imposed on the patients, are well documented in the literature.[12–18] Prostatectomy is still the only definite procedure that rids patients of their discomfort permanently. However, since BPH with urinary discomfort and retention is often a disease of elderly patients, coexisting severe diseases sometimes render surgery a life-threatening procedure. An alternative, offering relief of obstructive urinary symptoms without the high risk of infectious complications associated with the indwelling catheter, may be an excellent solution for those patients. Also, in the context of public medicine where the waiting period for surgery may be prolonged, patients could be temporarily relieved of the discomfort of an indwelling urinary catheter by the IUC. The IUC seems to give an appropriate solution to the patients in both groups.

Patients in whom the device has been successfully inserted do not have a urine collection bag, are free of the damage to body image, may continue sexual life (extremely difficult with the indwelling urinary catheter),[19] and have a much lower risk of developing severe infectious complications. In the group of patients who had the IUC for up to 4 weeks, bacteriuria was not observed, probably because of the antibiotic treatment before and after IUC insertion. Moreover, in patients with a long-term IUC, clinical UTI occurred in only three cases, with an overall clinical infection rate of 3.6%.[6]

When a patient is either temporarily or permanently unfit for surgery, or surgery has to be postponed for other 'technical' reasons other alleviating steps are required. Many patients ultimately have an indwelling Foley catheter for prolonged periods; others suffer the misery of nocturia, daytime frequency and possibly dribbling. The intra-urethral spirals or stents are intended to obviate the need for the Foley catheter, to reduce the infection rate and to restore a man's ability to undertake everyday tasks and to resume normal sexual activity. The correct insertion of each device allows a good urine stream, complete bladder evacuation and good continence. Fabian was the first to report on the use of a stent located in the prostatic urethra to relieve urinary retention.[2] Since then, several modifications have been made and put into clinical use.[3–6,20] Williams and colleagues[21] have successfully used an expandable tubular stent of stainless steel mesh in patients with infravesical obstruction. These stents are to remain permanently in the prostatic urethra and their structure allows epithelium to grow and cover the stent.[22,23] All other stents are basically designed to be changed periodically, although clinical experience is not long enough to allow conclusions to be made as to the exact time of replacement.

Metal spirals in use are intended not to cause local inflammation.[2,3,20–24] When such devices are correctly positioned, patients can achieve a good urinary stream, with good urine control.

The IUC, made from polyurethane, appears to be a simpler and more physiological prosthesis and is much more economical. It is easy to insert, either via the endoscope or without it, using the insertion set supplied. Its removal is undoubtedly easier to achieve, as nothing more than a pair of forceps is required. The IUC also provides a good stream, with no residual urine in the bladder and no clinical signs of infection. A total of 218 IUC insertions have been reported in the medical literature,[7,8,10] with a success rate of up to 84%[7] during a maximal period of 19 months.[10]

The endo-urethral metal devices do not allow a catheter to be inserted if obstruction does occur. The IUC can be pushed into the bladder by a catheter. Not all endo-urethral devices would enable an endoscope to pass into the bladder. This is in contrast to the expandable mesh stent,[21,22] which allows cystoscopic viewing and manipulation within the bladder.

The contraindications for the use of the devices are bladder tumours, bladder stones and probably the immediate post-ESWL (extracorporeal shock-wave lithotripsy) period.[6] The authors are not aware of any other contraindication and, in view of a relatively low price and the high success rate achieved, suggest the use of the IUC in any man in need of a temporary indwelling catheter for more than a few days. Patients who need an indwelling catheter for a longer period, such as patients temporarily unfit for surgery or those waiting for prostatic surgery, will probably benefit from all intra-urethral devices. Prostatic stents may also serve as a permanent viable alternative to surgery in poor-risk patients or those unwilling to undergo prostatectomy. In these cases they will have to be replaced within what seem to be the optimal period of 6–12 months if encrustations are to be prevented. The question of the relatively higher immediate cost in comparison to the standard Foley catheter has to be weighed with the known increased risks of infection and stricture formation while using the latter, as well as the need for a more frequent replacement of a Foley catheter. No doubt, extensive use, technical advances and free competition will make these devices more attractive to both patients and urologists.

The fact that an intraurethral catheter was found to preserve normal sexual activity in men with complete urinary retention[19] makes the IUC even more attractive to patients as an alternative to an indwelling catheter.

References

1. Sant G R, Long J P. Benign prostatic hyperplasia. In: Sant G R (ed) Pathophysiologic principles of urology. Oxford: Blackwell Scientific, 1994: 123–154
2. Fabian K M. Der intraporostatische 'Partiell Katheter' (Urologische Spirale). Urologe 1980; 236–238

3. Fabian K M. Der intraprostatische 'Partielle Katheter' (Urologische Spirale) II. Urologe 1984; 23A: 229–233

4. Nording J, Holm H H, Klarskov P et al. The intraprostatic spiral: a new device for insertion with the patient under local anesthesia and with ultrasonic guidance with 3 months of follow-up. J Urol 1989; 142: 756–758

5. Nissenkorn I. Experience with a new self-retaining intraurethral catheter in patients with urinary retention: a preliminary report. J Urol 1989; 142: 92–94

6. Nissenkorn I. A new self-retaining intraurethral device. Br J Urol 1990; 65: 197–200

7. Schulman C C. Intraurethral catheter (IUC). The Belgian Experience. First International Symposium on Urological Stents, Jerusalem, Israel. October 1996. Abstract O13.12

8. Ebert W, Ganz A, Walz P H. The temporary intraurethral catheter (IUC) as a diagnostic tool. First International Symposium on Urological Stents, Jerusalem, Israel, October 1996. Abstract O10.8

9. Chen Y, Greenstein A, Matzkin H et al. Treatment of urination difficulties in patients within benign prostatic hypertrophy (BPH) with an internal urethral catheter. J Urol 1989; 141: 4(2) 235A

10. Nissenkorn I. The intraurethral catheter (IUC) in the treatment of benign prostatic hyperplasia. First International Symposium on Urological Stents, Jerusalem, Israel, October 1996. Abstract O4.1

11. Sant G R, Meares E M Jr. Urinary tract infections. In: Sant G R (ed) Pathophysiologic principles of urology. Oxford: Blackwell Scientific, 1994; 271–298

12. Garibaldi R A, Burke J P, Dickman M L et al. Factors predisposing to bacteriuria during indwelling urethral catheterisation. N Engl J Med 1974; 291: 215–219

13. Harley R W, Hooton R M, Culver D H. Nosocomial infection in U.S. hospitals 75–76. Estimated frequency by selected characteristics of patients. J Med 1981; 70: 947–959

14. Jepsen O B, Larsen S O, Dankert J et al. Urinary tract infection and bacteraemia in hospitalized medical patients. A European multicentre prevalence survey on nosocomial infection. J Hosp Infect 1982; 3: 241–252

15. Culley C C. Nosocomial urinary tract infections. Surg Clin North Am 1988; 68: 1147–1153

16. Resnic M I. Preventing catheter-associated UTIs. Infec Urol 1988; 1: 18–21

17. Leidberg H. Catheter induced urethral inflammatory reaction and urinary tract infection. An experimental and clinical study. Scand J Urol Nephrol 1989; 124 (suppl): 1–8

18. Mincie H L, Warren J W. Reasons for replacement of long-term urethral catheters: implications for randomized trials. J Urol 1990; 143: 507–509

19. Richter S. Intraprostatic and intraurethral stents, and their impact on sexual function. Presented at the First International Symposium on Andrology, Bioengineering and Sexual Rehabilitation, Paris, France, July 1995; 226–229

20. Fabricius P G, Matz M, Zepnick H. Die endourethrospirale eine alternative zum dauercatheter? Z Arztl Forbild (Jena) 1983; 77: 482–485

21. Williams G, Jager R, McLoughlin J et al. Use of stents for treating obstruction of urinary outflow in patients unfit for surgery. Br Med J 1989; 298: 1429–1430

22. Milroy E J G, Chapple C, Eldin A et al. A new treatment for urethral strictures: a permanently implanted urethral stent. J Urol 1989; 141: 1120–1122

23. Chapple C R, Milroy E J G, Rickards D. Permanently implanted urethral stent for prostatic obstruction in the unfit patient. Br J Urol 1990; 66: 58–65

24. Nielsen K K, Klarskov P, Nordling J et al. The intraprostatic spiral. New treatment for urinary retention. Br J Urol 1990; 65: 500–503

Clinical and cost comparison of long-term catheterization and Memokath prostatic stenting

A. A. Chaudry and C. M. Booth

46

Introduction

Bladder outflow obstruction (BOO) due to benign prostatic enlargement is the commonest cause of lower urinary tract symptoms in the elderly male. Although transurethral resection of the prostate gland (TURP) is still accepted as the gold standard for the relief of moderate to severe obstruction, it is not without its dangers, particularly in men who have concomitant disease adding to the risk of complications or even death. With a growing elderly population, unfit males presenting with severe lower urinary tract symptoms or urinary retention due to BOO are likely to pose an increasing management problem. Thus a plethora of alternative less-invasive options (Table 46.1) has emerged in recent years. Despite these advances, many elderly men, perhaps fearing surgery, present late and are treated by long-term catheterization in the community with continuing care from the district nursing service (DNS). Contact with the urology team occurs only occasionally when major problems arise, but minor problems are frequent and can cause considerable suffering.

Table 46.1. *Alternative treatment options to TURP*

- Medication
- Transrectal hyperthermia
- Transurethral thermotherapy
- Balloon dilatation
- Laser therapy
- High-energy shock-wave therapy
- Focused ultrasound
- Prostatic spirals and stents

Use of the DNS

The burden placed on the DNS by community catheter care for elderly men may be enormous, especially in retirement areas such as the authors' district on the east coast of southern England. For example, in 1995 in their Health District alone, with a population of 320 000, a total of 607 male patients were seen by the DNS for catheter insertions, changes or continued catheter care. Although most patients required these services only temporarily, 161 patients required ten or more visits for long-term catheter care. In 1 year, the total number of visits paid to these patients by the DNS amounted to a huge total of 10 115. Furthermore, this total does not include patients seen by primary care doctors for the same purpose.

A detailed breakdown of the visits by the DNS to catheterized patients is shown in Table 46.2. While 1264 visits were for urethral/suprapubic catheterization, further attendance by the DNS to these patients merely to carry out bladder wash-outs or simply for catheter care amounted to 8682 visits. Several patients required more than 100 visits and two were visited almost twice every day, 698 and 764 times respectively. The District Nurses spent approximately 919 hours attending these two patients alone.

The cost of such an unexpectedly large number of DNS visits to patients with long-term catheters is consequently enormous and in the authors' district in 1995 totalled £428 141 (Table 46.2) — approximately £700 per patient per annum. Long-term catheterization is not a cheap treatment option.

Alternatives

Unfortunately, it is often difficult to assess the reason for, or the diagnosis leading to, the original catheterization. It may well be that the majority of these men failed to fulfil the basic criteria necessary to qualify for a TURP — the physical and/or mental ability to reach, recognize and utilize a toilet or even a bottle appropriately. Nevertheless, the suspicion exists that a significant number of men were catheterized because their primary carer considered they were not physically fit enough to undergo a TURP. However, the recent introduction of minimally invasive alternatives to TURP for treating BOO may now outdate this

Table 46.2. *District Nurse Service (DNS) activities and costs (1995)*

DNS activity (1995)	No of visits to 607 patients[*]	Catheters	Cost (£) DNS Visits[†]	Total
Catheterization	1093	10 099[≠]	44 813	54 912
Suprapubic catheterization	171	3271[§]	7011	10 282
Teaching intermittent catheterization	42	41[″]	1722	1763
Catherization to check post-op residual	1	9	41	50
Fitting initial Uro-Flo catheter	1	6	41	47
Catheter care	6135	–	251 535	251 535
Bladder wash-out	2547	–	104 427	104 427
Catheter removal	125	–	5125	5125
Total	10 115	13 426	414 715	428 141

[*]161 patients had >10 visits; [†]£41/visit; [≠]£9.24/catheter; [§]£19.13/catheter; [″]£0.98/catheter.

assumption in many cases. In particular, techniques that do not require general anaesthesia, such as thermo-ablation of the prostate and prostatic stents, may well offer an alternative to long-term catheterization with an improved quality of life at reasonable cost.

Use of prostatic stents

The authors approached prostatic stenting from the theoretical standpoint that the permanently implanted epithelializing stents were too risky to use in unfit patients. Their removal in the event of failure is difficult and requires general or regional anaesthesia, a complete contradiction to the concept of their use in frail patients. Opting to use 'temporary' non-epithelializing stents, the authors initially gained experience with the Prostakath® (Engineers & Doctors, Kvistgaard, Denmark).[1] This could be inserted under purely local urethral anaesthesia but, when complications arose, this stent, too, required removal under general anaesthesia.

Use of the Memokath

The introduction of 'shape memory' alloy technology to stenting in 1988 allowed a major advance, since the thermolabile properties of the nickel/titanium alloy used to make the Memokath® (Engineers & Doctors) for the first time allowed both easy insertion and removal under

local anaesthetic; indeed, insertion is almost as easy as catheterization.[2]

The Department of Urology at Colchester General Hospital has been involved from the onset in the clinical development of the Memokath®.[3] Since 1992, some 300 Memokaths have been inserted using three design developments aimed at simplifying insertion and removal and reducing the stent failure rate due to migration, mucosal blockage and encrustation.

During 1995, Memokaths were inserted into 57 patients aged 67–91 (mean 79) years presenting with symptomatic benign prostatic enlargement (34) or urinary retention (23) who were considered to be at varying risk from a conventional TURP (ASA III and IV).

The patients were monitored at 3 weeks then 6-monthly intervals after stent insertion using the International Prostate Symptom Score, urine culture and assessment of flow rate with an annual X-ray to exclude stent migration or encrustation.

The outcome in these patients is shown in Figure 46.1. Stent success is defined as a satisfactorily functioning stent to date (39), a functioning stent at death from a non-urological cause (6), or elective removal of a functioning stent (3). Five of these patients have required cystoscopic readjustment of the stent under local anaesthetic. Only four stents have failed during a minimum of 12 months follow up (Table 46.3).

Table 46.3. *Complications and failures of Memokath® stent (1995)*

Complication	Action	No. of patients	Outcome
Persistent UTI	Stent removed	1	Had TURP
Urinary incontinence	Stent removed	1	Had TURP
	Stent removed	1	Had TURP; still incontinent
	Stent readjusted	2	Happy with stent
Urinary retention	Stent readjusted	3	Happy with stent
	Stent removed	1	Had TURP; Hypocontractile bladder on urodynamics
Fear of possible complications	Working stent removed (patient's choice)	2	Long-term catheter
Severe immobility	Working stent removed (patient's choice)	1	Long-term catheter

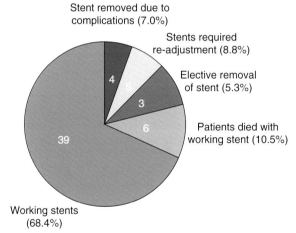

Figure 46.1. *Success rate for stents used in 57 frail patients in 1995.*

Costs

The total cost of Memokath® stent insertion in the authors' unit at 1995 prices is calculated as £771 per patient. Stent removal or readjustment costs £257 per patient; a detailed description of these costs and follow up is given in Table 46.4.

Perhaps because of the simplicity and low initial cost of catheterization a substantial number of high risk patients with BOO due to benign prostatic enlargement may be left in the community with long-term catheters. However, the true cost of catheterization and its several complications may be enormous, but appears to have been overlooked. Long-term catheterization and most catheter complications are dealt with mainly in the community and the cost of such services may not become noticeable as several agencies share the burden over a long time span. Yearly primary care and DNS block contracts may also mask the actual costs, and the authors' estimate of costs in this district does not include hospital costs incurred by emergency attendances and admissions.

Conclusions

Although prostatic stenting has maintained a role over recent years, it has been considered an expensive alternative to catheterization owing to its initial cost. Moreover, prostatic stenting as an alternative to TURP has gained only limited acceptance, probably because the complications experienced with 'permanent' stents have brought prostatic stenting in general into some disrepute. This assessment of male patients in the community, however, shows that long-term catheterization may not provide optimal care and is often very expensive. Prostatic stenting therefore appears to offer an improved clinical alternative that is also viable in terms of cost. Certainly this study requires further investigation and ultimately needs to be tested in a comparative clinical trial.

Table 46.4. *Cost of Memokath® stent insertion, removal and follow-up (1995)*

Activity	Materials, procedures and investigations	Expenses Cost (£)	Total (£)
Stent insertion	Memokath® stent	514	
	Cystoscopy	257	
	Consultation		771
Memokath® stent re-adjustment and/or removal	Consultation		
	Cystoscopy	257	257
Follow-up visit 1 (6 months)	Consultation		
	Flow-rate and ultrasound scan to check residual urine	70	
	Mid-stream urine for culture and sensitivity	5	75
Follow-up visit 2 (12 months)	Consultation		
	Flow rate and ultrasound scan to check residual urine	70	
	Mid-stream urine for culture and sensitivity	5	
	X-ray KUB* (to check any encrustation and position of stent)	13	88

KUB: kidney, ureter, bladder.

References

1. Booth C M, Alam A, Al-Dabbagh M A. The Prostakath®: an alternative to prostatectomy for acute retention, Irish J Med Sci 1992; 161: 21

2. Poulsen A L, Schou J, Ovesen H, Nordling J. Memokath®: a second generation of intraprostatic spirals. Br J Urol 1993; 72: 331–334

3. Booth C M, Al-Dabbagh M A, Lyth D R, Fowler C G. First medical application of 'memory alloys': a new prostatic stent. Harrogate, England: (Video presentation). British Association of Urological Surgeons, 1993

47

ProstaCoil in the non-surgical management of benign prostatic hyperplasia
D. Yachia

Introduction

A stent is a scaffold placed in a segment of a tubular organ. The term 'stent' is derived from the splint used to stabilize skin grafts, used by a 19th century London dentist, Charles Stent.[1]

In urology, the use of prostatic stents instead of indwelling catheters was introduced in 1980 in Germany by Fabian.[2] He developed a stainless steel coil instead of an indwelling catheter for the management of severe prostatic obstruction, and named this device a 'Partial Catheter' or 'Urologic Spiral'. Subsequently, this stent, and other new intraurethral devices that were introduced for urological use, gained increasing acceptance in daily urological practice, especially in Europe.[3–7] These were intraluminal devices that were left temporarily in the prostatic urethra and then either removed or replaced with a new one. Later, stents developed for vascular use were adapted for permanent implantation into the prostatic urethra.[8,9] Based on the same concepts, some of these stents were developed further for the treatment of urethral stricture disease. Today, the urethral stents available fall into two major categories – temporary stents and permanent stents (Tables 47.1, 47.2).

Initially all the temporary prostatic stents (Urospiral, Prostakath, ProstaCoil, Intraurethral catheter, Memokath 028, Barnes Stent, Trestle, Biofix) and the urethral temporary stents (UroCoil System stents, Urethrospiral, Memokath 044) were developed for use in the male prostatic or anterior urethra. The UroCoil/ProstaCoil stents were developed further to be used in various parts of the body, such as the biliary tract (EndoCoil), the oesophagus (EsophaCoil), the peripheral vascular system (VascuCoil) including the coronaries (CardioCoil) and the carotid (CarotidCoil).

All temporary stents hold the urethral lumen open by remaining in the urethral lumen and do not become incorporated into the urethral wall. All the permanent stents (Urolume, Memotherm, Ultraflex, Titan), which were initially developed as vascular stents and later adapted for urological use, are intended to be covered ultimately by the urethral epithelium and to remain permanently in the body. The characteristics of the temporary and permanent stents available and the sites of obstruction where they can be used in the urethra are summarized in Table 47.3.

This chapter covers the author's 10 years experience with the temporary ProstaCoil in the non-surgical management of benign prostatic hyperplasia (BPH). The results presented in this chapter are based on our experience using the ProstaCoil stents (Fig. 47.1a,b). Most probably, similar results can be obtained with other large caliber temporary prostatic stents.

Table 47.1. *Characteristics of temporary prostatic stents*

| Stent | Expansion | Sizes | | Material | Indwelling time (months) |
		Calibre (Fr)	Length (mm)		
Urospiral (Fabian stent)	Non-expanding	21	40–80	Stainless steel	≤12
Prostakath	Non-expanding	21	40–80	Gold-plated stainless steel	≤12
Intra-urethral catheter (IUC)	Non-expanding	16–18	25–80	Polyurethane	≤6
ProstaCoil	Self-expanding	24/30	40–80	Nitinol	≤36
Memokath 028	Heat-expandable	22/34	30–70	Nitinol	≤36
Biofix	Self-expanding	21	45–85	Polylactide polymer	≤6
Barnes stent	Non-expanding	16	50	Polyurethane	≤3
Trestle	Non-expanding	22	75	Polyurethane	≤6

Table 47.2. *Characteristics of permanent prostatic stents*

Stent	Expansion	Size Calibre (Fr)	Size Length (mm)	Material	Indwelling time (months)
Urolume/Wallstent	Self-expanding	42	20–40	Steel 'superalloy'	Permanent
Titan	Balloon expandable	33	19–58	Titanium	Permanent
Memotherm	Heat expandable	42	20–80	Nitinol	Permanent
Ultraflex	Self-expanding	42	20–50	Nitinol	Permanent

Table 47.3. *Urethral stents and their use in urethral obstruction*

Stent	Site of obstruction
Urospiral (Fabian stent)	Prostatic urethra
Prostakath	Prostatic urethra
Urethrospiral	Bulbar urethra
Intra-urethral catheter (IUC)	Prostatic and bulbar urethra
Barnes stent	Prostatic urethra*
Trestle	Prostatic urethra*
Memokath 028	Prostatic urethra
Memokath 044	Bulbar urethra
Titan	Prostatic urethra
Urolume (Wallstent)	Prostatic and bulbar urethra
Ultraflex	Prostatic and bulbar urethra
Memotherm	Prostatic and bulbar urethra
ProstaCoil	Prostatic urethra
UroCoil	Penile urethra
UroCoil-S	Bulbomembranous urethra
UroCoil-twin	Prostatic + bulbomembranous urethra

*After heat therapy.

Indications for ProstaCoil insertion

All patients with benign or malignant prostatic obstruction and who require insertion of an indwelling catheter are candidates for ProstaCoil insertion. Furthermore, in patients who have an absolute indication for transurethral resection of the prostate (TURP), such as those with a large volume of residual urine, or upper urinary tract deterioration, but who are not suitable for surgery because of concomitant conditions and thus fall into category ASA grade 5 (American Society of Anesthesiologists), the ProstaCoil can be used as an alternative to surgery. A distinct group of patients in whom the ProstaCoil can be used comprises those younger patients in whom prostate surgery is indicated but who refuse it because of fear of postoperative impotence.

Long-term stenting is contraindicated in the following conditions: urethral abscess or fistula; acute

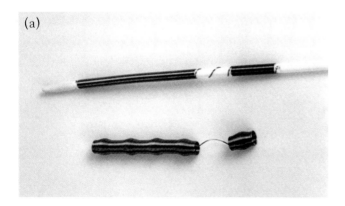

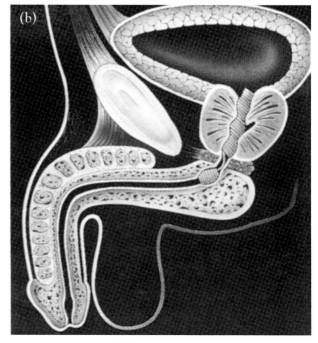

Figure 47.1. *The ProstaCoil. (a) ProstaCoil on its delivery catheter in its constricted form and after its release in its expanded wavy form. The ProstaCoil is composed of three segments: a long segment for stenting the prostatic urethra (prostatic segment); a short anchoring segment positioned in the bulbar urethra (bulbar segment), and a single helical wire connecting the two segments (trans-sphincteric spacer). (b) Position of the ProstaCoil after deployment.*

prostatitis or prostatic abscess; cystolithiasis; frequently recurring bladder tumours; purulent urethritis; and acute lower urinary tract infection. Insertion of a stent during the use of anticoagulants, such as warfarin and heparin, is contraindicated because of the risk of traumatic bleeding; in cooperation with the physician who prescribed them, these medications should be withdrawn for a week before insertion. They can be restarted when the voided urine becomes clear. Patients receiving low dose aspirin also may bleed during insertion of the stent; interruption of this medication for 5–7 days is also recommended in this group of patients.

Insertion technique

The ProstaCoil, in its present configuration, is inserted under fluoroscopic guidance. Trials of its endoscopic delivery failed because of design inadequacies of the endoscopic delivery device, causing high rates of malplacement. A step-by-step explanation of the entire procedure, during discussion of the stent option with the patient, helps to obtain his cooperation during the procedure and his compliance afterwards.

It is well known that insertion of any indwelling foreign body into the urethra causes irritative symptoms. Since the calibre of the released stent is much larger than that of an average indwelling catheter, in a patient who is without an indwelling catheter it is advisable to insert a 20 Fr Foley catheter a day before stent insertion, in order to accustom him to the feeling of a foreign body, and also to prepare the urethra to accept the stent. If the patient already has a smaller indwelling catheter, this should be replaced with one of 20 Fr. Antibiotic cover is also started a day before the procedure. In chronic urinary tract infection, appropriate antibiotics should be started 2–3 days before the procedure and continued for at least 2 weeks.

Strict adherence to the steps for insertion enables the best results to be obtained. Although the entire procedure is conducted under fluoroscopy, it is helpful to perform the procedure in a set-up that allows either rigid or flexible cystoscopy, which may be necessary in some cases. It is important to prepare all the necessary equipment before starting the insertion procedure and to have all sizes of the stent at hand. Also needed are 100 ml contrast, adequate amounts of anaesthetic lubricating gel,

an irrigation syringe (50–60 ml) and 5 ml and 10 ml syringes.

The ProstaCoil kit contains the following: a mounted stent; a special 14 Fr graduated balloon catheter marked with radiopaque dots at each centimetre, starting 1 cm from the base of the balloon and with a single opening at its tip (Fig. 47.2a,b,c); a 0.045 inch straight soft-tip guidewire, and radiopaque stickers to mark the anatomical landmarks.

The insertion procedure is started by removing the indwelling catheter and filling the urethra with 10–20 ml anaesthetic lubricating gel (i.e. 2% lignocaine). The patient is then prepared and draped. It is important to dry any excess antiseptic solution on the skin, because the marker stickers do not adhere to wet skin. As an alternative, the landmarks can be marked by using injection needles stuck transversely to the skin overlying the landmark. The ruler catheter is inserted 3–4 cm into the urethra and its balloon is inflated with 2–3 ml contrast for performing an ascending urethrogram. As a reaction to the retrograde injection of the contrast, patients usually contract the external sphincter. This is the first landmark that should be marked by sticking one of the radiopaque markers on to the skin at the level of the sphincter (Fig. 47.3a). The balloon is then deflated, and the ruler catheter is inserted into the bladder and, again, its balloon is inflated with 10 ml contrast. By gentle retraction of the ruler catheter, the balloon is positioned at the bladder neck. Counting the dots between the base of the balloon (bladder neck) and the external sphincter marker gives the exact length of the prostatic urethra (Fig. 47.3b). The bladder is then filled with 200–250 ml of diluted contrast and, under fluoroscopic control, the 0.045 inch guidewire is inserted through the ruler catheter until its soft tip makes one or two loops in the bladder. After deflation of the balloon the catheter is removed, leaving behind the guidewire. As 0.5–1.0 cm of the stent should protrude into the bladder, a stent 1 cm longer than the measured prostatic urethral length is chosen. After generous lubrication of the urethra, the stent is inserted over the guidewire, monitoring its advancement under fluoroscopy. Pushing of the stent is stopped when the trans-sphincteric spacer reaches the external sphincter marker (Fig. 47.3c). Although, at this point, the unreleased prostatic segment of the stent seems to protrude excessively into the bladder, this

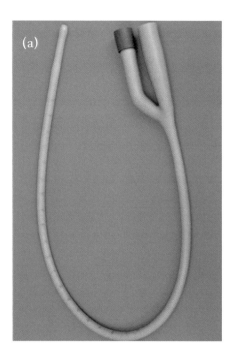

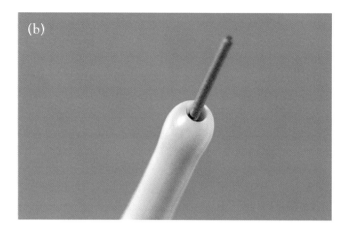

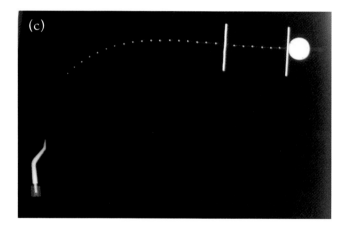

Figure 47.2. *(a) Foley-like 'ruler' catheter, showing radiopaque dots along the catheter. (b) The ruler catheter has a Council-type tip opening, allowing passage to a guidewire. (c) X-ray of the ruler catheter. The balloon is filled with contrast. The marker just below the balloon represents the bladder neck and the second marker the external sphincter. The radiopaque dots start 1 cm below the balloon. The distance between each dot is 1 cm. This ruler catheter, by coapting to the curves of the prostatic urethra, allows very accurate measurement of the distance between the bladder neck and the external sphincter.*

segment shortens when the stent is released. It is important to keep the bladder full, to prevent bladder perforation, and also to keep the trans-sphincteric part aligned with the sphincter marker. At this point, two or three half-turns of the locking handle of the stent will release the bladder end of the stent (Fig. 47.3d). The expansion and shortening of the stent can be followed by fluoroscopy. If necessary, it is still possible to make some minor positioning changes at this point, but it is impossible to remove and reinsert the stent after its distal end has been released. When the position of the stent is found to be satisfactory, the locking handle is given five or six full-turns, until the bulbar segment of the stent is also seen fluoroscopically to have been released. After its release, the stent continues to expand with a rotary movement. In fibrotic and cancerous prostates, in particular, where the tissue is more firm, it is important to wait 2–3 minutes (sometimes more) until the stent has fully expanded before the delivery catheter is gently removed, but

leaving the guidewire in place. Asking the patient to urinate and then stop the stream voluntarily enables the integrity of the external sphincter to be checked (Fig. 47.3e). If the patient cannot void at this moment, the ascending urethrogram is repeated to check the accurate placement of the stent. Another way to check the integrity of the sphincter is to ask the patient to cough: if the tubular part of the stent is within the external sphincter, the patient will leak. In such a case, some repositioning can be done using a grasping forceps mounted to a 17 Fr cystoscope. The cystoscope is passed along the guidewire, through the bulbar segment of the stent and, by grasping the trans-sphincteric wire, it can be pulled or pushed until it is correctly positioned. If the patient can void and control the stream, the guidewire is removed. Rarely, some bleeding can be caused during the insertion; this usually subsides within a few minutes. Since blood clots can obliterate the stent, in cases of prolonged bleeding, after a side hole has been opened above its balloon, the ruler

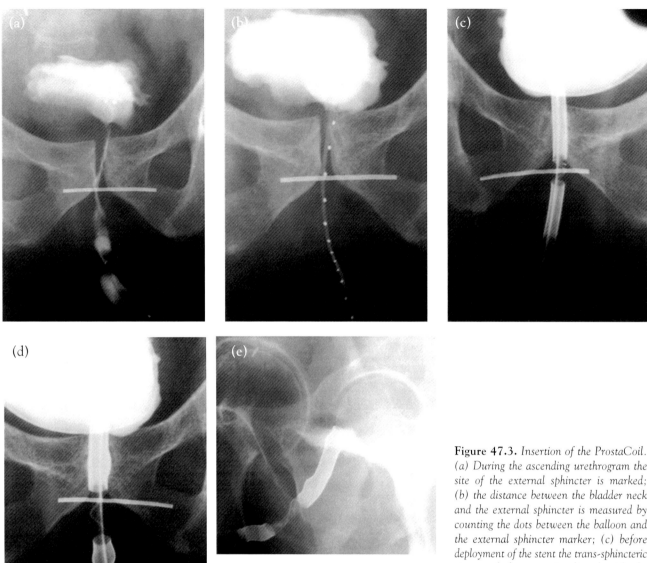

Figure 47.3. *Insertion of the ProstaCoil. (a) During the ascending urethrogram the site of the external sphincter is marked; (b) the distance between the bladder neck and the external sphincter is measured by counting the dots between the balloon and the external sphincter marker; (c) before deployment of the stent the trans-sphincteric spacer of the stent is aligned with the external sphincter marker; (d) the stent is completely released from the delivery catheter, resulting in a change in its diameter and shape; (e) voiding through the stent.*

catheter is reinserted over the guidewire, through the stent into the bladder. This catheter is left in place until the bleeding subsides completely and then it is removed carefully in order not to dislodge the stent.

The entire procedure can be conducted on an outpatient basis. In addition to antibiotic cover, it is advisable to prescribe a non-steroidal anti-inflammatory drug such as diclofenac sodium (100 mg) for 7–10 days to reduce the initial irritative symptoms caused by the stent.

Removal of the stent

The simplest removal technique is endoscopic. Using an endoscopic grasper on a 21 Fr cystoscope, the distal loop of the stent is grasped and the unravelled wire is pulled through the sheath of the endoscope to prevent trauma to the anterior urethra.

A second way to remove the stent is to pass a 12 Fr or 14 Fr Foley catheter through the entire lumen of the stent and inflate the balloon with 2–3 ml saline (or contrast if the procedure is done under fluoroscopy).

Gentle but constant pulling of the stent will dislocate it and bring its tip to the urethral meatus, from where it can be removed manually.

Troubleshooting

Almost all materials used for stent manufacture develop encrustation when in constant contact with urine. This problem can be reduced if the patient has an adequate water intake and, most importantly, an adequate urine output (minimum 1500 ml/day – or more in hot countries). The ProstaCoil stents are intended to be left indwelling for periods of 2–3 years (or more if the lumen remains open) and then replaced with a new one. During this period the stent occasionally may become obliterated, for two reasons: (1) severe encrustation along its lumen; and (2) reactive tissue proliferation below the external sphincter, occluding the entrance to the bulbar segment. In cases where encrustations are causing obliteration the best way to remove the obstruction and save the stent is to use a Lithoclast stone disintegrator. As the encrustations are soft and adhere loosely to the Nitinol wire, they break and peel off easily. The reactive hyperplastic tissue that may develop below the external sphincter in some patients usually does not obstruct the passage, and it disappears without any further treatment after the stent is removed. If this tissue causes obstruction, a 4 Fr ureteral catheter is passed under vision into the bladder and this tissue can be fulgurated using a small calibre cystoscope passed through the short bulbar segment of the stent. Because this tissue is just above the internal rings of the bulbar segment and around the helical trans-sphincteric wire, it is important to avoid touching the wires with the fulgurating ball. After fulguration, a 14 Fr catheter is inserted through the stent and left indwelling for 2–3 days.

Clinical experience and results

Because of the large calibre of the ProstaCoil stent and the possibility of endoscopic follow-up of its lumen, in patients who maintained a good diuresis it has been possible to leave the stent in place for as long as three or four years. This long indwelling time has significantly reduced the cost of its use and has also enabled it to be used instead of transurethral resection of the prostate (TURP) in 11 selected patients who refused surgery.

The ProstaCoil has been used in 199 patients with benign prostatic hyperplasia (BPH) and in 34 patients who had an obstructive prostate (CaP). The BPH patients were also divided into two categories, where 124 were permanently unfit for surgery and were classified as ASA grade 5 and 64 were temporarily unfit for surgery because of recent myocardial infarction or cerebrovascular accident. The use of the ProstaCoil in CaP is presented in Chapter 56 of this book. In the permanently unfit patients, the stent was left indwelling for 24–36 months and then changed to a new one if the patient was still living. However, a group of eight patients who entered the fourth year with the same stent are being followed to see if the same stent will remain unobstructed and can be left in place for four or more years. In the temporarily unfit patients, the stent was left in place until they became eligible for surgery.

The 11 young patients in whom the ProstaCoil was used as an alternative to TURP were aged 45–62 (mean 56) years. Despite having an absolute indication for surgery (such as upper tract deterioration, residual urine more than 200 ml, cystolithiasis, or severe trabeculation – with or without pseudo-diverticulum formation), these patients refused any surgical intervention on their prostate, fearing impotence. The follow-up of these patients is 2–28 (mean 14) months. Despite initial irritative symptoms (which resolved within 1 month), no patient requested removal of the stent. The maximal urinary flow (Q_{max}) increased from 2.2–8 (mean: 4.2) ml/s to 15–36 (mean 21.3) ml/s, with improvement in the patients' symptom score (international prostate symptom score – IPSS) and quality of life assessment (QOL) (Fig. 47.4a,b,c; Table 47.4).

Generally, major complications were not noted. Six patients developed urinary retention after stent insertion, because of blood clots obliterating the lumen; 10 patients complained of perineal burning for a few weeks; 20 patients found sitting on hard chairs uncomfortable. Migration of the ProstaCoil was observed in only one patient; this was due to malpositioning of the stent. Most patients complained of urgency for a few days and six patients noted stress incontinence, which resolved spontaneously within 2–3 weeks. No stent-induced clinical infection was noted; however, despite the antibiotic cover, 24 patients with a longstanding catheter before stent insertion continued to harbour an infection, but this was asymptomatic. Late

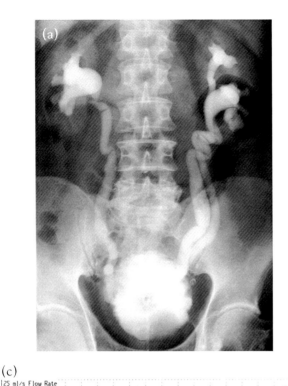

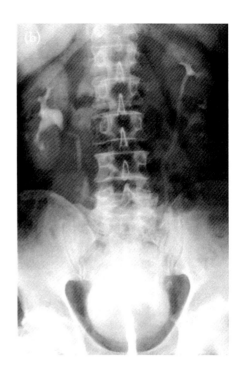

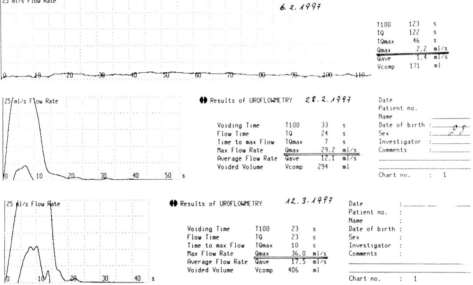

Figure 47.4. (a) IVP of a 62-year-old patient with severe bladder outlet obstruction; (b) complete disappearance of the obstruction, as seen 3 months after insertion of the ProstaCoil; (c) uroflow measurements of the patient before, and 3 and 5 weeks after, stent insertion; Q_{max} has increased significantly from 2.2 to 36 ml/s.

bleeding occurred in one patient for whom coumadine had been administered by his cardiologist. In six patients the stent became obliterated because of stone formation. The stone was disintegrated by Lithoclast in four patients and in two patients the stent was replaced with a new one.

Patients who were sexually active before the onset of the prostatic obstruction were able to resume their sexual activity after the stent had replaced the indwelling catheter. Some of these patients complained of transitory discomfort during orgasm and all of the sexually active patients reported retrograde ejaculation.

Follow-up cystoscopy was conducted in five patients who had transitional cell carcinoma and in two a small tumour could be fulgurated through a 15.5 Fr cystoscope passed through the stent.

Table 47.4. *(a,b) ProstaCoil as an alternative to TURP in healthy patients*

(a) Details of patients

Patients (n)	Age (years)	Prostate volume (cm³)	Residual urine (ml)	Indwelling time (months)
11	45–62 (mean 56)	24–62 (mean 38)	>200	2–26 (mean 10)

(b) Results before and after insertion of ProstaCoil

Symptom score (IPSS)		Uroflow (Q_{max} ml/s)		Quality-of-life assessment index (QOL)	
Before	After	Before	After	Before	After 6 months
26–31 (mean 28.2)	6–12 (mean 9)	2.2–8 (mean 4.2)	15–36 (mean 21.3)	3–5	0–2

Conclusions

Use of the large calibre ProstaCoil is a logical approach to the management of prostatic obstruction and also is an excellent alternative to the use of indwelling catheters or surgery in high-risk patients. The encouraging results obtained with the small group of patients who refused surgery show that the large calibre temporary stents can be a viable non-surgical alternative to TURP in selected patients.

References

1. Sigwart U. Introduction. In: Sigwart U (ed) Endoluminal stenting. London: W B Saunders, 1996: 2–5
2. Fabian K W. Der intraprostatische 'Partial Katheter' (urologische Spirale). Urologe A 1980; 19: 236–238
3. Fabricius P G, Matz M, Zepnick H. Die Endourethralspirale: eine Alternative zum Dauerkatheter. Z Arztl Fortbild (Jena) 1983; 77: 482–485
4. Reuter H J, Oettinger M. Las primeras experiencias con la espiral de acero en lugar del cateter permanente. Arch Esp Urol 1986; 39 (suppl): 65–68
5. Nordling J, Holm H H, Klarskov P et al. The intraprostatic spiral: a new device for insertion with the patient under local anesthesia and with ultrasonic guidance with 3 months followup. J Urol 1989; 142: 756–758
6. Yachia D, Lask D, Rabinson S. Self retaining intraurethral stent: an alternative to long term indwelling catheters or surgery in the treatment of prostatism. AJR 1990; 154: 111–113
7. Nissenkorn S, Richter S. A new self-retaining intraurethral device. An alternative to an indwelling catheter in patients with urinary retention due to intravesical obstruction. Br J Urol 1990; 65: 197–200
8. Milroy E, Chapple C, Eldin A et al. Permanently implanted urethral stent – two year experience and new indications (abstr). J Urol 1989; 141(2) 314A
9. Guazzoni G, Montorsi F, Coulange C et al. A modified prostatic Urolume Wallstent for healthy patients with symptomatic benign prostatic hyperplasia: a European multicenter study. Urology 1994; 44: 364

48

Urolume stents in the management of benign prostatic hyperplasia
J. C. D. Png and C. R. Chapple

Introduction

Benign prostatic hyperplasia (BPH) occurs histologically in approximately 50% of men at the age of 60 and in nearly 100% of men by 80 years.[1] It has been estimated that the prevalence of 'clinical' BPH, defined as an enlargement of the prostate gland to a weight of more than 20 g in the presence of symptoms and/or a urinary flow rate of less than 15 ml/s and without evidence of malignancy was 253/1000 in a sample of 705 men aged 40–79 registered with a group general practice in Scotland.[2] In the USA, Glynn et al.[3] calculated the chance of a 40-year-old-man subsequently requiring a prostatectomy as 29%.

Transurethral resection of the prostate (TURP) is still the traditional therapy of choice for symptomatic BPH and represents the gold-standard[4,5] against which other therapies need to be judged. Although mortality has been decreasing over the last decade, from 1.2% in 1984 to 0.77% in 1990, it is still significant[6–8] and increases with age from 0.39% in the 65–69 years age-group to 1.1% in the 75–79 years age-group and 3.54% in those older than 85 years.[9] This is associated with a significant morbidity of about 18%,[10] which includes a 1% risk of total incontinence, a 2.1% risk of stress incontinence, a 1.9% risk of urge incontinence, a 1.7% risk of vesical neck contractures and a 3.1% risk of urethral strictures.[11] This, coupled with increased public awareness of alternative non-surgical or minimally invasive treatment options, has raised a number of questions as to the appropriate therapy in contemporary practice.

One of the alternative surgical options is a minimally invasive approach using a permanent endoprosthetic stent to tackle the problem of bladder outlet obstruction secondary to BPH. The use of such prostatic stents appears to have a number of advantages: these include a short operating time, minimal blood loss, ease of insertion, a short hospital stay, no indwelling catheter after surgery and the absence of any of the expensive equipment that is often required in other alternative minimally invasive therapies.

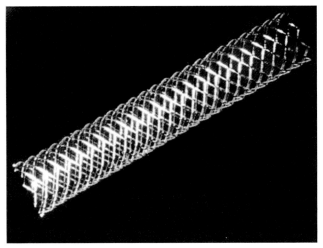

Figure 48.1. *Urolume stent.*

An example of such a stent is the Urolume stent (Fig. 48.1), which is a mesh of corrosion resistant nickel superalloy wire, woven into a flexible expandable tube. It was originally developed for endovascular use by Hans Wallsten, a Swiss national, for the prevention of stenoses after transluminal angioplasty,[12,13] but has been used successfully in the urinary tract for the treatment of urethral strictures[14,15] and, more recently, for the treatment of BPH in patients not fit to undergo TURP.

History of the Urolume stent

The Urolume stent was first used in urology, for the treatment of bulbar urethral strictures that were unresponsive to urethrotomy, by Milroy and Chapple, with fairly good results.[14] Given its success with bulbar strictures, it was used by the same authors[16] for the treatment of 12 patients with prostatic outflow obstruction who were in a high-risk group for surgery. This was successful in resolving the outlet obstruction in 11 patients, with good re-epithelialization of the stent in 6–8 months. In five patients, a length of stent protruded into the bladder, giving rise to encrustations in two. This study was extended 3 years later to include 54 unfit patients with prostatic outflow obstruction.[17] Four patients were unable to void after the procedure owing to chronic retention, leaving 50 patients who could void immediately postoperatively. A number of patients developed irritative urinary symptoms at 1–3 months after the procedure but this resolved after 9 months in the majority of patients. Symptom scores and peak flows were also significantly improved after stent insertion by more than twofold. Encrustation was a problem in 14 patients (25.9%) and occurred in those patients with either a protrusion of the stent into the bladder or with incomplete re-epithelialization. Only one patient developed incontinence as a result of stent encroachment over the distal sphincter mechanism; this was easily rectified. In all, six (11.1%) stents had to be removed — three because of problems with positioning, one because of distal obstruction secondary to prostatic adenocarcinoma and two because of severe urge incontinence in the presence of persistent detrusor instability.

Because of the relatively good results of the Urolume stent in unfit patients, a number of studies involving fit, healthy men with BPH was carried out both in Europe and in the USA.

A European series by Milroy et al.[18] in 140 patients with an 18-month follow-up showed similar findings to the earlier studies by Milroy and Chapple.[17] There were 94 patients with symptomatic BPH and 46 with acute urinary retention. Both groups showed significant improvements in peak urine flow and symptom score, from a preoperative mean peak flow of 9.3 ml/s to a postoperative mean peak flow of 17.3 ml/s in the symptomatic BPH group and 13.5 ml/s in the retention group. Symptom scores (Madsen–Iversen) were similarly reduced to a mean of 7.6 and 3, respectively. In 14 patients (10%) the stent was removed, in 11 because of malposition and in three because of persistent symptoms related to the stent.

The North American Urolume Prosthesis Study Group's experience with the Urolume prostatic stent was reported by Oesterling et al.[19] and involved 126 men, of whom 95 had symptomatic BPH and 31 had acute retention of urine. At 2-year follow-up, symptom scores (Madsen–Iversen) decreased from a mean of 14.3 preinsertion to 5.4 postinsertion in the non-retention group and to 4.1 postinsertion in the retention group.

Mean peak flows increased from 9.1 ml/s pre-insertion to 13.1 ml/s postinsertion in the non-retention group and to 11.4 ml/s in the retention group. Residual urine volumes were similarly improved, from 85 ml pre-insertion to 47 ml postinsertion in the non-retention group and to 46 ml in the retention group. Significant long-term complications that required stent removal were noted in 17 patients (13%); the stents were removed transurethrally without any subsequent effects. The most common causes of stent removal were stent migration (29.4%) and recurrent obstruction at the bladder neck or apex (29.4%). Two (11.8%) were removed because of persistent irritative symptoms, two because of perineal discomfort and two because of encrustation secondary to the exposed stents at the bladder neck.

Because of such complications with regards to protrusion of the stent into the bladder neck, modifications of the stent were studied in 135 fit men with prostate outflow obstruction by Guazzoni et al.[20] in a multicentre trial in Europe. The modifications allowed a reduction of the amount of shortening that occurs when the stent expands. This was thought to facilitate proper stent placement and was achieved by altering the crossing angles of the wires from 142 degrees to 110 degrees and using a greater wire diameter (0.17–0.20 mm). However, it also resulted in a decrease in the pressure applied per millimetre of urothelium, from 6972 to 2941 Pa. Long-term result with regards to improvements in symptom scores, uroflowmetry and residual urine volumes at 18 months did not differ from those of the earlier studies, but the modified less shortening (LS) Urolume stent had a much higher long-term complication rate (31.1%, n = 42) when compared with the commercially available (CA) Urolume stent. These complications included 11 (26.2%) cases of stent migration, 17 (40.5%) of understenting or malposition, four of severe epithelial hyperplasia, two of persistent irritative symptoms, two of subsequent regrowth of the median lobe and two of urethral stricture. These required the removal of the prostatic stents in 21 (15.5%) patients, with the authors commenting that some of the complications — particularly stent migration and epithelial hyperplasia — are related directly to the changes made in the modified LS Urolume stents. Use of this stent was subsequently terminated.

Stent insertion

The Urolume stent is designed for use with an introducer that is intended to be used like a cystoscope (Fig. 48.2). General, regional or local anaesthesia with urethral lignocaine and intravenous sedation are given and the patient is placed in the lithotomy position.

On the basis of the authors' previous experience with prostatic stent insertion, they have introduced a number of modifications to the original technique used for device implantation,[5] to ensure correct placement with maximum stenting of the prostatic urethra and, in particular, to avoid protrusion of the stent into the bladder when the bladder neck is funnelled open at the time of a full bladder.

The patient is subjected to cystoscopy and, using a purpose-designed measurement catheter with a Foley balloon at its proximal end, the length of the prostatic urethra is measured under direct vision from the bladder neck to the distal sphincter mechanism. A stent with a length 0.5 cm less than the measured length of the urethra is inserted. The stent insertion device is inserted under direct vision and the stent positioned at the bladder neck. The outer sheath is then withdrawn a little, allowing partial opening of the stent, which is then withdrawn distally to ensure that the stent lies distal to the bladder neck itself, checking particularly that this is the case at the 12 o'clock position. The outer sheath is then removed completely to the safety lock position and the position of the stent, relative to the bladder neck in particular, is then checked. At this stage the stent can be retracted into the device and repositioned as required. When the operator is happy with this position, the safety lock is removed and the stent fully deployed.

The stent can be removed by retrograde displacement back into the bladder followed by extraction by means of a purpose-designed extraction device. In the initial series the authors removed six stents, four at up to 1 month, because of initial problems related to placement. In two patients, removal was at longer intervals (11 months and 18 months) after insertion: one of these patients, with severe recalcitrant detrusor instability, had persistent incontinence; the other patient had Parkinson's disease. In these two patients it was necessary to resect the covering urothelium prior to removal.

Conclusions

Because of the relatively good results with the Urolume stent in patients with symptomatic BPH and because of the perioperative advantages (namely, a short operating time, minimal blood loss, ease of insertion, a reduced hospital stay and no indwelling catheter postoperatively), this stent appears to provide a suitable treatment alternative to TURP for the management of symptomatic BPH, especially in older patients.[9]

References

1. Isaacs J T. Importance of the natural history of benign prostatic hyperplasia in the evaluation of pharmacologic intervention. Prostate 1990; (suppl 3): 1–7
2. Garraway W M, Collins G N, Lee R J. High prevalence of benign prostatic hypertrophy in the community. Lancet 1991; 338: 469–471
3. Glynn R J, Campion E W, Bouchard G R, Silbert J E. The development of benign prostatic hyperplasia among volunteers in the normative aging study. J Epidemiol 1985; 121: 78–82
4. Chilton C P, Morgan R J, England H R. A critical evaluation of the results of transurethral resection of the prostate. Br J Urol 1978; 50: 542–546
5. Abrams P H, Farrar D J, Turner-Warwick R T. The results of prostatectomy: a symptomatic and urodynamic analysis of 152 patients. J Urol 121: 640–642
6. Roos N, Wenneburg J E, Fisher E S. Mortality and reoperation after open and transurethral resection of the prostate for benign prostatic hyperplasia. N Eng J Med 1989; 320: 1120–1124
7. Evans J W H, Singer M, Chapple C R et al. Haemodynamic evidence of per-operative cardiac stress during transurethral prostatectomy: preliminary communication. Br J Urol 1991; 67: 376–380
8. Evans J W H, Singer M, Chapple C R et al. Haemodynamic responses and core temperature changes during transurethral prostatectomy and non-endoscopic general surgical procedures in age matched men. Br Med J 1992; 304: 666–671

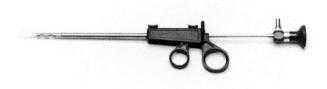

Figure 48.2. *Urolume stent with introducer.*

9. Lu-Yao G, Barry M J, Chang C H et al. Transurethral resection of the prostate among Medicare beneficiaries in the United States: time trends and outcomes. Urology 1994; 44(5): 693–699

10. Mebust W K, Holtgrewe H L, Cockett A T K, Peters P C. Transurethral prostatectomy: immediate and postoperative complications. A cooperative study of 13 participating institutions evaluating 3885 patients. J Urol 1989; 141: 243–247

11. McConnell J, Barry M, Bruskewitz R. Benign prostatic hyperplasia: diagnosis and treatment. Clinical Practice Guidelines, No 8. AHCPR Publication No 940582. Rockville, MD: Agency for Health Care Policy and Research, Public Health Service, US Department of Health and Human Services, 1994

12. Sigwart U, Puel J, Mirkovitch V, et al. Intravascular stents to prevent occlusion and restenosis after transluminal angioplasty. N Engl J Med 1987; 316: 701–706

13. Rousseau H, Puel J, Joffre F, et al. Self-expanding endovascular prosthesis: an experimental study. Radiology 1987; 164: 709–714

14. Milroy E J G, Chapple C R, Cooper J E et al. A new treatment for urethral strictures. Lancet 1988; 1: 1424–1427

15. Sarramon J P, Joffre F, Rischmann P, et al. Prosthèse endouréthrale Wallstent dans les stenoses recidivantes de l'urèthre. Ann Urol 1989; 23: 383–387

16. Chapple C R, Milroy J G, Rickards D. Permanently implanted urethral stent for prostatic obstruction in the unfit patient. Br J Urol 1990; 66: 58–65

17. Milroy E, Chapple C R. The Urolume stent in the management of benign prostatic hyperplasia. J Urol 1993; 150: 1630–1635

18. Milroy E, Coulage C, Pansadoro V et al. The Urolume permanent prostatic stent as an alternative to TURP: long-term European results. J Urol 1994; 151: 396A

19. Oesterling J E, Fefalco A J, the North American Study Group. The North American experience with the Urolume endoprosthesis as a treatment for benign prostatic hyperplasia: Long term results. Urology 1994; 44: 353

20. Guazzoni G, Pansadoro V Montorsi F et al. A modified prostatic Urolume wallstent for healthy patients with symptomatic benign prostatic hyperplasia: a European multicentre study. Urology 1994; 44: 364

49

Urolume endoprosthesis as an alternative treatment of BPH in inoperable patients

H.-J. Leisinger, M. Wisard and S. Gabellon

Introduction

The idea of using transluminally placed tube grafts to maintain the patency of stenotic arteries after balloon dilatation was first published in 1969.[1] Stents also have been utilized in the biliary ducts to maintain patency of the common bile duct.[2]

Fabian[3] in 1980 first described the use of a urological 'spiral' tube graft termed a 'partial catheter', which was placed endoscopically into the prostatic urethra in two patients, thus relieving their urinary retention. This spiral was considered as a temporary stent, and complications such as stent migration, urinary tract infection, stone formation, stent fracture and urethral stricture were quite frequent.[4] In search of an alternative treatment of benign prostatic hyperplasia (BPH), stenting of the urinary tract in prostatic outflow obstruction became an interesting field of research and many different devices have been developed.[5–7]

The Urolume endoprosthesis was developed originally by Wallsten in the authors' institution for endovascular use in the arterial system.[8] The authors introduced the Urolume endoprosthesis for the treatment of prostatic outflow obstruction, especially for patients with long-term indwelling urethral catheters who were unfit for prostatic surgery, to avoid long-term complications and problems in nursing care.

Patients and methods

From March 1993 to December 1996, 36 patients with obstructive BPH, unfit for regional or general anaesthesia, have been treated with the prostatic Urolume endoprosthesis. The mean age of the patients was 81 (70–94) years. Of the 36 patients treated, 31 had an indwelling catheter for almost 6 months and five presented with severe symptoms of prostatic outflow obstruction.

Preoperative assessment included physical examination, laboratory analysis, uroflowmetry, determination of residual urine volume and cystoscopy when indicated. To exclude prostatic cancer, digital rectal examination and prostate-specific antigen measurement have been used routinely. Transrectal sonography and biopsies were performed only when needed.

The associated pathological conditions responsible for the choice of the alternative stent treatment are presented in Table 49.1.

The nature and properties of the prostatic Urolume endoprosthesis and the specially developed deployment tool for placement of the device have been precisely described previously.[9] In the authors' department, the stent is placed in the endoscopic operation room under local anaesthesia by instillation of oxybuprocaine 1% in 10 ml distilled water. After cystourethroscopy, the distance from the bladder neck to the verumontanum is measured using an Eutrac balloon measuring catheter. A length of stent 5 mm less than the measured distance is selected.

In two cases in which the prostatic urethra was longer than 3 cm, two stents were placed with their ends overlapping by at least 0.5 cm (Fig. 49.1). It is extremely important that the endoprosthesis does not protrude into the bladder proximally and that the distal end does not extend to the verumontanum. After placement of the stent, its position is routinely checked by cystourethroscopy. X-rays of the pelvis are not routinely performed. For patients unable to void immediately after the procedure, a simple urethral 12 Fr catheter without

Table 49.1. *Associated pathological conditions in patients receiving the Urolume endoprosthesis*

Associated condition	No. of patients
Severe cardiac disease	18
Post-ictal	2
Thrombocytopenia or full anticoagulation	5
Pulmonary insufficiency	5
Senile dementia	6

The ASA score was 3–4 for all 36 patients.

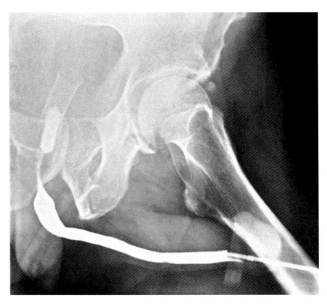

Figure 49.1. *Retrograde urethrography in a patient with two overlapping stents.*

balloon is placed through the stent into the bladder. All patients are given broad-spectrum antibiotics for almost 2 weeks.

Because of the major associated pathologies, patients have been hospitalized for 2–20 days (on average 7).

Follow-up visits are scheduled 3 months after the intervention and 6 months thereafter. The mean follow-up time is 35 (6–46) months.

Follow-up evaluation

The follow-up assessment has included urine examination, International Prostate Symptom Score (IPSS) evaluation, peak urinary flow rate, post-void residual urine volume and cystourethroscopy at 6 months. All patients, as well as nurses in charge of patients in social medical care homes, have been questioned with regard to urinary incontinence, local discomfort or bladder pain. According to the selection criteria of these patients, their sexual or erectile dysfunction has not been considered.

Results

All patients tolerated the endoscopic placement under local anaesthesia. No technical problems occurred, except in one patient where the first stent, because of inexact placement, had to be removed and replaced by another. Anticoagulation caused no technical problems,

except in one patient where heavy bleeding after cystoscopy prevented precise measurement of the length of the prostatic urethra; the intervention in this case was performed without complications 3 days later. Most patients, (30/36) complained of local discomfort and irritative symptoms during the first 3 weeks after the placement. One patient was particularly uncomfortable for 6 months because of bladder pain caused by stent wires protruding beyond the bladder neck (Fig. 49.2).

Migration of the stent occurred in two patients. In both cases the stents were removed and replaced by a new one. Urinary incontinence was noted in 4/36 patients. In two cases this incontinence improved spontaneously after 6 months and became socially acceptable; in the other two cases, a definitive percutaneous suprapubic catheter has been placed.

Temporary failures were observed in two patients treated for urinary retention with an indwelling urethral catheter for more than 12 months before the stent was placed. Both patients achieved spontaneous micturition and complete voiding after the first 8 weeks.

As shown in Table 49.2, the five patients who were not in urinary retention improved their IPSS considerably, although the peak urinary flow did not improve significantly. All five patients are satisfied with regard to the improvement of their quality of life.

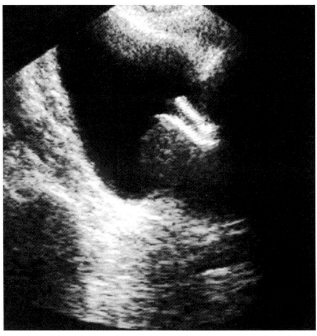

Figure 49.2. *Sagittal transabdominal ultrasound view in a patient with stent wires protruding slightly beyond the bladder neck.*

Table 49.2. *Results for five patients treated for severe symptoms of prostatic outflow obstruction*

Parameter		Pretreatment		Post-treatment	
IPSS	S	29.2	(23–33)	12	(6–17)
	Q	3.8	(3–4)	1.33	(1–2)
Flow: Q_{max} (ml/s)		5.6	(4–7)	9.67	(3–21)
Residual urine (ml)		175	(70–300)	30	(15–50)

For the 31 patients of the urinary retention group, no evaluation of the IPSS has been specially monitored, but all patients, as well as the nurses involved, were satisfied with the improvement in the quality of life. The peak urinary flow rates in this group do not differ from those in the non-retention group. Throughout the whole follow-up period, peak urinary flow rates, post-void residual urine and quality-of-life score did not change.

At the 6 months cystoscopy monitoring, all except two stents were noted to be covered with epithelium (Fig. 49.3). The one that was protruding slightly beyond the bladder neck was covered 3 months later.

During the long follow-up period, eight patients died. The minimal observation time for these patients was 15 months. No problems with regard to the endoprosthesis occurred in this group. None of the remaining 28 patients presented with late complications such as bleeding, stent migration, stent encrustation or

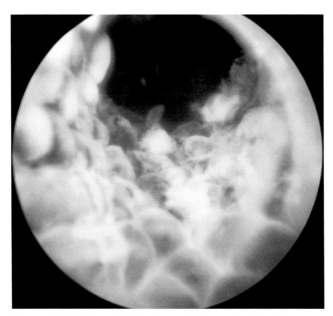

Figure 49.3. *Endoscopic view 1 month after stent implantation.*

urinary retention during an observation period of 6–46 months. No device had to be removed.

Symptomatic urinary tract infection occurred in six, three and two patients at 6, 12 and 18 months, respectively; appropriate antibiotic therapy was effective in all cases.

Discussion

Like McLoughlin et al.[10] in 1990 and Guazzoni et al.[11] in 1993, the authors used the Urolume endoprosthesis to treat prostatic outlet obstruction in high-risk patients unfit for locoregional or general anaesthesia. Most patients (31/36) were in urinary retention. All patients tolerated the procedure under local mucosal anaesthesia. No major technical problem was noted.

Although the majority of patients (30/36) complained of local discomfort and irritative symptoms during the first 3 weeks after stent insertion, all patients but two achieved spontaneous, painless and mostly complete bladder voiding without urinary incontinence. Of the 36 patients, two needed further urinary diversion by suprapubic percutaneous cystostomy because of intolerable incontinence of urine.

All patients, and especially all nurses caring for elderly handicapped men, were completely satisfied with the improvement in the quality of life achieved by the procedure.

These results are mainly in accord with those presented by other authors.[10–12] The poorer results with regard to the urinary flow rate in the patients in this series compared with the results of other authors could be explained by the selection of patients for this procedure: most were very old and presented with an aged and weak detrusor.

The first results are now known of various alternative treatments for the management of symptomatic BPH by minimally invasive methods such as visual laser ablation of the prostate (VLAP), transurethral thermotherapy (TUMT), transrectal high-intensity focused ultrasound (HIFU) and others that are introduced routinely. In view of the good results with the above-mentioned minimally invasive treatments, the authors continue to restrict the use of the Urolume endoprosthesis to a selected group of elderly surgical high-risk patients, although the results of extended follow-up show no complications after more than 3 years. Randomized clinical studies involving a large number of patients and a follow-up of more than 5 years will pinpoint the definitive place of the Urolume device in the treatment of BPH.

The authors' experience, as well as other reports,[9–12] confirm that the Urolume endoprosthesis is an appropriate device to relieve prostatic outlet obstruction and that it improves the quality of life for patients with indwelling bladder catheters, who are unfit for anaesthesia.

The stent placement is an easy, minimally invasive procedure (although the endoscopic technique requires a certain learning curve and should not be underestimated) that can be performed under local mucosal anaesthesia and gives good long-term results without complications.

As both the proximal and the distal ends of the prostatic urethra are often oblique in the sagittal plane, it is worth considering whether the incidence of irritative symptoms could be decreased by the use of a Urolume stent with one or two oblique ends.

References

1. Dotter C T. Transluminally-placed coilspring end-arterial tube grafts: long-term patency in canine popliteal artery. Invest Radiol 1969; 4: 329–332
2. Roddie M E. Metallic stents in biliary disase. Minimally Invasive Ther 1992; 1: 21–28
3. Fabian K M. Der intraprostatische 'Partielle Katheter' (Urologische Spirale). Urologe [A] 1980; 19: 236–238
4. Lewi H. The role of the intra prostatic spiral in 184 patients. Fifteen month follow-up. Paper presented at the 1992 Annual Meeting of BAUS, Bournemouth
5. Nissenkorn L. Experience with a new self retaining intraurethral catheter in patients with urinary retention. J Urol 1989; 142: 92–94
6. Gottfried H W, Schimers H P, Gschwend J et al. Erste erfahrungen mit dem memotherm-stent in der behandlung der BPH. Urologe [A] 1995; 34 (2): 110–118
7. Yachia D, Beyar M, Aridogan I A. A new, large calibre, self-expanding and self-retaining temporary intraprostatic stent (ProstaCoil) in the treatment of prostatic obstruction. Br J Urol 1994; 74 (1): 47–49
8. Rousseau H, Puel J, Joffre F et al. Self-expanding endovascular prosthesis: an experimental study. Radiology 1987; 164: 709–714
9. Oesterling J E, Defalco A J, Kaplan S A et al. The North American experience with the Urolume endoprosthesis as a treatment for benign prostatic hyperplasia : long-term results. Urology 1994; 44(3): 353–362
10. McLoughlin J, Jager R, Abel P D et al. The use of prostatic stents in patients with urinary retention who are unfit for surgery. An interim report. Br J Urol 1990; 66: 66–70
11. Guazzoni G, Bergamaschi F, Montorsi F et al. Prostatic UroLume Wallstent for benign prostatic hyperplasia patients at poor operative risk: clinical, uroflowmetric and ultrasonographic patterns. J Urol 1993; 150: 1641–1647
12. Milroy E, Chapple C R. The UroLume stent in the management of benign prostatic hyperplasia. J Urol 1993; 150: 1630–1635

Anatomical limitations of the prostatic urethra in using cylindrical stents

K. J. Ng and E. J. G. Milroy

50

Introduction

Metallic stents have been used in the prostatic urethra since 1980 as treatment for bladder outflow obstruction. Most are cylindrical in shape, and once deployed, some are left permanently in situ. Such permanent stents, over time, would then be covered by urothelium.

One of the complications of metal stents left exposed to urine is stone encrustation. At the time of deployment, some parts of the permanent stent may not be directly in contact with the prostatic urethra, resulting in poor coverage by urothelium. Over time, those parts of the stent that are exposed to urine are prone to stone formation.

To assess the probable success of using cylindrical permanent stents in individual patients, a precise knowledge of the geometry of the prostatic urethra is required. The authors have deployed a novel method of imaging at the Institute of Urology, London, UK[1] — three-dimensional (3-D) ultrasound imaging of the prostatic urethra.

Three-dimensional imaging of the prostatic urethra

This new method uses standard transrectal ultrasound scans to acquire a series of axial images of the posterior urethra during voiding. Scans were performed with either 7.0 MHz Acuson or 7.5 MHz Aloka transrectal probes. Patients were examined in a standing position with a comfortably full bladder. On commencement of micturition, 3-D scans were performed of the area of the bladder neck down to the external urethral sphincter. An average of 10 s was required to complete the scanning with 80 axial images captured during this period. The use of a positioning sensor (Polhemus System) that was attached to the scan probe obviated any error that may otherwise be introduced due to movement of the probe. More recently, this technique has been improved further by the use of sagittal sweeps, allowing mutiple 3-D urethral images to be recorded in a single voiding cycle.

A system specially developed by the Medical Physics Department, University College London[2] was used to record and subsequently process the images. A technique using grey-scale contrast was employed to define the margin between urethral wall and urethral cavity. The slices of images were then stacked together to form the urethral 3-D image (Fig. 50.1). Once reconstructed, the 3-D urethra can be rotated, tilted and viewed from any angle. It can also be re-sliced at any angle and any plane to reveal its geometric configuration (Fig. 50.2).

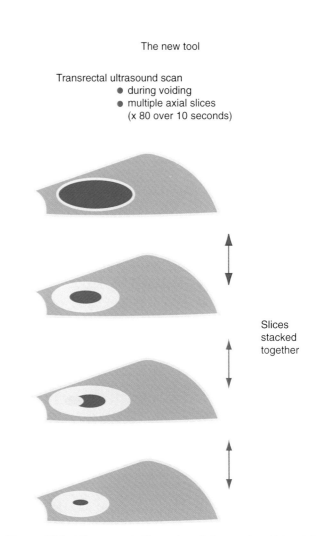

The new tool

Transrectal ultrasound scan
- during voiding
- multiple axial slices
  (x 80 over 10 seconds)

Slices stacked together

Figure 50.1. *Diagrammatic illustration of the way in which axial image slices are stacked electronically to produce the final 3-D urethra.*

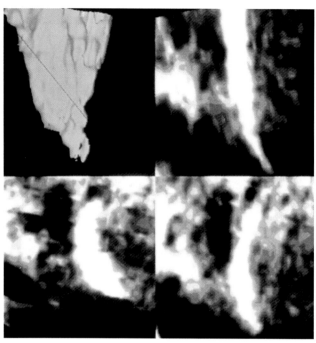

Figure 50.2. *A display of the re-slicing facility of the system. The urethra is re-sliced in different planes (clockwise from colour frame): longitudinal view of the urethral lumen demonstrating the appearance very much like a descending urethrogram; oblique view of the prostatic urethra; axial view showing the crescentic lumen in cross-section.*

The authors have identified two aspects of the prostatic urethra that are important in the long-term success of cylindrical stents: these are (1) shape in cross-section and (2) bladder neck–urethra angle.

The shape of the prostatic urethra varies markedly in bladder outflow obstruction. Fig. 50.3[2] illustrates the reconstructed urethra of a patient with benign prostatic hyperplasia (BPH). In this patient, the urethra was compressed by a right lobe adenoma of the prostate. This resulted in a crescentic-shaped top surface of the urethra (represented in grey colour in the diagram). The 3-D urethra in Fig. 50.3b has been rotated clockwise (viewed from above).

Figure 50.4 is a different 3-D prostatic urethra displayed in the stacked up multi-axial slice mode. The urethra in this case is more oval in cross-section.

When the technique is performed to include imaging of the bladder base, the bladder neck–urethra angle can be determined (Fig. 50.5). Knowledge of the bladder neck–urethra angle is particularly relevant in the management of BPH by deployment of prostatic stents (Fig. 50.6). One of the complications of current permanent prostate stents is stone formation on that

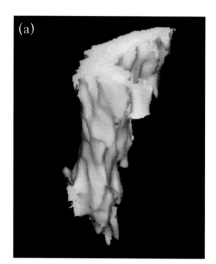

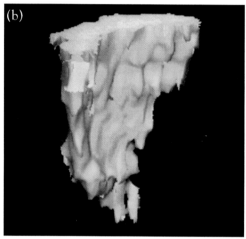

Figure 50.3 (a,b). *3-D urethra of a patient with BPH viewed from different angles. Note the crescentic top surface of the urethra due to right lateral lobe adenoma.*

part of the stent not covered with urothelium. If this bladder neck–urethra angle is not quite 90 degrees, then part of the end of a prostate stent would not be covered with urothelium and would be exposed directly to urine in the bladder, thus making it prone to stone formation. Perhaps a new series of stents should be produced with different angles of bevelling at the top end to help alleviate this problem.

As illustrated earlier, looking at the urethra in cross-section (bottom diagrams of Fig. 50.6), it may be crescentic or even hour-glass in shape. All current prostatic stents are cylindrical. Fitting a simple cylinder into these urethras would mean that certain areas would not be well covered with urothelium. New stent shapes, such as oval in cross-section, should perhaps be tried to allow better conformation within these urethras.

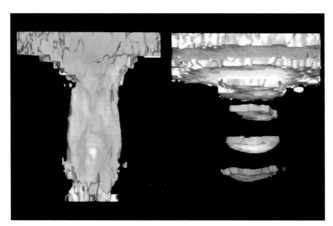

Figure 50.4. *Oval cross-section of a prostatic urethra.*

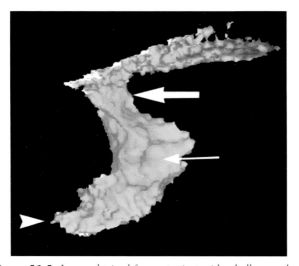

Figure 50.5. *Image obtained from a patient with a bulbar urethral stricture. Note the angle which the urethra made with the bladder neck. The urethra upstream of the stricture was seen to be ballooned out during voiding (bold arrow, level of verumontanum; slim arrow: proximal bulbar urethra, white arrow, site of stricture).*

New stent design

Importance of bladder
neck—urethra angle

Urethra not quite a simple cylinder

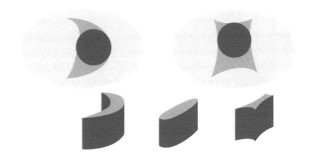

Figure 50.6. *Importance of the bladder neck–urethra angle is illustrated in the top diagrams (see text). The bottom diagrams demonstrate the poor conformation of a simple cylinder within urethras that have crescentic or hour-glass-shaped lumina.*

The future

Detailed morphological imaging of the urethra will assist in the design of future urethral and prostatic stents. All current prostatic stents are cylindrical; however, the authors' studies have confirmed that the prostatic urethra is variable in shape and in its relationship to the bladder neck, and conforms poorly to a simple cylinder. Such future 'customized' stents may well allow better ephithelial cover and minimize some of the complications, such as stone formation, currently encountered in clinical use.

References

1. Ng K J, Gardener J E, Rickards D et al. 3-Dimensional imaging of the prostatic urethra — an exciting new tool. Br J Urol 1994; 74(5): 604–608
2. Gardener J E. 3-D imaging for medicine: three-dimensional imaging of soft tissues using ultrasound. IEE Colloqu Dig 1991, 83

51

Is there a role for epithelizing stents in the treatment of BPH?

J. M. Glass and G. Williams

Introduction

Stenting of the prostatic urethra was first described by Fabian in 1980, who used a stainless steel coil to treat patients who would otherwise have faced long-term catheterization.[1] Initially, stents were designed for the temporary relief of bladder outflow obstruction secondary to benign prostatic hyperplasia (BPH). Their design was such that the stents did not become epithelialized and their use was associated with stent migration, recurrent infections and the development of encrustations on the stent.

Attempts to reduce the incidence of complications, and the drive to develop a day-case procedure for the treatment of bladder outflow obstruction (BOO), resulted in the development of the permanently implanted intraprostatic stent. These were initially made of a woven mesh of superalloy (AMS Urolume™) or titanium (Titan™), and offered as a treatment to those unfit for surgery. The ingrowth of urothelium reduced some of the complications associated with temporary stents but increased the difficulty in removal in patients already deemed unfit for surgery.

Williams observed in 1995 that long-term follow-up was becoming available for the so-called temporary stents, whereas the permanent stents — which, in many cases, were associated with poor outcome due to migration, pain, infection, calcification and excess epithelialization — were (with considerable difficulty) having to be removed.[2] A new design of stent made from nickel/titanium using shape metal technology was developed (Memotherm™). The early results of the Memotherm stent have also been disappointing.[3]

This chapter examines the data available on each of the permanently implanted stents that have been used in the treatment of BPH.

Urolume™

The Urolume™ stent (American Medical Systems, Minnetonka, MN, USA) was the first permanently implanted prostatic stent, introduced in 1987, originally for the treatment of urethral strictures.[4] It had been adapted from the original Urolume™ endoprosthesis developed by Hans Wallsten in Lausanne, Switzerland, which was designed for endovascular use.[5] It was made from a corrosion resistant superalloy wire woven mesh and manufactured in 1.5, 2.0, 2.5, 3.0, 3.5 and 4.0 cm lengths. [It is noteworthy that the other manufacturers of prostatic stents have produced stents up to 8 cm]. The original design has undergone at least two further modifications, and this limits the amount of long-term follow-up data available. It is often difficult, particularly in the American literature, to determine which stent is being described. The stents cost approximately US$1500.

Indications/contraindications

The original stent was first used in 1988 for the treatment of BOO in men unfit or unwilling to undergo major surgery.[6]

Insertion

Since 1990, after modification of the stent, it has been inserted on a specially designed disposable endoscopic delivery device. Safety locks ensure that the device is not released prematurely. Patients are sedated or given light anaesthesia and placed in the lithotomy position. Following cystourethroscopy, the length of the prostatic urethra is measured from the bladder neck to the external sphincter with the bladder full, using a graduated balloon occlusion catheter (Fig. 51.1); a stent 0.5 cm less than this length is used. The delivery device is introduced into the prostatic urethra under direct vision using a 0 degree cystoscope and water irrigation. When the stent is in position, the first safety lock is released and the stent is deployed into the urethra by pulling a trigger mechanism that allows the stent to expand. The cystoscope can then be used to check the position of the stent. If it is not placed appropriately, the stent can be resheathed and the position adjusted. The stent should not intrude beyond the bladder neck as the proximal part of the stent will not epithelialize

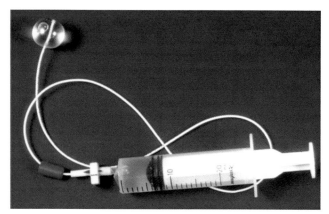

Figure 51.1. *Balloon occlusion catheter, used to measure the length of the prostatic urethra reliably.*

and will act as a focus for calcification. If the patient fails to void, a suprapubic catheter is inserted as a urethral catheter may dislodge the stent.

The procedure can be performed with the patient as a day case, but in the elderly and medically unfit a stay of a few days may be necessary because of the intense urgency and discomfort felt by some patients. These symptoms usually resolve in the first 3 months.

Results

A number of case series using the Urolume™ have been published.[5–7] The original Urolume™ was used in a study comprising 96 men who were unfit to undergo surgery,[6] 46 of whom came from the authors' centre; 53 stents 2 cm long and 43 stents 3 cm long were inserted; six patients needed insertion of a second stent because of persistent symptoms of BOO, and one patient required a total of three stents. Of these patients, 73 presented in acute retention, but all patients could void after stent insertion, 90 immediately. Follow-up at 3–30 months is reported. The peak flow rate was 15 ml/s at 12 months in the retention group (n = 23), and 18.1 ml/s in the non-retention group (n = 8). Using the Madsen–Iversen symptom score, in which 16 points are allocated for obstructed symptoms and 11 points for irritative symptoms,[8] the mean obstructive score was 0.26 (range 0–3) and the mean irritative score was 1.24 (0–9) in the non-retention group at 12 months. In the non-retention group at 12 months, the obstructive score was 0.63 (0–3) and the irritative score was 2.7 (0–7). Cystoscopy was performed 12 months after stent insertion on 27 patients: 15 patients had complete epithelialization, and a further 11 had >70% epithelialization. Complications included

urinary tract infection in 15 patients, associated in seven with stent encrustation. Eight stents were removed over the period of the study, three for persistent irritative symptoms, two owing to stent migration and two because the patient went into retention; the reason is not recorded in one case.

A contemporary multicentre study from North America,[5] using the original stent in 126 men, showed similar results in terms of improvement in urinary flow rate and symptom score and a similar complication rate, with stent removal being necessary in 16% of non-retention patients and 6% of patients in retention. Irritative voiding symptoms persisted in 10% of the patients in whom stent removal was not deemed necessary; 15% of patients suffered from urinary tract infections in the long term.

It became evident from these studies that no wires should project beyond the bladder neck into the bladder because of failure to epithelialize and calcification, and that, on release of the stent from the delivery system, the stent shortened to a variable degree. These observations resulted in the development of a new second stent, the subject of further study. Furthermore, the indications and contraindications were altered as a result of the first study. It was noted that antegrade ejaculation and potency were not significantly affected by stent placement and therefore stents could have a role in the treatment of BOO for men who were concerned about the potential loss of fertility as a result of retrograde ejaculation, or the possible loss of potency following a transurethral prostatic resection. Insertion was contraindicated in patients with BOO secondary to a large middle lobe or a large rigid prostate: the former resulted in the proximal stent lying within the bladder anteriorly resulting in encrustation (Fig. 51.2), whereas the latter would not allow full stent expansion.

A total of 135 men who were fit for surgery were entered into a European multicentre study using the modified 'less-shortening' stent:[7] 91 patients were obstructed and 44 had an indwelling catheter. In 19 patients the stent was removed immediately owing to mis-sizing or misplacement; ten patients had a new stent inserted at the same session, whereas six patients needed a second procedure to enable correct stent placement; the stent was not reimplanted in three patients, who subsequently underwent a prostatectomy.

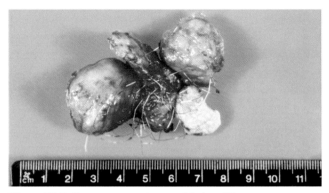

Figure 51.2. *Severe encrustation on a Urolume™ stent.*

The mean peak flow rate in the non-catheterized patients was 9.3 ml/s prior to stent placement. This improved to 16.5 ml/s in patients followed to 6 months (n = 76) and 17.1 ml/s at 18 months (n = 21). The mean obstructive score was 8.9 before treatment in the same non-catheterized patients, improving to 1.9 at 6 months, and the mean irritative score was 5.2, improving to 2.5 at 6 months. Symptoms of bladder irritability were initially almost universal, although settled in most men by 3 months, often with anticholinergic therapy. The irritability was particularly problematic in the elderly patients for whom the stent was designed to benefit.

In 51 patients (38%) long-term complications ensued, requiring stent removal in 21. Such complications included epithelial hyperplasia (Fig. 51.3), active urinary tract infection, understenting, migration, and distal misplacement requiring bladder neck resection or incision. As a result of these complications manufacture of both the original and this new stent was discontinued.

Removal of the Urolume™ can be exceedingly difficult, despite claims by others.[9] The epithelium needs to be resected and, if possible, the stent avulsed into the bladder and then pulled into the sheath of a resectoscope. The stent is often removed strand by strand in what can be a bloody and prolonged procedure. It is not always possible to remove the entire stent, owing to the epithelialization.

The Urolume™ has undergone a second modification as a result of the European study and has been subjected, without any initial studies, to a randomized trial comparing it with transurethral resection of the prostate (TURP).[10] Of 60 men, 34 have been allocated to the stent group, and 26 to the TURP group, with assessment of the flow rate and

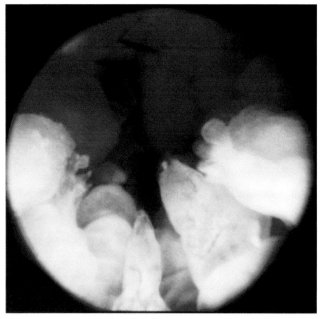

Figure 51.3. *Marked epithelial hyperplasia within the lumen of a Urolume™ stent.*

International Prostate Symptom Score (IPSS),[11] which rates seven symptoms on a 0–5 scale (with a score of 0 being symptom free and 35 being maximally symptomatic) at baseline and 3 months. The mean flow rate went from 8.0 and 8.4 ml/s to 16.7 and 16.0 ml/s and the IPSS from 19.0 and 21.6 to 11.2 and 11.0 in the TURP and stent groups, respectively. The Urolume™ was misplaced in two patients, resulting in these patients undergoing a TURP, and a slight increase in irritative symptoms was reported in the stented group. The mean length of stay was 2.4 days in the stented group and 4.0 days in those having a TURP. This study is dealt with in more detail in Chapter 40.

Memotherm™

The Memotherm™ stent (Angiomed, Wachhaus Str. 6, D-W 7500 Karlsruhe D-76227, Germany) was made from a woven nickel/titanium mixture termed nitinol, and was dependent on shape memory. This means that the stent is pliable and mouldable when cold, but assumes a predetermined 42 Fr cylindrical shape when warmed to body temperature. The Memotherm™ was marketed in 2–8 cm lengths and did not shorten when released from the delivery system. Removal of the Memotherm™ was usually easy, as the stent unravels when the terminal wire is pulled.

Indications/contraindications

The stents were used as an alternative to TURP in men with BOO. As these stents had not previously been studied in detail, there were no exclusion criteria.[3]

Insertion

Cystourethroscopy was performed and the distance from the bladder neck to the external sphincter measured, using a graduated balloon occlusion catheter. The stent was presented in an endoscopic delivery device (Fig. 51.4) and the proximal 1 cm of the stent was gold-plated to aid visualization. Using a 0-degree cystoscope and water for irrigation warmed to body temperature, the bladder neck was visualized, the safety catch removed and the stent expelled by repeatedly squeezing the trigger. Once the gold distal end was seen, the position of the stent was checked and adjusted. The Memotherm™ could not be replaced in the sheath, unlike the Urolume™: it became increasingly difficult to adjust the position of the stent, the more it was released from the introducer. The stent immediately expanded to 42 Fr with the warmed irrigation fluid.

If the patient failed to void, a suprapubic catheter was required.

Results

In a single-centre study, 49 stents were inserted in 48 men, with follow-up at 1, 3, 6 and 12 months with flow rates and Madsen–Iversen symptom scores.[3] Cystoscopy was performed at 6 and 12 months. Urinary retention developed immediately in 13 men following stent insertion; the remainder voided without difficulty. Ten stents were removed within the first year. Cystoscopy at 6 months showed distal migration in seven, proximal migration in two, and mucosal hyperplasia within the stent in 11. In 24 patients there was 75% epithelialization or less, and one patient had calcification. There was subjective improvement in both the obstructive and irritative components of the symptom score, but this was not matched by any marked improvement in the flow rates. In a further follow-up review at 2 years, 22 of the patients have now had their stents removed and more would have done so if they were fit enough to undergo the procedure.

This stent is no longer marketed. It is clear that major modifications to the stent are required before further clinical trials would be indicated.

Titanium stent (Titan)

A pure titanium mesh stent was developed by ASI (ASI Inc., San Clemente, California, USA), and called the ASI Prostate Dilatation System (PDS). Like many of the stents, the stent and the delivery system have undergone modifications. The stent has been modified to reduce the width of the bars of the mesh and the size of the fenestrations, which have become more numerous; this is known as the Titan™ stent. It is unclear in the published data which stent and delivery system have been employed in each study. Inappropriately, the results from two different stents are reported by Kaplan et al.[12] on patients treated with the PDS stent and 23 with the Titan™ intraprostatic stent. These stents differ little, except in the size of stent available, and in that the Titan™ stent has smaller, more numerous fenestrations; the stents have the same expanded diameter and wall thickness. In addition, the delivery system was changed during the period of the study, and the statement made that the new delivery system facilitates placement: 17 PDS stents had to be removed, whereas no Titan™ stents were removed; despite this, the results were combined. Of 25 patients followed for more than a year, only four had a flow rate greater than 15 ml/s.

In another study in which patients were followed for up to 21 months, (95 having been treated with the original stent and 45 with the modified stent), 86% were able to void but only 10 patients have undergone

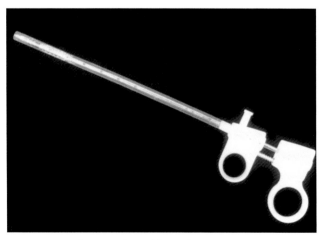

Figure 51.4. *The Memotherm delivery device.*

subsequent cystoscopic evaluation,[13] despite the fact that, in an in vitro study, titanium stents appeared the most likely to suffer encrustation (compared with steel, steel superalloy, and gold-plated stents).[14]

The manufacturers give data on 207 patients, of whom 170 were available for follow-up.[15] At 12 months the mean peak flow was only 10.9 mls/s; this would suggest that many patients were probably still obstructed.

Although this stent has been proposed as an alternative treatment of BPH in high-risk patients following a number of small studies,[16,17] this has not been borne out by longer-term follow-up and the stent has currently been withdrawn.

Conclusions

Since Fabian's report in 1980,[1] the prostatic stent has been modified in terms of the materials used to make the stent, the design of the structure of the stent, the way that the stent is delivered into the prostatic urethra and, finally, the way that it is held in position. If any stent has a role in the treatment of BOO it would ideally be a stent that can be delivered into the prostatic urethra through a system that requires local anaesthesia and completely relieves all symptoms in the patient. It would hold itself in position in the prostatic urethra in such a way that there was no risk of proximal or distal migration, and would either epithelialize without doing so excessively, or would not epithelialize but would not cause encrustation. It would be strong enough to withstand the compressive forces generated by the dynamic component of the prostate gland and permit the passage of a rigid endoscope.

It would have long-term follow-up data available with assessment of symptom and bother scores, flow studies and cystoscopic evaluation (although if the symptom scores and flow rate are satisfactory, follow-up cystoscopy is not essential). The stents should also be cheap, or any assessment must take into account the cost implications of treatment with the stent, including the cost of stent failures, compared with conventional therapy.

None of the permanent intraprostatic stents developed to date fulfil all of these criteria. Most fail because of encrustation, excessive tissue growth within the lumen of the stent or unacceptable irritability

resulting in stent removal, or because complete and satisfactory long-term follow-up is not available. Undoubtedly, some men fitted with a permanently implanted stent have had very satisfactory outcomes and in some men the stents have been very well tolerated. It is, however, impossible to predict who will do well following stent insertion. Stents are undoubtedly contraindicated in patients with a large middle lobe or high bladder neck and those with a large rigid prostate. Only one randomized controlled clinical trial has been performed, data from which are limited; the trial was conducted with a previously untried stent.

There is a need for a minimally invasive alternative treatment for BPH and the ideal stent, not yet designed, would be a possible alternative, but it must be shown to be cost effective and subjected to a rigorous, large, randomized controlled trial with long-term follow-up.

References

1. Fabian K M. Der interprostatiche 'partielle Katheter' (Urologische Spirale). Urologe 1980(A); 19: 236–238
2. Williams G. Urethral stents: history, surgical procedure, indication and results for treating BPH, urethral stricture and neurological voiding dysfunction. In: Buzelin J M (ed) Implanted and injected materials in urology. Oxford: Isis Medical Media, 1995: 74
3. Williams G, White R. Experience with the Memotherm™ permanently implanted prostatic stent. Br J Urol 1995; 76: 337–340
4. Milroy E J G, Cooper J E, Wallsten H et al. A new treatment for urethral strictures. Lancet 1988; 1: 1424–1427
5. Oesterling J E, Kaplan S A, Epstein H B et al. The North American experience with the Urolume endoprosthesis as a treament for benign prostatic hyperplasia: long term results. The North American Uroloume Study Group. Urology 1994; 44: 353–362
6. Williams G, Coulange C, Milroy E J G et al. The Urolume, a permanently implanted prostatic stent for patients at high risk for surgery. Br J Urol. 1993; 72: 335–340
7. Guazzoni G, Montorsi F, Coulange C et al. A modified prostatic Urolume wallstent for healthy patients with symptomatic benign prostatic hyperplasia. A European Multicentre Study. Urology 1994; 44: 364–370
8. Madsen P O, Iversen P. A point system for selecting operative candidates. In: Hinman F Jr (ed), Benign prostatic hypertrophy. New York: Springer-Verlag, 1983: 673
9. Parikh A M, Milroy E J. A new technique for removal of the urolume prostatic stent. Br J Urol 1993; 71: 620–621
10. Chapple C, Rosario D J, Wasserfallen M, Woo H H. A randomised study of the Urolume stent vs prostatic surgery. J Urol 1995; 153: 436A (abstr)
11. Walsh P C. Benign prostatic hyperplasia In: Walsh P C, Retik A B, Stamey T A, Vaughan E D (eds), 6th edn. Campbell's Urology, Philadelphia: Saunders, 1992: 1009
12. Kaplan S A, Merrill D C, Mosley W G. The titanium intraprostatic stent: the United States experience. J Urol 1993; 150: 1624–1629
13. Miller P D, Gillet D, Kirby R S et al. The ASI titanium stent — 3 years experience. Paper presented at the 1992 Annual Meeting of BAUS, Bournemouth, UK

14. Holmes S A V, Miller P D, Crocker P R et al. Encrustation of intraprostatic stents — a comparative study. Br J Urol 1992; 69: 383–387

15. ASI Clinical Update, May 1992. ASI Inc., San Clemente, California, USA

16. Abrams P, Gillat D, Chadwick D. Intraprostatic stent: experience with the ASI stent to treat bladder outflow obstruction. J Urol 1991; 145: 293A (abstr)

17. Parra R O. Titanium urethral stent an alternative to prostatectomy in the high risk surgical patient. J Urol 1991; 145: 239A (abstr)

52

Temporary prostatic stenting using the Barnes stent
D. G. Barnes and A. Yakubu

Introduction

Temporary prostatic stents/intra-urethral catheters have been used successfully to relieve bladder outflow obstruction, including retention of urine, in those considered unfit for surgery.[1,2] Advantages of this technique include the immediate relief of obstruction, the insertion and removal under local anaesthetic and the reversibility of the technique. An 80% success in acute retention has been reported and most patients eventually void if treated with a suprapubic catheter. Disadvantages include migration (usually proximal), irritative voiding symptoms, encrustation, infection and obstruction of the lumen.

Other indications for temporary prostatic stenting are a trial of stenting (prior to the insertion of a 'permanent' stent), temporary relief of obstruction while waiting for the effect of other therapies (such as coagulative treatments of the prostate,[3] or hormonal manipulation in carcinoma of the prostate[4]) and while waiting for other medical conditions to resolve.

The Barnes stent

The ideal stent for these combined procedures should be single-sized (to avoid measuring and the need for a large costly stock), easily inserted and removed (preferably under local anaesthetic), have a low migration rate, and be inexpensive. A suitable stent was designed and subsequently manufactured (Angiomed, UK, now Bard Limited). The stent is 75 mm in length, 16 Fr in diameter and made of polyurethane. The proximal end is similar to a urethral catheter in design; distally, a single preformed retaining basket is designed to sit at the verumontanum.

Insertion is by means of a curved introducer (Fig. 52.1). The stent is dislodged into the bladder using a pusher. Then, under cystoscopic control, the stent is pulled back (using the blue nylon threads) until positioned at the verumontanum (Fig. 52.2). The blue nylon strings can be shortened and left in situ to enable easy removal in the outpatient department. After insertion of a suitable local anaesthetic gel, removal is achieved by gentle traction on the strings.

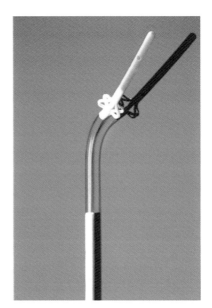

Figure 52.1. *Barnes stent on its introducer.*

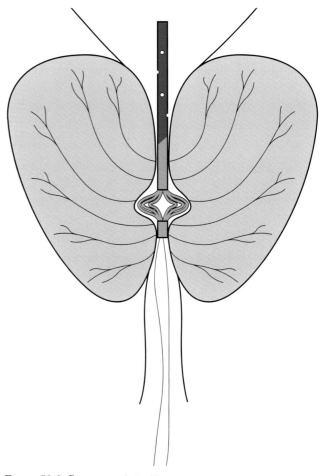

Figure 52.2. *Barnes stent in position.*

Combined techniques using the Barnes stent

Endoscopic laser ablation of the prostate

Endoscopic laser ablation of the prostate (ELAP) using a side-firing technique is becoming established as an alternative to endoscopic resection, transurethral resection of the prostate (TURP), in small and medium-sized glands (< 50 cm^3).[5-8] Several disadvantages of this technique have been established and are applicable to other coagulative techniques of the prostate. These include the use of a urinary catheter (urethral or suprapubic) for a minimum of 48 hours, the delayed improvement in flow and symptoms (6 weeks +), the poor reported results in the presence of urinary retention, and the frequently reported 'prostatitis' symptoms. These drawbacks, which reflect the delayed relief of the bladder outflow obstruction, must affect the patients' overall perception of the technique.

The rapid relief of the outflow obstruction, while maintaining the advantages of ELAP, can be achieved by two techniques: first, a bladder neck incision or resection could be executed using electric cautery or a laser technique; secondly, a temporary prostatic stent could be used.

This chapter presents the early results of the first 80 consecutive patients who underwent combined ELAP and temporary prostatic stenting using the Barnes stent. Preoperative assessment of these patients with symptomatic bladder outflow obstruction, including retention of urine (failed trial without catheter), included symptom score, flow rate, ultrasound residual volume estimation and prostate-specific antigen (PSA). Exclusion criteria included a peak flow greater than 15 ml/s, estimated prostate volume of more than 60 cm^3, or clinical suspicion of an underlying carcinoma of the prostate. Mean age was 72 (range 58–93) years and a median ASA grade 3. Of these 80 patients, 21 were on aspirin and 12 were fully anticoagulated on warfarin.

After preliminary cystoscopy, an 'anatomical' ELAP of the prostate was undertaken using a divergent side-firing fibre to achieve coagulation. No suprapubic catheter was inserted during the lasing. At the end of the procedure the single-sized prostatic stent was introduced, as described above. Postoperatively, patients were discharged once voiding had been re-established.

Postoperative assessment included a symptom score, flow rate and residual volume estimation at 6 weeks (stent in situ). At 8–12 weeks the stent was removed under local anaesthetic. Initially, stent removal was an endoscopic day-case procedure but latterly this has been achieved as an outpatient procedure by leaving the positioning 'strings' attached and applying gentle traction.

Results

Postoperatively, 59 patients (74%) voided immediately. In those who developed postoperative retention of urine, a suprapubic catheter was inserted and they were discharged home. Fourteen patients were in urinary retention preoperatively: 11 were in acute retention (failed trial without catheter) and three in chronic retentions (two already had temporary stents in situ, one a 980 ml residual). Of 14 patients, 11 (79%) voided immediately post-ELAP.

Mean peak flow rates at 6 weeks (stent in situ) rose from 8.5 ml/s preoperatively, in those voiding, to 16.9 ml/s overall. Residual volumes fell to less than 100 ml in 95% of patients. In the first 25 patients this flow rate increase corresponded to the subjective voiding score, with all but three patients describing their stream as normal by 6 weeks (see Figure 52.3 for details and exclusions). In the remaining 55 patients, international prostate symptom scores (IPSS) fell from 25 to 8 with the stent in position.

'Prostatitis' symptoms were experienced only in five patients and were reported as minor. Three had minor rectal discomfort on voiding, and two reported penile urethral discomfort for 1 week. No haematuria requiring hospitalization or transfusion occurred.

Stent migration occurred in five patients: in two, early migration at 48 hours resulted in acute retention of urine, requiring suprapubic catheterization; in three, late asymptomatic migration occurred between the 6-week and 3-month follow-up. Other postoperative complications included four cases of symptomatic lower urinary tract infections requiring antibiotic therapy.

At 8–12 weeks all stents were removed under local anaesthetic. No case of secondary retention has occurred following stent removal.

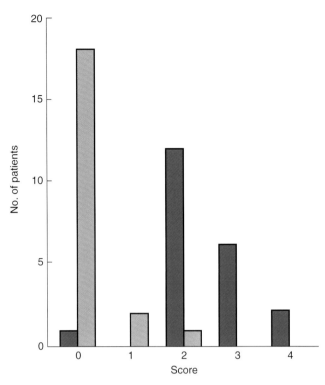

Figure 52.3. *Subjective voiding score (ad hoc scoring system; 4 = acute retention) in the first 25 patients to receive combined ELAP and temporary prostatic stenting using the Barnes stent:* ■ *preoperative score;* ■ *score at 6 weeks with stent in situ. There were four exclusions at 6 weeks: one patient had died (unrelated cause); there was one case of early stent migration; two patients were not available (clinical success).*

Discussion

The drawbacks of ELAP of the prostate using a side-firing technique are related to the delayed relief of outflow obstruction and postoperative oedema. The use of a temporary prostatic stent appears to overcome these, with rapid improvement of flow rate and improved bladder emptying. These objective measurements coincide with a rapid symptomatic improvement. The results recorded at 6 weeks with stent in situ were found to be comparable to those reported at 3 months following ELAP alone. Indeed, many patients considered that their urinary streams were normal within days of the procedure. This rapid improvement must be attributed to the temporary prostatic stent and is not surprising in view of the reported use of similar stents in retention of urine.[1,2]

Problems related to the stent were few, with only two early migrations, both resulting in retention of urine at 48 hours. This again supports the concept that it is the stent that is responsible for maintaining and improving the voiding pattern in the early postoperative period. How long the stent is needed is yet unknown. Certainly, with extensive ablation of the prostate on endoscopic examination at 3 months, the prostate is not healed but a cavity is seen. For this reason, the authors initially chose to remove the stents at 3 months. Three stents migrated between the 6-week follow-up and attendance for removal of the stent. On endoscopy, the surgical lateral lobes of the prostate were markedly reduced in size, allowing this late asymptomatic stent migration. Indeed, patients were warned that as the prostate shrank, migration into the bladder might occur. Further late migrations have not occurred, now that stents are removed at 8 weeks.

On removal of the stent, which was performed under local anaesthetic, no secondary retentions occurred. This process is now achieved in the outpatient department by simple traction on the positioning strings.

These results compare well with those obtained using biodegradable, self-reinforced, polyglycolic acid spiral stents.[9] These stents degrade into small fragments of polymer debris that are excreted on voiding. This process appears to be variable in urine, resulting in a reported late retention rate of 13%[10] and a deterioration in symptoms after 3 weeks.[9] This is not surprising, as these authors noted on endoscopy at 4 weeks that the entire prostatic urethra was lined with necrotic tissue in all patients but only some spiral stent fragments remained.

Conclusions

The use of temporary prostatic stenting, using the one-size Barnes stent, enables catheter-free ELAP with early improvement of flow and reduction of symptom score. The rapid reduction of outflow resistance, because of the prostatic stent, also permits treatment of cases of urinary retention without prolonged catheterization. Complications related to this combined treatment appear to be rare.

Locally advanced prostatic carcinoma

Bladder outflow obstruction secondary to locally advanced carcinoma of the prostate is usually treated by 'channel' TURP. These patients often are anaemic and may have disseminated intravascular coagulopathy. There is an increased morbidity in patients undergoing TURP compared with hormone therapy alone, with an increased incidence of incontinence and postoperative bleeding.

Alternatively, a urinary catheter may be inserted for 3+ months. At the Marsden Hospital, in combination with hormonal manipulation, 68–83% of those treated by these means eventually voided.[11]

Temporary prostatic stents have become popular in the treatment of outflow obstruction due to benign disease in those considered unfit for surgery. In 1993, the authors presented their initial results after treating bladder outflow obstruction in carcinoma of the prostate using temporary prostatic stenting (Porges Urospiral) and androgen suppression (flutamide). A successful result was achieved in eight of ten patients.[4]

The aims of the study reported here were to avoid TURP, to avoid an indwelling catheter and to provide voiding with minimal symptoms, while awaiting local tumour response.

Nineteen patients with a mean age of 75 (range 61–93) years were included, seven with severe outflow symptoms, six with acute urinary retention and six with chronic retention. All had locally advanced prostate cancer and many had metastatic disease at presentation. Spiral stents were inserted in eight (seven Memokath, Engineers and Doctors, Kvistgaard, Denmark) and Barnes stents in 11 (Bard, Crawley, UK).

Results

Of the 19 patients, 18 voided after stent insertion. In 12 patients (63%) the result was considered to be a success: six stents are still in situ (mean 11 months): three patients who died were still voiding with stents in situ (mean 3 months); three stents were removed as a planned procedure (mean 4.6 months) and those patients required no further treatment of their outflow obstruction. Overall, only four (21%) patients have required a TURP, of these, two required prolonged postoperative catheterization. Two patients (10.5%) have a long-term indwelling catheter in situ.

Conclusion

Temporary prostatic stenting and hormone manipulation provide a minimally invasive, catheter-free alternative treatment to outflow obstruction in locally advanced carcinoma of the prostate.

References

1. Nissenkorn I, Richter S. A new self-retaining intraurethral device. An alternative to an indwelling catheter in patients with urinary retention due to infravesical obstruction. Br J Urol 1990; 65: 197–200
2. Sassine A M, Shulman C C. Intraurethral catheter in high-risk patients with urinary retention: 3 years of experience. Eur Urol 1994; 25: 131–134
3. Barnes D G, Butterworth P, Flynn J T. Combined endoscopic laser ablation of the prostate (ELAP) and temporary prostatic stenting. Minim Invasive Ther Allied Technol 1996; 5: 333–335
4. Anson K M, Barnes D G, Briggs T P et al. Temporary prostatic stenting and androgen suppression. A new minimally invasive approach to malignant prostatic urinary retention. J R Soc Med 1993; 86 (11): 634–636.
5. Costello A, Bowsher W, Bolton D et al. Laser ablation of the prostate in patients with benign prostatic hypertrophy. Br J Urol 1992; 69: 603–608
6. Anson K, Watson G, Shah T, Barnes D. Laser prostatectomy: our initial experience of a technique in evolution. J Endourol 1993; 7: 333–336
7. Kabalin J. Laser prostatectomy performed with a right angle Neodymium:YAG laser fibre at 40 watt power setting. J Urol 1993; 150: 95–99
8. Costello A, Shaffer B, Crowe H. Second-generation delivery systems for laser prostatic ablation. Urology 1994; 43: 262–266
9. Petas A, Talja M, Tammela T et al. A randomised study to compare biodegradable self-reinforced polyglycolic acid spiral stents to suprapubic and indwelling catheters after visual laser ablation of the prostate. J Urol 1997; 157: 173–176
10. Petas A, Taari K, Talja M et al. SR-PGA urospiral compared to suprapubic and indwelling catheter in the treatment of postoperative urinary retention after VLAP. J Urol 1996; 155 (suppl): 706A (abstr 1581)
11. Hampson S S, Davies J H, Chang C R et al. LHRH analogues as primary treatment for urinary retention in patients with prostatic carcinoma. Br J Urol 1993; 71: 583–586

The Spanner™ temporary prostatic stent

A. P. Corica, F. Corica, A. Sagaz, M. Houlne,
A. G. Corica and T. Larson

53

Introduction

A stent acts as a scaffold spanning a segment of a tubular organ. Prostatic stents span the prostatic urethra from the bladder neck to urinary sphincter. Typically, they have been used either temporarily (three months or less) or permanently. Temporary stents may be either removable or biodegradable and are not designed to be incorporated into the urethral wall. Permanent stents become part of the urethral wall as they are invaded and covered by urothelium.

In the early 1980s, Fabian suggested the idea of partial urethral stents.[1–2] Further efforts by Nissenkorn,[3–4] and Yachia,[5–7] improved such devices. Thereafter, numerous studies have provided strong evidence that urethral stents are safe and effective as a minimally invasive option to relieve acute urinary retention.[8–25] They have been used either temporarily in patients in retention (particularly after one of the newer heat-based therapies) or permanently in patients who are deemed poor surgical risks.

Drawbacks of stent design include complex insertion/removal, proclivity for migration and patient discomfort. Biodegradable stents, in particular, degrade at an unpredictable rate that could result in recurrent retention or calcific encrustation of migrated bladder fragments.

Ongoing studies are evaluating temporary stents for patients with retention after non-urologic surgery and for patients temporarily unfit for transurethral resection of the prostate (TURP). These studies may expand the indications for use for prostatic stents.

The prostatic urethra is neither a cylindrical nor a straight tube. The shape of the prostatic urethra and its relation with the bladder neck show a wide range of variation depending on the architecture and size of the lateral and median lobes. These variations make the exact measurement of the length of the prostatic urethra somewhat difficult and can also compromise the stent's stability. On the longitudinal axis there is a bladder neck-urethra angle that varies primarily depending on shape and size of the median lobe. These wide variations in the prostatic urethral anatomy have been overlooked.

There has never been a time when a clinically useful temporary prostatic stent would be more welcomed by the urological community than today. Men in some nations are obliged to wait weeks or months for their TURP. New minimally invasive heat-based technologies are creating significant edema post treatment requiring Foley or clean intermittent catheterization. And cryotherapy and brachytherapy for prostate cancer can result in difficult recovery periods, sometimes involving extended catheterization times.

Criteria for a successful stent

During the Third International Consultation on Benign Prostatic Hyperplasia in 1995, criteria were established for the successful clinical performance of a prostatic stent.[26] Most importantly, the stent must provide disobstruction of the prostate. Further, the stent must be easy to insert and remove; it must not migrate from its position; and it must be well tolerated by the patient. Previous prostatic stent designs have failed to meet these criteria. The Spanner™ temporary prostatic stent may prove to effectively address these requirements.

If urologists were permitted to write the ideal performance standards for a temporary stent, these criteria would be included:

- Easy to insert and remove using standard catheter procedures, without imaging or visualization (blind placement).
- Bi-directionally stabilized to prevent migration or expulsion.
- Soft and flexible to provide for patient comfort.
- Thin-walled for minimal urodynamic resistance to improve voiding efficiency.
- Resistant to encrustation.
- Improves lower urinary tract symptoms (LUTS).
- Maintains continence.

- Causes minimal tissue irritation.
- Minimizes urinary tract infection (UTI) rate compared to Foley or clean intermittent catheterization.
- Cost-effective.

The Spanner™ temporary prostatic stent

The Spanner™ temporary prostatic stent (AbbeyMoor Medical, Inc., Miltona, Minnesota, USA) is a sterile, single use, disposable intra-urethral device. It is intended for temporary use (i.e. ≤ 30 days) in men with bladder outlet obstruction to reduce elevated post-void residual and relieve voiding symptoms. The Spanner™ is provided in 20 Fr and 22 Fr sizes in six lengths ranging from 4 cm to 9 cm.

The Spanner™ device description

The Spanner™ is designed to stent open the prostatic urethra to improve voiding efficiency and symptoms while allowing the bladder to continue to act as a reservoir and the external sphincter to maintain continence. The Spanner provides active bladder emptying versus the passive drainage achieved with a Foley catheter. The device (Fig. 53.1) is composed of three main parts:

1. a proximal stent and anchoring segment
2. a distal anchor
3. connecting sutures.

The proximal stent is positioned in the bladder neck and incorporates: (1) a balloon to prevent expulsion;

(2) a urine port situated proximal to the balloon; and (3) a stent of various lengths to span a portion of the prostatic urethra (Fig 53.2, 53.3).

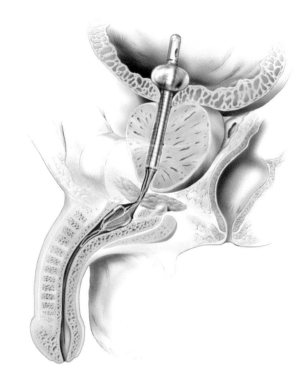

Figure 53.2. *Sagittal view of the Spanner™ in situ.*

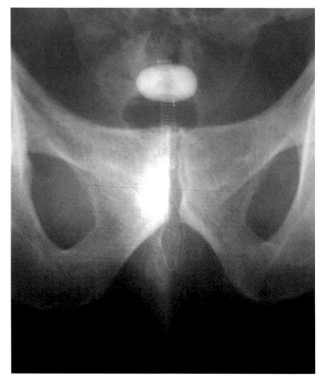

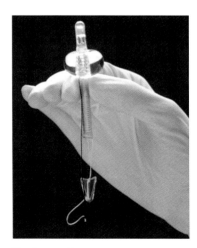

Figure 53.1. *The Spanner™ temporary prostatic stent.*

Figure 53.3. *X-ray of the Spanner™.*

The stent provides a tubular passageway for urine to drain from the bladder neck to the distal end of the prostate, thereby mechanically disobstructing the prostatic urethra, reducing urethral resistance to urine flow.

The distal anchor is seated in the bulbar urethra. Connecting sutures, which tether the proximal stent to the distal anchor, traverse the external sphincter and allow the sphincter to maintain continence.

A retrieval suture extends from the distal anchor through the urethra and terminates in the meatus. The retrieval suture is used to deflate the balloon and remove the device.

The prostatic-urethral portion is made of medical implant grade silicone embedded with a stainless steel wire coil to prevent stent lumen collapse.

Selecting the correct stent length: the Surveyor™

The length of the prostatic urethra varies among individuals, especially benign prostatic hyperplasia (BPH) patients who can present with prostate volumes ranging from as little as 20 cc to over 200 cc. To achieve effective use of the Spanner™, the appropriate length device must be selected to accommodate these anatomical differences. The length of the urethra from the bladder neck to the distal side of the external sphincter can be determined using the sterile, single-use Surveyor™ urethral measurement device (Figs 53.4, 53.5). The Surveyor™ consists of a 40 cm polymer tube with a silicone balloon on the proximal end and a hand piece on the distal end. A short Teflon probe (<1 cm length) encircles the tube and slides freely along the tube's length between the balloon and the handle. A stainless steel guidewire attached to the probe extends along the length of the tube through the Surveyor™ handpiece where it is attached to a small handle.

The Surveyor™ is positioned in the urethra with the proximal balloon anchored in the bladder neck. The probe is then gently advanced along the main tubing of the Surveyor™, until tactile changes in resistance indicate the location of the external sphincter. As the probe advances, the length of wire between the probe's handle and the Surveyor™ handle changes. When the external sphincter is reached, the length of wire

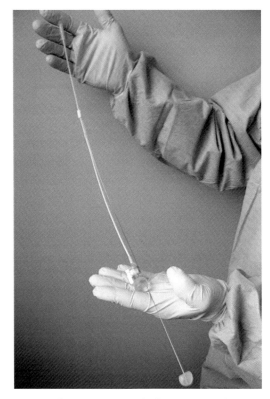

Figure 53.4. *The Surveyor™ urethral measurement device.*

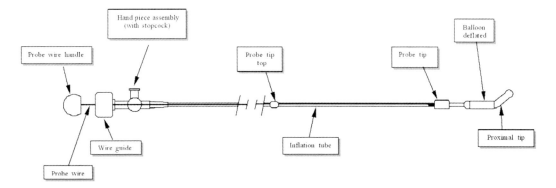

Figure 53.5. *Diagram of the Surveyor™ urethral measurement device.*

between the two handles represents the distance from the bladder neck to the distal side of the external sphincter. For many patients, the use of the Surveyor™ eliminates the need to measure with cystoscopy or transrectal ultrasound. However, a simple chart is provided to convert Surveyor™ measurements or transrectal ultrasound measurements to Spanner™ sizes (Figs 53.6, 53.7).

Insertion and removal procedure

The Spanner™ insertion procedure is performed without visual assistance, such as cystoscopy or ultrasound. In a sterile field, the urethra is injected with appropriate, topical anesthetic. The Spanner™ is mounted on a sterile, single-use insertion tool having either a straight tip or curved tip (Figs 53.8, 53.9 and 53.10a–d). The Spanner™ is inserted using standard catheter insertion procedures and is advanced slowly until the proximal tip and balloon are positioned in the bladder (Figs 53.8, 53.9). The balloon is then inflated with 5 cc of sterile water injected using a luer syringe connected to an inflation port on the insertion tool. Gentle traction applied to the coupled Spanner™ and insertion tool positions the balloon in the bladder neck. Further traction uncouples the insertion tool from the Spanner™ and leaves the stent in position in the

prostatic urethra and the distal anchor in position on the distal side of the external sphincter.

To remove the stent, an initial, gentle traction is applied to the retrieval suture. This action removes the

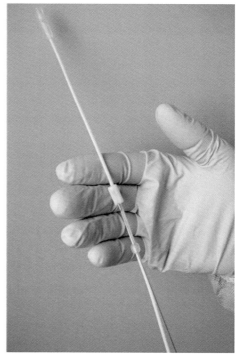

Figure 53.7. *Close-up of the proximal end of the Surveyor™.*

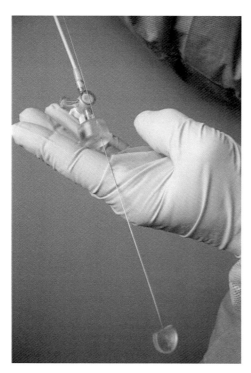

Figure 53.6. *Close-up of the distal end of the Surveyor™.*

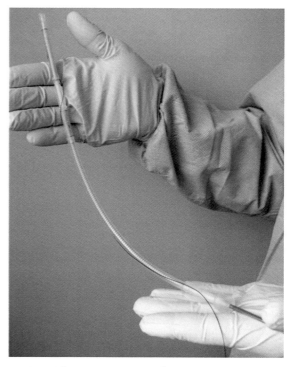

Figure 53.8. *The Spanner™ mounted on the insertion tool.*

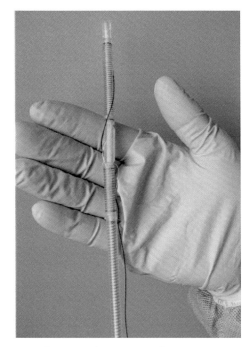

Figure 53.9. *Close-up of the Spanner™ device.*

plug from the proximal balloon, releases the 5 cc of sterile water and allows the balloon to deflate. After a brief pause, the stent is withdrawn by slowly pulling on the retrieval suture (Fig. 53.10e).

Clinical evaluation of the Spanner™

An early feasibility study on the Spanner™ was conducted at the University de Cuyo, Mendoza, Argentina. The objective of the study was to determine the impact of the temporary stent on parameters of voiding function and quality of life among patients diagnosed with severe lower urinary tract symptoms (LUTS). The Spanner™ was inserted into a series of 30 patients with LUTS. Subjects were excluded if they had prior surgery for prostate cancer, had any other urethral or bladder surgery, or if they were at high risk of developing bladder or kidney stones. The study was conducted under patient informed consent.

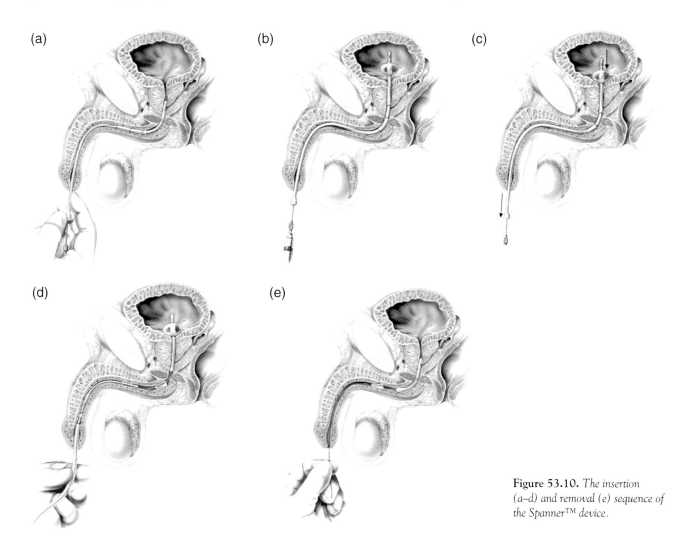

Figure 53.10. *The insertion (a–d) and removal (e) sequence of the Spanner™ device.*

The Spanner™ was inserted under topical anesthesia. Maximum flow rate (Q_{max}), voided volume (VV), post-void residual volume (PVR) and the international prostate symptom score (IPSS) were assessed. Patient tolerance to the device was assessed with the stent performance score developed by the author and with a visual-analog scale measuring patient quality of life. Patients were stratified into groups according to baseline PVR as follows: PVR ≤ 175 ml (Group 1; n = 13), PVR >175 ml and ≤ 500 ml (Group 2; n = 12) and PVR >500 ml (Group 3; n = 5). All data points collected for each patient were averaged to determine post-insertion values of Q_{max}, VV, PVR and IPSS.

Results

Stents remained in situ for a mean of 57 days (range 1–98 days; median, 63 days). Results are presented for the group as a whole in Table 53.1 and for the stratified patients in Table 53.2. All patient groups experienced a

Table 53.1. *LUTS patients, voided volume, PVR and Q_{max} results with the Spanner™*

	Q_{max} (ml/s)		Voided volume (ml/s)		PVR (ml)	
	Baseline	Post-insertion	Baseline	Post-insertion	Baseline	Post-insertion
Mean	8.2	11.6 (42%)	214.2	219.9 (2%)	312.1	109.4 (−65%)
Median	7	11.6	207.5	207.5	190	88.2
SD	3.6	3.3	109.2	72.9	360.9	138.3
Range	2.0–19.0	4.0–17.8	45.0–402.0	70.0–404.3	40.0–1500.0	15.0–812.8
p-value		0.0002		n.s.		0.004

One patient has two sets of data resulting from having a device inserted on two separate occasions. Thus, data are for 31 data points representing 30 individual patients. Percentage change from baseline in parentheses. n.s., not statistically significant; SD, standard deviation, LUTS, lower urinary tract infection; PVR, post-void residual volume.

Table 53.2. *LUTS patients, stratified by baseline PVR*

	Q_{max} (ml/s)		Voided volume (ml/s)		PVR (ml)	
	Baseline	Post-insertion	Baseline	Post-insertion	Baseline	Post-insertion
Group 1: Baseline PVR ≤175 ml (n = 13 patients)						
Mean	8	12.4 (55%)	189.8	222.8 (17%)	94.8	64.4 (−32%)
Median	8	12.9	174	207.5	100	53.4
SD	2.5	3.9	75.4	84.2	30.8	46.4
p-value		0.002		n.s.		n.s.
Group 2: Baseline PVR >175 ml ≤500 ml (n = 12 patients)						
Mean	9.5	11.2 (18%)	270.4	210.9 (−22%)	252.3	93.8 (−63%)
Median	9	9.7	316.6	208.4	243.5	95.6
SD	4.8	3.2	121.5	68.3	60.6	24.3
p-value		n.s.		n.s.		<0.001
Group 3: Baseline PVR >500 ml (n = 4 patients; 5 data points)						
Mean	5.9	10.5 (78%)	175.8	243.9 (39%)	1020.6	281.1 (−72%)
Median	7	11.1	228.8	260.5	1000	149.6
SD	2.2	1.9	109	55.5	373.9	299
p-value		0.007		n.s.	n.s.	0.008

Percentage change from baseline in parentheses. Data for one patient was omitted in Group 3 due to lack of baseline PVR data. Table represents data for a total of 29 patients. n.s., not statistically significant.

reduction in PVR and increase in Q_{max}. Group 3 patients experienced the most improvements over their baseline values for Q_{max}, VV and PVR. Groups 1 and 2 also experienced improvements. For the two groups, respectively, Q_{max} increased 55% and 18%, VV increased 17% for Group 1 but decreased 22% for Group 2 and PVR decreased 32% and 63%, respectively.

Mean overall baseline and post-insertion Q_{max} were 8.2 and 11.6 ml/s, respectively, representing a 42% improvement from the baseline ($p = 0.0002$). Q_{max} improved after stenting among all three patient groups: Group 1: 8.0–12.4 ml/s; 55%; $p = 0.002$; Group 2: 9.5–11.2 ml/s; 18%; $p = $ n.s.; and Group 3: 5.9–10.5 ml/s; 78%; $p = 0.007$.

Mean overall baseline and post-insertion VV were similar at 214.2 ml and 218.9 ml, respectively. Voided volume increased among Group 1 (17%) and Group 3 (39%), but decreased among Group 2 patients (22%) after stenting.

Mean overall baseline and post-insertion PVRs were 312.1 ml and 109.4 ml, respectively, representing a 65% decrease ($p = 0.004$). Decreases were seen in all three patient groups (32%, 63% and 72%, respectively).

Mean overall pre- and post-treatment IPSS scores were 22.3 and 7.1, representing a 68% improvement ($p<0.001$). All patients who completed the stent performance score were highly satisfied with the device.

In addition, a visual analog scale (Fig. 53.11) was used to assess patient tolerance of the Spanner™. Patients were asked to indicate on a horizontal scale of 0 to 10, with 0 being 'not at all' and 10 being 'very much'.

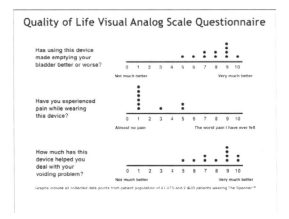

Figure 53.11. *A visual analog scale for patient quality of life.*

Minor complications

Adverse events experienced throughout the trial included urinary tract infection in 15 men, elevated PVR requiring removal of the stent after 8 weeks in one man, and intermittent hematuria, which resolved spontaneously in seven men. Five men experienced transient stress incontinence and six men had transient urgency incontinence. Eight men reported urgency symptoms in the first week after stent placement and 11 men complained of perineal discomfort that resolved during the first 2 weeks after stent placement. In most men, the discomfort was mild and was typically experienced during sitting. One man reported perineal discomfort that persisted until stent removal. In three men who wore the stent for 12 weeks, the retrieval suture broke and device removal was accomplished cystoscopically.

Tissue appearance after stent removal

The prostatic urethral tissue in 12 of 14 patients appeared normal when viewed cystoscopically after removing the Spanner™. In one patient, slight edema was observed at the location of the distal extremity of the distal anchor. In one patient, mild inflammation was recorded at the point of device contact.

Potential clinical applications for a temporary stent

The potential clinical utility for temporary prostatic stenting is varied. The specific role of stents will be better understood as more is learned about their ease of insertion and removal, patient comfort/satisfaction, stability, and how long they can function in a hostile environment (Table 53.3.)

From BPH to LUTS

Urologists have adopted the term 'LUTS' (lower urinary tract symptoms) to replace the term 'BPH' (benign prostatic hyperplasia), perhaps recognizing that symptoms of low flow/high PVR may not solely be caused by an obstructing prostate. The change of terminology indicates a need for better assessment of the bladder's contributions to symptoms. Jepsen and Bruskewitz suggest more attention and better measures should be developed to quantify the role of bladder dysfunction in BPH symptomatology.[27] They conclude:

Table 53.3. *Stent application based on stent longevity*

Application	≤30 days	30–90 days	≥90 days
AUR	X		
Post non-uro sx	X		
Adjunct to BPH drug therapy	X	X	
Chronic catheter usage			X
Differential diagnosis	X		
Nursing home patient			X
TURP waiting list			X
Comorbidity delaying TURP		X	
Post TUMT, TUNA, ILC, WIT	X		
Post-cryo, brachytherapy	X	X	X
Palliation of obstruction in prostate cancer			X
Stand alone BPH therapy		X	X
Poor surgical candidate			X
Drug delivery platform		X	
Bladder pressure transducer platform	X		

AUR, *Acute urine retention*; BPH, *benign prostate hyperplasia*; TURP, *transurethral resection of the prostate*; TUMT, *transurethral microwave thermotherapy*; TUNA, *transurethral needle ablation*; ILC, *interstitial laser coagulation*; WIT, *water-induced thermotherapy*.

'In the future, measuring bother due to LUTS and impact on the patient's quality of life with the BPH impact should be imperative and central to treatment decisions'.

Abrams and others have suggested urologists must better assess the bladder's contribution to LUTS rather than assume an obstructed prostate is the root cause of symptoms.[27–30] Abrams has shown that a significant percentage of men presenting with LUTS have impaired detrusor contractility as opposed to an obstructed prostate.[30] Do these impaired-detrusor patients comprise the approximate 20% of men who do not improve after TURP as reported by Emberton et al.? In 1958, Shields et al.[32] published what they described as 'differential uroflowmetry'.[32] Their goal was to investigate the two major variables contributing to the symptoms of LUTS: bladder outlet obstruction (BOO) and poor detrusor contractility. By holding the BOO variable constant with a urethral catheter, they recorded changes in uroflowmetry during volitional voiding through the catheter. Marked improvement in Q_{max} demonstrated both obstruction and, equally importantly, adequate detrusor contractility to efficiently empty the bladder. Javle, in a series of 53 patients, demonstrated that men with poor detrusor contractility did not benefit from surgery as compared to men with unequivocal obstruction and adequate detrusor contractility.[33]

The Spanner™ may be an innovative method to evaluate the LUTS patient. The urologist may gain greater insight into the root causes of LUTS by comparing baseline data (Q_{max}, PVR, IPSS and voiding diaries) with changes seen while the patient is wearing the Spanner. A pronounced improvement in Q_{max} and other uroflowmetry parameters might demonstrate not only the presence of obstruction, but also the bladder's ability to contract sufficiently to adequately empty the bladder. A reduction in PVR would be further evidence. The converse should also hold. Mechanical disobstruction of the patient without material improvement in uroflowmetry and PVR, may point to impaired bladder contractility rather than BOO as the underlying cause of LUTS. Perhaps wearing the Spanner™ for two to four weeks before undergoing a prostate disobstructing surgery will provide the patient the opportunity to experience disobstruction and the impact on his symptoms, before his surgery. This patient experience has been observed in our early investigation of the Spanner for both LUTS and AUR patients.

TUMT, TUNA, ILC, WIT: *minimally invasive therapies (MIT) for LUTS*

The data suggests high-temperature therapies for LUTS (transurethral thermal therapy or TUMT; transurethral needle ablation or TUNA; interstitial laser coagulation or ILC; water-induced thermotherapy or WIT) cause coagulation necrosis of prostatic tissue to improve voiding efficiency and symptoms. The general degree of improvement attained by these minimally invasive treatments (MIT) falls somewhere between medical therapy and TURP, the gold standard. The major advantages of MITs, as opposed to surgery, are lower morbidity and fewer anesthesia requirements, but they are not without their limitations. The edema caused by these heat-based technologies requires post-treatment catheterization times unfavorable to patient and urologist alike. Five to ten days of catheterization are not uncommon. An additional problem arises after the Foley has been removed when a significant number of these men re-present in acute retention, often requiring an emergency room visit. Nearly all MIT patients see a worsening of their flow rates and symptoms until the edema and thermal injury resolve over a period of 8–12 weeks. The Spanner™ may play a useful role during this recovery phase. The same useful role may be found post-brachytherapy and post-cryosurgery for localized prostate cancer.

Long waiting lists for TURP

In countries where socialized medicine is practiced, men may have to wait weeks, and in some cases, months, for their TURP. The Spanner™ might provide a better alternative to Foley catheterization or clean intermittent catheterization while patients await their treatment. It is this waiting list population where the Spanner's™ usefulness as a differential diagnostic tool might be seen, particularly if it is proven that the changes in uroflometry and symptoms will help predict the outcomes of TURP.

Bladder rehabilitation

Tubaro et al. discuss the association of increased bladder wall thickness with prostatic obstruction, using a new transabdominal ultrasound technology.[34] This research may further evidence the role of the compensating bladder in the presence of BOO. If the Spanner™ were left in situ for 2–3 months to relieve the prostatic obstruction, would the thickness of the bladder wall decrease over time? Intuitively, many urologists prescribe a 30–60 day use of a Foley catheter in acute retention patients before TURP. Dubey et al. suggest a period of adequate bladder rest (approximately 3 weeks)

to improve the outcomes of TURP.[35] Such methods perhaps give the bladder a chance to rest, recuperate and rehabilitate prior to TURP, resulting in a chance for even greater symptomatic improvement after TURP. In such a role, the Spanner™, which provides active volitional voiding compared to passive bladder drainage with a Foley catheter, might give the bladder the opportunity to strengthen (recycle) in the presence of low urethral resistance.

Conclusions

Temporary prostatic stenting has been envisioned for nearly 25 years. However, technical, as well as clinical limitations, have relegated stents to limited use. Ease of insertion and removal, migration issues and patient acceptance have been the major limiting factors.

In the Argentina study outlined above, the Spanner™ effected symptomatic relief and urodynamic improvements while preserving volitional voiding and continence. Post-insertion urodynamic variables indicated the device ameliorated bladder outlet obstruction and improved symptoms. The residual urine was reduced in nearly all patients, often remarkably. The results of the questionnaire regarding patient comfort/acceptance of the device appear to confirm a patient's willingness to wear the Spanner™. It remains to be seen how long the stent can function in a hostile environment. The answer to this question will help determine the Spanner's™ place in the urologist's armamentarium for the assessment, management and perhaps, treatment of bladder outlet obstruction.

The Spanner™ seems to meet the previously outlined criteria for a successful stent. Further clinical studies are warranted to determine the stent's safety and efficacy and expand its current indications.

References

1. Fabian K M. The intraprostatic, partial catheter (urological spiral) (in German). Urologe A 1980; 19: 236–238
2. Fabian K M. The intraprostatic "partial catheter" (urological spiral II) (in German). Urologe A 1984; 23: 229–233
3. Nissenkorn I, Slutzker D, Shalev M. Use of an intraurethral catheter instead of a Foley catheter after laser treatment of benign prostatic hyperplasia. Eur Urol 1996; 29: 341–344
4. Nissenkorn I. The intraurethral catheter – three years of experience. Eur Urol 1993; 24: 27–30
5. Yachia D, Beyar M, Aridogan I A. A new, large caliber, self-expanding and self-retaining temporary intraprostatic stent

(ProstaCoil) in the treatment of prostatic obstruction. Br J Urol 1994; 74: 47–49

6. Yachia D, Lask D, Rabinson S. Self retaining intraurethral stent: an alternative to long term indwelling catheters or surgery in the treatment of prostatism. AJR 1990; 154: 111–113

7. Yachia D, Beyar M. Preservation of sexual function by insertion of 'ProstaCoil' instead of indwelling catheter in surgically unfit BPH patients. In: Proceedings of the Second International Congress in Therapy in Andrology. Bologna; Monduzi Editore, 1991: 399–402

8. Devonec M, Dahlstrand C. Temporary urethral stenting after high-energy transurethral microwave thermotherapy of the prostate. World J Urol 1998; 16(2): 120–123

9. de la Rosette J, Beerlage H P, Debruyne F M J. Role of temporary stents in alternative treatment of benign prostatic hyperplasia. J Endourol 1997; 11(6): 467–472

10. Isotalo T, Talja M, Valimaa T, et al. A pilot study of a bioabsorbable self-reinforced poly L-lactic acid urethral stent combined with Finasteride in the treatment of acute urinary retention from benign prostatic enlargement. BJU Int 2000; 85: 83–86

11. Vincente J, Salvador J, Chechile G. Spiral urethral prosthesis as an alternative to surgery in high risk patients with benign prostatic hyperplasia: prospective study. J Urol 1989; 142: 1504–1506

12. Rosenkilde P, Pedersen J F, Meyhoff H H. Late complications of Prostakath treatment for benign prostatic hypertrophy. Br J Urol 1991; 68: 387–389

13. Gesenberg A, Sintermann R. Management of benign prostatic hyperplasia in high risk patients: long-term experience with the Memotherm stent. J Urol 1998 (July); 160: 72–76

14. Badlani G H. Role of permanent stents. J Endourol 1997; 11(6): 473–475

15. Anjum M I, Chari R et al. Long-term clinical results and quality of life after insertion of a self-expanding flexible endourethral prosthesis. Br J Urol 1997; 80: 885–888

16. Bailey D M, Foley S J, McFarlane J P et al. Histological changes associated with long-term urethral stents. Br J Urol 1998; 81: 745–749

17. Petas A, Isotalo T, Talja M, Tammela T L, Valimaa T, Tormala P. A randomized study to evaluate the efficacy of a biodegradable stent in the prevention of postoperative urinary retention after interstitial laser coagulation of the prostate. Scand J Urol Nephrol 2000; 34(4): 262–266

18. Laaksovirta S, Talja M, Valimaa T, Isotalo T, Tormala P, Tammela T L. Expansion and bioabsorption of the self-reinforced lactic and glycolic acid copolymer prostatic spiral stent. J Urol 2001; 166(3): 919–922

19. Laaksovirta S, Isotalo T, Talja M, Valimaa T, Tormala P, Tammela T L. Interstitial laser coagulation and biodegradable self-expandable, self-reinforced poly-L-lactic and poly-L-glycolic copolymer spiral stent in the treatment of benign prostatic enlargement. J Endourol 2002; 16(5): 311–315

20. Petas A, Talja M, Tammela T L, Taari K, Valimaa T, Tormala P. The biodegradable self-reinforced poly-DL-lactic acid spiral stent compared with a suprapubic catheter in the treatment of post-operative urinary retention after visual laser ablation of the prostate. Br J Urol 1997; 80(3): 439–443

21. Petas A, Talja M, Tammela T, Taari K, Lehtoranta K, Valimaa T, Tormala P. A randomized study to compare biodegradable self-reinforced polyglycolic acid spiral stents to suprapubic and indwelling catheters after visual laser ablation of the prostate. J Urol 1997b; 157(1): 173–176

22. Talja M, Tammela T, Petas A, Valimaa T, Taari K, Viherkoski E, Tormala P. Biodegradable self-reinforced polyglycolic acid spiral stent in prevention of postoperative urinary retention after visual laser ablation of the prostate-laser prostatectomy. J Urol 1995; 154(6): 2089–2092

23. Traxer O, Anidjar M, Gaudez F, Saporta F, Daudon M, Cortesse A, Desgrandchamps F, Cussenot O, Teillac P, Le Duc A. A new prostatic stent for the treatment of benign prostatic hyperplasia in high-risk patients. Eur Urol 2000; 38(3): 272–278

24. Isotalo T, Talja M, Hellstrom P, Perttila I, Valimaa T, Tormala P, Tammela T L. A double-blind, randomized, placebo-controlled pilot study to investigate the effects of Finasteride combined with a biodegradable self-reinforced poly L-lactic acid spiral stent in patients with urinary retention caused by bladder outlet obstruction from benign prostatic hyperplasia. Br J Urol 2001; 88(1): 30–34

25. Cooper K, Te A, Kaplan S. Long term safety and efficacy in 147 patients treated with prostatic stents for BPH: 12 year results: J Urol 2003; 169(4): 466

26. Cockett A T, Aso Y, Denis L, et al. Recommendations of the International Consensus Committee concerning: 4. Treatment recommendations for Benign Prostatic Hyperplasia (BPH). Proceedings of the Third International Consultation on Benign Prostatic Hyperplasia. Monaco, 1995: 625–650

27. Jepsen J V, Bruskewitz R C. Comprehensive patient evaluation for benign prostatic hyperplasia. Urology 1998; 51 (suppl 4A): 13–18

28. McConnell J D. Epidemiology, etiology, pathophysiology, and diagnosis of benign prostatic hyperplasia. In: Campbell's urology: 1440–1452

29. Kaplan S A, Te A E. Uroflowmetry and urodynamics, advances in benign prostatic hyperplasia. Urol Clin North Am 1995; 22, 2: 309–320

30. Abrams P. Objective evaluation of bladder outlet obstruction. Br J Urol 1995; 76 (suppl 1): 11–15

31. Emberton M, Neal D E, Fordham M, Harrison M, Blandy J P, McBrien M P, Williams R E, McPherson K, Black N, Devlin H B. The National Prostatectomy Audit. Morbidity, mortality and adverse events. J Urol 1994; 1121(5): 508A

32. Shields J R, Baird R A, McDonald D F. Differential uroflowmetry. J Urol 1958; 79(3): 580–588

33. Javle P, Jenkins S A, Machin D G, Parsons K F. Grading of benign prostatic obstruction can predict the outcomes of transurethral prostatectomy. J Urol 1998; 160: 1713–1717

34. Tubaro A, Anthonijs G, Avis M, Snijder R. Effect of Tamsulosin on bladder wall hypertrophy in patients with lower urinary tract symptoms suggestive of bladder outlet obstruction: results of a multicentre, placebo-controlled trial. Abstract 1798. Presented at the 2003 AUA, Chicago, USA

35. Dubey D, Kumar A, Kapoor R, Srivastava A, Mandhani A. Acute urinary retention: defining the need and timing for pressure-flow studies. Br J Urol 2001; 88: 178–182

54

Role of temporary stents after minimally invasive treatment for benign prostatic hyperplasia

H. Leenknegt and J. J. M. C. H. de la Rosette

Introduction

During the past decades an increasing number of less invasive treatment modalities have been introduced in the management of benign prostatic hyperplasia (BPH). Currently, the open prostatectomy is still considered to be the most efficient BPH treatment for relieving symptoms and improving uroflow for large prostates, but it is also the most invasive and morbid.

For moderately enlarged prostates, on the other hand, transurethral resection of the prostate (TURP) is the first treatment of choice but not without possible complications.[1,2] These may include intraoperative and postoperative blood loss, urethral or bladder neck strictures, erectile dysfunction, urinary incontinence, retrograde ejaculation, urinary tract infection and epididymitis. Patients who prefer to avoid surgery or no longer respond to medication, or with high comorbidity may undergo an alternative, less invasive therapy. These less invasive therapies are applied more and more often, mainly in an outpatient setting, without the need for general anesthesia or intensive patient monitoring.

Less invasive therapies include visual laser ablation of the prostate (VLAP), high intensity focused ultrasound (HIFU), transurethral needle ablation (TUNA),[3] and transurethral microwave thermotherapy (TUMT). VLAP delivers photothermal energy resulting in ablation of prostatic tissue. HIFU transrectally induces prostatic tissue ablation through focused ultrasound,[4] and TUNA delivers low radio-frequency energy via needles to the hyperplastic prostate tissue, producing coagulation necrosis and subsequently shrinking of the prostate gland. TUMT delivers heat through microwave energy.[2]

These thermal therapies all generate coagulation necrosis of prostate tissue with edema which may result in acute retention (Table 54.1). Subsequently, this can be treated with clean intermittent catheterization, a prolonged indwelling catheter or suprapubic catheterization. However, all of these may be inconvenient to the patient, and provide a possible route for bacterial infection of the bladder. Transient urinary retention and voiding difficulty resulting from these procedures may be managed with the temporary placement of a stent positioned in the prostatic urethra.

Fabian initially described the use of a nonexpandable metal coil stent in the urethra for bladder outlet obstruction as a result of BPH. His original design

Table 54.1. *Retention with need for catheterization after minimal invasive therapy*

Series	No. pts	Treatment	No. retention	Duration of catheterization (days)
Dahlstrand et al.[20]	38	TUMT	NA	3–5
Dahlstrand et al.[19]	15	TUMT	NA	14
De la Rosette et al.[21]	116	TUMT	116	16
Devonec et al.[22]	37	TUMT	7	7
Djavan et al.[16]	91	TUMT	10	7–14
Norris et al.[23]	108	VLAP	NA	2–7
Kabalin et al.[24]	13	VLAP	NA	5
Petas et al.[9]	22	VLAP	NA	6.5
Foster et al.[25]	15	HIFU	11	1–4
Madersbacher et al.[26]	50	HIFU	NA	6
Eberle et al.[27]	27	HIFU	NA	11
Schulman et al.[28]	25	TUNA	4	2
Sirls et al.[29]	68	TUNA	NA	1

is marketed as the Urospiral®, and a similar but gold-plated design is available as the Prostakath® but both have problems, such as encrustation and displacement.[5] Therefore, these are not suitable for prolonged use. Some of the more recently introduced stents for temporary use include a biodegradable spiral stent, the Trestle® prostatic bridge, the Prosta Coil®, the Conticath® , the Memokath® and the Barnes® stent.[6,7] The advantage of these stents is easier positioning and removal, preferably under local anesthesia. These devices are discussed elsewhere in this book and are only considered briefly here.

The design of the stents and the choice of the material are based on different concepts and are related to ease of application, ease of removal and risk of migration.

A blind method of application is being investigated in the Trestle® stent. The Trestle® silicone stent comprises three parts: two tubes, and a compressible connection. The connection lies at the level of the sphincter without disturbing its normal function. The upper tube bridges the prostate and has an external diameter of 22 Fr. After placement of the stent the proper position of each part may be confirmed by flexible cystoscopy. If necessary, the stent can be repositioned. The removal of the stent is easily performed by pulling a string connected to the distal part of the stent end that can be grasped at the level of the meatus. In addition, the special design of the stent, consisting of two parts, is meant to avoid possible migration.

The ProstaCoil® is designed based on a similar concept. This catheter is made of a nickel and titanium alloy (Nitinol/NiTi) which has a shape memory.[8] The coil is wound onto a delivery catheter and after expansion it has a wavy form with a diameter of 24–30 Fr. Like the Trestle® it has a trans-sphincteric, helical part, maintaining normal sphincter function. This stent is placed under fluoroscopy.

Another shape memory prostate stent is the Memokath®. The Memokath® stent is a coil of a nickel-titanium alloy (NiTi), the lower end expands when heated. It is inserted with a flexible cystoscope.

In summary, all the above stents can be easily inserted and attempt to avoid migration by including a part that crosses the external sphincter. However, the removal is easier in some types of design than others.

A different type of design is the Conticath® stent. This stent has a proximal curl that is positioned in the bladder and prevents distal migration, a prostatic segment, a narrow sphincteric segment ending with a small plastic cage that prevents proximal migration.

The 16 Fr Barnes® stent is 75 mm long, of which 15 mm is a 'basket' that opens in the prostatic cavity for anchoring.

Finally, one has to mention the biodegradable stents. These stents are composed of self-reinforced polyglycolic acid and its geometry is that of a simple helical spiral. This spiral tends to expand so that the outer diameter increases by half. Degradation into glycolic acid occurs through hydrolysis and is generally at week 3 or 4. After 4–6 months all the components cease to exist.

Results

The application of laser energy for the treatment of benign prostatic hyperplasia (BPH) was very popular about 10 years ago. In a follow-up to the blinded application using the transurethral laser induced prostatectomy (TULIP) device, the visual laser ablation of the prostate (VLAP) came to be used. Later, interstitial laser coagulation (ILC) was introduced and more recently, Holmium laser resection has become available. The main disadvantage of most later applications is the prolonged need of bladder drainage because of post-treatment retention. The use of temporary stents following laser treatment seems an excellent solution.

Petas et al. used a biodegradable stent in the prostatic urethra.[9] Following VLAP with placement of a suprapubic catheter they compared stenting with a suprapubic catheter with a combined suprapubic and indwelling catheter. Voiding began 1 or 2 days postoperatively in 20 of 27 stented patients, 8 of 23 patients with a suprapubic catheter, and 16 of 22 men after removal of their indwelling catheter, which occurred after an average of 6.5 days. The patients with only a 1 or 2 day catheterization period had fewer infections. In a more recent study, they demonstrated that the mean peak urinary flow rate increased significantly in the stented group only after a 1 month follow-up.[10] Some patients reported decreased urinary flow after 3–4 weeks, probably due to the degradation of the stent.

Laaksovirta et al. also evaluated a biodegradable stent after ILC. Of 39 patients all but one voided on the first postoperative day.[11] One stent was located too proximally. When it was repositioned, this patient also voided.

Barnes et al. used another type of stent following laser ablation. Postoperatively, 88% of patients voided immediately.[12] When postoperative retention occurred, a suprapubic catheter was placed. More recently, a Barnes® stent was placed by Yakubu et al. Of 55 men, 37 (67%) voided immediately.[13] One early stent migration resulted in urinary retention for 48 hours. This supports the concept of a prostatic stent maintaining and improving voiding in the early postoperative period.

Transurethral microwave thermotherapy (TUMT) is considered to be the most promising minimal invasive therapy for BPH.[14] However, following TUMT urinary retention is significant and several stents have been applied to prevent acute retention. In one study, the Trestle stent was used in 42 patients.[15] Six patients had their stent replaced for a suprapubic catheter due to clot formation while under oral anticoagulants. They had their catheter changed for a stent after 2 days, after which they also could void freely. Following TUMT, they also compared a Foley catheter with placement of a biodegradable polyglycolic stent. The mean duration of Foley catheterization was 14 days. One of the 16 patients receiving a stent showed retention, which resolved after it was replaced. After this he voided freely. Another patient developed retention after 14 days. He received a suprapubic catheter until the edema resolved. None of the patients experienced secondary retention as a result of degradation of the spirals.

Another study also used a Trestle stent after TUMT.[16] None of these 54 patients experienced acute retention that lasted more than 1 week, while 10 of 91 patients who only underwent TUMT required catheterization. Three stents had to be removed due to clot formation with subsequent impairment of patency. Three were removed due to migration.

In addition to the two minimal invasive therapies described above (VLAP and TUMT) that have been demonstrated to be satisfactory alternatives for the management of BPH there have been more therapeutic developments. Transrectal high intensity focused ultrasound (HIFU) is capable of decreasing the degree of bladder outflow obstruction, but the most important side-

effect is transient urinary retention requiring suprapubic catheterization. The suprapubic catheter was removed after a mean of 5.8 days, but may be required for up to 19 days.[4] Results indicate that transurethral needle ablation (TUNA) is also effective in relieving symptoms in patients with BPH.[3] However, Oesterling et al. reported that up to 40% of patients treated with TUNA required transient catheterization.[17] Most probably, these two groups of patients would also benefit from temporary stenting of the prostatic urethra following these minimally invasive therapies (Table 54.2).

Discussion

Numerous modern heat therapies, including laser ablation and transurethral microwave thermotherapy (TUMT), have have shown to be effective in the management of bladder outlet obstruction from prostatic hyperplasia. It offers an appealing treatment option for those that for some reason can or will not undergo more demanding therapies, such as transurethral resection of the prostate (TURP). While these minimal invasive therapies are safe procedures with a positive effect on voiding difficulties from BPH, significant morbidity is introduced through the need for transient catheterization following these therapies.

The early trials support the concept that temporary stenting of the prostatic urethra is very useful after minimally invasive therapies using heat. They maintain the urethral lumen, which immediately results in adequate voiding and prevention of the long-term use of an indwelling or suprapubic catheter. One month after stent removal, symptoms and flow rates remain stable to 1 year of follow-up.[16]

Some studies reported some minor discomfort in the first few days after stent placement, but provide effective relief from retention. In an outpatient setting, these stents are straightforward and non-traumatic to position, under a local anesthetic. Removal is performed in the same setting, and is usually carried out by administration of a local anesthetic and gently pulling out the device, avoiding causing any damage to the urethra.

However, these temporary stents also have their disadvantages. In addition to some difficulty in delivering and positioning these stents, migration resulting in incontinence or retention, retention from blood clots may also occur.[9] Biodegradable stents may

Table 54.2. *Morbidity of temporary stenting of the prostate after minimal invasive therapy*

Series	No. pts	Treatment	Type stent	Problems				
				discomfort	retention	migration	infection	bloodclotting
Nissenkorn et al.[18]	15	Laser	prostate bridge	2/15	3/15	0/15	0/15	NA
Talja et al.[30]	22	Laser	biodegradable	5/22	4/22	0/22	3/22	NA
Yakubu et al.[13]	55	Laser	Barnes® stent	3/55	18/55	3/55	2/55	NA
Barnes et al.[31]	80	Laser	Barnes® stent	5/80	21/80	5/80	4/80	NA
Petas et al.[9]	27	Laser	biodegradable	NA	7/27	2/27	7/27	1/27
Petas et al.[10]	21	Laser	biodegradable	2/21	3/21	1/21	3/21	0/21
Laaksovirta et al.[11]	39	Laser	biodegradable	2/39	1/39	1/39	3/39	NA
Devonec et al.[15]	42	TUMT	prostatic bridge	NA	6/42	0/42	0/42	6/42
	16	TUMT	biodegradable	NA	2/16	1/16	NA	0/16
Djavan et al.[16]	54	TUMT	prostatic bridge	NA	0/54	3/54	2/54	3/54
Dahlstrand et al.[19]	15	TUMT	biodegradable	4/15	0/15	1/15	NA	NA

cause voiding to be more obstructed between the third and fourth weeks following minimally invasive therapy or even late urine retention.[9,11] None of the authors showed that stents remained in the urethra at 6 months. However, some necrotic tissue was still seen in the prostatic urethra at that time. There were also patients with prolonged irritative symptoms during at least 3 months postoperatively.[18] Patients receiving a biodegradable stent needed more nursing care than those given a Foley catheter.[15]

Some patients may have problems with additional interventions that may be required following stent placement in order to confirm adequate positioning, such as using transrectal ultrasound and cystoscopy.[19] Problems should be prevented by carefully selecting patients eligible for temporary stenting.

What is the future for temporary stents in combination with minimal invasive therapies? Obviously, these stents should meet several requirements. The ideal stent should be easy to insert and remove, usually under a local anesthetic. It should also be able to conform to the shape of the prostate and urethra. It should not extend beyond the prostatic urethra into the bladder, should not migrate or cause any local reaction or encrustation. When positioned, it should allow spontaneous voiding while maintaining continence. Importantly, it should be relatively inexpensive. Finally, biodegradable stents seem the most attractive, however, they should have a longer degradation time of a minimum of 6 weeks.

Multi-center studies will confirm that the intraprostatic stent is a valuable addition to the armamentarium of the urologist treating elderly or frail men with advanced bladder outlet obstruction, and complements existing technologies.

References

1. Jespen J, Bruskewitz R C. Recent developments in the surgical management of benign prostatic hyperplasia. Urology 1998; (suppl.4a): 23–31
2. Williams J H, Chilton C P. New therapeutic options in prostatic enlargement. Br J Hosp Med 1994; 51: 477–481
3. Beduschi M C, Oesterling J E. Transurethral needle ablation of the prostate: a minimally invasive treatment for symptomatic benign prostatic hyperplasia. Mayo Clin Proc 1998; 73: 696–701
4. Madersbacher S, Klingler C H, Schatzl G, Schmidbauer C P, Marberger M. The urodynamic impact of transrectal high-intensity focused ultrasound on bladder outflow obstruction. Eur Urol 1996; 30: 437–445
5. Fabian K M. Der intraprostatische 'Partielle Katheter' (urologische Spirale). Urologe A 1980; 19: 236
6. Kletscher B A, Oesterling E. Current perspectives for the management of benign prostatic hyperplasia. Urol Clin North Am 1995; 22: 423–430
7. Khoury S. Future directions in the management of benign prostatic hyperplasia. Br J Urol 1992; 70 (suppl 1): 27–32
8. Yachia D, Beyar M, Aridogan I A. A new, large calibre, self-expanding and self-retaining temporary intraprostatic stent (ProstaCoil) in the treatment of prostatic obstruction. Br J Urol 1994; 74: 47–49
9. Petas A, Talja M, Tammela T et al. A randomized study to compare biodegradable self-reinforced polyglycolic acid spiral stents to suprapubic or indwelling catheters after visual laser ablation of the prostate. J Urol 1997; 157: 173–176
10. Petas A, Isotalo T, Talja M, Tammela T L J, Valimaa T, Tormala P. A randomised study to evaluate the efficacy of a biodegradable stent in the prevention of postoperative urinary retention after interstitial

laser coagulation of the prostate. Scand J Urol Nephrol 2000; 34(4): 262–266

11. Laaksovirta S, Talja M, Valimaa T, Isotalo T, Tormala P, Tammela T L J. Expansion and bioabsorption of the self-reinforced lactic and glycolic acid copolymer prostatic spiral stent. J Urol 2001; 166: 919–922

12. Barnes D G, Butterworth P, Flynn J T. Combined endoscopic laser ablation of the prostate (ELAP) and temporary prostatic stenting. Minim Invasive Ther Allied Technol 1996; 5: 333–335

13. Yakubu A, Barnes D. Catheter-free endoscopic laser ablation of the prostate using a 1-size prostatic stent. J Urol 1998; 159: 1974–1977

14. de la Rosette J J M C H, Beerlage H P, Debruyne F M J. Role of temporary stents in alternative treatment of benign prostatic hyperplasia. J Endourol 1997; 11: 467–472

15. Devonec M, Dahlstrand C. Temporary urethral stenting after high-energy transurethral microwave thermotherapy of the prostate. World J Urol 1998; 16: 120–123

16. Djavan B, Ghawidel K, Basharkhah A, Hruby S, Bursa B, Marberger M. Temporary intraurethral prostatic bridge-catheter compared with neoadjuvant and adjuvant alpha-blockade to improve early results of high-energy transurethral microwave thermotherapy. Urology 1999; 54: 73–80

17. Oesterling J E, Issa M M, Roehrborn C G, Bruskewitz R, Naslund M J, Perez-Marrero R et al. Long-term results of a prospective, randomized clinical trial comparing TUNA to TURP for the treatment of symptomatic BPH (abstr). J Urol 1997; 157 (suppl): 328

18. Nissenkorn I, Slutzker D, Shalev M. Use of an intraurethral catheter instead of a Foley catheter after laser treatment of benign prostatic hyperplasia. Eur Urol 1996; 29: 341–344

55

Use of biodegradable stents after visual laser ablation of the prostate

A. Pétas

Introduction

In 1980, Fabian introduced a urological spiral to keep the prostatic lobes from compressing the urethra, thus allowing spontaneous voiding.[1] Since then, permanent and temporary stents have been used to relieve infravesical obstruction. Permanent stents have been described as incorporated into tissue and temporary stents as removable, although nowadays the difference between these has become less clear, because temporary stents have been left for long periods, semi-permanently. As a result of active research for better stents, new stent materials and designs have been introduced. Although the idea of stenting the male urethra seems quite simple and attractive, stents have had many side effects and technical problems, such as encrustation, migration and irritative symptoms. Progress in manufacturing biodegradable materials has enabled helical spirals to be produced that can be used as biodegradable stents. The major advantage of a biodegradable spiral stent is that there is no need for removal of the implanted material. This chapter deals with experiences with the use of a biodegradable spiral stent combined with visual laser ablation of the prostate (VLAP).

Materials and methods

VLAP has become one alternative for the treatment of benign prostatic hypertrophy (BPH); it was first introduced in clinical use in Australia in 1990.[2] The therapy is based on photothermal coagulation of the prostate tissue with a neodymium:yttrium aluminium garnet (Nd:YAG) laser and right-angle side-firing free-beam delivery system. There are, however, several problems associated with VLAP, including postoperative urinary retention due to oedema following coagulation necrosis and requiring brief (up to 2 days) catheterization in the majority of patients and prolonged catheterization in up to 38%.[3]

Biodegradable materials have been used for sutures for more than 20 years and for bone fixation for more than 10 years.[4] They are based on polymers, which in

this study were glycolic acid and lactic acid. Biodegradation is defined as disintegration of the polymer in any biological environment by hydrolysis, enzymes or bacteria. The benefits of biodegradable stents are (1) there is no need for a second removal procedure, (2) the flexible spiral construction, and (3) the property of expansion at body temperature thus fixing the implant in place.

Self-reinforced, poly-L-lactide (SR-PLLA) spirals showed good biocompatibility in the anterior urethra.[5,6] Biodegradable spiral stents were first designed for strictures in the anterior urethra. In an experimental study in rabbits[5], SR-PLLA implanted for 6 months showed minimal tissue reaction and good biocompatibility. It also showed that its mechanical properties are suitable for supporting tubular structures such as the urethra. After VLAP was introduced for the treatment of bladder outlet obstruction (BOO) due to BPH, it became apparent that it carried a high risk of postoperative urinary retention. As a natural consequence, a biodegradable spiral stent was designed for the prostatic urethra based on the stent described by Fabian. The degradation time of a self-reinforced polyglycolic acid (SR-PGA) spiral stent was about 3–4 weeks and of self-reinforced poly-DL-lactic acid (SR-PLA 96) about 3–4 months in vitro (Fig. 55.1). Several

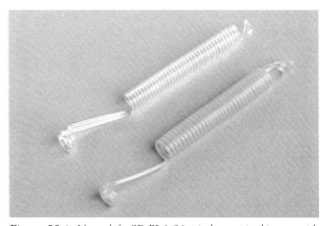

Figure 55.1. *Upper left, SR-PLA 96 spiral stent, in this case with double helix configuration; lower right, SR-PGA spiral stent.*

other investigators have reported good results with similar metal spirals for transient or definitive therapy of prostatic obstruction.[7–9]

Studies with biodegradable stents

The author has studied the efficacy and safety of an SR-PGA spiral stent in the treatment of postoperative urinary retention after VLAP. In the first pilot study, an SR-PGA spiral stent was inserted in 22 patients after VLAP.[10] After encouraging results had been obtained, a second randomized study in three arms was performed with 72 patients.[11] In the third study, the efficacy and safety of a SR-PLA 96 spiral stent, which had a degradation time of about 3–6 months, were evaluated.[12] Patients with symptomatic BOO due to BPH, who underwent VLAP, were accepted for these studies. Follow-up studies were performed at 1, 3, and 6 months in all three studies.

Insertion technique

After laser therapy, a 5–7 Fr ureteral catheter was inserted into the urinary bladder. The ureteral catheter performed as a guidewire to prevent the flexible spiral stent from kinking or bending during its deployment into the prostatic urethra, especially in the case of a large median lobe. A suture thread was looped to the distal ring or to the few distal loops of the prostatic part of the stent for use as a pulling device. The urethra was lubricated with gel, then the spiral stent was pushed into the urethra over the ureteral catheter. Using the tip of the cystoscope, the spiral stent was pushed into the prostatic urethra. The correct location of the stent was verified endoscopically (Fig. 55.2). By pulling the suture thread, the spiral stent could be moved distally for repositioning. First the ureteral catheter was removed, then the thread and finally the cystoscope. The patients were allowed to void immediately.

SR-PGA spiral stent: pilot study

This study involved 22 patients aged 55–81 (mean 68.5) years. The mean prostatic volume was 43 (range 26–92) cm^3. All patients completed the 6-month follow-up period. All patients voided freely on postoperative day 1 or 2. Four patients experienced late retention due to early degradation of the spiral at 3–4 weeks postoperatively. The median dose of laser energy used

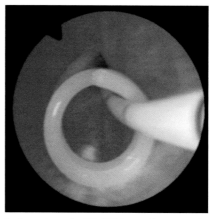

Figure 55.2. *Insertion: the SR-PGA spiral stent is placed over the catheter. Then the stent is pushed along the catheter with the tip of the cystoscope into the correct position. The distal ring of the stent is at the bulbous urethra near the external urethral sphincter.*

was 656 (range 273–1083) J/cm^3. The peak urinary flow rates increased and symptom scores decreased significantly during the 6-month follow-up (Table 55.1); post-void residual volume also decreased significantly, from 176 to 75 ml. There was no significant change in the sexual symptom score. About half of the patients stated that the urinary stream became poorer at 3–4 weeks. The obstructive symptoms also increased for some weeks. Cystoscopy at 4 weeks showed remains of spiral fragments in the prostatic urethra (Figs 55.3 and 55.4). No stones or foreign bodies were found at 6 months follow-up.

SR-PGA spiral stent: randomized study

A total of 72 patients aged 52–83 (mean 68.5) years with symptomatic BPH entered the study. Six patients had urinary retention. Mean prostatic volume was 44 (range 12–92) cm^3. The patients were randomized into three groups (Fig. 55.5): group A (n = 27) received an SR-PGA spiral stent and suprapubic catheter; group B (n = 23) received suprapubic catheter, and group C (n = 22) received a suprapubic catheter and indwelling catheter. In all groups the suprapubic catheter was inserted prior to laser therapy and was removed when the patient was able to void. In the indwelling catheter group (group C) a 20 Fr silicone indwelling catheter was removed after a median of 6.5 days.

All but one patient completed the 6-month follow-up period. The mean dose of laser energy used was 957 J/cm^3 in group A, 950 J/cm^3 in group B, and 983 J/cm^3

Table 55.1. *Results of studies using biodegradable spiral stents with VLAP*

Reference	No. of patients	Treatment group	Peak urinary flow rate (ml/s)		DAN-PSS score		Mean residual volume (ml)	
			Preop.	6 months[*]	Preop.	6 months[*]	Preop.	6 months[*]
Talja et al.[10] SR-PGA	22	SR-PGA	8.1	14.1	16.4	3.0	176	75
Pétas et al.[11] SR-PGA	27	SR-PGA	8.4	15.8	23.3	4.7	164	40
	23	Suprapubic catheter	7.5	16.4	22.1	4.4	139	40
	22	Suprapubic catheter and indwelling catheter	8.4	11.3	18.4	6.0	138	40
Pétas et al.[12] SR-PLA 96	22	SR-PLA 96	6.9	15.2	27.0	9.1	132	45
	23	Suprapubic catheter	7.5	16.4	22.1	4.4	139	40

[*]All values at 6 months were statistically significant compared with preoperative value.

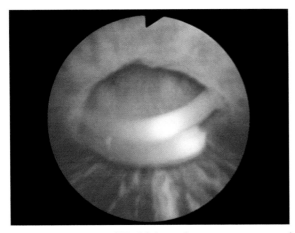

Figure 55.3. *Fragments of SR-PGA spiral stents in prostatic urethra at 1 month follow-up.*

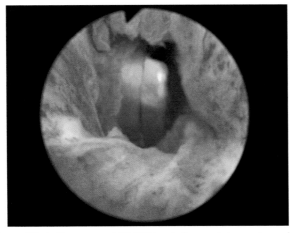

Figure 55.4. *Fragments of SR-PGA spiral stents in prostatic urethra at 1 month follow-up.*

in group C. Of the 27 patients, 20 voided freely on the first or second postoperative day in group A, compared with 8/23 in group B ($p < 0.001$). In group C, 16 of the 22 patients were able to void within 2 days after removal of the indwelling catheter.

In group A, bleeding from the prostate during laser therapy caused blood clots postoperatively and delayed the beginning of voiding in one patient. In two patients, the spiral stent was pushed proximally because of too-distal placement; the first patient had urinary leakage and the second had urinary retention. Alternatively, the positioning could be checked by transrectal ultrasound (Fig. 55.6). Another patient had a thin, membrane-like stricture at the external sphincter area at the 1 month follow-up; this was treated by internal urethrotomy and no further strictures were noted during follow-up. In one patient a suprapubic catheter was re-inserted for 7 days because of preperitoneal urine leakage after removal of the suprapubic catheter.

In group B, four cases of postoperative urinary retention (range 4–29 days) were treated after the beginning of voiding and removal of the suprapubic catheter. Transurethral incision of the prostate was performed 3 months postoperatively in one patient in this group because of bladder neck stenosis.

In group C urinary retention developed 10 days postoperatively in one patient and 2 months postoperatively in a second patient, including haemorrhage requiring bladder irrigations. In one

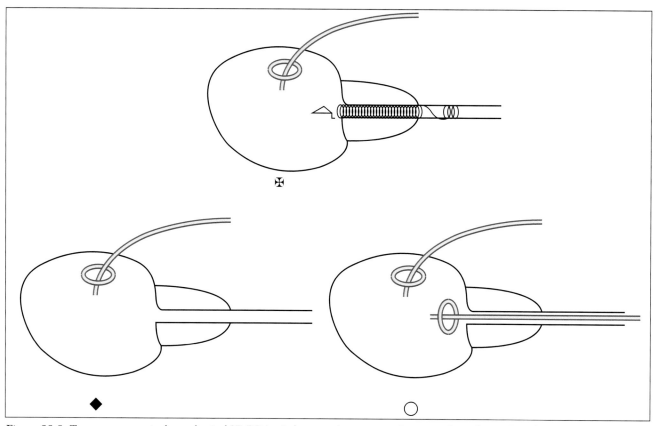

Figure 55.5. *Treatment groups in the randomized SR-PGA spiral stent study:* ✠, *stent;* ◆, *suprapubic catheter;* ○, *indwelling catheter.*

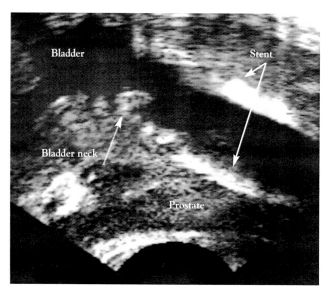

Figure 55.6. *The SR-PGA spiral stent is clearly visualized on transrectal ultrasound (TRUS) examination, here at postoperative day 5, showing the bladder neck opening and the lumen of the proximal end of the stent in the correct position.*

patient, stricture developed at the external sphincter area 3 months postoperatively; this was treated by urethrotomy and self-dilatation.

The peak urinary flow rates increased significantly during the 6-month follow-up ($p < 0.001$, Table 55.1) in all groups. In addition, the mean residual urine volume decreased significantly in all groups during the follow-up period. The prostatic symptom score had also decreased significantly at the 6-month follow-up ($p < 0.001$, Table 55.1) in every group. No significant change in the sexual symptom score occurred in any of the groups.

Some patients experienced a decrease in the force of their urinary stream after 3 weeks and an increase in their obstructive symptoms for some weeks, as in the pilot study. At 4 weeks, patients still had some spiral stent fragments in the posterior urethra. No foreign bodies or urinary stones were noted in the bladder at 3 or 6 months. The entire prostatic urethra was lined with

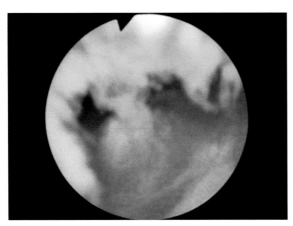

Figure 55.7. *Image of prostatic urethra in a patient with SR-PGA spiral stent at 1 month follow-up. Between 7 and 2 o'clock, white necrotic sloughing tissue can be seen; at the 3–6 o'clock position, the urethral wall is covered with epithelium. No stent fragments are visible.*

necrotic tissue 4 weeks postoperatively in all patients (Fig. 55.7). At 3 months in half of the patients the lased prostatic surface was still covered with necrotic tissue. In one-third of the patients a few small necrotic areas in the prostatic urethra at 6 months after VLAP could still be noted.

The rate of infection was 7/27 (26%) in Group A, 8/23 (35%) in Group B and 8/22 (36%) in Group C. The infection rates between treatment groups did not differ significantly. However, when patients were divided into new groups according to suprapubic catheterization time, infections were noted in 6/28 patients (21%) in the group catheterized for 1–2 days and 17/44 infections (38%) in those catheterized for more than 2 days. The rate of infection was significantly ($p = 0.0046$) lower in those catheterized for 1–2 days. Pressure–flow studies were not conducted.

SR-PLA 96 spiral stent

A total of 45 patients were randomized into the study. All patients completed the 6-month follow-up. The mean dose of laser energy used was 1032 (range 570–2670) J/ml. Mean prostatic volume was 35 (range 12–60) ml. The patients were randomized into groups receiving the SR-PLA 96 spiral stent or a suprapubic catheter.

Postoperatively, voiding began in 18 patients at day 1 or 2 (range 0–10) in the SR-PLA 96 spiral stent group. In contrast, eight patients in the suprapubic

catheter group were able to void at day 1 or 2 (range 1–13) ($p < 0.001$). The peak urinary flow rates had increased significantly ($p < 0.001$) in the SR-PLA 96 spiral stent group at 1, 3 and 6 months follow-up; in the suprapubic catheter group, peak flow rates had increased significantly at 3 and 6 months follow-up ($p < 0.001$). The mean residual urine volume decreased significantly in both groups during follow-up. The prostate symptom score (DAN-PSS) decreased significantly at 6 months ($p < 0.001$) in both groups. There were no significant changes in the sexual symptom scores. The differences between these groups in peak flow rate, symptom score or mean residual volume were not significant at any given follow-up period.

Urethroscopy showed that the stents were intact and accurately positioned at the 1-month follow-up. At 3 months the stents were found to be partially degraded in all patients. At the 6-month follow-up the fragments were still in the prostatic urethra or urinary bladder in 20 of 22 patients. Stone formation was seen in two patients in the spiral stent group at 6 months. The first patient had an asymptomatic stone in the urinary bladder, whereas the second patient had many irritative symptoms, with a stone in the prostatic urethra and five stones in the urinary bladder. These patients had recurrent urinary tract infections but no evidence of the spiral stent fragments was found.

Fragmentation of the SR-PLA 96 spiral stent took the same general course: first, the neck between the distal ring and prostatic part of the stent tended to break; then the helical prostatic part broke into large circular fragments (Fig. 55.9); finally the fragments broke further into smaller curved pieces 2–4 mm in length (Fig. 55.8). The stent fragments migrated into the urinary bladder or were voided with the urine. The fragments were not removed during cystoscopy at follow-up.

The rate of infection was 9/22 (41%) in the SR-PLA 96 spiral stent group and 8/23 (35%) in the suprapubic catheter group. Infection was judged to be a bacterial count, in culture, of 10^5. When infections were divided into groups according to suprapubic catheterization time, the infection rates were 3/20 (15%) in those with a catheter for up to 3 days compared with 14/25 (56%) in those with a catheter for more than 3 days ($p = 0.002$).

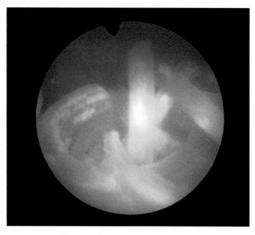

Figure 55.8. *Small curved fragments of SR-PLA 96 spiral stent at 6 months follow-up.*

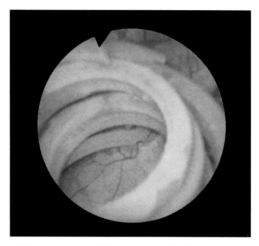

Figure 55.9. *Large helical fragments of SR-PLA 96 spiral stent at 6 months follow-up.*

Discussion

Transurethral resection of the prostate (TURP) is still the gold standard for the treatment of BPH, although VLAP has some benefits over TURP. VLAP is a fast and safe procedure and hospitalization is shorter. The biodegradable self-reinforced polyglycolic acid spiral stent is a unique method for the temporary stenting of the male urethra for prevention of urinary retention after VLAP.

VLAP induces high temperatures in the prostatic tissues, which leads to acute tissue swelling due to burn oedema which obstructs the prostatic urethra and causes transient urinary retention for several days. This retention is conventionally treated by use of an indwelling catheter or suprapubic catheter. A suprapubic catheter was used in every patient because the laser procedure is easier to perform with continuous irrigation, and because the patient could test the onset of voiding by closing the suprapubic catheter. Indwelling catheterization times of 24 h to 7 days have been reported.[13,14] Prolonged urethral or suprapubic catheterization after VLAP is inconvenient for the patient, and both the suprapubic and the urethral catheter provide a route for bacterial infection into the bladder.[15] Bacterial contamination of the necrotic prostatic tissue may even lead to prolonged urinary tract infection. After VLAP, infection rates up to 30% (and up to 50% without antibiotic prophylaxis) have been reported.[16,17] The incidence of postoperative infection in the study reported here was significantly lower in those patients with a short catheterization period (1–2 days). This suggests that infections associated with VLAP are due to catheter contamination and ascending infection. Presumably, by use of the spiral stent, the incidence of postoperative urinary retention and infections could be decreased.

Many patients given an SR-PGA spiral stent noted that voiding became more obstructed at 3–4 weeks postoperatively. There were also four cases of late retention in the pilot study. This problem was probably due to the degradation and sloughing of the spiral stent at a time when oedema and necrotic debris still obstructed the prostatic urethra. This transient voiding problem might be avoided by use of a spiral stent with a longer degradation time of up to 6–8 months, achieved by selecting more slowly degrading molecules. On the other hand, the degradation time of SR-PLA 96 turned out to be much longer than the period of tissue oedema, when used in combination with VLAP. The authors, therefore, do not recommend the SR-PLA 96 spiral stent for use after VLAP.

There was no need to remove the device because the spiral stent broke down into small fragments that were excreted with the urine. Many patients did not notice softened fragments in the urine, although some commented on them. The fragments passed without causing discomfort. If SR-PGA fragments remained in the bladder, they degraded completely within a few weeks without stone formation, whereas SR-PLA 96 fragments moved partially into the bladder, where they were still noted in 20 of 22 patients at 6 months.

The outcome of VLAP in this study was thus in line with the results reported by others. Overall, the decrease in voiding symptoms was highly significant. The patient-assessed symptom score system was useful in the author's study, since it included a 'bother' score in addition to the symptom score, and therefore is considered to provide a more reliable estimate of symptoms than other scoring systems.

The lasing technique used was similar to that in other VLAP studies, with a comparable energy dose.[18] The mean dose of laser energy in the pilot study was 656 J/ml, in the randomized SR-PGA study 963 J/ml and, in the SR-PLA study, 1032 J/ml. Cystoscopic examination revealed much remaining adenoma in many patients at 6 months. The laser dose in the pilot study was probably too low to induce enough necrotic tissue, which led to urinary retention at the time of degradation. Nowadays, much higher energy levels, of 2000 J/ml and more, have been recommended.

SR-PGA and SR-PLA 96 spiral stents are so rigid that they cannot be closed by compression of the prostatic side lobes in the early phase. The short length of the spiral stent may be the most important reason for delayed voiding in the author's patients. The spiral shortens, when it dilates, by about 0 to 4% of its original length. Nowadays it is recommended that the length of the spiral may exceed 10–15 mm in the urinary bladder to ensure adequate length. Sloughing tissue and blood clots can obstruct the spiral stent. Migration of the spiral stents was not detected; the expanding property of about 50% in diameter secures fixation of the stent. In these studies there was no need to remove the device; polymer fragments, if retained in the bladder, degraded completely within 6–8 months. Encrustation and stone formation on metallic stents is a frequent occurrence;[19,20] however, this had a low incidence in the study reported here: two cases of stone formation occurred in patients with recurrent urinary tract infection. Infection accelerates degradation of the spiral stent because of the increase in urine pH.

Biodegradable spiral stents could be used with other treatment modalities that cause prostatic oedema, such as transurethral microwave therapy (TUMT), transurethral needle ablation of the prostate (TUNA), high intensity focused ultrasound (HIFU), interstitial laser coagulation of the prostate (ILC), and cryotherapy. Other indications for the spiral stent might be recurrent bladder neck stenoses and temporary treatment of patients with urinary retention awaiting surgery, or in early-phase resolution of BOO in patients waiting for medical therapy to take effect and as a temporary supporting device in reconstructive surgery of the urethra.

Future prospects

Further controlled studies are needed to compare the biodegradable spiral stents with other methods of preventing urinary retention. New properties are being examined; such as shorter expansion time, and various degradation times and configurations. Research is needed to modify the spiral stent and to assess the most suitable materials for various demands. New properties, such as radiopacity, modifications in configuration, tailored degradation sequence and stents with rapid expansion times, are to be studied in the future.

Conclusions

The biodegradable SR-PGA spiral stent was safe and effective in the treatment of postoperative urinary retention after VLAP. The SR-PLA 96 spiral stent is not the best choice for use in combination with VLAP because of its excessively long degradation time. Other treatment modalities, such as ILC and TUNA, may require different optimal degradation times. The results are promising, but more randomized studies in other combination methods including medical treatment are still needed.

References

1. Fabian K M. Der Intraprostatische 'Partielle Katheter' (Urologische Spirale). Urologe A 1980; 19: 236–238
2. Costello A J, Bowsher W G, Bolton D M et al. Laser ablation of the prostate in patients with benign prostatic hypertrophy. Br J Urol 1992; 69: 603–605
3. Norris J P, Norris R D, Lee R D, Rubenstein M A. Visual laser ablation of the prostate: clinical experience in 108 patients. J Urol 1993; 150 (part 2): 1612
4. Törmälä P. Biodegradable self-reinforced composite materials; manufacturing structure and mechanical properties. Clin Mater 1992; 10: 29–34
5. Kemppainen E, Talja M, Riihelä M et al. Bioresorbable urethral stent. Urol Res 1993; 21: 235
6. Rokkanen P, Böstman Ö, Vainionpää S et al. Biodegradable implants in fracture fixation: early results of treatment of fractures of the ankle. Lancet 1985; 1: 1422

7. Nordling J, Holm H H, Klarskov P et al. The intraprostatic spiral: a new device for insertion with the patient under local anesthesia and with ultrasonic guidance with 3 months of follow-up. J Urol 1989; 142: 756–758

8. Ala-Opas M, Talja M, Tiitinen J et al. Prostakath in urinary outflow obstruction. Ann Chir Gynaecol Suppl 1993; 206: 14–18

9. Thomas P J, Britton P J, Harrison N W. The prostakath stent: four years experience. Br J Urol 1993; 71: 430–432

10. Talja M, Tammela T, Pétas A et al. Biodegradable self-reinforced polyglycolic acid spiral stent in prevention of postoperative urinary retention after visual laser ablation of the prostate-laser prostatectomy. J Urol 1995; 154: 2089–2092

11. Pétas A, Talja M, Tammela T et al. A randomized study to compare biodegradable self-reinforced polyglycolic acid spiral stent to suprapubic catheter and indwelling catheter after visual laser ablation of the prostate. J Urol 1977; 157: 173–176

12. Pétas A, Talja M, Tammela T L J et al. Biodegradable self-reinforced poly-DL-lactic acid (SR-PLA 96) spiral stent compared to suprapubic catheter in the treatment of postoperative urinary retention after visual laser ablation of the prostate. Br J Urol 1997; 80: 439–443

13. Kabalin J N. Laser prostatectomy performed with a right angle firing neodymium:YAG laser fiber at 40 watts power setting. J Urol 1993; 150: 95–99

14. Costello A J, Schaffer B S, Crowe H R. Second-generation delivery systems for laser prostatic ablation. Urology 1994; 43: 262–266

15. Nickel J C, Grant S K, Costerton J W. Catheter associated bacteriuria. Urology 1985; 26: 369

16. Boon T A, de Gier R P E, van Venrooij G E P M et al. Clinical and urodynamic results six months after 'TULIP' laser prostatectomy. In: Proceedings of the XIth Congress of the European Association of Urology, 13–16 July 1994, abstr 149

17. le Rolland B, Barthelemy Y, Colombel M et al. TULIP laser in the treatment of benign hypertrophy of the prostate (BPH). In: Proceedings of the XIth Congress of the European Association of Urology, 13-16 July 1994 abstr 152

18. Costa F J. Lomefloxacin prophylaxis in visual laser ablation of the prostate Urology 1994; 44: 933–936

19. Costello A J, Crowe H R. A single institution experience of reflecting laser fibre prostatectomy over four years. J Urol 1994; 151: 229A

20. Holmes S A V, Miller P D, Crocker P R, Kirby R S. Encrustation of intraprostatic stents — a comparative study. Br J Urol 1992; 69: 383–387

Prostatic stents in prostate cancer

Relief of bladder outlet obstruction caused by prostate cancer using a long-term intra-urethral stent (ProstaCoil)

I. A. Aridogan and D. Yachia

Introduction

Prostate cancer is a major factor in the health of the ageing male population and, in terms of incidence, it is the most common cancer among American men.[1] With regard to prevalence, prostate cancer probably represents the most common malignancy in males. Incidental, unsuspected or latent carcinoma has been detected in about 10–20% of prostate tissue specimens examined following prostatectomy performed because of lower urinary tract symptoms due to benign prostatic hyperplasia (BPH).[2]

Although radical prostatectomy offers a patient with locally confined disease an excellent opportunity for cure, unfortunately large numbers of newly diagnosed prostate cancer cases are found in the advanced stage of the disease, which is usually not considered amenable to radical surgery. Hormonal manipulation is usually the treatment of choice in these patients.

Occasionally, prostate cancer patients who have metastatic or locally advanced disease present with urinary retention. Moul and associates found that 13.3% of patients with acute retention had adenocarcinoma of the prostate.[3] In both groups of patients conventionally an indwelling catheter is inserted and hormone manipulative treatment is started. However, despite the potential operative morbidity and postoperative sequelae,[4] another alternative is to combine transurethral resection of the prostate (TURP) with hormonal manipulation. The advanced age of the patients may also increase the surgical risk. After hormonal manipulation, regression of the prostatic mass may take several months. When deciding on the use of an indwelling catheter until the prostatic mass reduces, the complications caused by the indwelling catheter, its acceptability to the patient, and interference with his social and personal life, should also be taken into consideration.[5]

Use of intraprostatic stents

The first application of an intraprostatic stent to relieve urinary obstruction is credited to Fabian in the early 1980s, following his report on the temporary placement of the Urological Spiral 'Partial Catheter' in men with urinary retention due to BPH.[6] Since then, the use of intra-urethral stenting devices has gained acceptance and others have applied similar devices successfully in the interim management of symptomatic BPH and urethral strictures. These first-generation stents, because of their high spontaneous migration rates (reaching to 30–35%) and occlusion by clots or stone formation, gave way in the late 1980s to new, larger calibre, temporary or permanent expandable stents allowing access to the bladder. Although permanent self-expandable mesh stents have been used in BPH with relative success, their use in malignant disease has been less successful because of tumoral tissue proliferation through the openings of the mesh.

The use of a temporary intraprostatic stent in patients with urinary retention due to adenocarcinoma of the prostate was reported by Anson and associates in 1993, for the first time.[7] They used a combination of the Porgés Urospiral with the oral anti-androgen flutamide in ten patients with urinary retention or severe bladder outflow obstruction. The mean age of their patients was 72 years. The stent was inserted on an inpatient basis under direct vision. In their series one patient developed persistent dysuria and urinary frequency necessitating early stent removal and TURP 2 weeks later. Another patient spontaneously voided his stent at 4 weeks postoperatively. The remaining eight stents were removed under sedoanalgesia, with the patients as day cases, 3 months after insertion. The authors reported that at the 3 month follow-up all patients successfully voided after stent removal and had adequate flow rates and low post-micturition residuals; they mention only the failure rate and the cost of this combination as disadvantages of the procedure.

In 1994, Guazzoni and associates used the Urolume Wallstent in 16 patients with stage D prostate cancer and urinary retention unrelieved by total androgen blockade with goserelin and flutamide.[8] The stent, which is permanent, was inserted endoscopically on an inpatient basis. In their 1-year follow-up, only ten patients were evaluated: all but one patient were relieved of obstruction at 1 year. Furthermore, the subjective response was satisfactory and showed a progressive amelioration with time, probably related to the increasing re-epithelialization. In the series of Guazzoni and associates, improvement was more evident in the obstructive than the irritative symptoms, which confirms previously reported data.[9]

Use of the ProstaCoil in malignant obstruction

After successfully using intraprostatic stents (the Prostakath and the ProstaCoil) for some years for BPH,[10,11] the authors decided to use the self-expanding ProstaCoil in malignant obstruction. The aim in using the ProstaCoil in such cases was to allow patients to void spontaneously during hormone manipulative treatment until reduction of the size of the prostatic mass. The ProstaCoil was used in 34 patients with advanced carcinoma of the prostate who had an indwelling catheter and failed to void at repeated trials. Their mean age was 78 (range 52–91) years. All patients underwent surgical (subcapsular orchiectomy) or non-surgical (anti-androgens) hormone manipulative treatment concomitantly or shortly after insertion of the stent. Bilateral subcapsular orchiectomy was performed in 19 patients and the other 15 patients received 250 mg oral flutamide every 8 h and 3.6 mg goserelin was administered subcutaneously once every 4 weeks for total androgen blockade.

The ProstaCoil stent is a large-calibre, self-expanding and self-retaining coil stent, made of nitinol (nickel–titanium alloy) which is a biocompatible alloy with a shape memory. This property of the alloy allows the insertion calibre of the stent to be reduced to 17 Fr and then to expand to its maximal calibre of 24/30 Fr when deployed.[11] The technique for the insertion is an easy procedure and is described in Chapter 39.

The follow-up period was 3–66 months (mean 31 months). A total of 21 patients are voiding with adequate flow rates and their residual urine is less than 100 ml, 3–60 months (mean 32 months) after removal of the stent. During the follow-up period none of the 16 patients who had sterile urine developed urinary

infection with the stent in place or after its removal. Because of their tightly closed coils, none of the stents were occluded by tumour growth into their lumen. In eight of the patients who did not respond to hormonal manipulation and could not void spontaneously, a new stent was inserted; a ninth patient underwent TURP to relieve the obstruction. Four patients are waiting for stent removal.

Advantages of combined hormonal manipulation and a temporary intraprostatic stent

A review of the various reports of different authors who combined intraprostatic stents with androgen-suppressive treatment, together with the present authors' experience, indicates that the combination of a temporary prostatic stent and medical androgen suppression offer a number of advantages over conventional treatment methods. Major surgery is avoided with its attendant morbidity and mortality. This combination significantly decreases inpatient stay and reduces bed occupancy. The patient is free of a catheter and can go home voiding naturally, thus reducing demands on the district nurse and general practitioner time associated with community catheter care. Since the beginning of the decade it has been found that in the long run, intra-urethral stents are more economical than indwelling catheters, saving costs on catheters, urine bags, antibiotics, trained personnel and probably hospitalization for severe infections and their complications.[10] In addition the ProstaCoil can be left in place, in patients who have not responded to the treatment, for long periods (3 years or more) instead of indwelling catheters. Unlike mesh stents, use of the ProstaCoil carries no risk of occlusion of the lumen by tumoral tissue growth through the coil, because of its tightly closed coils.[12] Such occlusion through the mesh of permanent stents was reported by Guazzoni and associates.[13]

Conclusions

The combination of a temporary ProstaCoil and androgen-suppression therapy is an alternative to palliative TURP in patients with prostate cancer who present with urinary retention, and avoids indwelling catheterization during the period of hormone-manipulative treatment. In patients who do not respond to hormonal manipulation, this stent can be a long-term alternative to indwelling catheters or repeated TURP.

References

1. Wingo P A, Tong T, Bolden S. Cancer statistics 1995. Cancer 1995; 45: 8
2. Kozlowski J M, Grayhack J T. Carcinoma of the prostate. In: Gillenwater J Y, Grayhack J T, Howards S S, Duckett J W (eds) Adult and pediatric urology. St Louis: Mosby 1996: 1575–1713
3. Moul J W, Davis R, Vaccaro J A et al. Acute urinary retention associated with prostatic carcinoma. J Urol 1989; 141: 1375
4. Kassabian V S, Scardino P. Management of local recurrence of prostate cancer. In: Lepor H, Lawson R K, (eds) Prostate diseases. Philadelphia: Saunders, 1993: 378–390
5. Ouslander J G, Greengold B, Chen S. Complications of chronic indwelling catheters among male nursing home patients: a prospective study. J Urol 1987; 138: 1191–1195
6. Fabian K M. Der intraprostatiche 'Partielle Katheter' (Urologische Spirale). Urologe A 1980; 19: 236–238
7. Anson K M, Barnes D G, Briggs T P et al. Temporary prostatic stenting and androgen suppression: a new minimally invasive approach to malignant prostatic retention. J R Soc Med 1993; 86: 634–636
8. Guazzoni G, Montorsi F, Bergamaschi F et al. Prostatic Urolume Wallstent for urinary retention due to advanced prostate cancer: a 1-year followup study. J Urol 1994; 152: 1530–1532
9. Oesterling J E. Urologic applications of a permanent, epithelializing urethral endoprosthesis. Urology 1993; 41 (suppl 1): 10
10. Yachia D, Lask D, Rabinson S. Self-retaining intra-urethral stent: an alternative to long-term indwelling catheter or surgery in the treatment of prostatism. AJR 1990; 154: 111–113
11. Yachia D, Beyar M, Aridogan I A. A new, large calibre, self-expanding and self-retaining temporary intraprostatic stent (ProstaCoil) in the treatment of prostatic obstruction. Br J Urol 1994; 74: 47–49
12. Yachia D, Aridogan I A. The use of a removable stent in patients with prostate cancer and obstruction. J Urol 1996; 1956–1958
13. Guazzoni G, Montorsi F, Coulange C et al. A modified prostatic Urolume Wallstent for healthy patients with symptomatic BPH: a European multicenter study. Urology 1994; 44: 364–370

57

Permanent prostatic stent in the management of obstructive prostate cancer in high-risk patients

H. W. Gottfried

Introduction

Prostatic carcinoma is the most common malignant tumour in men in the US and most European countries.[1] At the time of diagnosis a considerable proportion of patients already have an advanced carcinoma with voiding difficulties.[2,3] Furthermore, because of the patient's advanced age, there are increasing numbers of patients who present serious surgical risks because of multiple concurrent diseases not related to the cancer. Ablative hormonal therapy is the classical mode of management for such patients:[3-7] this form of treatment gives satisfactory results within 3 months in roughly two-thirds of all patients with bladder voiding disorders due to their carcinoma;[8,9] however, the remaining one-third of patients require further treatment to relieve their subvesical obstruction.[8,9] The conventional approach in such cases is palliative transurethral resection of the prostate (TURP), which, although known to carry only a low mortality, has an approximately 20% morbidity.[10-12] For patients in whom anaesthesia presents serious risks, the only therapeutic alternative has been an indwelling catheter with all its associated problems. The author has therefore evaluated the results achieved by insertion of a permanent prostatic stent system (Memotherm®) in high-risk patients with advanced prostatic carcinoma and subvesical obstruction.

Materials and methods

Patients

From May 1992 to December 1995, a total of 35 patients (Table 57.1), all with carcinoma of the prostate with subvesical obstruction, were treated. Their mean age was 75.3 (53–89) years. Of these 35 patients, 21 (60%) had bone metastases demonstrated by bone scan. Because of their age (> 75 years) or serious concurrent diseases, 14 of the 35 (40%) patients were not amenable to surgical curative treatment.

All patients received anti-androgen therapy for a mean of 4.3 (3–5.6) months. In 19 (54.3%) of the

Table 57.1. *Details of 35 high-risk patients who received a Memotherm® stent for subvesical obstruction caused by prostatic carcinoma*

No. of patients	Age (years)	Prostate volume (ml)	Stent length (mm)	Follow-up (months)
35	75.3 (53–89)	51.0 (± 20.5)	36.4 (20–55)	15.2 (3–38)

patients, androgen ablation was achieved by bilateral orchiectomy, and in 16 (45.7%) by administration of a gonadotrophin-releasing hormone (GnRH) analogue.

Mean prostatic volume determined by transrectal sonography (TRUS) was 51.0 (± 20.54) ml. Of the 35 patients, 18 (51.4%) were still able to void spontaneously; however, they had substantial volumes of residual urine and obstructive symptoms. A total of 17 patients (48.6%) with chronic retention were treated with an indwelling catheter.

The patients had major concurrent cardiopulmonary or cerebrovascular diseases. As defined by the guidelines of the American Association of Anesthesiology, 17 (48.6%) of the patients were classified under ASA 3 risk status, and 18 (51.4%) under ASA 4.

The mean follow-up period of the patients is 15.2 (3–48) months. Eight (22.9%) patients have died since the commencement of the trial: four of these deaths (11.4%) were due to the cancer and four (11.4%) to concurrent diseases. In all patients, the ability to void before the procedure was documented by determination of post-micturition residual urine, maximum urinary flow rate (Q_{max}) and AUA-6 symptom score. Other preprocedural investigations performed in all patients were digital rectal examination (DRE), TRUS, measurement of prostate-specific antigen (PSA) and bone scintigraphy.

Stent system

For these patients the Memotherm® stent system, specially constructed for urological use, was employed. This stent consists of a self-expanding knitted mesh tube (Fig. 57.1) made of heat-sensitive material

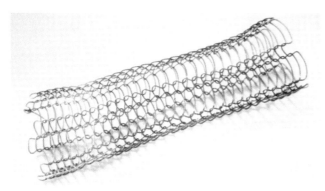

Figure 57.1. *Memotherm® prostatic stent system.*

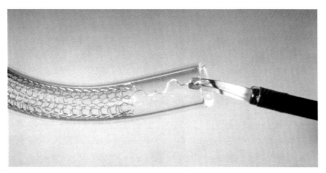

Figure 57.2. *Unravelling of a Memotherm® prostatic stent.*

(Nitinol). For use in the prostatic urethra, the Memotherm® stent has a diameter of 42 Fr in its expanded state. Maximal expansive force is reached at body temperature (36.5C°). The knitted mesh stent can be unravelled like a knitted sweater when necessary (Fig. 57.2). It is available in lengths of 20–70 mm in 5 mm steps. The insertion system consists of a single-use cystoscope with the disposable applicator integrated into it.

Surgical technique

Stent insertion was carried out under spinal anaesthesia in 19 (54.3%) of the patients and under topical mucosal anaesthesia in 16 (45.7%).

In all patients, the first step was to insert a 10 Fr suprapubic catheter. The urethra was then inspected through a 21 Fr cystoscope with a 5-degree lens; then the bladder was inspected with a 70-degree lens. Again using the 5-degree lens, the length of the prostatic urethra — from bladder neck to the apex of the prostate — was measured. A stent having the same length as the obstructed prostatic urethra was then selected. The stent was fitted to the single-use cystoscope, and this system was passed into the bladder.

The next step was to withdraw the applicator to the level of the bladder neck, and to deploy the stent, starting from the bladder neck, without pushing the stent forward into the bladder. Using the cystoscope, the position of the stent in relation to the external sphincter was checked. (If the stent projects beyond the external sphincter the stent should be pushed forward with the cystoscope until the external sphincter is left free.)

The suprapubic catheter was left open for 24 hours. Then the patient's spontaneous voiding was observed, residual urine being checked by means of the indwelling suprapubic catheter.

Statistics

All results are expressed as mean ± standard deviation. Statistical comparisons between measurements at different times were performed by variance analysis, the preoperative result being compared with the postoperative results. In the event of a significant F-value ($p < 0.05$) the means were further analysed by the Student t-test.

Results

Of the 35 patients treated, 33 (94.3%) were able to void spontaneously (Figs 57.3–57.5). Reassessment of the two patients (5.7%) who could not void spontaneously showed that too-short a stent was incorrectly positioned. After insertion of a second stent, overlapping the first, the patients were able to void. In two other patients (5.7%), stent occlusion by the tumour occurred within 6 months. Because of serious concurrent diseases, these patients were fitted with a suprapubic catheter. In two other patients (5.7%) — in one case 13 months and in the other 18 months after stent implantation — renewed subvesical obstruction occurred due to cancer tissue growth proximal to the stent. In these patients the obstructing tumoral tissue was destroyed by Nd:YAG laser inserted through an endoscope passed through the stent. Both patients were able to pass urine after the procedure.

Postoperative dysuria was noted in 12 (34.3%) patients. This lasted for a mean of 7.8 (4–31) days and

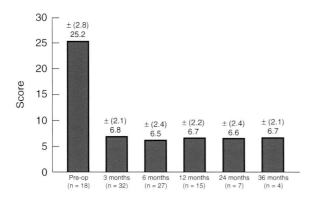

Figure 57.3. *Improvement in AUA 6 Symptom Score after Memotherm® stent insertion.*

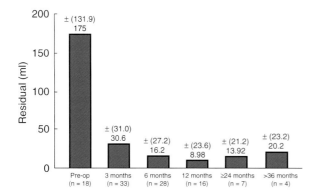

Figure 57.4. *Residual urine before and after stent placement.*

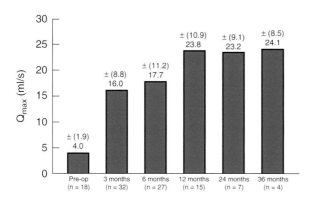

Figure 57.5. *Uroflowmetry before and after stenting.*

was made tolerable in all cases by giving anticholinergic drugs. There were no serious complications arising from stent implantation. During the first 6 months after stent implantation, three of 27 patients (11.1%) developed

significant urinary infections. After 12 months, 2 of 15 patients (13.3%) who had urinary tract infections required treatment. Endoscopic examination of the stent was carried out in eight patients within the first 12 months postoperatively: this showed epithelialization in seven (87.5%) (Fig. 57.6). One patient (12.5%) had non-epithelialized areas within the stent zone, but there was no evidence of any encrustation.

Among patients who had been able to pass urine preoperatively, statistical analysis of postoperative micturition parameters revealed statistically significant improvement. This was true for residual urine at all times postoperatively ($p < 0.001$). The corresponding figure for maximal urine flow rate was $p < 0.01$ and for AUA 6 symptom score it was also $p < 0.01$ at all times postoperatively.

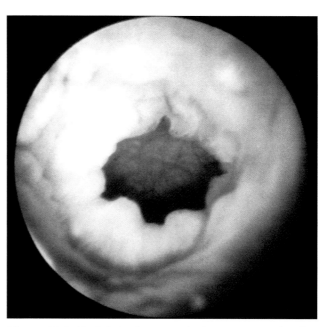

Figure 57.6. *Epithelialized stent inside the prostatic urethra (12 months after application).*

Discussion

For patients with obstructive carcinoma of the prostate who are unsuitable for curative treatment, hormone ablation is the therapy of choice.[3,7,8] However, 3 months after the begining of the ablative hormone therapy, one-third of all patients continue to show peristent obstruction.[8,9] The standard treatment for this group of patients is palliative TURP. However, TURP is not without its problems, first because of the possible risk of disseminating the cancer,[13,14] and also because its morbidity — roughly 20% — cannot be disregarded.[10–12] For patients in poor general condition because of concurrent diseases, other than the cancer, an indwelling catheter is often the only therapeutic option; this, of course, seriously impairs their quality of life.

For some years, subvesical obstruction due to benign prostatic hyperplasia in high-risk patients has been managed with good results by implantation of a permanent metal stent.[15–21] using various stent systems.[17,19,22] The use of a permanent metal stent for subvesical obstruction in advanced prostatic carcinoma was first advocated by Guazzoni et al.[22] In a small series of 11 patients he achieved lasting subjective and objective improvement in the obstructive symptoms by using the Urolume® Wallstent. In the present author's larger series of 35 patients, with follow-up times of up to 38 months, it is now possible to confirm Guazzoni's results. The Memotherm® stent system appears to have certain advantages over the Urolume Wallstent, in particular the ease of its removal because of the knitted structure of the stent. Furthermore, the Memotherm® stent system is available in lengths of 20–70 mm, so that a stent of adequate length is available for every prostatic urethra. The Memotherm® stent is made of non-magnetic metal, and investigations by magnetic resonance imaging remain feasible (Fig. 57.7).

In the majority of patients with subvesical obstruction due to advanced prostatic carcinoma, stent

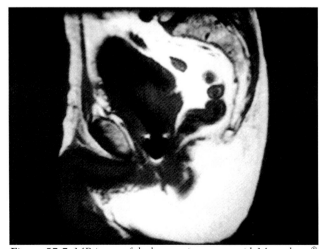

Figure 57.7. *MR image of the lower urinary tract with Memotherm®*

treatment successfully restored satisfactory micturition. This minimally invasive mode of therapy can be performed without problems, even under topical mucosal anaesthesia, and is of particular benefit for high-risk patients. Furthermore, insertion of a permanent metal mesh stent of large diameter permits further transurethral procedures if these become necessary. For example, in the author's case of renewed obstruction due to prostatic carcinoma growing proximal to the stent, it was possible by transurethral laser ablation, to overcome the obstruction for a second time. In the light of the results reported here, stent insertion for the relief of subvesical obstruction is regarded as a valuable treatment not only for benign prostatic hyperplasia, as advocated by many workers,[15–22] but also for obstructive prostatic carcinoma.

Despite the admittedly high costs of all stent systems, their use appears to be justifiable, especially in high-risk patients, because permanent catheter drainage so seriously impairs their quality of life. Another advantage of stent insertion is that it avoids the theoretical risk of tumour dissemination entailed by transurethral resection.[1,22] One further point in favour of stent insertion is the fact that the relief of subvesical obstruction by stent implantation is long term: a small group of the author's patients have had functioning stents for more than 3 years.

Despite the excellent results obtained after stent placement in these patients, the expense of this treatment must be mentioned. All permanent stent systems are rather expensive (about US$1500). The indication to insert one of the permanent stents has to be decided on an individual basis, such as a life expectancy of at least 1 year. It is also necessary to verify that the continence region (external sphincter) is intact and there is no evidence of sphincteric infiltration by the cancer.

Last but not least, although the insertion procedure looks very simple on all videos prepared by all stent manufacturers, in reality it is not. Correct measurement of the length of the prostatic urethra and correct placement of the stent should be an easy procedure, but it is not. For successful permanent prostatic stent insertion, a skilled endoscopic surgeon is recommended who will also have to traverse the individual learning curve.

References

1. Parker S L, Tang T, Bohler S, Wingo P A. Cancer statistics (1996). CA 1996; 46 (1): 5–27

2. Enstein J I, Pizou G, Walsh D C. Correlation of pathologic findings with progression after radical retropubic prostatectomy. Cancer 1993; 71: 3582–3593

3. Labrie F, Belanger A, Simand J et al. Combination therapy for prostate cancer Cancer 1993; 71: 1059–1067

4. Chute R, Willetts A T, Gens J P. Experiences in the treatment of carcinoma of the prostate with stilbestrol and with castration by the technique of intra-capsular orchiectomy J Urol 1942; 48: 682–692

5. Fleischmann J D, Catalona N J. Endocrine therapy for bladder outlet obstruction from carcinoma of the prostate J Urol 1985; 134: 498–500

6. Huggins C, Hodges C V. Studies of prostatic cancer: I. Effect of castration, estrogen and androgen injections on serum phosphatases in metastatic carcinoma of the prostate. Cancer Res 1941; 1: 293-297

7. Montie J E. The management of bladder outlet dysfunction due to prostate cancer, untreated and after endocrine treatment Prostate 1992; 54 (suppl 4): 153

8. Mommsen S, Petersen L. Transurethral catheter removal after bilateral orchiectomy for prostate carcinoma associated with acute urinary retention Scand J Urol Nephrol 1993; 28: 401–404

9. Moul J W, Davis R, Vaccaro J A et al. Acute urinary retention associated with prostatic carcinoma J Urol 1989; 141: 1375–1377

10. Doll H A, Black N A, McPherson K et al. Mortality, morbidity and complications following transurethral resection of the prostate for benign prostatic hypertrophy. J Urol 1992; 147: 1566–1573

11. Holtgrewe H L, Mebust W K, Dowd J B et al. Transurethral prostatectomy: practice aspects of the dominant operation in American urology. J Urol 1989; 141: 248–253

12. Mebust W K, Holtgrewe H L, Cockett A T K, Peters P C. Transurethral prostatectomy: immediate and postoperative complications. A cooperative study of 13 participating institutions evaluating 3,885 patients. J Urol 1989; 141: 243–247

13. Arcangeli G, Micheli A, Verna L et al. Prognostic impact of transurethral resection on patients irradiated for localized prostate cancer. Radiother Oncol. 1995; 35(2): 123–128

14. Sandler H M, Hanks G E. Analysis of the possibility that transurethral resection promotes metastases in prostate cancer. Cancer 1988; 62: 2622

15. Chapple C R, Milroy E J, Rickards D. Permanently implanted urethral stent for prostatic obstruction in the unfit patient — preliminary report. Urology 1990; 66: 58

16. Gottfried H W, Schimers H P, Gschwend J et al. Initial experiences with the Memotherm® stent in treatment of benign prostatic hyperplasia. Urologe [A] 1995; 34(2): 110–118

17. Kaplan S A, Merrill D C, Mosely W G et al. The titanium intraprostatic stent: the United States experience. J Urol 1993; 150: 1624–1629

18. Kirby R.S, Heard S R, Miller P et al. Use of the ASI titanium stent in the management of bladder outflow obstruction due to benign prostatic hyperplasia. J Urol 1992; 148: 1195–1197

19. Milroy E, Chapple C R. The urolume stent in the management of benign prostatic hyperplasia. J Urol 1993; 150: 1630–1635

20. Oesterling J E, Kaplan S A, Epstein H B et al. The North American experience with the Urolume endoprothesis as a treatment for benign prostatic hyperplasia: long term results. The North American Urolume Study Group. Urology 1994; 44(3): 362–363

21. Williams G, Coulange C, Milroy E J G et al. The Urolume, a permanently implanted prostatic stent for patients at high risk for surgery. Results from 5 collaborative centres. Br J Urol 1993; 72: 335–340

22. Guazzoni G, Montorsi F, Bergamaschi F. et al. Prostatic Urolume-Wallstent for urinary retention due to advanced prostate cancer: A 1 year follow-up. J Urol 1994; 152: 1530–1532

58

External irradiation for prostate cancer in patients with urethral stents
E. Gez and M. Cederbaum

Introduction

External irradiation is an effective treatment for patients with localized prostate cancer. The results (i.e. local control and survival) depend mainly on tumour grade, tumour stage and serum prostatic specific antigen level.[1,2] Total tumour dose has an important role in local control and may affect survival.[3]

Conformal radiotherapy is a new method of treatment in which the volume of irradiation is made to conform to the tumour volume in size and configuration. Studies with conformal radiotherapy in patients with prostate cancer have shown that the radiation dose to the prostate can be increased safely up to 84 Gy without increasing the toxicity to the rectum and the urinary bladder, and also that the local control and survival improve significantly.[4,5]

Most patients with prostate cancer present urinary obstructive symptoms that require immediate treatment. Indwelling catheter plus transurethral resection of the prostate comprise the traditional treatment for this condition, but it is accompanied by complications, such as urinary incontinence.[6,7] The insertion of a temporary metallic intraprostatic stent is a new alternative treatment for this problem.[8,9]

Because of the importance of external irradiation in prostate cancer, the question arises whether the presence of a metallic stent in the prostatic urethra changes the dose distribution in the gland.

To investigate this issue the authors conducted a study in vitro to simulate the effect of a urethral intraprostatic metallic stent on the dose absorbed by the surrounding tissue.

Materials and methods

A metallic urethral stent was used that was composed of a nickel and titanium alloy, made of 0.4 mm diameter wire coiled into an undulating spring with a mean diameter of 9 mm (donated by Medtronic Instent, MN, USA).

The dose perturbation was expected to occur within a very limited range of a few millimetres from the surface of the stent.[10] It was, therefore, imperative to employ a dosimetric method that has a correspondingly small spatial resolution. Radiographic film was selected as a medium of relative dosimetry. Although the film itself has an excellent spatial resolution that is inherently determined by its grain size, it needs to be read out with a densitometer. The densitometer's resolution is limited by its aperture size, which in this case was 1 mm in diameter — too large to give any reasonable accuracy within the expected range of position measurement. It was, therefore, decided to place a pack of films perpendicularly to the beam axis, effectively limiting the spatial resolution to the thickness of a single film, 0.18 mm.

The experimental set-up is shown schematically in Figure 58.1. The stent was embedded in a 1 cm thick tissue-equivalent material made of oil-jelly (bolus). Sheets of Kodak X-Omat V film were cut to a size slightly larger than the radiation field size and stacked one on the other in a light-proof paper envelope. These film stacks were placed directly above and below the stent. In order to simulate a real treatment situation, 10 cm of nearly tissue-equivalent plastic were placed above and below the stent and the film packs.

The whole set-up was irradiated in a Varian 600C accelerator using a single 6 MV beam with a field size of 7×7 cm, indicative of the small fields used in prostate-only irradiation. The stent was at the rotational centre of the accelerator (isocentre). The dose was choosen to give maximal contrast, as determined by previous pilot experiments.

All films were developed at the same time in a Kodak X-Omat developer together with an unexposed film, the level of transparency of which was taken as the fogging level for all other films. The optical density (OD) was measured in the middle of the image of the stent and in the area surrounding it, the latter reading being the OD that would have been obtained in the absence of the stent. The fogging level was deducted from the readings, but no correction was made for film non-linearity. Thus, the OD of the film was directly proportional to the relative dose received by the film at the point of measurement. The OD was measured in an optical densitometer with an aperture of 1 mm. The accuracy of a single OD measurement was 0.01.

The distance from the stent surface was given for the first point by the thickness of the paper envelope plus half the film thickness. Subsequent measurement points were separated by 0.18 mm — the film thickness. The distances were not corrected for water equivalency.

Results

All dose measurements are relative and are normalized to the dose as it would have been in the absence of the stent. Figure 58.2 shows two typical films just above and below the respective stent surface after being irradiated by a single field. These are positive radiographs; thus, the whiter the area the higher the dose. Note that in the film above the stent the image of the stent is whiter than its surroundings and the other way around below the stent. This corresponds to an enhanced relative dose 'upstream' of the stent and a reduction of dose just below it.

The changes in the absorbed dose above and below the stent are shown graphically in Figure 58.3. There

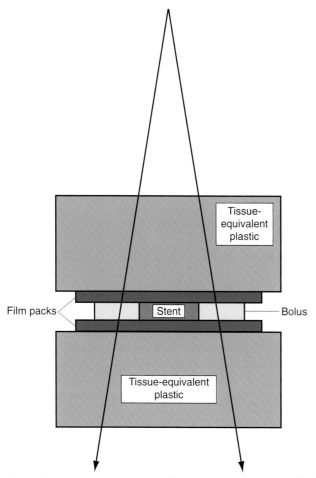

Figure 58.1. *Experimental set-up. The stent is completely embedded in tissue-equivalent material with film packs 'upstream' and 'downstream' of the radiation field.*

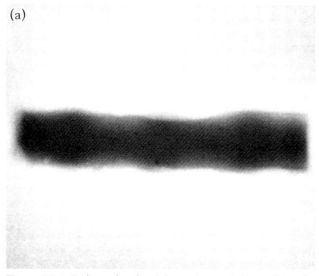

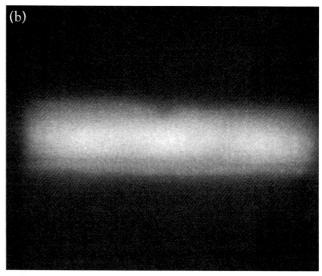

Figure 58.2. *Radiographs taken (a) just above and (b) just below the stent. These are positive films so that the dose enhancement above the stent is whiter than the surroundings and vice versa. The pictures are contrast enhanced.*

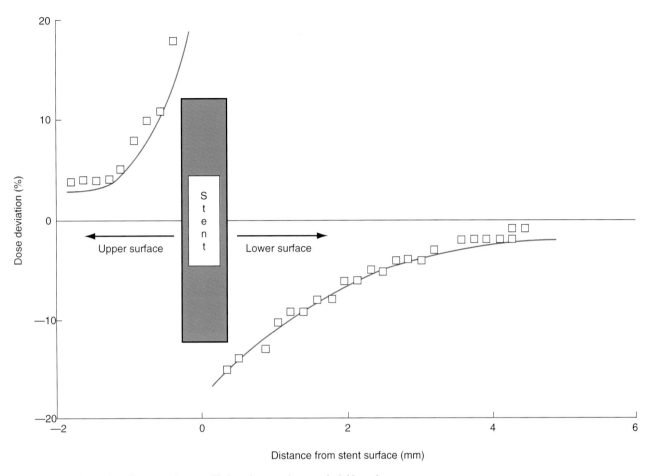

Figure 58.3. *Relative dose deviation above and below the stent for a single field irradiation.*

was a significant dose enhancement starting at about 1 mm above the stent, increasing to about 20% at the upper surface. On the other hand, there was a dose reduction immediately below the stent of about 18% that then increased gradually to the normal value at about 3 mm. It should be noted that these changes in the absorbed dose occurred when radiation was given in one single field.

Discussion

The results of the measurements described show that, when radiation was given in one single field, there was a 20% increase in the dose immediately above the stent and an 18% decrease immediately below it. These changes occurred within 1–3 mm from the stent. This increase at the upper stent surface is caused by electrons backscattered from the high-atomic-number metallic stent.[11] The radiation is attenuated slightly more by the

stent than by the replaced tissue and, in addition, the scattering power of the stent is higher than the surroundings, causing electrons to be scattered out at large angles from the stent. This will result in a reduction of relative dose just below the lower stent surface.

In practice, radiotherapy for prostate cancer is given in at least four fields: two opposed coaxial A/P and P/A fields and two opposed lateral fields. The composite dose distribution for a pair of mutually opposed coaxial fields was calculated from the single-beam data and is shown in Figure 58.4. The effects partially cancel out and the resultant deviation is considerably less than for the single field. The dose variation is confined to ± 4 % within 2 mm of the upper and lower stent surface. In a real four-field treatment these deviations would tend to be even smaller because of the contribution of scattered electrons from the additional fields.

In conclusion, the presence of a urethral stent in

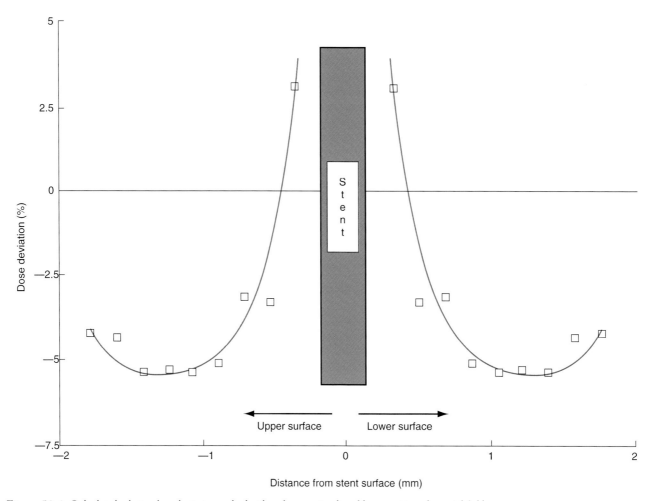

Figure 58.4. *Calculated relative dose deviation on both sides of a stent irradiated by two opposed coaxial fields.*

patients receiving radiotherapy for prostate cancer causes a small and insignificant change in the absorbed dose and, therefore, should not influence the radiation treatment planning. The issue of dose perturbation due to a high-density material in patients receiving radiotherapy to the pelvis has so far been studied only in patients with femoral head prostheses.[12,13] These studies have shown a more profound change in the absorbed dose pattern due to the much larger metallic mass of the prostheses.

Two questions remain to be answered: (1) what is the biological effect of the urethral stent on the surrounding normal tissue and (2) is the toxicity, both acute and chronic, of pelvic irradiation influenced by the presence of a metallic urethral stent?

References

1. Perez C A. Prostate. In: Perez C A, Brady L W (eds) Principles and practice of radiation oncology, 2nd edn. Philadelphia: JB Lippincott, 1992; 1067
2. Ennis R D, Peschel R E. Radiation therapy for prostate cancer. Long-term results and implications for future advances. Cancer 1193; 72: 2644
3. Leibel S A, Fuks Z, Zelefsky M J, Whitmore W F G. The effects of local and regional treatment on the metastatic outcome in prostatic carcinoma with pelvic lymph node involvement. Int J Radiat Oncol Biol Phys 1994; 28: 7
4. Sandler H M, McLaughlin P W, Ten Haken R K et al. Three dimensional conformal radiotherapy for treatment of prostate cancer: low risk of chronic rectal morbidity observed in large series of patients. In J Radiat Oncol Biol Phys 1995; 33: 797
5. Hanks G E, Lee W R, Hanlon A L et al. Conformal technique dose escalation for prostate cancer: biochemical evidence of improved cancer control with higher doses in patients with pretreatment prostate-specific antigen ≥ 10 ng/ml. Int J Radiol Biol Phys 1996; 35: 861

6. Ouslander J G, Greengold B, Chen S. Complications of chronic indwelling catheters among male nursing home patients: a prospective study. J Urol 1987; 138: 1191

7. Mazur A, Thompson I. Efficacy and morbidity of 'channel' TURP. Urology 1991; 38: 526

8. Yachia D, Lask D, Rabinson S. Self-retaining intraurethral stent: an alternative to long-term indwelling catheters or surgery in the treatment of prostatism. AJR 1990; 154: 111

9. Yachia D, Aridogan A. The use of removable stent in patients with prostate cancer and obstruction. J Urol 1996; 155: 1956

10. Tatcher M, Kuten A, Helman J, Laufer D. Pertubation of cobalt 60 radiation doses by metal objects implanted during oral and maxillofacial surgery. J Oral Maxillofac Surg 1984; 42: 108

11. Spiers F W. Transition-zone dosimetry. In: Attix F H, Roesch W C, Tochilin E (eds) Radiation dosimetry, Vol III. New York: Academic Press, 1969; 809

12. Hudson F R, Crawley M T, Samarseker M. Radiotherpy treatment planning for patients fitted with prostheses. Br J Radiol 1984; 57: 603

13. Biggs P J, Russel M D. Effect of femoral head prosthesis on megavoltage beam radiotherapy. Int J Radiat Oncol Biol Phys 1988; 14: 581

Stents in urethral strictures

Stenting after urethral surgery
E. J. Wright and G. D. Webster

Overview

In the adult male, urethral surgery is performed primarily for managing injury or stricture disease. Following either of these endeavours, urethral catheterization and stenting is customary, both to support the repair and to achieve urinary drainage. The spectrum of surgical procedures available is considerable, as is the spectrum of philosophies regarding catheter or stent material, size, configuration, function and duration.

It seems appropriate that an answer to these questions should be based on an understanding of the process of epithelialization and urethral wound healing. Re-epithelialization probably occurs within days of a superficial mucosal injury. Work in canines demonstrates that 7–10 days is necessary for a strong mucosal bridge to form following urethral transection.[1] Regeneration of the spongiosum is observed after 3–5 weeks with formation of a stable healing union. Certainly, the healing characteristics of any organ are affected by additional factors such as vascularization and the presence of infectious or inflammatory agents. Urine may pose such an inflammatory risk and lead to unpredictable scar formation.[2] Stricture-free healing is most likely to occur with a well-approximated, water-tight anastomosis,[3] enhanced by diversion or reduction of the urine stream by stent or catheter.

Catheters: materials, size, configuration

The use of catheters and stents following injury or urethral surgery is predicated on a balance between risk and benefit: whereas the effects of urine diversion, wound drainage and stabilization of a given repair may aid healing, the presence of a foreign body can potentiate infection. The catheter material itself may act as an inflammatory agent, and luminal diameter treads a line between adequacy of drainage and ischaemic compression. These factors must be weighed in the selection and use of urethral stents and catheters.

Material

Currently, standard urethral catheters are manufactured from rubber, latex and various silicon-based materials. Numerous studies have examined the effects of these agents on urethral mucosa and healing. Although many researchers indicate that siliconized materials are the least reactive,[4,5] agreement is not universal.[6,7] On a microscopic level, the in vivo friction coefficient for silicone is less than that of rubber,[8] a fact that may contribute to improving mucosal healing to the extent that surface abrasion may be deleterious.

Size

The luminal diameter of urethral catheters affects drainage and mucosal compression in an inverse relationship. Urinary flow rates through catheters of variable diameter demonstrate that a size greater than 12 Fr is adequate for drainage.[4] The effects of compression with increasing size are not well studied, but the potential for catheter-induced ischaemia and stricture is certainly minimized with selection of narrow-calibre tubes.

Configuration

Design configuration is another parameter of catheters and stents that can be manipulated. Whereas the standard Foley catheter has two lumina, one for terminal drainage and one for balloon activation, other configurations exist. Turner-Warwick originally described modification of a standard Foley catheter with fenestrations to provide localized urethral drainage[9] (Fig. 59.1). Similar attempts at providing specific urethral drainage were made by manufacturing a catheter ribbed along its shaft and by employing a standard three-way Foley with intra-urethral fenestrations in a dedicated lumen that could be placed to a separate collection device, or even suction.[10] Each of these tubes is placed across the sphincter-active region of the urethra and, as such, requires a drainage port for bladder contents. Borrowing from a concept

(a)

(b)

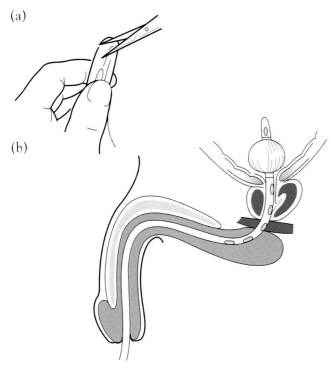

Figure 59.1. *The fenestrated urethral catheter stent is optimal following urethroplasty. Either a balloon or straight catheter may be used. The fenestrations allow debris and exudate to be washed away from the site of repair. Bladder irrigation cannot be performed unless the catheter is inserted all the way in to the bladder so that the most distal fenestration is above the bladder neck. (a) Use of scissors to fashion fenestrations taking care not to disrupt the balloon inflation port if Foley catheter is used. (b) The fenestrated catheter in place across the bulbar and sphincter-active urethra. (Adapted from ref. 9, with permission).*

often employed in children following hypospadias repair, a urethral 'splint' has been described[11] that resides distal to the sphincter mechanism, leaving the patient continent and voiding through the urethral tube when necessary. It is clear that this configuration requires a tube of large calibre to prevent perisplint extravasation at high flow rates. A 22 Fr tube was originally described, though this size may be larger than is otherwise necessary.

Suprapubic drainage represents an alternative in urethral catheter and stent configuration. This route provides adequate urine diversion and avoids the potential deleterious effects of urethral infection, inflammation and compression attendant on catheter placement. Standard techniques use 10–14 Fr catheters placed through the anterior abdominal wall into the bladder for both continuous and intermittent drainage. Relative contraindications include prior abdominal surgery.

Endoprostheses represent a newer alternative to managing urethral stricture.[12,13] These self-retaining devices can be deployed cystoscopically or fluoroscopically across any portion of the urethra to provide a 24–42 Fr internal diameter lumen. The most widely used intra-urethral prostheses are fashioned from self-expanding wire mesh. More recently, polyurethane and thermoexpansile materials have been used for stent construction.[14,15] These endoprostheses can be used on both a temporary and permanent basis, and may be especially suitable for patients who are either unfit or unwilling surgical candidates. Early experience seems favourable, and one series indicates that 93% of patients had satisfactory outcomes when followed up to 6 years.[16] Re-treatment rate for men with recurrent strictures improved from 75 to 14% following wire-mesh stent placement in the North American Multicenter Urolume trial.[17]

Intra-urethral stents are generally well tolerated. Epithelial overgrowth follows placement of the device and this, together with material biocompatibility, minimizes infection and encrustation. Complications can occur, however; the most common cause of device failure is fibrotic overgrowth with stricture recurrence. This complication can often be treated with endoscopic resection of the obstructing tissue, but occasionally requires stent removal. In selected situations, placement of an additional stent of slightly smaller calibre through the existing device has been successful.[18] Stent migration and extrusion can also occur secondary to poor placement and deployment errors. Extensive dense fibrotic strictures have the poorest outcome with indwelling stents and may represent a relative contraindication to placement.

It is clear that endoprostheses offer an additional treatment option for a wide range of urethral strictures. As follow-up continues to mature and both the materials and design of these devices improve, intra-urethral stents may find their role expanding.

Urethrography

The use of any catheter or stent following urethral surgery or injury requires an initial assessment of severity. Retrograde urethrography is the gold standard for this evaluation, and should be done when urethral injury has occurred or when stricture is suspected. The retrograde urethrogram (RUG) is performed with the patient in the 45-degree oblique position with the dependent knee slightly flexed. To minimize operator exposure and instil adequate contrast material, a 12 Fr Foley catheter is advanced into the meatus and the balloon is inflated with 1–2 ml water in the fossa navicularis. Fluoroscopy can be used to monitor the examination but this is not essential. Sufficient water-soluble contrast should be instilled into the urethra to allow passage into the bladder (15–20 ml).

In addition to the initial assessment of injury or stricture disease, retrograde urethrography can be incorporated into the postoperative evaluation by instilling contrast alongside an indwelling catheter to ensure an absence of extravasation at the repair site prior to catheter removal. If extravasation is present, a decision to delay catheter removal can be made without additional insult.

Retrograde urethrography carries minimal risk. Concerns over the introduction of infection or injury from extravasation of contrast material during the RUG are unfounded, provided that an aseptic technique is used and instillation pressures are not excessive.[19] Systemic complications, even in the setting of extravasation, are, likewise, exceedingly rare.[20]

Urethral injury

Urethral injury is most commonly seen in the setting of blunt external trauma or iatrogenic instrumentation. Straddle injury and instrumentation commonly affect the bulbar segment, while pelvic fracture accompanies 95% of posterior urethral distraction injuries.

These injuries are classified as (1) stretch or contusion, (2) partial tear and (3) complete disruption. Although they may be further stratified, these categories are the most clinically relevant in determining therapy, and are easily assessed by a RUG. A stretch or contusion is present when the RUG shows passage of contrast into the bladder without evidence of extravasation. It should be treated by placing a 14–16 Fr Foley catheter for 24–72 h, and rarely results in stricture. A partial tear is suggested by extravasation of contrast with incomplete passage of contrast into the bladder. Blind catheter placement carries significant risk for extending the underlying injury and should be avoided. Instead, partial urethral tear should be managed by placing a suprapubic

tube for 2–3 weeks and no attempt made to place a urethral catheter. The majority of these injuries will heal spontaneously. When strictures occur in this setting they are usually short (< 2 cm) and more easily managed. Stage 3 injuries are complete disruptions; consequently, a RUG demonstrates significant extravasation and an absence of bladder contrast. As with stage 2 injuries, complete disruptions warrant placement of a suprapubic tube for immediate urine drainage and diversion.

Further management strategies employ immediate exploration, delayed primary repair or secondary repair, and may involve endoscopic or open surgical techniques. The relative merits of these alternatives are beyond the scope of this chapter; regardless of the approach, however, the authors generally favour a 3-week period of 14–16 Fr catheterization following any of these repairs, with a pericatheter RUG prior to removal.

Use of catheters by urethroplasty type

The interval, size and configuration of any urethral catheter or stent should be guided by an understanding of the time necessary for regeneration of the urethral epithelium and the underlying spongiosum. Along with an understanding of urethral surgery and the intent of various repair strategies, these devices can be used to enhance healing while minimizing further insult. A generalized approach to urethral stricture repair is reviewed here and catheterization strategies based on this schema are recommended.

Dilatation, calibration and endoscopic urethrotomy

In the treatment of urethral stricture, properly performed techniques of dilatation and endoscopic incision are essentially equivalent in outcome.[21] Much has been written regarding the concomitant use of catheters following these procedures, with large variance of opinion. Some researchers recommend a period of 5–14 days of catheterization following urethrotomy; however, few studies support any benefit derived after the first day,[23] or use of a catheter at all.[23]

The purpose of urethrotomy is to create a cleft through the spongiofibrosis at the stricture site. Epithelialization of the cleft leads to a larger luminal diameter. Only through stabilization of the underlying scar are results successful in the long term. The same is true for dilatation, which is intended either to stretch or to fracture an area of spongiofibrosis. In the absence of significant trauma induced in the application of these procedures, it is unlikely that catheterization contributes to the healing process. It may, in fact, be deleterious following urethrotomy if abrasion of the healing cleft results.

It is with this understanding that the degree of injury incurred at the time of dilatation or urethrotomy dictates the use and duration of catheterization. If significant bleeding is induced with urethrotomy and the risk of urinary extravasation is high, a standard Foley catheter of 16–20 Fr may be used to limit the hydrostatic force of voiding on the urethra and to provide some element of tamponade for a period not exceeding 3–5 days. In the absence of significant trauma to the urethra a catheter need not be used, as the distending force of voiding carries no risk of extravasation and may enhance scar stabilization.

The exception in endoscopic urethral surgery is the case of 'core-through' procedures following obliteration of the urethrovesical anastomosis after radical prostatectomy or failed posterior urethral repair. In these special situations, a long length of densely scarred tissue often remains. It seems optimal to leave a 22 Fr silastic catheter for a period of 3–6 weeks to act as a template for scar stabilization, with a longer defect requiring the longer interval. Following stent removal, a course of self-calibration with a catheter up to 22 Fr will help preserve the lumen. The authors often employ a simultaneous suprapubic tube in this setting, following removal of the urethral catheter and the early period of resumed voiding.

Anterior urethroplasty

A number of principles guide the authors' use of stenting catheters following anterior urethroplasty. To allow luminal drainage of debris, secretions or haematoma, they favour locally fenestrated catheters; however, fenestrations must only be in the bulbar portion of the catheter. Silicon-based materials are used for any interval greater than 7 days. A pericatheter RUG is obtained prior to catheter removal and, if extravasation is present, the catheter is left in place for an additional 7 days.

Anastomotic repair

In the case of short bulbar urethral strictures (≤ 1 cm), anastomotic repair is highly successful. With a watertight approximation of healthy urethral tissue, a conservative period of 10–14 days of urine diversion allows adequate epithelial regeneration. A lateral stenting force is unnecessary, and the authors generally employ a 14–16 Fr silastic Foley catheter fenestrated in the bulbar region for a period of 14 days.

Substitution repair

Bulbar strictures in excess of 1 cm, or strictures of any length in the pendulous urethra, require the addition of preputial or penile shaft skin, or buccal or bladder mucosa, for successful repair. This substitution can be in the form of a flap or a graft used as an onlay patch or tube interposition. In general, onlay repairs fare better than tube interposition.

Flap repair

Skin flaps are more reliably applied to the pendulous urethra where the spongiosum is thin and offers little support for a graft. In this location, flaps minimize chordee formation associated with the 15–20% shrinkage that accompanies grafts. With regard to postoperative stenting, the authors advocate the use of a 14–16 Fr Silastic Foley catheter to minimize abrasion and pressure at the anastomotic line. The majority of these island pedicle repairs are placed distally on the urethra, and intraluminal wound drainage can egress along the catheter without the need for fenestration. A 10–14 day period of catheterization followed by a pericatheter RUG is adequate in the majority of these repairs.

Graft repair

As noted previously, graft repair finds optimal use in the bulbar urethra proximal to the suspensory ligament of the penis. Graft shrinkage in this area has a lesser effect on curvature, and the processes of imbibition and inosculation are best supported by the surrounding spongiosal tissue. Previous tradition held that these graft repairs required a large-bore (22–26 Fr) catheter to foster graft adherence to the bed, thereby minimizing shrinkage. This reasoning may have foundation for grafts applied to the ventral aspect of the bulbar urethra, where there is rich vascular spongiosum but little anchorage against contraction and local trauma. It must be accepted that using a large-lumen catheter in this situation shifts the balance between risk and benefit, raising the potential for remote urethral injury and graft abrasion.

Newer techniques applying grafts to the dorsal aspect of the urethra make use of the underlying corporal bodies and tunica albuginea, for fixation.[24] With anchorage to the tunica albuginea shrinkage is minimized and the graft stabilized for subsequent inosculation. A 14–16 Fr Silastic catheter can be used effectively for urine diversion following this repair. Additional fenestrations in the bulbar region of the catheter allow egress of wound secretion and prevent dislocation of the graft. A catheterization period of 3 weeks is adequate for graft healing, with a pericatheter RUG performed as confirmation prior to removal.

Staged repair

The technique of staged urethroplasty marsupializes the strictured portion of the urethra to the surface at the first stage. This technique either approximates scrotal skin to the urethral margins, or grafts fenestrated full- or split-thickness skin alongside the open urethra. At this first stage, the proximal and distal urethral ostia open to the surface at the repair limits. A small 14 Fr silastic catheter placed across both ostia for 10–14 days is adequate for stenting. Following its removal, the patient may void through a perineal urethrostomy. Optional is the placement of a suprapubic tube, allowing for continued urinary diversion after stenting urethral catheter removal. This may be advantageous in cases where perineal flap healing is delayed or graft take is suspect, and an attempt is being made to avoid the adverse affects of urine contact.

Prior to completing the second-stage closure, revising one or both ostia is often necessary.[25] Rarely is a stent required following revision of the distal ostium, as it is separate from the urine stream. Following revision of the proximal ostium, usually accomplished with a Y–V plasty, a standard 14 Fr latex Foley catheter is left in place for 5–7 days to divert the urine stream until healing has occurred.

At the time of final urethral reconstruction, a 24 Fr rubber catheter is used as a template to facilitate urethral sizing and neo-urethral tubularization. This tube is exchanged for a 14 Fr Silastic Foley at the end of surgery, and the stent remains in place for 14–21 days. This catheter is again fenestrated in the proximal portion of the repair to allow intraluminal secretions to drain without compromising the suture line.

Fossa navicularis repair

As these repairs most commonly employ rotational flaps, they are treated similarly to other, more proximal, flap repairs.

Conclusions

The nature of urethral surgery and the many forms it takes make it difficult to dictate a strategy for catheter and stent use. The authors have had success with the practices outlined here and consider that they are based on principles of urethral healing as well as on a measure of experience and practicality. Others may have reasonable success with different approaches. As understanding of the interactions between catheters, stents and wound healing advances, so, too, will the effective application of these devices.

References

1. Weaver R G. Experimental urethral regeneration. Surg Gynecol Obstet 1962; 115: 729
2. Abol-Enein H, el-Baz M, Ghoneim M A. Optimization of uretero-intestinal anastomosis in urinary diversion: an experimental study in dogs. II. Influence of exposure to urine on the healing of the ureter and ileum. Urol Res 1993; 21: 131–134
3. McRoberts J W, Ragde H. The severed canine urethra: a study of two distinct methods of repair. J Urol 1970; 104: 724
4. Edwards L E, Lock R, Powell C, Jones P. Post-catheterisation urethral strictures. A clinical and experimental study. Br J Urol 1983; 55: 53–56
5. Talja M, Korpela A, Jarvi K. Comparison of urethral reaction to full silicone, hydrogen-coated and siliconised latex catheters. Br J Urol 1990; 66: 652–657
6. Robertson G S, Everitt N, Burton P R, Flynn J T. Effect of catheter material on the incidence of urethral strictures. Br J Urol 1991; 68: 612–617
7. Anderson R U. Response of bladder and urethral mucosa to catheterization. JAMA 1979; 242: 451–453

8. Nickel J C, Olson M E, Costerton J W. In vivo coefficient of kinetic friction: study of urinary catheter biocompatibility. Urology 1987; 29: 501–503

9. Turner-Warwick R. Observations on the treatment of traumatic urethral injuries and the value of the fenestrated urethral catheter. Br J Surg 1973; 60: 775–781

10. Smith P J, Ball A J. Combined bladder and urethral drainage catheter. Urology 1984; 24: 190–191

11. Fair W R. Internal urethrotomy without a catheter: use of a urethral stent. J Urol 1982; 127: 675–676

12. Milroy E J G, Chapple C, Eldin A. A new treatment for urethral strictures: a permanently implanted urethral stent. J Urol 1989; 141: 1120

13. Saporta L, Beyar M, Yachia D. New temporary coil stent (urocoil) for treatment of recurrent urethral strictures. J Endourol 1993; 7: 57–59

14. Nissenkorn I. A simple nonmetal stent for treatment of urethral strictures: a preliminary report. J Urol 1995; 154: 1117–1118

15. Ricciotti G, Bozzo W, Perachino M et al. Heat-expansible permanent intraurethral stents for benign prostatic hyperplasia and urethral stricture. J Endourol 1995; 9: 417–422

16. Milroy E, Allen A. Long-term results of Urolume urethral stent for recurrent urethral strictures. J Urol 1996; 155: 904–908

17. Badlani G, Press S, Defalco A et al. Urolume endourethral prosthesis for the treatment of urethral stricture disease: long-term results of the North American Multicenter Urolume trial. Urology 1995; 45: 846–856

18. Pansadoro V, Scarpone P, Emiliozzi P. Treatment of a recurrent penobulbar urethral stricture after Wallstent implantation with a second inner Wallstent. Urology 1994; 43: 248–250

19. Jakse G, Marberger M, Simonis H J, Paulini K. Urethrography in urethral trauma: tissue reaction to extravasation of contrast dye and iatrogenic infection. Eur Urol 1981; 7: 178–183

20. McCallum R W, Colapinto V. Urological radiology of the adult male lower urinary tract. Springfield, Illinois: Charles C. Thomas, 1976

21. Steenkamp J W, Heyns C F, De Kock M L S. Internal urethrotomy versus dilation as treatment for male urethral strictures: a prospective, randomized comparison. J Urol 1997; 157: 98

22. Iversen Hansen R, Reimer Jensen A. Recurrency after optical internal urethrotomy. A comparative study of long-term and short-term catheter treatment. Urol Int 1984; 39: 270–271

23. Dahl C, Hansen R I. Optical internal urethrotomy with and without catheter. A comparative study. Ann Chir Gynaecol 1986; 75: 283–284

24. Barbagli G, Selli C, Tosto A, Palminteri E. Dorsal free graft urethroplasty. J Urol 1996; 155: 123–126

25. Carr L K, Macdiarmid S A, Webster, G D. Treatment of complex anterior urethral stricture disease with mesh graft urethroplasty. J Urol 1997; 157: 104–108

60

Appropriate stenting in hypospadias surgery
A. J. Kirsch and J. W. Duckett*

Introduction

The dicta of contemporary hypospadias surgery focus on sound principles of plastic reconstructive surgery. These include the use of optical magnification and micro-instrumentation with fine suture material, as well as delicate tissue handling. In order to achieve a leak-free tissue closure that heals with minimal scarring or deformity, stenting the urethra following hypospadias surgery has been a standard adjuvant manoeuvre. Three functions are accomplished: these are (1) avoidance of obstruction secondary to oedema formation which may last for up to 1 week, (2) maintenance of luminal continuity until epithelialization and tensile strength is obtained in the healing wound, and (3) prevention of forceful urination with leakage through suture lines into the surrounding tissues. Other functions include immobilization of suture lines, reduction of tissue reaction, and the avoidance of painful urination.

History of stenting for hypospadias surgery

During the 19th century, complicated and incomplete healing following surgery for hypospadias was the rule rather than the exception. In 1874, the French surgeon Simon Duplay reported the first successful ventral skin tube after a five-stage operation.[1] Although the 1900s saw dramatic improvements in surgical outcomes, poor healing and infection remained frequent complications.

The use of the buried skin strip, first described by Denis Browne in 1953,[2] forms the groundwork for the stenting philosophy. In his original description, a stenting catheter was left in place for up to 6 weeks to allow the buried strip to epithelialize around the catheter. This was not a successful operation, yet was very popular owing to Denis Browne's charisma. In 1964, Van der Meulen[3] advanced the Denis Browne repair by spiralling dorsal skin to the ventrum to cover the buried skin strip without the need for 'beads and stops'. He did not use stenting catheters and allowed

urine to leak through the repair with generous drains in the subcutaneous space. Interestingly, no fistulas were reported using this technique.[4] In addition to urethral stents, many surgeons utilized urinary diversion by suprapubic catheters or perineal urethrostomy tubes. However, poor wound healing, loss of catheter access and painful bladder spasms for the patients limited their acceptance.

Wound healing and stent use

Knowledge of normal wound healing is essential in understanding the appropriate use and timing of stent use in hypospadias surgery. Wound healing is divided into three phases — inflammatory, fibroplasia and maturation. The *inflammatory phase* begins immediately following incision and lasts for up to 7 days. During this phase, little tensile strength is gained in the wound. However, as the wound epithelializes (3–7 days) water-tightness is achieved. The *fibroplasia phase* occurs between 7 and 10 days postoperatively with the synthesis and accumulation of collagen by activated fibroblasts. Intra- and intermolecular cross-linking of collagen fibres allows the healing wound to gain tensile strength rapidly. Increased deposition, continued cross-linking and remodelling of collagen allow wounds to increase their tensile strength further. This final *maturation phase* begins at about 10 days.[5] Depending on the tissue, this phase lasts for up to several months. Unlike skin, which gains 30% tensile strength by 3 weeks, the bladder and urethra gain 70% tensile strength by 2 weeks.[6] For this reason, mucosal grafts are likely to heal more rapidly than skin grafts, decreasing the necessity for slowly degrading sutures and prolonged stenting.

The biology of free grafts must be understood when considering the duration of urethral stenting and/or urinary diversion. Under ideal conditions, free grafts initially survive on nutrient diffusion between the graft bed and recipient site by a process termed 'imbibition'. During the next 4 days, new blood vessels form and

*Deceased. (1936–1997). The author would like to dedicate this chapter to the memory of J.W.D. Jr.

nourish the graft. This revascularization phase is known as inoscultation. By 7 days, lymphatic drainage of the graft is also restored. Thus, it can be appreciated that a free graft requires a longer period of diversion than other graft types: in general, a period of 10–14 days is adequate.

Over the past decade, tissue sealants, such as methyl-methacrylate (Krazy Glue®) and fibrin glue[7] have been employed to minimize urinary leakage in urologic surgery. However, problems with tissue reactivity, biological contamination or proven efficacy have limited their usefulness. Recently, laser tissue soldering with human albumin-indocyanine green dye solder, in conjunction with a low power diode laser, has been used for hypospadias repair.[8] Using this technique, a leak-free anastomosis is achieved with minimal sutures. However, currently the use of laser soldering does not preclude the use of stents following hypospadias surgery.[9]

Today, despite improved surgical technique and advances in the understanding of wound healing, complications such as fistula and stricture formation remain consequences of proximal and reoperative hypospadias repair, and continue to occur in a small percentage of patients with anterior and middle hypospadias. With the development of proper stent management at home, virtually every hypospadias repair may be performed on an outpatient basis today. This has been enhanced by preoperative parental teaching regarding home care. Effective dressing treatments are also critical. These measures serve to minimize the acute complications of oedema and haematoma, and urinary extravasation that may lead to complications. Avoidance of collecting devices prevents unexpected tube removal.

Urinary diversion systems

The stents and catheters referred to in this section are listed in the Table 60.1. Except where indicated for historical interest, these catheters represent the most commonly used in contemporary hypospadias surgery.

Table 60.1. *Commonly used catheters and stents for hypospadias repair*

Catheter name	Material*	French sizes	Company name	Cost (US$)
Foley catheter	Silastic Silicone	8, 10, 12, 14 and up	CR Bard, Covington, GA Kendall Health Care Products, Mansfield, MA	8.60 6.90
Cystostomy catheter (suprapubic tube)	Silicone	8, 10, 12	Cook Urological, Spencer, IN	52.50
Stamey percutaneous suprapubic catheters	Polyethylene	8, 10, 12, 14, 16	Cook Urological	29.00
Kendall catheter	Polyurethane	6	Kendall Health Care Products	10.05
Zaontz urethral stent	C-Flex	8, 10	Cook Urological	18.00
Firlit–Kluge urethral stent	Silicone	8, 10	Cook Urological	20.75
Pediatric urethral C-stent	C-Flex	10, 13	Cook Urological	18.20
Fair Pediatric urethral stent	Polyurethane	10	Cook Urological	15.90
Tarkington urethral stent	C-Flex	8	Cook Urological	28.35
Medical grade tubing for 'home-made' stents	Elastomer Silicone	4, 8, 10, 12	Bentec Medical, Sacramento, CA	0.60 (60.00 for 50 feet)

* The materials listed above have chemical properties that give them rigidity. The softest material listed is silicone and the most rigid is polyurethane. C-Flex (trademark of Cook Urological) is an intermediate material. The cost is the amount per catheter in US dollars as of December 1996.

Suprapubic tubes

Suprapubic tubes have provided an effective form of urinary diversion, although currently used only in selective circumstances. The Pediatric Cystostomy Catheter™ is placed within the bladder through a stylet or steel trocar, depending on its size, and is sutured to the skin (Fig. 60.1); an adhesive-backed faceplate is not effective. Similarly, the line of the Stamey Percutaneous Suprapubic Catheters™ is placed within the bladder with a sharp stylet, and maintained in the bladder by either a Malecot (Fig. 60.2a) or loop distal tip (Fig. 60.2b). These catheters are primarily for emergency situations of urinary retention from acute urethral stricture and are rarely needed

Perineal urethrostomy tubes

This form of urinary diversion was used in the 1950s and involved grasping a urethral catheter through the perineum where a cut-down was made in the bulbar region.[10] Sometimes diverticula or fistulas developed at this site. Currently, there do not appear to be any advantages to this technique over contemporary forms of stenting the urethra.

Indwelling bladder catheters

The 'drip stent' concept was introduced by Duckett and Snyder in 1985[11] and initially utilized a very soft 6 Fr silastic tube (cerebroventricular shunt tubing) sutured to the glans. This was left dripping into a diaper (nappy) making tubing and drainage bags unnecessary. It was amazing how little these soft tubes irritated the bladder, causing few bladder spasms. However, problems with early removal or migration into the urethra led to the development of the currently preferred 6 Fr Kendall catheter™, a polyurethane tube with multiple perforations distally and with a Luer-lock end

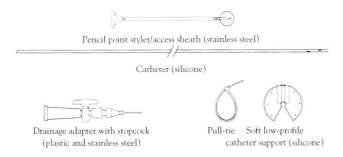

Figure 60.1. Pediatric Cystostomy Catheter.

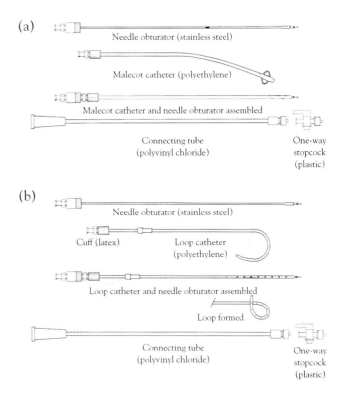

Figure 60.2. (a) Stamey percutaneous malecot suprapubic catheter; (b) Stamey percutaneous loop suprapubic catheter.

proximally. The smooth end makes passage into the bladder more certain than with the silastic tubing.

Snyder prefers to use medical grade silicone tubing (100 cm) which is cut into 15 cm lengths prior to surgery. It is placed into the bladder and sutured to the glans to prevent migration. This material has the advantage of being available in small (4 Fr) and large (12 Fr) calibre sizes.

To overcome the problem of proximal stent migration, other catheters were developed with a bulb into which to place a stitch to fix the stent in the glans (Firlit–Kluge Urethral Stent™ (Fig. 60.3). As a variation of the Firlit–Kluge stent™, Zaontz designed a urethral stent that was kept in position by a funnel-shaped distal end that is sutured to the glans, which prevents retrusion into the urethra (Fig. 60.4). The distal tip of the catheter was designed to terminate just within the bladder and serves to minimize bladder spasms.

The Tarkington Urethral Stent™ was designed to be stabilized in the urethra without use of sutures at the meatus (Fig. 60.5). It is introduced into the bladder with a stylet and is maintained in position by a coil in the bladder.

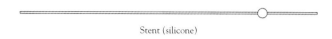

Figure 60.3. *Firlit-Kluge urethral stent.*

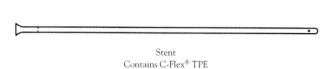

Figure 60.4. *Zaontz urethral stent.*

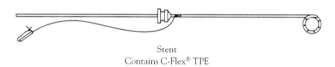

Figure 60.5. *Tarkington urethral stent.*

Partial urethral stents

Small-calibre urethrovesical stents and urethra-only stents ('splents') have been developed that allow the patient to be continent between voidings through the splents. Partial urethral stents have been used in urethral surgery for over 40 years. Hodgson[12] used a 9.4 Fr silicone tube with side holes passed into the bulbar urethra for hypospadias repair; King[13] described a silicone urethral stent for meatotomy, while Fair[14] utilized a similar urethral stent for urethrotomy. The Fair™ a paediatric urethral catheter has multiple side-holes and is useful in hypospadias repair using buccal mucosa grafts (Fig. 60.6).

'Home-made' cystourethral and urethral stents

Individual preferences have led several surgeons to construct their own catheters from commercially

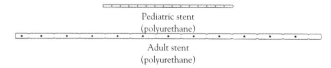

Figure 60.6. *Fair urethral stent.*

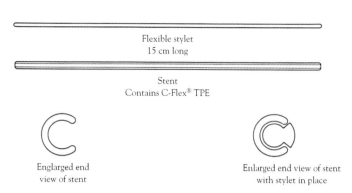

Figure 60.7. *Urethral C-stent.*

available materials. In general, these catheters are less expensive and have the advantage of being tailored to the individual patient at the time of surgery.

Mitchell[15] has utilized medical grade silastic tubing cut into segments which at the time of surgery have a longitudinal strip cut out measuring one-quarter of the circumference of the tube. The advantages of this 'pleated stent' are that it is easy and inexpensive to construct, prevents bladder spasm by virtue of its position distal to the external sphincter, and allows its edges to fold inward during oedema formation without losing its lumen. The commercially available paediatric urethral C-Stent™ is similar to that described by Mitchell (Fig. 60.7).

Special considerations for hypospadias stent placement

The extent of the surgery and an assessment of the healing process may encourage the consideration of urethral stents in any form of hypospadias repair. It should always be kept in mind that postoperative urinary retention may lead to traumatic catheterization and subsequent fistula formation following hypospadias repair.

MAGPI, Arap and urethral advancement repairs

Meatoplasty and glanuloplasty (MAGPI) and Arap (colocystoplasty) repairs and urethral advancement procedures are usually managed without urethral stents.

Parameatal-based skin flap (Mathieu procedure)

Meatal-based flaps (e.g. Mathieu or flip-flap, Snodgrass) have been studied with and without postoperative urinary diversion. In 37 consecutive meatal based repairs without stents reported by Buson and co-workers,[16] seven patients (19%) required early postoperative catheterization for urinary retention and two of these developed urethrocutaneous fistula. In contrast, of the 16 boys who underwent the Mathieu repair with stents, only one patient (6.3%) developed a fistula and meatal stenosis. Pike et al.,[17] utilizing indwelling Foley catheters or suprapubic catheters, have had a similar experience. It was the conclusion of these studies that the use of a stent for urinary diversion was advantageous for the success of anterior hypospadias repair. In general, urinary diversion is used for 5–7 days, but others have shown that no diversion is needed.

In a series of 59 patients undergoing catheterless Mathieu hypospadias repair reported by Rabinowitz,[18] no fistulas were noted by 18 months postoperatively. In a small prospective study comparing stented and non-stented Mathieu repairs, McCormack and co-workers[19] found no difference in complication rates and concluded that urethral stents had no beneficial effect on surgical outcome. Wheeler et al.[20] have had a similar experience.

Megameatus intact prepuce (MIP)

In this complex variant of anterior hypospadias, the prepuce is intact and a megameatus exists.[21] Since the repair usually involves tapering and refashioning of urethral tissue, urinary diversion for 5 days is all that is needed.

Onlay island flap

In this procedure, the urethral plate is left intact and the ventral urethral wall is formed by a U-shaped closure of a vascularized island flap of inner preputial skin fashioned over the urethral plate.[21] Since this repair involves skin-to-skin wound healing, 7–10 days of urethral stenting is usually required to ensure adequate epithelialization and tensile strength.

Free grafts and tubularized grafts

Free grafts, whether placed as an onlay or tubularized, require longer periods of stenting (up to 3 weeks). The neccessity for these repairs often arises in patients who have undergone previous hypospadias surgery and in whom chronic inflammation may exist. In these complex situations, urethral stents serve several functions including alignment of the urethra, prevention of leaks and provision of a scaffolding for repair.

Buccal mucosa is the preferred graft material today, owing to its rapid 'take' and healing.[22] Specialized staining of the buccal mucosa with an antibody with the basement membrane of blood vessels (type IV) shows that the lamina propria is rich with vascularity, compared with skin and bladder mucosa.[22] Bladder mucosa is too thin for good healing and leads to meatal eversion in 24%,[23] and thus has been abandoned. Results with extragenital skin also are unacceptable, with a 60% failure rate.[24]

The authors prefer to stent buccal mucosa grafts for 12–14 days. When a suprapubic tube is used, a trial of voiding is given before removal, and low-dose antibiotics are given throughout the period of urinary diversion.

Complications from urethral drainage catheters

Untoward effects resulting from short-term catheter drainage are mainly limited to plugged catheter and unintentional removal with secondary bladder spasms or bladder irritation, and may result in haematuria, bacteriuria or erosion if prolonged. Simple irrigation relieves a plugged catheter, and oxybutynin (Ditropan) is helpful in relieving pain associated with bladder spasms. Banthine and opium suppositories (B & O Supprettes) have been used in the past but dosage inconsistencies in children make them unsafe.

The most significant advantages of postoperative dressings are to prevent haematoma, with compression and immobilization of the repair for 3 days. Equally as important is to protect the urinary stent from unintentional removal. The authors prefer to use a 'sandwich dressing' (Fig. 60.8) composed of a Telfa pad and gauze sponge laid on top of the penis and covered with a bio-occlusive dressing (Tegaderm, 3M Medical–Surgical Division, St Paul, MN, USA). A single or double diaper (nappy) system affords even more protection. The dressing is left on for 72 hours.

Hypospadias repair in the prepubertal child does not pose any significant risk factors for infection and may be

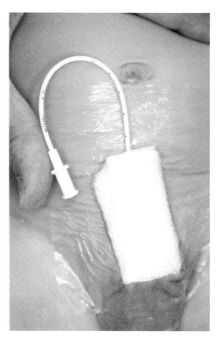

Figure 60.8. *'Sandwich dressing' after hypospadias repair.*

performed without the use of antimicrobial agents in nearly all cases. In Montagnino's retrospective review,[25] comparing the incidence of urinary tract infection in 100 children managed with a closed or open urinary drainage system, no significant difference was identified. In this study the open-drainage system utilized a double-diapering technique. The incidence of urinary tract infection was 24%, regardless of whether open or closed systems were employed or whether antibiotics were used postoperatively. All infections were asymptomatic and resulted after approximately 12 days of drainage. The authors prefer to use prophylactic sulphatrimethoprim to cover the open drainage of the 'drip stent', but it may not be necessary.

Conclusions

In the majority of cases, the authors prefer to use a No. 6 Kendall stent placed through the urethra and sutured with a 5/0 Prolene stitch to the glans. The free end drips urine constantly into a single nappy, or, in the older child, the Luer-lock may be closed for several hours to permit periods of social continence. The authors prefer to avoid drainage bags, which are likely to get caught and exert traction on the meatus. In their experience, simple dressings and simple drainage systems usually work best.

References

1. Murphy L J T. The urethra. In: Murphy L J T (ed) The history of urology, 1st edn. Springfield, Illinois: Charles C. Thomas 1972: 454–455
2. Browne D. A comparison of the Duplay and Denis Browne techniques for hypospadias operation. Surgery 1953; 34: 787–793
3. Van der Meulen J C. Hypospadias monograph. Leiden, The Netherlands, A.G. Stenfert, Kroese NV, 1964
4. Van der Muelen J C. Correction of hypospadias: types I and II. Ann Plastic Surg 1982; 8: 403–411
5. Foster L S, McAnnich J W. Suture material and wound healing: An overview. AUA Update Series 1992; Vol. XI, Lesson 11
6. Van Winkle W Jr, Hastings J C. Considerations in the choice of suture materials for various tissues. Surg Gynecol Obstet 1972; 135: 113
7. Holmes S A V, James M, Whitfield H N. Potential use of tissue adhesives in urinary tract surgery. Br J Urol 1992; 69: 647–650
8. Kirsch A J, Miller M I, Chang D T et al. Laser tissue soldering in urinary tract reconstruction: first human experience. Urology 1995; 46(2): 261–266
9. Kirsch A J, de Vries G M, Chang D T et al. Hypospadias repair by laser tissue soldering: intraoperative results and followup in 30 children. Urology 1996; 48: 261
10. Matthews D N: Method of Matthews using Denis Browne technique. In: Horton C E (ed) Plastic and reconstructive surgery of the genital area, 1st edn. Boston: Little, Brown and Co, 1973: 341
11. Duckett J W, Snyder H M. Hypospadias 'pearls'. Soc Pediatr Urol Newslett 1985; 7: 4
12. Hodgson N B. A one-stage hypospadias repair. J Urol 1970; 104: 281
13. King L R. Overview: Hypospadias repair. In: Whitehead E D, Leiter E (eds) Current operative urology, 2nd edn. Philadelphia: Harper and Rowe, 1984: 1265
14. Fair W R. Internal urethrotomy without a catheter: use of a urethral stent. J Urol 1982; 127: 675
15. Mitchell M E, Kulb T B. Hypospadias repair without a bladder drainage catheter. J of Urology 1986; 135: 321–323
16. Buson H, Smiley D, Reinberg Y, Gonzalez R. Distal hypospadias repair without stents: is it better? J Urol 1994; 151: 1059–1060
17. Pike J G, Brzezinski A, Kiruluta G H. Use of a urethral splent in one-stage hypospadias repair. Can J Surg 1991; 34: 507–509
18. Rabinowitz R. Outpatient catheterless modified Mathieu hypospadias repair. J Urol 1987; 138: 1074–1076
19. McCormack M, Homsy Y, Laberge Y. 'No stent, no diversion' Mathieu hypospadias repair. Can J Surg 1993; 36: 152–154
20. Wheeler R A, Malone P S, Griffiths D M, Burge D M. The Mathieu operation: is a urethral stent mandatory? Br J Urol 1993; 71: 492–493
21. Duckett J W, Baskin L S. Hypospadias. In: Gillenwater J Y, Grayhack J T, Howards S S, Duckett J W (eds) Adult and pediatric urology, 3rd edn. Chicago: Mosby Year Book, 1996; 2549
22. Duckett J W, Coplen D, Ewalt D, Baskin L S. Buccal mucosa urethral replacement. J Urol 1995; 153: 1660–1663
23. Keating M A, Duckett J W. Bladder mucosa in urethral reconstructions. J Urol 1990; 144: 827–834
24. Secrest C L, Jordan G H, Winslow B H et al. Repair of the complications of hypospadias surgery. J Urol 1993; 150: 1415.
25. Montagnino B A, Gonzales E T, Roth D R. Open catheter drainage after urethral surgery. J Urol 1988; 140 (part 2): 1250

61

How do temporary urethral stents work in recurrent urethral strictures?

D. Yachia

Introduction

Urethral stricture is the result of scar tissue development after either traumatic or inflammatory injury of the urethra. Urethral stricture has confounded the urologist in the past and is still one of the most challenging situations for the surgeon and a most troublesome condition for the patient.[1,2]

Treatment of urethral stricture has one main aim – to allow the patient to void with a satisfactory stream and control. To achieve this, a urethra with an adequate calibre must be created, either by dilatation or endoscopic incision of the stricture or by one of the many urethroplasty techniques developed for this purpose. About 80% of urethral strictures recur after dilatation or urethrotomy because of new stenotic scar development. Conventionally, after such treatment a latex, silicone or polyurethane urethral catheter is left indwelling for a few days to three weeks, for urine drainage and help in remodelling of the stenotic urethra. Unfortunately, at the time that the catheter is removed, the tissue-healing process is still active, making the outcome of the treatment unpredictable and, in many cases, a recurrent stricture. The cost of this recurrence to the health care system is tremendous, not to mention the loss of quality of life that often accompanies the recurrent stricture. Although marked progress in restoration of the structure and function of damaged tissues has been achieved over the last decades, the reason for stricture recurrence is still not clearly understood. To understand better the reason for the high rates of recurrence of urethral strictures, the physiopathology of human wound healing should be reviewed briefly.

It is known that wound-healing is a highly dramatic and integrated series of cellular, physiological and biochemical events occurring in the tissues. In humans, as in most mammals, the capacity of regeneration is limited to tissues, such as the liver, bone and skeletal muscle. Research in the emerging field of regenerative biology is attempting to identify the cellular and molecular differences that distinguish tissue embryogenesis (regeneration) from wound repair (scarring). Some limited success in stimulating the regeneration of some tissues has been achieved by bridging the lesions with artificial or natural biomaterial 'scaffolds' for promoting migration, proliferation and differentiation of cells.[3] In the coming decades it will probably be possible to regenerate a number of vital tissues, which may include the urethra. This not only will increase the quality of life of these patients but also will substantially reduce health costs.

Until tissue-regenerative technologies are available, new approaches are being developed for the management of diseases where natural wound repair takes place by scarring. The use of stents in these diseases, in general, and in recurrent urethral stricture disease, in particular, are such novel approaches. Figure 61.1 is a flow chart of the management of urethral stricture disease that was conventional until 1990. Figure 61.2 depicts the addition of this novel alternative and minimally invasive approach. Until recently, the most definitive way to treat a urethral stricture was to perform a urethroplasty when the less invasive treatments failed. Urethroplasty is performed either by replacing or patching the stenosed segment of the urethra, using tissues taken from other parts of the body, such as skin, bladder or buccal mucosa; alternatively, if the stenosed segment is short, it is performed by resection and reanastomosis, being successful in up to 90% of cases in experienced hands. There is no doubt that for performing a good and successful urethroplasty, hands capable of neat work, technological perfection and sufficient experience are all necessary. Unfortunately, the number of urethral strictures is much greater than the number of urologists performing this type of surgery. Fearing failure, most urologists still manage their stricture patients with repeated dilatation or urethrotomies, which are non-curative methods.

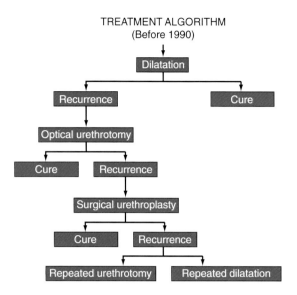

Figure 61.1. *Flow chart of conventional management of urethral stricture before stent era.*

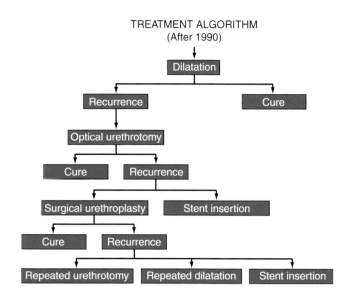

Figure 61.2. *New flow-chart in the management of urethral stricture after introduction of stents.*

Why do most urethral strictures recur?

Although all wounds heal by the same basic process, there are some basic differences between the healing of an acute and a chronic injury wound. This difference is also seen during the treatment of urethral strictures. Endoscopically, an incised or dilated urethra may appear to be healed within a few weeks; however, in most cases the stricture will recur, despite the complete epithelial coverage of the wound, because of the ongoing scarring process in the deeper layers of the urethra. Although short and superficial strictures occurring after transurethral surgical manipulation may disappear after a single treatment, when the traumatized urethra becomes infected – with its deeper layers involved – the stricture will almost always recur.

Wound-healing is a phased and complex process requiring the collaborative efforts of the contributory cell types during the phases of proliferation, migration, matrix synthesis and contraction, as well as the growth factor and matrix signals present at the wound site.[4] Basically, in every wound a fibrin clot forms to plug the defect for initiating the repair. Within minutes of injury, inflammatory cells begin to arrive at the site, attracted by a variety of chemotactic signals that include growth factors released by degranulating platelets and the by-products of proteolysis of fibrin. The neutrophils arriving at the wound counteract the initial rush of contaminating bacteria. Recent studies have shown that

they are also a source of pro-inflammatory cytokines that probably serve as early signals to activate the local fibroblasts.[5] The neutrophil infiltration ceases after a few days and those expended are phagocytosed by tissue macrophages. Macrophages accumulating at the wound site are essential for effective wound-healing; however, if macrophage infiltration is disrupted by severe wound infection, the healing process is severely impaired.[6] Repeated manipulations, such as follow-up cystoscopies for bladder tumours, repeated dilatations and the insertion of an indwelling catheter after such procedures, cause an ascending infection at the wound. After the inflammatory cells, fibroblasts and capillaries invade the fibrin clot to form a contractile granulation tissue that draws the wound margins together and the epithelial edges migrate forward to cover the wound surface. This is made easier by the underlying contractile connective tissue, which shrinks to bring the wound margins towards one another. As an early response to injury, fibroblasts in the neighbourhood of the wound begin to proliferate and, 3–4 days later, they begin to migrate into the provisional matrix of the wound clot where they start to lay down their own collagen-rich matrix. About a week after wounding, the wound clot is fully invaded and replaced by activated fibroblasts that are stimulated by growth factors to synthesize and remodel the new collagen-rich matrix.[4]

In undisturbed tissue healing, programmed cell death occurs in some of the wound fibroblasts, probably the myofibroblasts, after wound contraction has ceased,[7] marking the stabilization of the scarring process. Under normal conditions there is an equilibrium between collagen synthesis and collagen degradation during the wound-healing process. Repeated trauma and infection cause a disequilibrium in this process. This disequilibrium is responsible for the increase in collagen synthesis and the decrease in its degradation, resulting in stricture recurrence, a process similar to that of other hypertrophic scar tissues developing in any other organ. In the urethra, as in other cylindrical organs, this scar usually involves the entire circumference of the injured segment.

It is known that the wound-healing process depends on genes that are too rapid in their action. Theoretically, slowing this process might give better long-term results; however, in practice, pharmaceutical means – such as steroid injections into the scar – have failed to change this course substantially.

Role of stents in urethral strictures

A chronic wound in the urethra usually fails to heal primarily, as would an acute wound. The chronic wound heals up to a point and then, usually, the healing process turns toward contraction. As it is impossible to predict this course and change this process effectively, the way to prevent stricture recurrence is to interfere mechanically, in order to prevent the scarring process ending in contraction.

The introduction of stents for use in the urinary tract opened up the possibility of a new approach to the treatment of urethral strictures. The mode of action of stents in the treatment of urethral stricture is based on this mechanical interference.

Stents used in the treatment of urethral strictures are either permanent or temporary. Tables 61.1 and 61.2 list the different urethral stents available for use in urethral stricture disease.

The mode of mechanical interference differs between permanent and temporary stents. Permanent stents act as a reinforcement, like the iron bars in concrete used in buildings, and remain permanently in the wall of the urethra. Clinical experience with these stents is also detailed in Chapter 62.

The rationale behind the mode of action of temporary stents is also based on interference but differs completely from that of permanent stents. A temporary stent is left as a mould in the urethra until stabilized scar tissue forms a cast around it under the regenerated urethral epithelium; the stent also prevents scar contraction. When the stent is removed, it leaves behind a remodelled large-calibre urethra that does not contain any foreign body.

Table 61.1. *Temporary urethral stents used in the treatment of urethral stricture*

Stent	Expansion	Size		Material	Indwelling time (months)
		Calibre (Fr)	Length (mm)		
Urethrospiral	Non-expanding	21	40–70	Stainless steel	≤ 12
UroCoil	Self-expanding	24/30	40–80	Nitinol	≤ 36
UroCoil-S	Self-expanding	24/30	40–80	Nitinol	≤ 36
UroCoil Twin	Self-expanding	24/30	40+50/50+50	Nitinol	≤ 36
Memokath 044	Heat-expandable	22/34,22/44	30–70,30–50	Nitinol	≤ 36

Table 61.2. *Permanent stents used in the treatment of urethral stricture*

Stent	Expansion	Size		Material	Indwelling time (months)
		Calibre (Fr)	Length (mm)		
Urolume Wallstent	Self-expanding	42	20–40	Steel 'superalloy'	Permanent
Memotherm	Heat-expandable	42	20–80	Nitinol	Permanent
Ultraflex	Self-expandable	42	20–50	Nitinol	Permanent

The results presented in this chapter are based on our experience using the three different configurations of the UroCoil-System stents (Figs 61.3–61.9. Most probably, similar results can be obtained with other large calibre temporary stents.

Insertion technique

A prophylactic antibiotic, such as a cephalosporin, is administered, starting 1 day before the procedure and continuing for at least 5 days. In cases where the urine culture shows an infection, the antibiotic is chosen according to the sensitivity.

An ascending urethrogram is performed in the operating room. Under fluoroscopy, the beginning and the end of the stricture are marked, using radiopaque skin markers (provided with the stent) or metal skin-staples. If the stricture is in the bulbar urethra or near the external sphincter, or if it is a combined stricture, the site

of the external sphincter is also marked (Fig 61.10). Performing the ascending urethrogram before general or spinal anaesthesia eases the identification of the external sphincter by asking the patient to contract the sphincter. With a cooperative patient, the entire procedure, including urethrotomy and insertion of the stent, can be performed under topical anaesthesia using 2% lignocaine gel left for not less than 15 minutes in the urethra.

For insertion of the stent, access is gained by balloon or gradual dilatation or by visual urethrotomy. The author prefers urethrotomy to gradual dilatation or balloon dilatation because it enables the site and number of incisions to be decided and their depth to be controlled visually. In cases where the depth of the spongiofibrosis is partial, a single incision at the 12 o'clock position usually suffices. This incision is deepened until healthy tissue is reached. This depth is important for allowing epithelialization over healthy spongious tissue around the stent. Where the entire thickness of the corpus spongiosum has become fibrosed, the incisions are made in an inverted Y-shape, in three

(a)

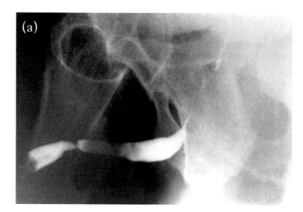

(a)

(b)

Figure 61.3. *(a) UroCoil mounted on its delivery catheter in its constricted form and after its release in its expanded wavy form; (b) the UroCoil is intended for use in post-bulbar strictures along the entire penile urethra.*

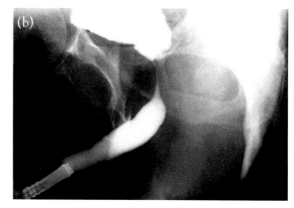

Figure 61.4. *(a) Mid-penile urethral anastomotic stricture; (b) UroCoil stenting the stricture.*

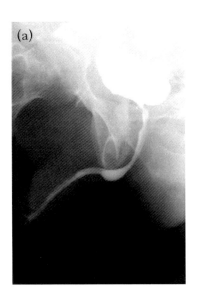

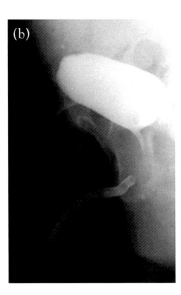

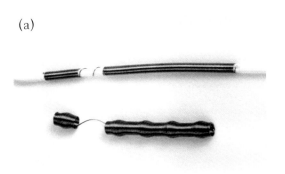

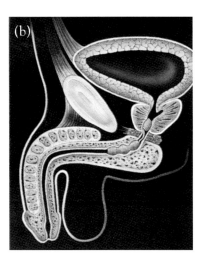

Figure 61.5. (a) Anterior urethral stricture 14 cm in length, which developed in a patient after long-term catheterization; (b) the entire stricture could be stented by overlapping one 80 mm and one 70 mm UroCoil.

Figure 61.6. (a) UroCoil-S mounted on its delivery catheter in its constricted form and after its release in its expanded form. The UroCoil-S is composed of three segments: a long segment for stenting the bulbomembranous urethra (bulbar segment), a short anchoring segment positioned at the prostatic urethra (prostatic segment) and a single helical wire connecting the two segments (trans-sphincteric spacer); (b) UroCoil-S is intended for use in cases of bulbomembranous strictures.

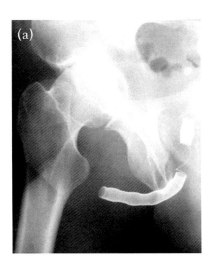

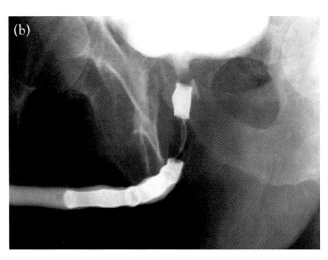

Figure 61.7. (a) UroCoil-S in place; (b) ascending urethrogram with the UroCoil-S in place. Note the position of the segments of the stent conforming to the anatomy of the urethra.

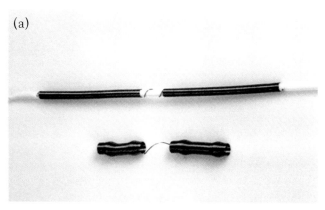

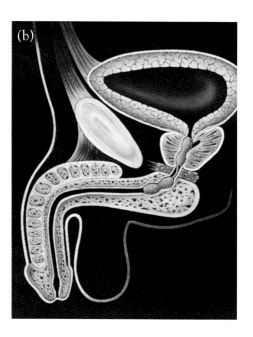

Figure 61.8. *(a) UroCoil-Twin mounted on its delivery catheter in its constricted form and after its release in its expanded wavy form. The UroCoil-Twin is composed of three segments: two long segments for stenting the prostatic and the bulbomembranous urethra and a single-helical wire connecting the two segments (trans-sphincteric spacer); (b) UroCoil-Twin is intended for use in combined strictures below and above the external sphincter.*

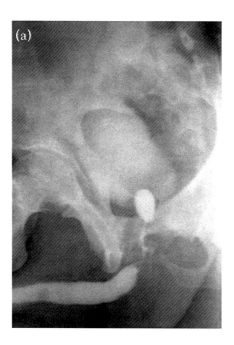

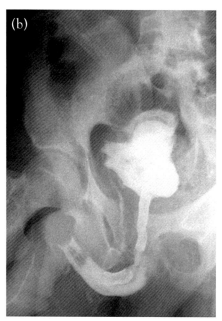

Figure 61.9. *(a) Combined strictures at the level of the membranous urethra, mid-prostatic urethra and bladder neck (this patient, who was involved in a severe traffic accident and had pelvic fractures, underwent several interventions before stent insertion); (b) UroCoil-Twin in place; the long segments of the device are stenting the membranous and prostatic urethra as well as the bladder neck.*

directions, as deep as possible but taking care not to enter the corpora cavernosa. If serious bleeding occurs and cannot be controlled satisfactorily during urethrotomy, a large calibre catheter is left indwelling and insertion of the stent is postponed for a few days in order to prevent stent blockage by clots. Opening up of the stricture to more than 22 Fr may cause stent migration. As the radial force exerted by the stent during its expansion is quite strong, a dilatation of 20–22 Fr is adequate. Before the urethrotome is

removed, a 0.038 inch or 0.045 inch guidewire is inserted into the bladder through the sheath of the urethrotome. After the endoscope has been removed, a Council-type Foley-like special measuring catheter (fluoroscopic ruler catheter) is inserted over the guidewire (Figs. 61.11 and 61.12) and the balloon is inflated with diluted (15%) contrast. The distance between the beginning and the end of the stricture (and the distance between the external sphincter to the proximal marking of the stricture) is measured by

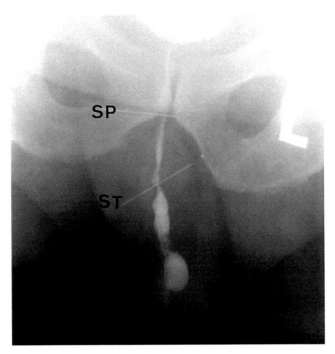

Figure 61.10. *Ascending urethrogram at the beginning of the procedure, before dilatation or urethrotomy. The anatomical landmarks and the stricture are marked at this stage. SP, external sphincter; ST, stricture.*

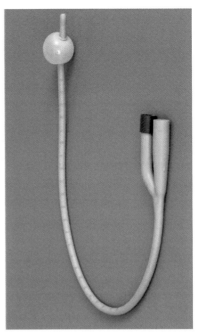

Figure 61.11. *Council-type Foley-like fluoroscopic ruler catheter. The radiopaque dots start 1 cm below the balloon. The distance between each dot is 1 cm.*

counting the dots (graduations) between the markers. If a UroCoil is to be used, the appropriate length for insertion is calculated by adding 2 cm to the measured length of the stricture, because 1 cm of the stent should be in the healthy part of the urethra at either side of the stricture. If a UroCoil-S is to be used, 2 cm is added to the distance between the external sphincter and the distal end marker. If a UroCoil-Twin is going to be used, 1 cm is added to the distance between the bladder neck and the external sphincter and 1 or 2 cm is added to the distance between the external sphincter and the distal marker. Then the ruler catheter is removed and the appropriate stent is inserted over the guidewire. As in the UroCoil, after its release from the delivery catheter, shortens from its upstream end by about 40% of its pre-release length, it is important to position the distal end (downstream) of the stent 1–2 cm below the proximal marker. When using the UroCoil-S or UroCoil-Twin, it is important to position the trans-sphincteric spacer at the level of the external sphincter before releasing the stent. When the unreleased stent is seen on fluoroscopy as adequately positioned, the locking handle is turned clockwise by 1–2 full-turns to release the upstream end of the stent. The released end of the stent starts to

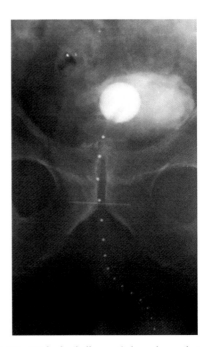

Figure 61.12. *With the balloon of the ruler catheter filled with contrast and pulled to the bladder neck, the radiopaque dots are counted in order to measure the distance between the externally applied markers. Since the catheter is very flexible, it coapts itself to the curves of the urethra. Counting the dots on fluoroscopy allows very accurate measurement.*

expand. At this stage, minor adjustments of positioning can be made by manipulating the delivery catheter. If the positioning is found to be satisfactory, clockwise turning of the locking handle is continued until the entire stent is released. Then the delivery catheter is gently pulled out, taking care not to dislodge the stent. If a UroCoil-S or a UroCoil-Twin is used, it is important to check the patency of the external sphincter before completing the procedure. In a patient who has undergone transurethral resection of the prostate, asking him to cough may demonstrate the integrity of the external sphincter. If the sphincter is disturbed by the tubular part of the stent, the patient will immediately leak and will not be able to stop the stream. In a patient with an intact bladder neck mechanism, success in starting to void and then stopping the stream indicates that the external sphincter mechanism is not impaired. If the patient cannot void when asked, an ascending urethrogram will show the relation between the external sphincter and the trans-sphincteric helical wire. If repositioning is necessary, a 17 Fr cystoscope with a grasping forceps is used. The endoscope is passed under vision through the lumen of the stent and, with the operator holding the trans-sphincteric wire, the stent is manipulated until it is properly positioned. If a UroCoil needs to be repositioned, the stent is held by one of its ends with the forceps and is gently pulled or pushed. These manipulations allow only minor repositioning (1–2 cm). As the stent, once released, cannot be removed and reinserted, for major repositioning the malplaced stent should be removed and a new one should be inserted.

A day after the insertion, uroflow is measured to mark the baseline urinary outflow of the patient.

Removal of the stent

Because of their tightly closed coils, these stents do not allow tissue ingrowth into their lumen; removal of the stent is, therefore, very easy, even after a year or more.

The urethra is filled with 10–20 ml 2% lignocaine gel, which is left in place for 10 minutes.

A UroCoil stent in the penile urethra is removed by holding the last loop of the coil with an endoscopic grasping forceps, and the uncoiled wire is pulled out gently until the entire stent emerges. To ensure that the entire stent has been removed, it is important to see the miniature balls at each end of the wire.

To remove a UroCoil-S or a UroCoil-Twin, a large calibre cystoscope (19 Fr or larger) is used. Again, by holding the last loop of the coil with the endoscopic grasping forceps, the wire is pulled out through the sheath of the cystoscope to prevent injury of the distal urethra.

Immediately after removal of the stent it is advisable to perform a urethroscopy to observe the healing of the stricture. In most cases the slight pressure marks left by the coil can be seen on the mucosa (Fig. 61.13a).

Follow-up

During the indwelling period of the stent (12 months or more) it is advisable to acidify the urine (pH below 6) and maintain a urine output of 1500–2000 ml/day to prevent urinary tract infection (UTI) and reduce encrustations. Monthly urine cultures and appropriate antibiotics are prescribed, especially to patients who had a chronic infection before stenting or who develop clinically significant UTI.

Uroflow measurements 1, 3, 6 and 12 months after stent insertion enable the patency of the stent lumen to be assessed. A significant decrease in Q_{max} generally indicates partial stent occlusion by encrustation, which is seen mostly in chronically infected patients.

One day after removal of the stent, the first uroflow measurement is made, to mark the post-removal Q_{max} baseline; this then is repeated 1, 3, 6, 12 and 24 months after removal. A decrease of 15% in Q_{max} from the baseline is accepted as normal, but a decrease of more than 20% on two consecutive measurements is regarded as pathological. In such a case, either a urethroscopy or a urethrogram is performed to establish the cause of the obstruction.

Urine culture is performed immediately after stent removal and, where positive, it is repeated until the urine becomes sterile after appropriate treatment.

Clinical experience and results

Since 1990, 172 patients with recurrent urethral strictures have been treated with the three configurations of the UroCoil-System stents. The strictures were situated all along the urethra, from the urethral meatus up the posterior urethra (Table 61.3). The initial results of the use of this removable temporary stent in 18 patients were published in 1991, opening a new era in the treatment of urethral stricture disease.[8] All patients had undergone at least three urethral dilatations

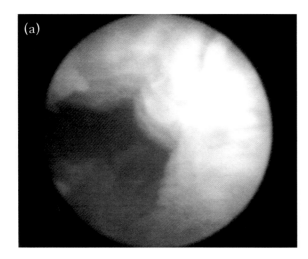

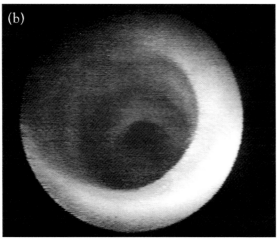

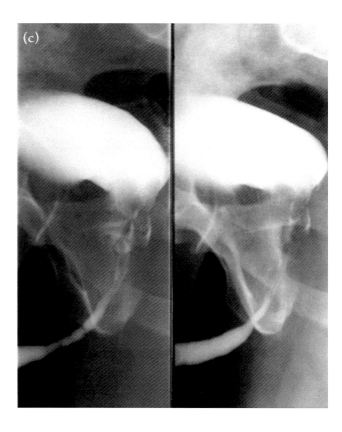

Figure 61.13. *(a) Endoscopic view of the urethra immediately after removal of the stent (note the complete epithelialization of the urethra and the transient pressure marks left by the stent on the epithelium); (b) endoscopic view of the urethra of the same patient after 3 years; (c) pre- and post-procedural urethrograms of the same patient.*

Table 61.3. *Location of strictures treated with UroCoil system stents*

Stent	Location	No. of patients
UroCoil	Penile urethra	27
	Membranous urethra	8
	Urethral meatus	4
UroCoil-S	Bulbomembranous urethra	53
	Bulbar urethra	72
UroCoil-Twin	Prostatic and bulbar urethra	8
Total		172

or two optical urethrotomies during the year preceding the procedure. Patients with urethral diverticula or fistula were not eligible for this treatment. Patients with acute urethral infections received intensive antibiotic treatment before the procedure. Patients with persistent infection were warned that they might develop acute exacerbation of the infection or stone formation on the stent. The average indwelling time of the stent was 12 (range 9–14) months and average follow-up after stent removal is 36 (range 8–50) months. At the end of the second year, 83% of the patients had a patent urethra and were voiding with a stream that was found to be within the normal range.

Only 17% of the patients were diagnosed as developing recurrent strictures; either they received another stent (not included in this group of patients) or they were periodically dilated. The recurrence rate rose to 20% in year 3 but stayed at the same level during year 4 (Table 61.4).

Table 61.4. *Results obtained with the use of UroCoil stents in cases of recurrent urethral strictures*

Indwelling time (months)	9–14 (av. 12)
Follow-up (months after stent removal)	8–50 (av. 36)
Percentage recurrence: 2 years	17
3 years	20
4 years	20

Conclusions

Management of recurrent urethral strictures with a temporarily inserted UroCoil-System stent is a simple and satisfactory procedure. The 6 year experience presented in this chapter, with more than 80% success rates obtained after failure of all conventional treatments, indicates that the use of stents can replace repeated urethral manipulation for maintenance of an adequate urethral calibre. In many cases, this approach may replace some of the complicated urethroplasties performed today. The smoothness and ease of removal of these stents allow their use all along the urethra, even in young patients, without interfering with their sexual life. As the stents remain in the urethral lumen without becoming epithelialized, they can be used in patients who underwent urethroplasty using skin.

The various lengths (40–80 mm) and configurations of the UroCoil-System stents allow a more economical and more tailored approach to strictures along the entire urethra between the bladder neck and the urethral meatus.[9,10]

The results obtained in recurrent post-traumatic posterior urethral strictures are also very promising. However, a larger series of patients and longer follow-up are needed to confirm the effectiveness of this approach.

On the basis of this experience, it can be concluded that large calibre temporary urethral stents enable most urethral strictures to be treated in a minimally invasive way. This experience also shows that the results obtained using stents are comparable to those of urethroplasty. A more extensive use of stents in the treatment of urethral strictures will reduce the number of repeated dilatations or urethrotomies, which are non-curative procedures.

The accumulating experience indicates that, in the near future, stenting will become the primary treatment of urethral strictures, superseding urethroplasty.

References

1. Kropp K A. Male urethral strictures. In: Gillenwater J Y, Grayhack J T, Howards S S, Duckett J W (eds) Adult and pediatric urology. Chicago: Year Book Medical, 1978; 1297–1314
2. McAnnich J W. Disorders of penis and urethra. In: Tanagho A E, McAnnich J W (eds) Smith's general urology, 13th edn. London: Prentice-Hall (Lange Medical Books), 1992; 602–605
3. Stocum D L. Editorial. Science 1997; 276 (5309): 15
4. Martin P. Wound healing — aiming for perfect skin regeneration. Science 1997; 276 (5309): 75–81
5. Hubner G, Brauchle M, Smola H et al. Differential regulation of pro-inflammatory cytokines during wound healing in normal and glucocorticoid-treated mice. Cytokine 1996; 8: 548–556
6. Leibovich S J, Ross R. The role of the macrophage in wound repair. A study with hydrocortisone and antimacrophage serum. Am J Pathol 1975; 78: 71–100
7. Desmouliere A, Redard M, Darby I, Gabbiani G. Apoptosis mediates the decrease in cellularity during the transition between granulation tissue and scar. Am J Pathol 1995; 146: 56–66
8. Yachia D, Beyar M. Temporarily implanted urethral coil stent for the treatment of recurrent urethral strictures: a preliminary report. J Urol 1991; 146: 1001–1004
9. Yachia D. The use of urethral stents for the treatment of urethral strictures. Ann Urol 1993; 27: 245–252
10. Yachia D, Beyar M. New, self-expanding, self-retaining temporary coil stent for recurrent urethral strictures near the external sphincter. Br J Urol 1993; 71: 317–321

62

Long-term results of Urolume stents in recurrent urethral strictures

E. J. G. Milroy

Introduction

The use of permanently implanted metallic stents in the urinary tract started after it was demonstrated that woven mesh stents constructed of small-diameter biocompatible wire in the dog urethra would become covered with urothelium in exactly the same way that Sigwart et al.[1] had earlier demonstrated the rapid covering of endovascular stents by endothelium when placed in the lumen of blood vessels. The early experimental work on the dog urinary tract was carried out jointly by Milroy[2] and Sarramon,[3] and this important finding of stent epithelial covering opened the way for the use of these devices in the human urinary tract, in the knowledge that, once the metallic stent had become covered with epithelium, there would be no contact of the metal wires with urine, and thereby avoiding the inevitable consequence of the encrustation, stone formation and infection that occurs when any foreign material is left in contact with urine.

Following these encouraging experimental results, further developments to the stent and delivery system were made and the first metallic mesh stents were implanted into recurrent urethral strictures in 1987, with the early results of the first eight patients treated being published the following year.[2,4] These results, and those subsequently reported by Sarramon,[3] led to a European multicentre study of this urethral stent in 71 patients with recurrent urethral strictures followed for up to 3 years.[5] The authors of this study stated that 'implanting this urethral stent was a simple endoscopic procedure and offered effective treatment for many recurrent bulbar urethral strictures'. A similar multicentre trial of the device in recurrent bulbar strictures in the United States and Canada showed good results in 175 patients with a follow-up to 2 years, with few side effects and excellent relief of obstruction.[6] The stent used in all these studies was originally designed and manufactured by Hans Wallsten in Lausanne, Switzerland and was known as the Wallstent. It is now called the Urolume and is manufactured by American Medical Systems, Minnetonka, Minnesota, USA.

Urolume stent

The stent is manufactured as a woven self-expanding tubular mesh of small-diameter biocompatible superalloy wire available in lengths of 20 and 30 mm with an unconstrained diameter of 14 mm (42 Fr). The wire diameter is 0.17 mm and there are 24 wires in each stent. The stent is supplied by the manufacturers, American Medical Systems, sterile and pre-loaded on a stent delivery system (Fig. 62.1). When the stent was first used, a different delivery system developed from the endovascular stent delivery device was employed. In this original system the stent was held in a compressed and elongated form by a rolling plastic membrane which, once the stent was correctly positioned, peeled back to allow the stent to expand. Because of problems in correct positioning of the stent in the urethra using this device, the new and currently available delivery system was developed. This uses a standard direct vision (0-degree) telescope inserted down the centre of the delivery system, allowing complete visualization of the urethra and stent as it is deployed within the area of the urethral stricture.

These stents have been used in urethral strictures occurring in the bulbomembranous urethra. It is, of course, important to keep the stent away from the

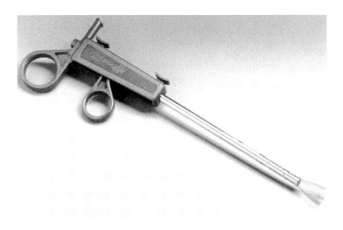

Figure 62.1. *Urolume permanent urethral stent with delivery device. (Reproduced with permission from Journal of Urology.)*

sphincter active area of the urethra: implanting a Urolume stent in this position will result in urinary incontinence. Recurrent strictures in this area have, in fact, been treated by using the Urolume in combination with an artificial urinary sphincter, but very careful patient selection is necessary for these cases.[7] Care should be taken to avoid stenting the penile urethra in sexually active patients, for two reasons: first, the stent diameter is too large for most penile urethras, although for the more distensible bulbar urethra the large diameter is acceptable; secondly, the stented urethra will not elongate during erection and this may cause painful erections. At least two endoscopic urethrotomies or dilatations should have failed before stent implantation is considered for any patient. All patients in the author's series were candidates for urethroplasty and all gave their fully informed consent to undergo stent insertion, on the understanding that, should the stent fail, a urethroplasty (with removal of the unsuccessful stent) would be carried out as had originally been planned before the stent was available.

Technique

Insertion of the Urolume stent is easy. A pretreatment urethrogram with ascending and descending (voiding) views is essential in order to identify and document areas of urethral abnormality. If suitable, the urethral stricture is then dilated. It makes little difference whether bougie dilatation or urethrotomy is used. Disadvantages of urethrotomy are that bleeding may make accurate positioning difficult and, if a single deep urethrotomy is made, the stent may lie off-centre in the urethra, causing subsequent difficulties and possible urethral distortion. For this reason, if urethrotomy is necessary because of dense fibrosis, the author prefers to carry out three separate radial incisions to ensure that the stent lies centrally within the urethra. The urethra should be dilated to 26–30 Fr, depending on the size of the penile urethra. Overdistension of the penile urethra should, of course, be avoided. The length of strictured urethra may be measured either from the preoperative urethrogram or at the time of endoscopy using a calibrated endoscope or ureteric catheter, and an appropriate length of urethral stent selected. It is important that the stent overlaps onto healthy urethra

at least 0.5 cm at each end of the stricture. This allows for some shortening of the stent as it expands and also ensures good positioning of the device within the urethra and encourages rapid epithelial covering of the wires of the stent.

With the appropriate stent length already mounted on its delivery system with a 0-degree telescope inserted down the centre of the device, the delivery tool is passed down the penile urethra into the area of the stricture. The delivery system is provided with two release catches. Releasing the first allows deployment of the stent to commence: as the outer metal sheath of the delivery tool is withdrawn the stent will open. This procedure should be commenced well upstream of the stricture in order to allow for shortening of the stent as it expands from the delivery tool. As the outer sheath is pulled back it reaches the second safety catch: at this point the stent is still held within the delivery system and correct positioning of the stent within the stricture can be checked by sliding the telescope up and down the length of the stent. The stent, still attached to the delivery system, may be drawn gently down the urethra if necessary but cannot be pushed further up the urethra. If the stent has been deployed too far downstream the outer sheath can be pushed forwards, enclosing the stent once more within the delivery tool; the whole system can then be repositioned and the stent redeployed. This allows for accurate positioning of the stent without difficulty. When it is decided that the position is correct, the second safety catch can be pressed and the outer sheath pulled back to its limit, whereupon the stent will spring free from the delivery tool. Complete release of the stent from the delivery tool can be checked by gentle rotation within the urethra. The final position of the stent can be reviewed endoscopically without difficulty, and the delivery tool can then be passed through the stent into the bladder in order to empty the bladder before the delivery device is finally removed. No catheter is necessary and the patient can undergo this procedure as an outpatient or on a day-stay basis without difficulty. Although, with most patients, the author has used a light general anaesthetic, is is certainly possible to insert this stent using local or regional anaesthetic, depending on the difficulty of dilating the stricture.

Once the stent has been released from the delivery system it is not possible to reposition it, although it can be removed by grasping its distal end firmly with alligator forceps. As the stent is pulled it elongates and narrows, enabling it to slide out of the urethra with little damage to the urethral epithelium. Once the stent has become completely covered with epithelium it is impossible to remove endoscopically. Removal would then require open excision of the stent with urethral reconstruction.

Results

The first 50 patients with recurrent urethral strictures treated with this device have been reported in detail elsewhere.[8] As stated earlier, all patients had recurrent strictures, in many cases with numerous previous treatments for up to 50 years before stent insertion. In this first series of patients all types of bulbomembranous urethral stricture were treated (Table 62.1), although patients younger than 30 years were excluded. The mean age was 58.2 (range 30–89) years with a mean duration of stricture history of 9.94 (± 10.8) years range 1–50 years.

All the stents in this series of 50 patients were inserted between May 1987 and December 1989. Four of the 50 patients had an additional overlapping stent inserted at the time of the first implant in order to cover the strictured area completely. All the patients were followed with regular assessment of symptoms, urine flow rate and urethroscopy until the stents were fully covered with epithelium. Subsequent urethrograms and urethroscopies were carried out only if patients experienced problems or if their flow rate deteriorated.

Four patients have been followed for 6 years, 23 for 5 years, five for 4 years and one was lost to follow-up. Follow-up was limited to 1–3 years in six cases because of patient death, to 1–3 years in another six cases because of serious unrelated ill-health, to 1 year in one patient because of stent excision and to 3 years in two patients because of subsequent urethroplasties. Two patients refused further follow-up after 1 and 2 years, respectively, because all was well and they could not afford the time for further hospital attendance! Mean follow-up was 4 (± 2) years. All patients unable or unwilling to attend for further investigation were contacted by means of a postal questionnaire.

Mean maximum urine flow rate at last follow-up was 19.7 (± 6.9) ml/s. Patient satisfaction was good, with 91% of patients being moderately or very satisfied with the final result, 2% somewhat satisfied and only 7% unsatisfied (Fig. 62.2).

The overall objective results of the 50 patients in this study are summarized in Table 62.2. Of these unselected strictures, 31 (63%) were satisfactorily treated with no stricture recurrence at endoscopy or urethrogram review, with a normal urine flow rate and no obstructive symptoms (Fig. 62.3). Stricture recurrence at one or other end of the stent occurred in nine patients. These were all the result of incorrect positioning of the stent which, as it expanded and shortened, pulled away from one end of the stricture

Table 62.1. *Aetiology of stricture in 50 patients*

Aetiology	No.
Catheter stricture	15
Post-TURP*	13
Failed urethroplasty	8
Infective	6
Traumatic	4
Unknown	4
Total	50

* TURP, transurethral resection of the prostate.
(Reproduced with permission from Journal of Urology.)

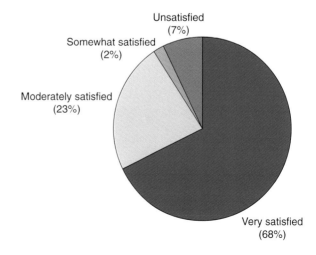

Figure 62.2. *Patient satisfaction (Reproduced with permission from Journal of Urology.)*

Table 62.2. *Overall results*

Result	No.*	
Objective relief of stricture	31	(63)
Recurrent stricture **outside** stent (misplaced)	9	
Significant narrowing **inside** stent	8	(16)†
Slight narrowing inside stent	1	
Lost to follow-up	1	
Total	50	

* Percentages in parentheses.
† True failure.
(Reproduced with permission from Journal of Urology.)

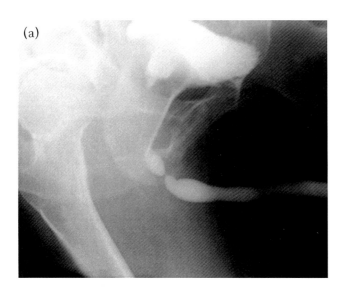

(a)

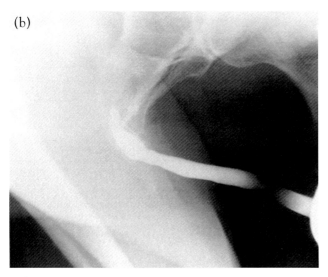

(b)

Figure 62.3. *(a) Recurrent bulbar stricture after two failed urethrotomies; (b) ascending urethrogram 6 years after Urolume insertion. (Reproduced with permission from Journal of Urology.)*

causing partial recurrence of the original stricture beyond the stent. All nine patients were successfully treated by the later insertion of an overlapping Urolume stent. These treatment failures could be considered part of the learning curve of using this new device. In eight patients (16%), significant narrowing developed within the lumen of the stent itself and in one there was insignificant narrowing that did not cause symptoms or reduction of urine flow rate. The eight patients can be regarded as the true failures of the series, because of the dense fibrosis that occurred within the lumen of the stent as the scar tissue of the original stricture grew through the mesh of the stent, despite attempts at normal epithelial covering of the wire. This complication occurred in two of the four cases of post-traumatic urethral rupture stricture and in four of the eight patients whose strictures had recurred following scrotal or penile inlay urethroplasty. This intrastent fibrosis also occurred in one of the six cases of post-inflammatory stricture and one of the 15 cases of catheter stricture. Although this finding suggests that traumatic and posturethroplasty strictures are more at risk of failure, it is also of interest that the mean duration of stricture history in the stent failure cases was 23.8(± 14.3) years whereas the mean duration of strictures in the entire series was 9.94 (± 10.8) years. It seems likely, therefore, that the length of time that a stricture has been present, with the related periurethral fibrosis and scar tissue associated with multiple endoscopic treatments, is at least as important in stent failure as the cause of the original stricture itself.

In three of these eight stent failures, excision of the stent was carried out at open surgery with subsequent urethral reconstruction (in one of the cases of post-traumatic rupture and in two cases of posturethroplasty failure) after only temporary relief of obstruction following endoscopic resection of the fibrosis. In the other five patients, fibrosis was resected endoscopically on one or two occasions with relief of obstruction and no recurrence of the narrowing at follow-up. These stricture recurrences, described above, all occurred within 6 months of stent insertion, with one exception — a patient developed narrowing within the lumen of the stent 4.5 years after stent insertion into a long-standing chronically infected stricture.

All the stents in this series became completely covered with epithelium on urethroscopic examination.

In most, this occurred within the first 3 months of stent insertion, although, in a few patients, complete covering of the wire took 6–9 months, particularly in those with posturethroplasty stricture. In many patients a hyperplastic reaction of the epithelium was noted in the first 4–6 weeks after stent implantation as the epithelium grew over the wires of the stent. This hyperplasia was particularly noticeable in cases of posturethroplasty stricture, presumably because of the presence of squamous rather than normal urethral epithelium; the reaction resolved spontaneously during the subsequent 6–12 months. Most patients noticed some postmicturition dribbling incontinence during the first 6–8 weeks after stent insertion. This problem seems to be related to a combination of serous exudate from the hyperplastic epithelium covering the stent, together with the small residual amount of urine left in the stent after finishing micturition. As the hyperplastic reaction to the stent resolves, this post-micturition dribbling tends to improve in the majority of patients: however, it persisted in nine patients (18%). It is noticeable that this problem is greater in those with 3 cm or more of stented urethra. The amount of incontinence was rarely more than a few drops of urine and was not often of any real significance to the patient. It is of note that, if patients are closely questioned, post-micturition dribbling is frequently found in patients with chronic urethral stricture and particularly in those who have undergone substitution urethroplasties.

Several patients noticed a minor degree of discomfort for a short time after stent insertion and with one patient this discomfort persisted, although further questioning revealed that the pain was identical to the discomfort he had felt before stent insertion as a result of chronic prostatitis. Two patients experienced pain with erections for the first 2 months after stent insertion when the stents were inserted at the penoscrotal junction partially into the penile urethra in sexually active men. The pain resolved spontaneously and subsequent erections were normal and painless. Several patients, when questioned, noted that the ejaculate fluid was somewhat more watery than before stent insertion, as seminal fluid was diluted with the small amount of residual urine contained within the stent lumen. No stent became infected, although five patients noticed a continuation of stricture-related urinary infections in spite of stent insertion and adequate relief of obstruction. No evidence of stent encrustation or stent displacement after insertion of the device was found.

Discussion

Since the first reports of the Urolume stent for the treatment of recurrent urethral strictures, this device has gained considerable popularity in Europe. A successful multicentre investigation of the device has been completed in the United States, with excellent medium-term results,[6] and the Urolume device has recently been passed by the FDA for use in recurrent bulbar stricture in the USA.

These long-term results demonstrate that the treatment is effective and, although further follow-up is necessary, the results seem to be stable up to 5 or 6 years. The failure rate is higher in strictures resulting from post-traumatic urethral rupture and in patients who have failed an earlier substitution urethroplasty, presumably because of the amount of periurethral scar tissue associated with these cases. If these two groups of patients are excluded from the original 50 patients in this study (four cases of traumatic stricture, eight of urethroplasty stricture and one failed follow-up) the failure rate (defined as intrastent fibrosis) falls from 16% to 5.4% (2/37 patients). This success rate of 94.6% is certainly comparable to, if not better than, other available treatments for recurrent strictures, whether by means of repeated urethrotomy or urethroplasty, and certainly justifies more extensive use of this device in carefully selected cases of urethral stricture. The problem of intrastent fibrosis has been reported by a number of urologists using the Urolume stent, but care in selecting patients, by excluding those with a long history of multiple stricture treatments and those with extensive fibrosis of the corpus spongiosum and periurethral tissues, will significantly reduce the incidence of these problems. Treatment of intrastent fibrosis by careful limited endoscopic resection of the fibrosis can result in satisfactory stabilization of the scar tissue in a number of patients, although, if this fails, stent excision and urethral reconstruction may be necessary. It is interesting to note that other urologists experienced in the use of the Urolume stent have not found this increased incidence of intrastent fibrosis in strictures following urethral trauma or failed urethroplasty.

The history of the treatment of urethral strictures includes many new techniques that offer the promise of long-term cure for this disabling condition. The existence of so many techniques and procedures is indication enough that all involve failures as well as successes. The Urolume is certainly no different in this regard. It is by no means a guaranteed cure for every stricture in the bulbar urethra and should be used only as one of the many available treatment options in carefully selected patients by experienced urologists. Longer follow-up, to 10 years at least, of larger groups of patients is necessary before the definitive place of this device in the treatment of urethral strictures can be determined.

References

1. Sigwart U, Puel J, Mirkovitch V et al. Intravascular stents to prevent occlusion and restenosis after transluminal angioplasty. N Engl J Med 1987; 316: 701–706
2. Milroy E J G, Chapple C R, Cooper J E et al. A new treatment for urethral strictures. Lancet 1988; 1: 1424–1427
3. Sarramon J P, Joffre F, Rischmann P et al. Prosthèse endouréthrale "Wallstent" dans les stenoses recidivants de l'urèthra. Ann Urol 1989; 23: 383–387
4. Milroy E J G, Chapple C R, Eldin A, Wallsten H. A new treatment for urethral strictures: a permanently implanted urethral stent. J Urol 1989; 141: 1120–1122
5. Ashken M H, Coulange C, Milroy E J G, Sarramon J P. European experience with the urethral Wallstent for urethral strictures. Eur Urol 1991; 19: 181–185
6. Badlani G H, Press S M, Defalco A et al. Urolume endourethral prosthesis for the treatment of urethral stricture disease: long term results of the North American multicentre Urolume trial. Urology 1995; 45: 846–856
7. Milroy E J G. Treatment of sphincter strictures using permanent Urolume stent. J Urol 1993; 150: 1729–1733
8. Milroy E J G, Allen A. Long term results of Urolume urethral stent for recurrent urethral strictures. J Urol 1996; 155: 904–908

63

Role of permanent stents in the management of complex urethral strictures

D. K. Shah and G. H. Badlani

Introduction

Stenting of the urinary system is one of the most common urologic procedures. The concept of using a permanent stent to maintain the patency of a lumen was first described in the vascular surgery literature by Wallsten, who used the technique to prevent restenosis after balloon angioplasty.[1] Since these initial experiments with dogs, many studies have been performed in human patients, demonstrating the efficacy of stents in large arteries with rapid flow.[2,3]

Despite advances in endoscopic and reconstructive urology, about one third of patients with urethral strictures remain a therapeutic challenge.[4] Strictures treated by optical urethrotomy or urethroplasty often remain resistant to relief. Multiple urethral dilations and self-catheterization are disappointing, if not unacceptable, alternatives.

Fabian was the first to describe use of a stent or spiral coil to maintain the patency of the prostatic urethra in patients with retention secondary to benign prostatic hyperplasia.[5] In 1988, Milroy and associates described the use of stents for the treatment of recurrent bulbar urethral strictures.[6] This use was a natural extension of the general concept of vascular stenting. In the same way that incorporation of a stent into a vessel wall helps prevent restenosis and clotting, incorporation of a stent into the urethral wall helps prevent migration, encrustation, and closure.

Urethral and stricture anatomy

To understand the role of the permanent stents in urethral stricture disease, knowledge of urethral anatomy is crucial.

The urethra is conceptually divided into five regions: prostatic, membranous, bulbar, and penile and the fossa navicularis. The *prostatic urethra* lies proximal to the verumontanum and is surrounded by the prostatic glandular tissue. The *membranous urethra* is a short segment surrounded by the external urethral sphincter.

The *bulbar urethra* is covered by the bulbospongiosus muscles and lies distal to the external sphincter and proximal to the suspensory ligament of the penis. The *penile urethra* lies distal to the suspensory ligament and centrally in the corpus spongiosum. The *fossa navicularis* is within the glans penis and terminates at the junction of the urethral epithelium and the skin of the glans. The posterior urethra comprises both the prostatic and membranous portions, while the anterior urethra consists of the bulbar and penile portions.

Posterior urethral strictures are generally associated with external trauma (i.e. pelvic fracture [95%]) in which the membranous urethral segment is displaced with a piece of the pelvic bone. Anterior urethral strictures are usually the result of straddle-type injuries, inflammation (e.g. sexually transmitted disease), or instrumentation (including catheters), although a few are idiopathic.[7]

Unlike vascular lesions, urethral strictures are composed of inelastic scar tissue. Their depth may be measured with real-time ultrasonography with the urethra filled with lubricating jelly.[8] Devine and colleagues have classified urethral strictures on the basis of the depth of invasion of scar into the surrounding spongiosum (Table 63.1).[9]

Classic treatment

Prior to the development of stents, the urologist had three options for treating urethral stricture disease:

Table 63.1. *Classification of urethral strictures*

Stage	Description
A	Mucosal fold
B	Small iris constriction not involving spongiosum
C	Full-thickness involvement of urethra without spongiosum inflammation
D	Full-thickness stricture with spongiofibrosis
E	Inflammation and fibrosis outside of spongiosum
F	Complex stricture complicated by fistula

From Devine et al. (1992).[9]

dilatation, internal urethrotomy, and formal open urethroplasty. Urethral dilatation gradually stretches the stricture to a size that will permit an adequate urine flow. However, repeated dilatation can result in overstretching and shearing of scar tissue, as well as trauma that may ultimately intensify the inflammatory process and worsen the stricture.[10] Thus, although dilatation is considered to therapeutic, it is not curative: patients may need to return for another session every 6 to 12 months.

The goal of optical internal urethrotomy is to incise the stricture visually and open up the urethra for subsequent epithelialization and healing with a larger diameter. A urethrotome is used to cut the stricture at some point, commonly the 12 o'clock position. Urethrotomy is useful for stages A, B and C strictures, for which it can be curative. However, more often than not, the stricture reappears, and sometimes, the inflammation from the urethrotomy makes the recurrent stricture even more extensive.

Urethroplasty has traditionally been the last line of therapy for strictures failing to respond to internal urethrotomy or dilatation, and it is the first choice for strictures in stages D through F.[9]

The final options are lifelong self-catheterization or a perineal urethrostomy. These measures are psychologically unacceptable to most patients and not feasible for others.

Stents have been recommended for use only to manage complex bulbar urethral strictures, as this region contains rich spongiofibrous tissue that resists erosion. Furthermore, in a bulbar location, the stent does not affect penile lengthening during erection; and because of its shape, the bulbar urethra has uniform radial forces, leading to better stent fixation and epithelialization.[11] However, the quality of the local tissue is more important for epithelialization than is the site of stent placement.

Permanent urethral stents

Various types of urethral stents are used for both diagnostic and therapeutic purposes. These stents provide mechanical endoluminal support and thereby maintain patency.

Fabian introduced the first spiral stent to be used for lower urinary tract obstruction. This stent is made of two stainless steel wire coils connected by a short straight wire. The proximal coil is placed in the prostatic urethra with its tapered proximal end resting in the bladder. The distal coil sits in the bulbar urethra with the connecting wire extending through the external sphincter. As metal coils do not become epithelialized and remain in the urethral lumen, this stent has high incidence of dislodgment, encrustation, and urinary tract infection (UTI).[12]

The UroLume Wallstent (American Medical Systems, Minnetonka, MN, USA) is the only permanent stent approved by the Food and Drug Administration (FDA) for urethral use in the United States. It is made from a biocompatible non-magnetic super-alloy (nickel and titanium) woven into a tubular mesh. The prosthesis is flexible and self-expanding. The stent is dispensed loaded in an endoscopic deployment tool. It is currently available in 1.5 cm, 2 cm, 2.5 cm, and 3 cm lengths; all have a 42 F internal diameter when fully expanded. The expandable nature of the stent keeps it in place until epithelialization anchors it firmly to the tissue. Urothelium will grow through the interstices of the stent and, in most patients, completely bury it (see below).[4] Epithelialization prevents exposure to urine, which can cause encrustation and encourage infection, which, along with migration, compromised earlier attempts at permanent urethral stenting.[6]

In the North American Urolume Trial, patients with strictures longer than 2.5 cm or strictures in two separate regions received more than one stent at the time of initial treatment.[13] Other patients required more than one stent owing to misplacement, restricturing adjacent to the stent, migration, separation of two previously placed stents, underestimation of stricture length, or ingrowth of hyperplastic tissue within the stent.[13] However, there is considerable debate as to whether more than one stent should be used, both because of cost and because of the possibility of increasing the complication rate.

Indications and contraindications

There are no universally accepted indications for urethral stenting, but many urologists accept the following as reasons to place a permanent stent:

1. Multiple failed internal urethrotomies (in poor surgical candidates).

2. Multiple failures of both internal urethrotomy and urethroplasty.
3. Multiple failed urethroplasties.

Ideal candidates for UroLume stent placement have a bulbar urethral stricture <3 cm long and at least 5 mm of healthy urethra distal to the external sphincter.

The relative contraindications for stent placement are:

1. Meatal stricture.
2. Coexistent pathology that may interfere with stent action (e.g. prostate cancer, bladder tumor, hydronephrosis, neurogenic bladder dysfunction, active urinary tract infection).
3. Age less than 21 years.
4. Strictures extending beyond the bulbar scrotal junction.
5. Inability to dilate the urethra to at least 26 Fr.

Preoperative preparation

Before patients provide informed consent, they should be told that they will be undergoing a surgical procedure, albeit a minor one. We explain the three most common postoperative complaints: postvoid dribbling, perineal discomfort and light bleeding. Patients should be informed that they may feel some dysuria and perineal discomfort for the first week after surgery but that it is normal and abates over time. Pain on erection usually resolves within 6 months. The reason for dribbling (see below) is explained. Patients are informed of the possibility of urethral restenosis necessitating subsequent retreatment, although the incidence of this problem is much lower after insertion of a urethral stent than it is without any treatment. Patients who have had urethroplasties are told that they are at higher risk for restenosis.

Urethroscopy or urethrography is performed in the office a few days before the procedure to examine the bladder and urethra and identify the site, length, and number of strictures. Urine flow is measured, and the AUA symptom score is determined.

Stent placement is performed as an ambulatory procedure. Our preference is to begin prophylactic administration of fluroquinolone 48 hours before stent insertion.

Technique

The instruments for UroLume stent insertion are listed in Table 63.2. The disposable endoscopic insertion tool houses the stent and the lens, provides a port for irrigation, and permits observation and control of device deployment (Fig. 63.1). If necessary, the device may be retracted into the sheath and repositioned before release.

We use 2% lidocaine jelly as an anesthetic lubricant. Most patients benefit from some mild sedation as well. A cystoscope is inserted into the urethra, and a 6 Fr open-ended catheter with a guidewire is passed across the stricture. The catheter is removed, leaving the guidewire in place. It is helpful (not absolutely essential) to have an image intensifier available to check the position of the guidewire. Cold-knife internal urethrotomy may be performed at the 12 o'clock position. Alternatively, dilatation is carried out sequentially over the guidewire using an 8 Fr Teflon catheter and an Amplatz dilator. In

Table 63.2. *Instruments and materials for UroLume stent insertion*

- Cystoscopy table with fluoroscope (optional)
- 50% Hypaque solution (optional)
- 20 Fr and 17 Fr cystoscope sheath
- Optical urethrotome with semicircular blade
- 30° and 0° lenses
- 0.038 inch Bentson guidewire
- 16 Fr open-ended urethral catheter (optional)
- Amplatz dilator system to 28 Fr
- UroLume endoscopic insertion tool

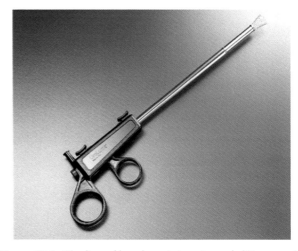

Figure 63.1. *The disposable endoscopic insertion tool. (Courtesy of American Medical Systems, Inc., Minnetonka, MN.)*

either case, the urethral stricture should be dilated to 26–28 Fr before insertion of the stent.

The stent should be at least 0.5 cm longer than the stricture. The 2 cm or 3 cm insertion tool is selected on this basis. We tend to overestimate the stricture length slightly to compensate for the tool's less than ideal accuracy: 5 mm is added to each end of the estimated stricture length. This obviates the occasional second procedure to place an additional stent overlapping the device already in place.

A 0° lens is then inserted into the tool. The outer sheath of the tool is heavily lubricated, and the entire assembly is advanced gently to the stricture under direct vision (Fig. 63.2). The sheath is then moved through the stricture so that its length and the external sphincter beyond can be viewed. One must be careful not to overdistend the bladder during this procedure. The lens is moved back and forth within the insertion tool until the proximal portion of the stent is visible. At this point, the outer safety stop that prevents premature deployment is removed, and the second safety stop is rotated to a vertical position for easy reach. The thumb ring of the device maintains the position in the urethra while the forefinger grip pulls the sheath back to release the stent; the thumb grip should remain stationary during stent deployment.

The stent is slowly deployed 5 mm distal to the external sphincter. We have found that it is easier to have the device positioned a few millimeters distal to

the sphincter and to pull the stent down in a more distal direction than it is to move the stent to a more proximal position once it has been deployed, as moving the stent proximally requires retracting it into the sheath and redeploying it. A number of attempts with the deploy-retract maneuver will quickly reassure the operator that he or she can easily control the device during this early positioning phase (Fig. 63.3). It must be kept in mind that the stent will shorten as the device expands to its full diameter.

Once the surgeon is comfortable with the stent position, the outer sheath is retracted with the forefinger while holding the thumb fixed. The lens must be pulled back to observe the progress of deployment as the sheath is moved back. The lens is then advanced to confirm the relative positions of the external sphincter and the proximal position of the stent. If the stent is not positioned correctly, it may be retracted into the sheath and repositioned.

Once the position of the stent is deemed adequate, the second safety lock, which prevents final release of the stent, is removed. The sheath is then slowly retracted, and the stent pops off the insertion tool to lie free across the stricture (Fig. 63.4). If the stent gets hung up on the end of the deployment tool, gentle rotation of the assembly should release it. If the stent is not released, the sheath is not fully retracted.

Once the stent is deployed, the finger grips of the deployment tool are extended again to withdraw the stent-holding prongs back into the sheath and prevent

Figure 63.2. *Deploying and retracting of the device confirms easy control. (Courtesy of American Medical Systems, Inc., Minnetonka, MN.)*

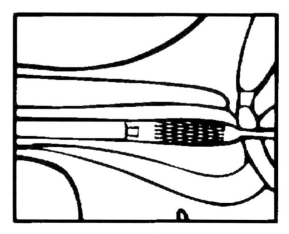

Figure 63.3. *When the stent is correctly positioned, the second safety lock is removed, and the sheath is slowly retracted. The stent will detach from insertion tool to lie free across the stricture. (Courtesy of American Medical Systems, Inc., Minnetonka, MN.)*

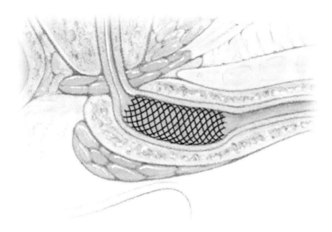

Figure 63.4. *final stent position across the stricture. (Courtesy of American Medical Systems, Inc., Minnetonka, MN.)*

urethral injury during sheath removal. At this point, the sheath should not be passed back into the expanded stent because of the risk of dislodging it. It is much better to inspect the distal end of the stent with a cystoscope of 17 Fr or smaller using a 0° lens. Care is taken not to strike the end of the wires during this maneuver. Once insertion is completed, a retrograde urethrogram will confirm that the stent is patent. If confirmation is needed then a uroflow assessment may be attempted in patients who are not too sedated.

Strategic placement is very important in patients who have had prostate surgery. If the stent transgresses the external sphincter, these patients will become incontinent, as the internal sphincter has been destroyed.

Postoperative care

No urinary catheter is required postoperatively. We advise patients to drink generous amounts of fluids for 48 hours to flush the urethra. We instruct them to avoid sexual activity for 2 weeks and to continue taking ciprofloxacin for the same period. For postoperative dysuria and perineal discomfort, we prescribe a mild analgesic, such as ibuprofen. A lateral radiograph is obtained immediately after the procedure and again at 24 hours to confirm the proper position and full expansion of the device. We advise patients that they may have some dribbling of the urine that remains in the distended portion of the urethra after voiding. Several weeks after the procedure, we allow patients to milk the urethra to get rid of this urine. Earlier attempts at this maneuver may dislodge the stent.

We observe two precautions to prevent displacement of the stent in the early postoperative period. First, if at all possible, we do not catheterize the patient. If catheterization is unavoidable, we insert a Council-tip catheter over a guidewire placed with a flexible cystoscope. Second, we avoid endoscopy; when this procedure is necessary, we do not let the endoscope touch the stent.

Follow-up is required at 6 weeks, 6 months, and 12 months and annually thereafter. At 6 weeks, uroflow reassessment and retrograde urethrography are performed. At this first visit, some distance may be noted between the wall of the stent and the contrast column on urethrography. This is caused by hyperplastic tissue reaction, which abates with time.

Results

Our experience with the UroLume stent stems from our involvement in the North American UroLume Trial, which was a multi-center, prospective, controlled trial of the prosthesis leading to its FDA approval for the treatment of recurrent urethral strictures. The 22 investigators at 12 sites in the United States and 3 sites in Canada enrolled 179 patients between March 1989 and April 1996. All patients had recurrent strictures in the bulbar urethra. Most had been treated for more than 5 years and had undergone five or more dilatations or urethrotomies. The exclusion criteria were those listed above under Contraindications.

The stent was inserted endoscopically after internal urethrotomy or sequential dilatation of the stricture to 30 Fr over a guidewire. A total of 158 patients (90%) underwent one insertion procedure, 16 (9%) underwent two, and three patients (1%) underwent multiple procedures.[4] The rate of patient compliance with follow-up was 79% at 2 years.

Insertion of the UroLume prosthesis decreased retreatment rates for urethral strictures at 1 year, an effect that was sustained at 2 years and thereafter. The retreatment rate decreased from 75.3% before insertion to 14.3% after insertion in the 105 patients followed for at least 1 year.[4] Moreover, no urethroplasties were required, so the morbidity of any necessary retreatment was significantly less than in patients who had not received stents.

Of the patients stented, 16 out of 179 were reported as deceased secondary to causes unrelated to stent placement and nine patients had undergone permanent stent removal. Eleven patients, implanted late in the pre-approval phase of the study, completed their five years of post-approval follow-up before reaching the 11 year mark, and thus did not become eligible for 11 year follow-up. The remaining 121 patients were discontinued due to their early exit from the pre-approval study or opted not to participate in the post-approval study. The 24 patients who consented to further follow-up were evaluable at 11 years.

Paired uroflow data before and after UroLume insertion were available for 21 of the 24 patients followed for 11 years. Prior to stent placement, the mean peak flow rate for these 21 patients was 8.7 ml/s (range 3.0–16.0 ml/s). At 11 years, the mean peak urinary flow rate had improved to 19.7 ml/s (7.6–46.0 ml/s) (Table 63.3). Improvement can be seen by 1 year that was maintained throughout the study. ANOVA testing on the data from the 21 patients indicated significant improvement (P <0.0001) at all eight time points.

Paired symptom score data were available for 23 patients at 11 year follow-up (Table 63.4). Improvement was seen at 1 year that was maintained throughout the study. At 11 years, the mean symptom score had improved to 3.0 from 11.3. ANOVA testing indicated significant improvement at all eight time points. The P-values were <0.0001 through 7 years' follow-up, <0.0335 at 9 years, and <0.0002 at 11 years.

At 11 years, 16 patients (73%) had mild or no tissue change while 5 (23%) had moderate and one (7%) had marked tissue change (Table 63.5). Complete epithelialization (≥90% coverage) of the endoprosthesis was seen by 1 year in more than 90% of patients and was sustained throughout 11 years of follow-up (Fig. 63.5).

Among the 179 patients in the pre-approval multicenter trial, 9 stent removal procedures were required during 11 years of follow-up. Seven of those nine patients (78%) underwent stent removal during the first year after placement. Of the remaining two removals, one occurred 4 years after stent placement and the other at 5 years and 3 months. The reasons for stent removal were pain/discomfort (three cases), pain/discomfort

Table 63.3. *Uroflow rates before/after UroLume placement*

Follow-up (yrs)	Mean peak flow rate	SD	Minimum	Maximum	No. of patients
1	9.7/22.7	6.6/11.9	1.0/4.5	35.4/63.4	122
2	8.6/22.5	5.6/11.5	1.3/3.6	31.0/62.0	85
3	8.8/20.1	5.8/12.5	1.0/3.9	35.4/63.2	75
4	9.2/21.0	5.4/11.9	2.0/6.4	31.0/62.0	57
5	8.8/19.7	4.3/10.6	2.0/4.6	22.0/51.0	41
7	9.1/20.4	4.7/12.1	2.0/3.7	22.0/58.0	31
9	8.3/18.9	4.1/11.4	2.0/5.3	16.0/44.8	26
11	8.7/19.7	3.7/11.0	3.0/7.6	16.0/46.0	21

Table 63.4. *Symptom scores before/after UroLume placement*

Follow-up (yrs)	Mean	SD	Minimum	Maximum	No. of patients
1	12.5/2.5	5.4/3.0	2.0/0	28.0/19.0	137
2	12.4/2.5	5.1/3.4	2.0/0	25.0/18.0	87
3	12.4/3.2	5.4/4.5	2.0/0	25.0/20.0	90
4	12.5/2.5	5.2/3.4	3.0/0	25.0/16.0	67
5	12.2/2.9	5.2/3.2	2.0/0	25.0/10.0	47
7	12.0/3.5	5.9/3.1	2.0/0	25.0/12.0	22
9	11.7/4.1	5.6/5.3	2.0/0	25.0/27.0	31
11	11.3/3.0	4.8/3.6	4.0/0	25.0/15.0	23

Table 63.5. *Extent of tissue change*

Evaluation period (yrs)	None	Mild	Moderate	Marked	No. of patients
1	52	20	7	1	80
2	54	25	9	3	91
3	49	22	10	3	84
4	36	24	3	3	66
5	24	10	3	0	37
7	14	9	5	1	29
9	14	8	3	0	25
11	7	9	5	1	22

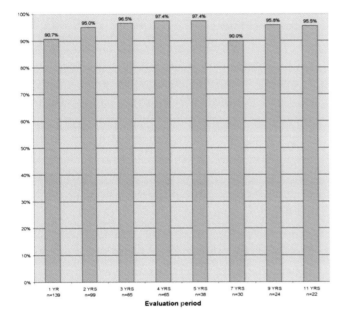

Figure 63.5. *The percentage of patients having ≥90% epithelialization of the stent.*

associated with distal migration (two cases), pain/discomfort associated with tissue changes and infection (one case), chronic urinary tract infection (one case), encrustation and recurrent stricture (one case), unrelated health problem (two cases).

During 11 years of follow-up, 27 of the 179 patients (15.1%) underwent a total of 30 retreatment procedures within the stented area. The time ranged from less than 2 months to 11.2 years. Retreatment procedures included transurethral resection (11 cases), dilatation (9 cases), additional stent placement (5 cases), resection and additional stent insertion (1 case), resection and dilatation (1 case), and dilatation and laser treatment (1 case).

In 1997, we studied the 41 patients who required placement of multiple stents to determine whether they achieved the same efficacious and durable results as the rest of the group.[13] Of these patients, 61% required placement of multiple stents as part of the primary procedure because of stricture length (>3 cm), and 39% later received additional stents because of recurrent stricture adjacent to the original stent,[4] gaps between two previously placed stents, or hyperplastic tissue within the stent lumen. The peak flow rates and symptom scores for the patients who required multiple stents showed improvement comparable to that of the overall study group. At 2 years, the mean symptom score had decreased from 14.3 to 3.1 (compared with 12.5 to 2.6 in the total study group), and the peak flow rate had increased from 8.2 to 22.0 ml/s (compared with 8.98 to 23.56 ml/s).

Ashken and associates reported on 71 patients with up to 3 years' follow-up at four European sites.[14] The mean peak flow rate increased from 6 ml/s before stent insertion to 22 ml/s at 15 months' follow-up. Sixty-eight patients were happy with their results. Three patients with traumatic strictures experienced recurrences. Complications included postvoid dribbling and transient urethral or perineal discomfort. Sertcelik and colleagues described an 87% success rate with a mean follow-up of 4.3 years in their experience with UroLume placement for recurrent bulbar urethral stricture.[15]

Adverse events

In only one patient in the study did a stone form on an exposed surface of the stent. This was found 3 years after insertion and was easily removed with stone-crusher forceps with no complications or recurrence. No patient developed encrustation of the stent within the 2 year follow-up period regardless of the percentage of epithelialization of the stent. The few patients with inadequate epithelialization at 2 years after insertion did not have a higher risk of encrustation. Additionally, other postoperative complications (e.g. urinary tract infection, restenosis, pain, and incontinence) were not more common in these patients, nor were the complications these patients experienced any more severe than those in patients with adequately epithelialized stents. It is possible that with extended follow-up, more patients with exposed stents will develop encrustation; however, to date, this has not been the experience.

During the 2 year follow-up, hyperplastic tissue growth along the lumen of the stent was noted in 74 of 179 patients (41.3%) at one or more follow-up visits. This growth resulted from growth of the urethral endothelium through the openings between the wires of the stent. Of these cases 62 (83%) were mild, whereas 12 patients (16%) had moderate to severe hyperplasia that necessitated removal of tissue from within the lumen. Most often (75% of the patients), removal was achieved by transurethral resection. In total, 12 of 175 patients (7%) required excision of tissue from the lumen of the stent. Biopsies in four patients yielded a combination of squamous metaplasia, fibrosis, mild inflammation, and local fibroblastic reaction. No significant association between hyperplastic tissue growth and the cause of the original stricture was demonstrated (P >0.7). Of the 16 patients requiring removal of tissue, in only 3 (19%) was the cause of the hyperplasia found to be traumatic injury (P >0.3).[13] When hyperplastic tissue ingrowth was noted, transurethral resection was usually curative. Some patients required more than one transurethral resection to achieve patency.

In comparison, 43 of 179 patients (24.2%) receiving the UroLume stent had a history of urethroplasty. Of these patients, 17 (40%) required secondary treatment for restenosis after insertion of the device. Only 14 (11%) of the 130 patients who had not had a previous urethroplasty required secondary treatment (P <0.001); 8 of 17 patients (47%) requiring secondary treatment underwent transurethral resection of tissue within the stent. The incidence of resection among urethroplasty patients compared with non-urethroplasty patients was 8 of 43 (18%) versus 3 of 127 (2%) (P<0.001). Put another way, of the 16 patients (9%) in the study who

required transurethral resection to remove tissue from within their stents, 8 (50%) had previously undergone urethroplasty. The two urethroplasty patients who ultimately required stent removal accounted for 29% of the patients requiring stent removal during the study.

The incidence of hyperplastic tissue ingrowth associated with the UroLume stent has been widely discussed in the literature of late. Numerous case reports have documented tissue growth between the wires. Although the incidence of hyperplastic tissue ingrowth is indeed relatively high, the growth usually is not clinically significant. Many investigators feel that it occurs more frequently in posttraumatic strictures.[16,17]

The data from the North American UroLume Trial show that prior failed urethroplasty, not traumatic injury, is the major risk factor for restenosis within the UroLume prosthesis. A majority of patients (62%) will not require treatment beyond transurethral resection, although a portion may ultimately require removal of the stent because of frequent restenosis. However, the use of the UroLume stent in patients with traumatic strictures is not contraindicated as long as the higher risk of failure is recognized.

Urine cultures were positive before stent insertion in 15 of 161 patients (9.3%). There was no statistical difference between the preinsertion infection rate and the infection rate at 6 months (15/139 [10.8%]) and at 2 years (10/72 [13.9%]) (P = 0.1). The only preoperative variable that was independently predictive of postinsertion infection was a positive urine culture preoperatively.

Migration of the stent was seen in 2 of the 179 patients (2.5%). Incontinence was evaluated by questionnaire; no pad testing was performed. Severe incontinence was noted at 2 years in 2.5% of patients, whereas 4.3% of patients had severe incontinence at 6 weeks. Mild incontinence was also noted in 16 of 80 patients (20%) at 2 years. There was an improving trend with time in both of these complications. The degree of incontinence was not evaluated preoperatively, so in some patients, incontinence might have been present before insertion of the stent. Also, the true incidence of incontinence is lower that these figures suggest, as many patients report postvoid dribbling as incontinence. Postvoid dribbling remained a problem for as long as 2 years after insertion in 41 of 80 patients (51%), although it was mild in most cases. In summary, the available data indicate that the use of the UroLume does not increase the risk of incontinence.

Local pain/discomfort that followed stent insertion decreased progressively with time. Thus, 102 of 164 patients (62%) reported some degree of pain at 6 weeks, but the number decreased to 9 of 80 (11%) patients at 2 years. In most patients, these symptoms were mild.

Conclusions

The results from the North American UroLume Study Group and its European counterpart validated the use of the UroLume endourethral prosthesis in the treatment of recurrent bulbar urethral strictures. At 11 years of follow-up, the improvement persisted, with endoscopy showing good epithelial cover with little tissue change. The stents were well tolerated, as judged by the incidence of pain and changes in sexual function. Problems with insertion were minimal. Perhaps most important is that the need for retreatment for urethral stricture disease was markedly reduced after insertion of the UroLume stent. This result suggests that the better outcomes are result of stenting and not simply of internal urethrotomy or dilatation at the time of stent insertion.

References

1. Dotter C. Transluminally placed coil spring endarterial tube grafts: long term patency in canine popliteal artery. Investig Radiol (Berl) 1969; 9: 252–255
2. Mass D. Transluminal implantation of intravascular 'double helix' spiral prosthesis: Technical, bological consideration. Proc Eur Soc Artif Organs 1982; 9: 252–258
3. Wright K, Wallace S, Charnsangavej C, Carrasco C, Gianturco C. Percutaneous endovascular stents: an experimental evaluation. Radiology 1985; 156(1): 69–72
4. Badlani G, Press S, Defalco A. Urolume endourethral prosthesis for the treatment of urethral stricture disease: long term results of the north American multicenter Urolume trial. Urology 1995; 45: 846–856
5. Fabian K. Der intraprostatische 'Partielle Katheter' (urologische Spirale). Urologe A 1980; 19: 236–242
6. Milroy E, Cooper J, Wallsten H, Chapple C. A new treatment for urethral strictures. Lancet 1989; 25: 1424–1427
7. Press S, Badlani G. Urethral stents. In: Smith A (ed) Smith's textbook of endourology. Philadelphia: W B Saunders, 1995
8. McAninch J, Laing F, Jeffrey R. Sonourethrography in the evaluation of urethral strictures: A preliminary report. J Urol 1988; 139(2): 294–297
9. Devine C, Jordan G, Sclossberg S. Surgery of the penis and urethra. In: Jr V E. (ed) Campbells urology (6th edn). Philadelphia: W B Saunders, 1992: 2986
10. Ballentine Carter H. Instumentation and endoscopy. In: Wein A (ed) Campbell's urology. Philadelphia: WB Saunders, 1998: 162–164
11. Curujo M, Badlani G. Epithelialization of permanent stents. J Endourol 1997; 11: 477–481
12. Nielsen K, Klarskov O, Nordling J, Holm H, Andersen J. The prostate coil. A new form of treatment of urinary retention in men. Clinical experiences during a 6 month observation period. Ugeskr Læger 1989; 151(44): 2888–2889
13. Tillem S, Press S, Badlani G. Use of multiple Urolume endourethral prosthesis in complex bulbar urethral strictures. J Urol 1997; 157: 1665–1668
14. Ashken M, Coulange C, Milroy E. European experience with the urethral wallstent for urethral strictures. Eur Urol 1991; 19: 181–186
15. Sertcelik N, Sagnak L, Imamoglu A, Temel M, Tuygun C. The use of self expanding metallic urethral stents in the treatment of recurrent bulbar urethral strictures: Long term results. BJU Int. 2000; 86: 686–689
16. Sneller Z, Bosch R. Restenosis of the urethra despite indwelling Wallstent. J Urol 1992; 148: 145–149
17. Verhamme H, Van Poppel H, Wan DeVoorde W. Total fibrotic obliteration of urethral stent. Br J Urol 1993; 72: 389–390

Treatment of recurrent anastomotic stenoses after radical prostatectomy or radical cystoprostatectomy and orthotopic bladder replacement with temporary stents

D. Yachia

64

Introduction

A patient with newly diagnosed bladder or prostate cancer faces not only psychological stress and the prospect of major surgery he also has to learn to live with either a continence mechanism with which he is not familiar or, where an orthotopic bladder replacement is necessary, he has to learn how to void spontaneously with the neobladder. In addition, one in five of these patients will also suffer from voiding disturbances arising from strictures developing at the anastomosis site, between the bladder/neobladder and urethra. An incidence of 0.8–20% of urethrovesical anastomotic stenoses after radical prostatectomy[1–3] and of 2–30% of urethro-neobladder anastomotic stenoses after radical cystoprostatectomy have been reported.[4–8] Conventionally, these strictures ara managed either by dilatation or by optical urethrotomy. Most mild strictures are amendable to dilatation. In many cases the proximity of the external sphincter to the stenotic area prevents the surgeon from resecting the fibrotic tissue endoscopically to obtain a large channel. The most that the surgeon can do is to incise the stenotic area, taking great care to protect the external sphincter. Unfortunately, despite these manipulations, some strictures recur. In some recurrent cases the patients have to be trained in self-catheterization in order to keep the vesico-urethral anastomosis open.

Clinical experience and results

In view of the good results obtained with the use of UroCoil/ProstaCoil stents in the management of prostatic and urethral obstructions, ten patients were fitted with a short ProstaCoil stent. Recurrent anastomotic strictures had developed between the urethra and the bladder after radical prostatectomy in nine of these patients (Fig. 64.1) and in one patient between the urethra and neobladder after orthotopic bladder substitution (Fig. 64.2).

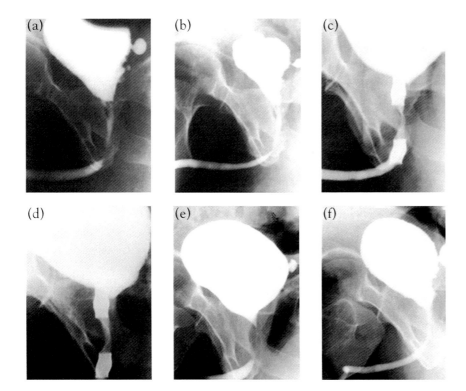

(a) (b) (c)

(d) (e) (f)

Figure 64.1. *Anastomotic stenosis after radical prostatectomy: (a) stenosis 1 cm in length at the level of the vesico-urethral anastomosis; (b) recurrent anastomotic stenosis after six dilatations and one endoscopic incision; (c) ascending urethrogram after balloon dilatation of the stenosis and insertion of a 40 mm ProstaCoil into the stenotic area (note the contraction of the external sphincter around the trans-sphincteric spacer of the stent); (d) voiding through the ProstaCoil; (e) ascending urethrogram 7 months after removal of the ProstaCoil, which was left indwelling for 9 months (note the smooth funnel at the bladder neck and the normal configuration of the external sphincter); (f) voiding urethrogram of the same patient.*

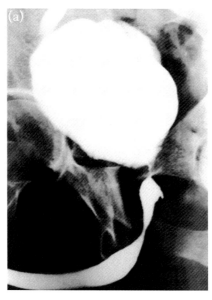
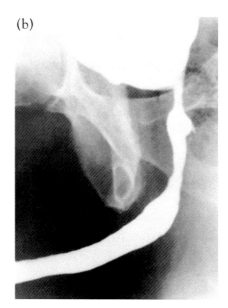

Figure 64.2. *Anastomotic stenosis after radical cysto-prostatectomy and orthotopic neobladder: (a) Neobladder-urethral anastomotic recurrent stenosis after four dilatations; (b) large-calibre passage 4 months after removal of the ProstaCoil, which was left indwelling for 6 months.*

The stent used in these cases was the shortest available ProstaCoil (40 mm), which was inserted after endoscopically guided balloon dilatation of the stenotic anastomosis. (The insertion procedure is detailed in Chapters 39 and 52) The ProstaCoil was left in place for 6–13 (mean 11) months. With a follow-up of 1–10 (mean 7) months, in seven patients the anastomotic stricture has disappeared; in six patients (one with the orthotopic bladder), continence is excellent and one has stress incontinence that is a continuation of the stress incontinence that he displayed after the orignal surgery. Three patients are voiding through their stents and awaiting stent removal.

Discussion

The urethrovesical and neobladder-urethral anastomotic stenoses may recur because of the same mechanism, causing the recurrence of traumatic complete posterior urethral strictures where fibrosis surrounds the traumatized urethra. In both cases urethrotomy fails to cure the stenosis because of the depth of fibrosis.

Anastomotic stenoses differ from bladder neck stenoses occuring after transurethral resection of the prostate (TURP) or open prostatectomy. In such cases, endoscopic deep incisions at the stenotic bladder neck

usually achieve an open bladder neck. In post-TURP bladder neck stenoses, the fibrotic ring starts from the edge of the new bladder neck and obstructs the passage; it usually takes the form of a membrane 1–1.5 mm thick, in which, at the level of the bladder, the tissues surrounding the fibrotic ring are natural. In anastomotic stenotic rings, the fibrotic process continues through the tissues surrounding the vesico-urethral anastomosis, as part of the scarring process. In anastomotic stenoses, if this thick fibrotic tissue is incised, normal healthy tissue cannot be reached, thus resulting in a restenosis. Stenting of this area, after incising it and waiting until the scarring process has stabilized, may create a tubular fibrotic segment large enough to allow the patient adequate voiding. As in some traumatic urethral strictures where the fibrotic process is dense and the open surgical approach is extremely difficult or impossible, in anastomotic stenoses also the aim is to create a cast of fibrotic tissue tube covered by healthy epithelium, replacing a short segment of the urethra. The role of the stent in these cases is as a mould placed in the stenotic area to reshape the urethral passage with a tube of fibrotic tissue that forms a cast around it.

Unlike mesh stents, in which the fibrotic tissues can grow through the interstices of the meshwork and remain permanently in the body, closed-coil stents can be inserted temporarily for a period of a few months and then removed easily. This approach is based on the same concept of using temporary stents for the treatment of recurrent urethral strictures, especially traumatic strictures. Currently, the only available self-expanding temporary stents are the ProstaCoil, the Memokath and the Horizon. The design of the current Memokath precludes the use of this stent at the bladder neck because it lacks a reliable anchoring mechanism. Although the available ProstaCoil is not specially designed for such a purpose, its shortest size (40 mm) can be used for this purpose. If, in the future, a shorter stent (25–30 mm) should become available, it would be a better fit for the short distance between the bladder neck and the anastomosis, and would be anchored by its bulbar segment, which is positioned below the external sphincter. However, because of the proximity of the external sphincter to the anastomotic stricture, in most cases the presence of a large calibre stent in such a situation disturbs the function of the external sphincter, rendering the patient more incontinent than the usual incontinence observed in the early months after radical prostatectomy. This disturbance is the result of the foreign body irritation, coupled with the mechanical interference. The author personally explains this phenomenon to the patient before inserting the stent and also requests the patient to activate (contract) the sphincter voluntarily with the stent in place, in order to preserve (or even develop) the sphincter tone. A second important recommendation for these patients is to avoid using external urine-collecting devices but to use a penis clamp in order to stay dry. This allows the patient to preserve his bladder capacity during this incontinent period and also encourages him to activate the sphincter in the middle of his voiding, trying to stop the stream.

Conclusions

Although this series is small and the follow-up too brief, the initial results of complete success in all the 7 patients in whom the stent was removed are very impressive and promising. Larger, multicentre series with a longer follow-up are needed to evaluate the effectiveness of this treatment.

References

1. Surya B V, Provet J, Johanson K E, Brown J. Anastomotic strictures following radical prostatectomy: risk factors and management. J Urol 1990; 143: 775–758

2. Rossignol G, Leandri P, Gautier J R et al. Radical retropubic prostatectomy: complications and quality of life (429 cases, 1983–1989) Eur Urol 1991; 19: 186–191

3. Fowler F J Jr, Barry M J, Lu-Yao G et al. Patient reported complications and followup treatment after radical prostatectomy. The National Medicare experience, 1988–1990 (updated June 1993). Urology 1993; 42: 622–629

4. Mandressi A, Bernasconi S, Zaroli A et al. 100 orthotopic neobladders in men after cystectomy: a 5-year experience. Arch Ital Urol Androl 1996; 68(5) 323–331

5. Samodai L, Zamoti A, Kelemen I, Kovacs L Continent urinary diversion after radical cystectomy: 3 years experience. Int Urol Nephrol 1996; 28(4) 511–516

6. Ghoneim M A, Atallah A S, Mahran R M, Kock N G. Further experience with the urethral Kock pouch. J Urol 1992; 147: 361–365

7. Boyd S D, Esrig D, Stein J P et al. Undiversion in men following cystoprostatectomy and cutaneous diversion. Is it practical? J Urol 1994; 152: 334–337

8. Narayan P, Broderick G A, Tanagho E A. Bladder substitution with ileocaecal (Mainz) pouch; clinical performance over 2 years. Br J Urol 1991; 68: 588–595

Histological changes associated with stenting the urinary tract
D. Bailey

65

Introduction

The majority of studies documenting histological changes found in association with stenting in general are based on stenting of the biliary tree[1–5] and the arterial system,[6–12] particularly the coronary arteries. The earliest biliary tract studies date from the mid-1980s and document mucosal proliferation through the wall of the stent mesh resulting in partial or complete blockage of the lumen. Squamous metaplasia was also noted. Most of these studies were based around endoscopic biopsies that were subjected to electron microscopy and/or light microscopical observations.

Some studies of coronary artery stents were carried out using intravascular ultrasound[11,12] and as such were not truly histological in nature. The results were largely based upon subjective interpretation of ultrasonographic information without histological interpretation of biopsies; however, several studies documented light-microscopical changes,[6–10] including intimal hyperplasia, reversible proliferation of vasa vasorum and accumulation of thrombus around the stent wires.

Investigation of urinary tract stenting[13–22] began in 1985 with ureteric stenting,[13] and studies of the pathological effects of urethral stenting followed from the late 1980s.[23] Reviewing the literature shows that the changes associated with stenting in part depend on the nature of the stent used. The earliest studies investigated effects of double-J stents of the ureter,[13] whereas most recently, the first study of patients with long-term, self-expanding urethral stents documented histological changes in a group of 18 patients.[24] The numbers investigated are very small when compared with some of the larger histological studies carried out in the field of histopathology and the information gleaned can thus only be regarded as anecdotal. Several trends have emerged, however, and further long-term studies in larger groups of patients would provide a welcome correlation for these papers, which can be regarded as pilot studies at best.

Ureteric stenting

Few papers detailing the histological effects of ureteric changes are available.[13,18,19,22] Most are based upon animal studies.[13,18,19] Porcine urodynamic studies[13] show an increase in intrapelvic pressures, hydroureter, vesicorenal reflux and generalized thickening of the ureteric wall; the histological changes must, at least in part, be due to these factors. El Deen et al:[18] documented changes in 34 male rabbits that had internal stents inserted, which included dilatation of the pelvicalyceal system and renal tubules, inflammatory infiltration of the kidney and ureter, mucosal ulceration and muscular hypertrophy of the ureter. The bladder mucosa showed evidence of severe inflammation, numerous von Brunn nests and ulceration with focal squamous metaplasia. These changes were found to be reversible if the stent was removed within 1 week. Further studies also noted thickening of the wall of the ureter, mainly due to muscular hypertrophy.

Few other examples are available,[22] particularly from humans, but a single case from the archives of University College Hospital, London (Dr M. C. Parkinson, personal communication), showed polypoid hyperplasia of the urothelium with intense chronic inflammation of the underlying connective tissue. The stent was of the self-expanding type and the wires had become embedded into the suburothelial connective tissue, forming pseudo-diverticula surrounded by invaginations of urothelium. These clefts were further emphasized when the stent wires were dissected out by the pathologist at cut-up of the specimen, and were surrounded by micro-abscesses and foreign body giant cells.

Urethral stenting

Urethral stents have been in use since the early 1980s with a great deal of success in alleviating obstructive symptoms due to stricture,[23,25–29] benign prostatic hyperplasia (BPH)[30-32] as a low risk, minimally invasive alternative to transurethral resection, or to neurological injury.[33-36] Currently, 15–20 000 Urolume stents alone have been sold world-wide (personal communication, American Medical Systems, Minnetonka, MN, USA), although how many of these have actually been used in patients is not known.

Baert et al.[37] and Verhamme et al.[38] showed fibrotic obliteration of the stent lumen after 22–31 months in a total of four patients with urethral stents. Milroy et al.[23] showed hyperplastic urothelial covering of the stent with little underlying inflammation or fibrosis in a study of four dogs with prostatic (Urolume) stents in situ for 2–12 months. Bosnjakovic et al.[39] used scanning electron microscopy (EM) to demonstrate subtotal hyperplastic urothelial covering of Strecker stents in artificially created urethral strictures in eight dogs between 4 and 12 months after insertion.[39] Latal et al.[40] also used scanning EM to demonstrate urothelial hyperplasia protruding into the lumen through Strecker stents inserted into 18 normal dog urethras for up to 18 months.[40] Until recently therefore, there had been few studies documenting light-microscopic changes in humans subjected to urethral stenting.

A recent study of 18 patients with long-term urethral stents[24] looked at biopsy or resection specimens and assessed the associated histological changes. All 18 patients had Urolume stents. Three had external sphincter stents for detrusor–sphincter dyssynergia (DSD) secondary to spinal injury; eight had prostatic stents for obstruction secondary to BPH and seven had urethral stents for recurrent strictures, either traumatic or infective in origin. The mean age for all patients was 62.22 (range 22–90) years, for DSD patients 43 (range 38–47) years, for stricture patients 54.6 (range 22–78) years and for BPH patients 76.12 (range 60–90) years. The patients with DSD had their stents in situ for 2–6 (mean 3.75) years; the prostatic stents had been present for 2–7 (mean 4.2) years; the urethral stents had been in place for 2–4 (mean 2.7) years.

The changes observed include polypoid hyperplasia (Fig. 65.1) of the urothelium and underlying connective tissue (11/18 patients), between and around the stent mesh wires, non-keratinizing (2/18, Fig. 65.2) or keratinizing (7/18) squamous metaplasia (Figs. 65.3 and 65.4), chronic inflammation (Fig. 65.5,

15/18) with prominent plasma cell infiltrates (11/18), and variable foreign body granuloma (2/18) and microabscess formation (5/18). The wires of most of the stents, being of the self-expanding variety, had embedded themselves into the urethral wall and were surrounded by invaginations of urothelium, in a manner similar to the ureteral stent described above. These pseudo-diverticula were usually surrounded by the microabscesses and/or foreign body granulomas (3/5, Fig. 65.6). The incidences of polypoid hyperplasia, non-keratinizing and keratinizing squamous metaplasia with respect to clinical reason for stenting are noted in Table 65.1. The stents had become at least partially incorporated into the urethral wall in the majority of cases. In ten cases, this had led to failure of the stent due to luminal obstruction with

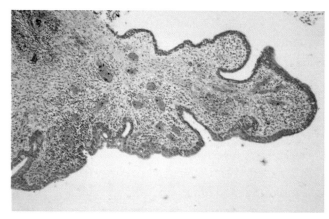

Figure 65.1. *Polypoid hyperplasia of the urothelium and suburothelial connective tissue associated with a urethral stent.*

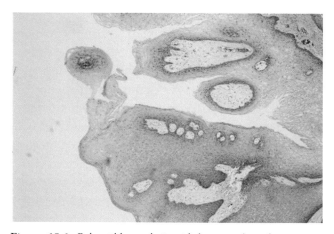

Figure 65.2. *Polypoid hyperplasia with features of non-keratinizing squamous metaplasia.*

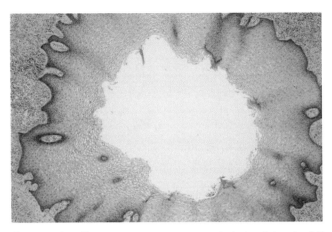

Figure 65.3. *Keratinizing squamous metaplasia involving the full urethral circumference with keratotic tiers.*

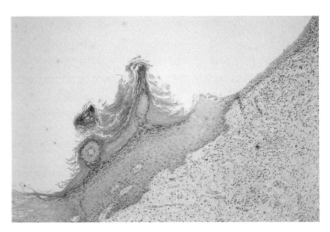

Figure 65.4. *High-power view of a keratotic tier (same case as Figure 65.3).*

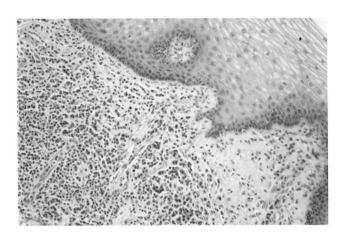

Figure 65.5. *Dense chronic inflammatory infiltrate underlying metaplastic squamous epithelium.*

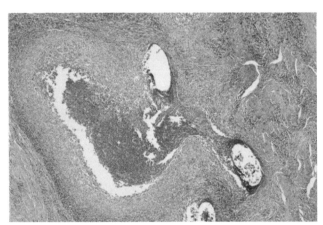

Figure 65.6. *Stent cleft (pseudodiverticulum) surrounded by microabscess and foreign body granuloma formation.*

Table 65.1. *Histological changes in the urothelium of patients with long-term urethral stents, according to patient group*

Reason for stenting	Histological changes		
	Polypoid hyperplasia	Non-keratinizing squamous metaplasia	Keratinizing squamous metaplasia
DSD	3/3	0/3	2/3
Stricture	4/7	1/7	5/7
BPH	4/8	1/9	0/9

associated infection and retention of urine, although in the remaining eight cases the stents were functioning normally and the biopsies were taken incidentally at the time of cystoscopy to investigate other symptoms or conditions.

Much discussion has taken place regarding the role of squamous metaplasia in the development of squamous carcinoma in the urinary tract. Some authors deny this link, citing the incidence of squamous metaplasia of the vaginal (non-keratinizing) type in otherwise healthy bladders at post-mortem examination, particularly in women.[41,42] Others feel that both non-keratinizing and keratinizing metaplasia are an indication of a 'sick mucosa', within which squamous carcinoma and other types of neoplasia may develop.[43] Keratinizing squamous metaplasia in the bladder[44–46] and urethra[46] has been reported as a premalignant condition, predisposing to squamous cell or transitional cell carcinoma. In studies by O'Flynn and Mullaney,[44] Walts and Sacks[45] and Benson et al.,[46] these lesions developed over a period ranging from 3 months to 30 years, mean 9.85 years for squamous cell carcinoma and 19.5 years for transitional cell carcinoma. None of the patients documented in this study had their stents in situ for more than 7 years. Urethral squamous metaplasia is reported to be more common in patients with urethral strictures[47,48] and both squamous metaplasia and squamous carcinoma of the bladder have been reported in spinal cord injury patients,[49,50] particularly those with long-term, indwelling catheters.[44] It is interesting that the chronic irritation presumably associated with the presence of a calculus in one patient was not associated with squamous metaplasia in the subsequent biopsies.

As ten of the 18 stents had failed, this may have biased the changes observed; however, it is important to note the changes seen in the remainder of the patients who had normally functioning stents. It is probably not possible to say whether the high incidence of squamous metaplasia in the DSD and stricture patients is due to the presence of the stents, to the primary underlying pathology or to infective complications. The roughly equivalent incidence of changes in both functioning and failed stricture stents should be noted; however, in all cases the numbers of patients assessed meant that the results failed to reach statistical significance.

Further long-term studies of larger patient groups are necessary to assess the likelihood of developing carcinoma, as well to determine the true incidence of pathology in patients with stents.

Miscellaneous stenting

Stenting of the vas deferens,[51–52] particularly as treatment for prepubertal injury,[52] has been carried out. The effects of the stent on the vas deferens itself have not been studied; however, one study by Urry et al.,[51]

documented testicular changes including reduced numbers of spermatocytes, spermatids and spermatozoa in association with the use of chromic stents.[51] No such changes were found in association with Silastic stents.

Conclusions

In conclusion, stenting of the urinary tract gives rise to a number of changes that seem to be predictable, depending on the type of stent used. The self-expanding stent seems to bury itself in the wall of the site stented with pseudo-diverticulum formation, sometimes associated with micro-abscess and/or foreign body giant cell formation. The surrounding connective tissue and overlying urothelium become infiltrated by inflammatory cells and the urothelium commonly undergoes squamous metaplasia. Further long-term study of larger patient groups would appear to be indicated to assess the true incidence of pathology in these patients and to assess the possibility of development of malignancy in the long-term.

References

1. Karsten T M, Coene P P, van Gulik T M et al. Morphologic changes of extrahepatic bile ducts during obstruction and subsequent decompression by endoprosthesis. Surgery, 1992; 111: 562–568
2. Vorwerl D, Kissinger G, Handt S, Gunther R W. Long-term patency of Wallstent endoprostheses in benign biliary obstructions: experimental results. J Vasc Intervent Radiol 1993; 4: 625–634
3. Hunt J B, Sayer J M, Jacyna M et al. Combined percutaneous transhepatic and endoscopic placement of biliary stents. Surg Oncol 1993; 2: 293–298
4. Karsten T M, Davids P H, van Gulik T M et al. Effects of biliary endoprostheses on the extrahepatic bile ducts in relation to subsequent operation of the biliary tract. J Am Coll Surg 1994; 178: 343–352
5. Cardella J F, Wilson R P, Fox P S, Griffith J W. Evaluation of a second generation tantalum biliary stent in a canine model. J Vasc Intervent Radiol 1995; 6: 397–403
6. Yoshioka T, Wright K C, Wallace S et al. Self-expanding endovascular graft: an experimental study in dogs. AJR 1988; 151: 673–676
7. Buchwald A, Unterberg C, Werner G et al. Initial results with the Wiktor stent: a new balloon-expandable coronary stent. Clin Cardiol 1991; 14: 374–379
8. Van Beusekom H M, Van der Giessen W J, Van Suylen R et al. Histology after stenting of human saphenous vein bypass grafts: observations from surgically excised grafts 3 to 320 days after stent implantation. J Am Coll Cardiol 1993; 21: 45–54
9. Pisco J M, Correia M, Esperanca-Pina J A, de Sousa L A. Vasa vasorum changes following stent placement in experimental arterial stenoses. J Vasc Intervent Radiol 1993; 4: 269–273

10. Van Beusekom H M, Serruys P W, Post J C et al. Stenting or balloon angioplasty of stenosed autologous saphenous vein grafts in pigs. Am Heart J 1994; 127: 273–281

11. Peacock J, Hankins S, Jones T, Lutz R. Flow instabilities induced by coronary artery stents: assessment with an in vitro pulse duplicator. J Biomech 1995; 28: 17–26

12. Gorge G, Ge J, Haude M et al. Intravascular ultrasound for evaluation of coronary arteries. Herz 1996; 21: 78–89

13. Ramsay J W, Payne S R, Gosling P T et al. The effects of double J stenting on unobstructed ureters. An experimental and clinical study. Br J Urol 1985; 57: 630–634

14. Cronan J J, Horn D L, Marcello A et al. Antibiotics and nephrostomy tube care: preliminary observations. Part II. Bacteremia. Radiology 1989; 172(3 pt 2): 1043–1045

15. Van Arsdalen K N, Banner M P, Pollack H M. Radiographic imaging and urologic decision making in the management of renal and ureteral calculi. Urol Clin North Am 1990; 17: 171–190

16. Tschada R, Mickisch G, Rassweiler J et al. Success and failure with double J ureteral stent. Analysis of 107 cases. J Urol (Paris) 1991; 97: 93–97

17. Abdel-Razzak O M, Bagley D H. Clinical experience with flexible ureteropyeloscopy. J Urol 1992; 148: 1788–1792

18. El Deen M E, Khalaf I, Rahim F A. Effects of internal ureteral stenting of normal ureter on the upper urinary tract: an experimental study. J Endourol 1993; 7: 399–405

19. Selmy G I, Hassouna M M, Begin L R et al. Long-term effects of ureteric stent after ureteric dilatation. J Urol 1993; 150: 1984–1989

20. Ryan P C, Lennon G M, McLean P A, Fitzpatrick J M. The effects of acute and chronic JJ stent placement on upper urinary tract motility and calculus transit. Br J Urol 1994; 74: 434–439

21. Cormio L, Koivusalo A, Makisalo H et al. The effects of various indwelling JJ stents on renal pelvic pressure and renal parenchymal thickness in the pig. Br J Urol 1994; 74: 440–443

22. Cormio L. Ureteric injuries. Clinical and experimental studies. Scand J Urol Nephrol Suppl. 1995; 171: 1–66

23. Milroy E J, Chapple C R, Cooper J E et al. A new treatment for urethral strictures. Lancet 1988; 1(8600): 1424–1427

24. Bailey D M, Foley S J, McFarlane J P et al. Histological changes associated with long-term urethral stents. Br J Urol 1998: in press

25. Milroy E J, Chapple C R, Eldin A, Wallsten H. A new stent for treatment for urethral strictures. Br J Urol 1989; 63: 392–396

26. Milroy E J, Chapple C R, Eldin A, Wallsten H. A new treatment for urethral strictures: a permanently implanted urethral stent. J Urol 1989; 141: 1120–1122

27. Sarramon J P, Joffre F, Rischmann P et al. Use of the Wallstent endourethral prosthesis in the treatment of recurrent urethral strictures. Eur Urol 1990; 18: 281–285

28. Milroy E J. Treatment of sphincter strictures using permanent Urolume stent. J Urol 1993; 150(5 part 2): 1729–1733

29. Milroy E J, Allen A. Long-term results of Urolume urethral stent for recurrent urethral strictures. J Urol 1996; 155: 904–908

30. Harrison N W, De Souza J V. Prostate stenting for outflow obstruction. Br J Urol 1990; 65: 192–196

31. Chapple C R, Milroy E J, Rickards D. Permanently implanted urethral stent for prostatic obstruction in the unfit patient. Preliminary report. Br J Urol 1990; 66: 58–65

32. Kletscher B A, Oesterling J E. Prostatic stents. Current perspectives for the management of benign prostatic hyperplasia. Urol Clin North Am 1995; 22: 423–430

33. Shaw P J R, Milroy E J G, Timoney A G et al. Permanent external striated sphincter stents in patients with spinal injuries. Br J Urol 1990; 66: 297–302

34. Soni B M, Vaidyanatham S, Krishnan K R. Use of Memokath, a second generation urethral stent for relief of urinary retention in male spinal cord injured patients. Paraplegia 1994; 32: 480–488

35. Sauerwein D, Gross A J, Kutzenburger J, Ringert R H. Wallstents in patients with detrusor–sphincter dyssynergia. J Urol 1995; 154: 495–497

36. McFarlane J P, Foley S J, Shah P J R. Long-term outcome of permanent urethral stents in the treatment of detrusor–sphincter dyssynergia. Br J Urol 1996; 78: 729–732

37. Baert L, Verhamme L, Van Poppel H, Vandeursen H. Long term consequences of urethral stents. J Urol 1993; 150: 853–855

38. Verhamme L, Van Poppel H, Van de Voorde W. Total fibrotic obliteration of urethral stent. Br J Urol 1993; 72: 389–390

39. Bosnjakovic P, Ilic M, Ivkovic T et al. Flexible tantalum stents: effects in the stenotic canine urethra. Cardiovasc Intervent Radiol 1994; 18: 280–284

40. Latal D, Mraz J, Zerhau P et al. Nitinol urethral stents: long term results in dogs. Urol Res 1994; 22: 295–300

41. Goertchen R, Schiche I, Modelmog D, Kunze K. The epidemiology and importance of metaplasia and dysplasia of the urinary bladder mucosa in autopsy material from a middle-size industrial city (study of Gorlitz). Zentralbl Allg Pathol 1990; 136: 663–670

42. Wiener D P, Koss L G, Sablay B, Freed S Z. The prevalence and significance of Brunn's nests, cystitis cystica and squamous metaplasia in normal bladders. J Urol 1979; 122: 317–321

43. Mostofi F K, Davis C J Jr. Epithelial abnormalities of urinary bladder. Prog Clin Biol Res 1984; 162A: 81–93

44. O'Flynn J D, Mullaney J. Leukoplakia of the bladder. A report on 20 cases including 2 cases progressing to squamous cell carcinoma. Br J Urol 1967; 39: 461–471

45. Walts A E, Sacks S A. Squamous metaplasia and invasive epidermoid carcinoma of bladder. Urology 1977; 9: 317–320

46. Benson R C Jr, Swanson S K, Farrow GM. Relationship of leukoplakia to urothelial malignancy. J Urol 1984; 131: 507–511

47. Chambers R M; Baitera B. The anatomy of the urethral stricture. Br J Urol. 1977; 49: 545–551

48. Colapinto V, Evans D H. Primary carcinoma of the male urethra developing after urethroplasty for stricture. J Urol 1977; 118: 581–584

49. Kaufman J M, Fam B, Jacobs S C, et al. Bladder cancer and squamous metaplasia in spinal cord injury patients. J Urol 1977; 118: 967–971

50. Broecker B H, Klein F A, Hackler R H. Cancer of the bladder in spinal cord injury patients. J Urol 1981; 125: 196–197

51. Urry R L, Thompson J, Cockett A T. Vasectomy and vasovasostomy. II. A comparison of two methods of vasovasostomy: silastic versus chromic stents. Fertil Steril. 1976; 27: 945–950

52. Pryor J L, Fusia T, Mercer M et al. Injury to the pre-pubertal vas deferens. II. Experimental repair. J Urol. 1991; 146: 477–480

Stents in detrusor–sphincter dyssynergia

66

Memokath™ stent in the treatment of detrusor external sphincter dyssynergia following spinal cord injury

R. Hamid and J. Shah

Introduction

The sacral spinal micturition centre is located at the level of T12/L1 vertebrae. Spinal cord injury (SCI) above this level results in neurogenic detrusor overactivity (NDO) with detrusor external sphincter dyssynergia (DESD).

'Dyssynergia' means loss of coordination between two groups of muscles, which generally work together. DESD generally implies either lack of relaxation or involuntary contraction of the external striated urethral sphincter when the detrusor contracts. The degree of dissociation is worse in males with complete lesion and prolonged continuous detrusor contractions.[1]

Historically, stents have not been used as a first-line treatment for DESD. However, the advantages of urethral stenting compared to more invasive procedures, that is, external sphincterotomy is that it is minimally invasive, with fewer complications (minimal bleeding) or side-effects (erectile dysfunction).

Memokath™ (Engineers & Doctors A/S Hornbaek, Denmark) is a temporary urethral stent, first used in the prostatic urethra to treat bladder outflow obstruction.[2] Subsequently, it has been utilized in the treatment of DESD.[3,4] This stent has the advantage of being easily removable, with minimal trauma to the urethra.

Characteristics of the Memokath™ stent

The Memokath™ stent is made from an alloy of nickel and titanium with two forms: martensite and austenite. It consists of a floppy and a rigid component. This structure gives it a 'shape memory' (i.e it will return to a preformed shape after deformation when heated to 45–50°C). The stent prevents urothelial ingrowth by virtue of having a closed, tight, spiral structure. This aids in ease of removal, when required. Importantly, it is magnetic resonance imaging (MRI) compatible.[5]

The stent is supplied in lengths from 35 mm to 95 mm and can admit a flexible cystoscope (calibre 22 Fr). It is a temporary stent and can be left in situ for 3 years.[6]

Insertion technique

The Memokath™ stent has been inserted under direct vision with cystoscopy, ultrasound guidance and using an image intensifier.[7] We perform the insertion of the Memokath™ stent under general anaesthesia or sedation (depending on the completeness of SCI) and all patients receive intravenous gentamicin at induction. A cystourethroscopy is performed with a 17 Fr rigid cystoscope to exclude any associated abnormality (i.e. urethral strictures or bladder stones). The length of stent to be deployed is then measured. This is calculated by withdrawing the cystoscope to the level of the bladder neck and placing a marker at this level. The cystoscope is withdrawn and a second marker is placed at the level of the verumontanum. A Memokath™ stent 10 mm longer than the measured length is selected for insertion. The stent is supplied premounted (Fig. 66.1) and is deployed with a 0° telescope. When the stent is just beyond the level of bladder neck 150–200 ml of normal saline, prewarmed to 50°C is instilled leading to its expansion within the urethra (Fig. 66.2).

Removal technique

Removal of stents, when necessary, can easily be performed by instillation of cold saline at 5–10°C, which leads to uncoiling and softening thus resulting in non-traumatic stent retrieval. Simple endoscopic graspers are used to retrieve the stent. This can be

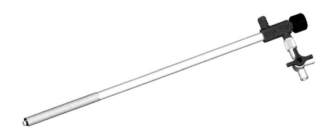

Figure 66.1. *Memokath™ mounted on a delivery tool.*

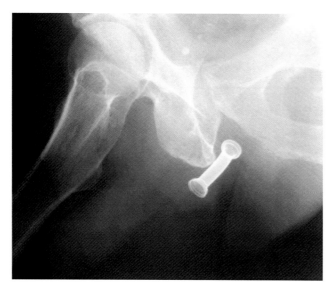

Figure 66.2. *The deployed Memokath™ stent.*

accomplished within 2–3 minutes and can be performed in day surgery. However, we prefer to perform this procedure in the operating room under supervision of an anaesthetist, in order to control autonomic dysreflexia if this complication arises.

Stent care

The potential complications of the Memokath™ stent must be explained to the patient. It is difficult to pass even a small calibre catheter into the bladder through the stent. Hence, if retention occurs a suprapubic catheter is preferred. The insertion of a urethral catheter for urodynamic studies requires great care and should preferably be done under fluoroscopic control. Finally, manual evacuation of bowels can dislodge the Memokath™ stent, so patients and their carers should exercise great caution whilst performing this procedure.

Publications on the Memokath™ stent on the treatment of DESD

The Memokath™ stent has been available for almost a decade, but only a handful of publications have been reported in the literature on its efficacy. All are retrospective studies. The majority of these are in prostatic or ureteric obstruction.[5,8] The first use of the Memokath™ stent in the treatment of DESD was reported by Soni et al. in 1994.[3] A total of 10 patients had a Memokath™ stent inserted for the treatment of

DESD. All were functioning adequately at a follow-up of 3–7 months. However, they have recently reported a longer-term follow-up of these patients with 9/10 stents being removed at a mean of 13 months (range 4–30 months).[9] The reasons for removal included encrustation with stone formation, autonomic dysreflexia, stent migration and mucosal proliferation. In 1997, Shah et al. reported a series of 14 patients with a follow-up of 2 years.[4] Seven of these patients had a functioning stent at 2 years. They reported resolution of preoperative hydronephrosis and dysreflexic episodes with a significant reduction in residual volume. Three were classified as failures due to stent migration whilst the remaining 3 were removed due to other reasons. This group has recently presented a longer-term follow-up with 25 patients. There was a significant reduction in maximum detrusor pressure, duration of contraction and residual urine volume ($P<0.05$) on videourodynamics (VCMG) 6 months after insertion of the stent. Six patients have a functioning Memokath™ stent at a mean follow-up of 34.7 months (range 6–86 months). Nineteen stents in this group were removed for several reasons at a mean of 20.3 months (range 0.25–41 months). The reasons for failure are summarized in Table 66.1. Low and McRae in 1998 reported their experience of Memokath™ stent in 24 patients (26 stents).[7] Nineteen had to be removed at a mean of 7 months (range 2–18 months), whilst 7 were functioning adequately at a mean follow-up of 16 months (range 12–24 months). The reasons of failure in this group were similar to that of others. Unlike external sphincterotomy, none of the authors have reported any significant change in erectile function after stent placement. However, no validated questionnaires have been used to substantiate this assumption.

Probable explanations for stent failure

Stent migration. It is suggested that migration of the stent is more likely to occur if an external sphincterotomy has been performed before stent insertion.[7] The likely explanation is dilatation of the prostatic urethra that reduces the 'grip' of the stent.

Encrustation and stone formation. A history of stone disease may predispose to encrustation. A possible reason can be recurrent urinary tract infections with biofilm formation.

Table 66.1. *Causes of failure of the Memokath™ stent*

Cause	No.	Mean time (mths) of stent removal (range)
Autonomic dysreflexia	3	3.6 (0.25–10)
Entry into fertility programme	1	23
Encrustation and stone formation	5	17.6 (6–33)
Proximal migration of stent	7	20.4 (6–25)
Incomplete emptying (without obstruction)	3	25 (22–29)
Total	19	20.3 (0.25–41)

Autonomic dyreflexia. The Memokath™ stent may lead to constant stretch of the urethral wall resulting in autonomic dysreflexic symptoms.

Perspectives on the Memokath™ stent in the treatment of DESD

We feel that the ease of insertion and removal makes the Memokath™ stent an attractive option for recently injured quadriplegics who are likely to regain manual dexterity for performing clean intermittent self-catheterization. It is a suitable option for patients still contemplating sphincterotomy as a method of bladder management. Additionally, it can also be used for patients in a fertility programme. All authors agree that the Memokath™ is a temporary stent that is effective in relieving the symptoms of DESD in the short term. The majority of these will have to be removed within 2 years due to the complications described above.

Future directions

The Memokath™ stent is a useful addition to the treatment options available for the management of DESD following spinal cord injury. Multi-centre, prospective long-term studies are needed to establish the place of the Memokath™ stent in the treatment of DESD. Moreover, improvement in design by the manufacturers may lead to a lower incidence of migration and encrustation and make it a more acceptable option for both short- and intermediate-term usage.

References

1. Linsenmeyer T A, Bagaria S P, Gendron B. The impact of urodynamic parameters on the upper tracts of spinal cord injured men who void reflexly. J Spinal Cord Med 1998; 21: 15–20
2. Poulsen A L, Schou J, Ovesen H, Nordling J. Memokath: A second generation of intraprostatic spirals. Br J Urol 1993; 72: 331–334
3. Soni B M, Vaidyanatham S, Krishnan K R. Use of Memokath, a second generation urethral stent for relief of urinary retention in male spinal cord injured patients. Paraplegia 1994; 32: 480–488
4. Shah N C, Foley S J, Edhem I, Shah P J. Use of Memokath temporary urethral stent in treatment of detrusor-sphincter dyssynergia. J Endourol 1997; 11: 485–488
5. Perry M J, Roodhouse A J, Gidlow A B, Spicer T G, Ellis B W. Thermo-expandable intraprostatic stents in bladder outlet obstruction: an 8-year study. BJU Int 2002; 90: 216–223
6. Fitzpatrick J M, Mebust W K. Minimally invasive and endoscopic management of benign prostatic hyperplasia. In: Walsh P C, Retik A B, Vaughan E D, Wein A J (eds) Campbell's urology, 8th edn. Philadelphia: WB Saunders, 2002: 1379–1422
7. Low A I, McRae P J. Use of the Memokath for detrusor-sphincter dyssynergia after spinal cord injury—a cautionary tale. Spinal Cord 1998; 36: 39–44
8. Kulkarni R, Bellamy E. Nickel-titanium shape memory alloy Memokath 051 ureteral stent for managing long-term ureteral obstruction: 4-year experience. J Urol 2001; 166: 1750–1754
9. Vaidyanathan S, Soni B M, Oo T, Sett P, Hughes P L, Singh G. Long-term result of Memokath urethral sphincter stent in spinal cord injury patients. BMC Urol 2002; 2: 12
10. Hamid R, Arya M, Mohashiri R, Shah P J R. The use of Memokath stent in the treatment of detrusor sphincter dyssynergia following spinal cord injury. A 7 year review. Abstract. World Congress of EndoUrology, September 2002, Genoa, Italy, 25: 18

67

Complications related to Urolume sphincter stent used for the management of detrusor–sphincter dyssynergia

M. B. Chancellor and D. A. Rivas

Introduction

External sphincterotomy has been the treatment of choice for over 30 years for those afflicted with spinal cord injury (SCI) or other neurological impairment associated with detrusor hyperreflexia (DH) and detrusor–external sphincter dyssynergia (DESD) who are unable to perform clean intermittent catheterization. The procedure permits low-pressure urinary drainage, often significantly reducing post-void residual urine volumes.[1] Urinary collection is accomplished using an external condom catheter after sphincterotomy, although total dribbling incontinence is unusual unless the bladder neck and prostatic urethra have been previously surgically compromised. The complications associated with external sphincterotomy include a reoperation rate ranging from 12 to 26%, haemorrhage requiring blood transfusion in 5–23% of cases, and erectile dysfunction (either complete or partial loss of erection) in 2.8–64% of patients.[2–8]

The complications, hospitalization requirement and cost of irreversible surgical external sphincterotomy has prompted investigation of placement of an intra-urethral wire-mesh stent prosthesis at the level of the membranous urethra as an alternative to defeating the function of the external sphincter.[9,10] A major potential advantage of the sphincter stent is that the treatment is reversible: sphincter function returns when the stent is removed. In this chapter, the results of the multicentre North American clinical experience of UroLume sphincter stent placement are briefly presented and, the complications encountered, their treatment, and the reversibility of sphincter stent therapy for DESD are discussed.

Multicentre North American Trial

A total of 153 men with a stable neurological SCI and urodynamically confirmed DESD were entered into this experimental study at 15 North American centres.[11] Each patient underwent a preoperative evaluation that included a medical history, physical examination, urine analysis and culture, serum chemistry evaluation, complete blood count, urodynamic study, and upper tract imaging with either renal ultrasound, intravenous pyelogram, or radioisotope renal scan.

The presence or absence of subjective symptoms of autonomic dysreflexia was recorded prior to stent insertion and at each postoperative period. The patients were generally aware of their history of autonomic dysreflexia as manifested by headache, diaphoresis and previously documented paradoxical hypertension and bradycardia, especially during urological manipulation.

Urodynamic evaluation included measurement of voiding pressure, urethral pressure, maximal cystometric capacity, residual urine volume, and electromyography. Patients who demonstrated electromyographic evidence of DESD during an involuntary detrusor contraction were considered as candidates for sphincter stent placement. Concomitant documented bladder neck dysfunction or prostatic enlargement resulting in bladder outflow obstruction served as exclusion criteria. The Urolume™ Prosthesis (American Medical Systems, Minnetonka, MN, USA) was inserted using lengths of 2, 2.5, and 3 cm with a standard technique presented elsewhere in this volume (Chapter 53).

Trial results

Patient demographics

The patients ranged in age from 16 to 74 (mean 36) years. Neurogenic lower urinary tract dysfunction was attributed to SCI in 144 patients (94.1%), multiple sclerosis (MS) in eight patients (5.2%), and spinal cord tumour in one (0.7%). The mean duration of SCI or neurological disease was 8.9 ± 9.6 years. Of the 153 patients, 44 (28.8%) had undergone at least one previous external sphincterotomy, with a mean number of 1.7 ± 1.0 sphincterotomies. In addition, nine patients (5.9%) had been treated with a previous transurethral prostatectomy, nine patients (5.9%) had undergone bladder neck resection and two patients (1.3%) a bladder neck incision.

Urodynamic results

A statistically significant decrease in voiding pressure occurred in the patients with matched data from preinsertion to postinsertion values at each follow-up period (Figs. 67.1–67.3). The data were reanalysed with respect to the two subgroups, specifically those patients with or without a prior sphincterotomy. No statistically significant differences were evident between the two groups regarding their preoperative urodynamic parameters, except that the patients without previous sphincterotomy demonstrated a higher voiding pressure (81 ± 27 cmH$_2$O) than those with prior sphincterotomy (64 ± 28 cmH$_2$O), $p = 0.001$. During the follow-up period (3, 6, 12 and 24 months), all the urodynamic parameters were similar between the two groups, except for two isolated data points, the voiding pressure at 3 months and the residual urine volume at 12 months. At 24 months of follow-up, no differences were documented between patients with and without prior external sphincterotomy when all three urodynamic parameters were compared.

Stents required

Of the 153 patients, 126 (82.4%) have required a single insertion procedure to ensure patency of the entire external sphincter; 26 (17.0%) required two, and one patient (0.6%) required three insertion procedures. A total of 105 patients (68.6%) required a single 3 cm stent to bridge the external sphincter adequately, while 43 patients (28.1%) required two, four patients (2.6%) required three, and one patient (0.6%) required four stents.

Epithelialization and hyperplasia

Cystoscopically, epithelialization of the device appears to be initiated shortly after sphincter stent placement. At 3 months, 45.9% of patients demonstrated 90–100% stent epithelialization, while only 9.1% epithelialized less than 50%. At 1 year, 87.5% of patients had established 90–100% epithelialization.

At 3 months, cysto-urethroscopy revealed epithelial hyperplasia within the lumen of the endoluminal stent in 42 patients (27.5%). This ingrowth was considered minor in 36 of the 42 patients (85.7%), moderate in five

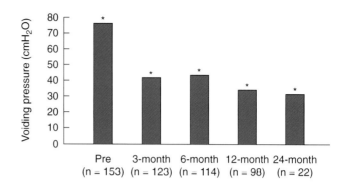

Figure 67.1. *Voiding pressure 3, 6, 12 and 24 months after prosthesis placement versus preoperative values. Asterisk indicates significant difference between value pre-insertion and those for each follow-up period (*p < 0.05; ANOVA).*

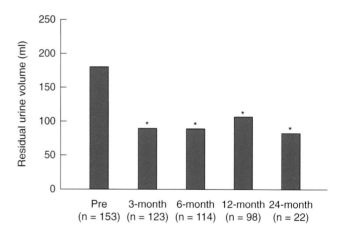

Figure 67.2. *Residual urine volume 3, 6, 12 and 24 months after prosthesis placement versus preoperative values. Asterisk indicates significant difference between value pre-insertion and those for each follow-up period (*p < 0.05; ANOVA).*

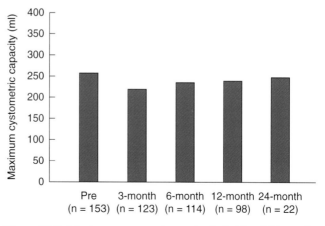

Figure 67.3. *Maximum cystometric capacity 3, 6, 12 and 24 months after prosthesis placement versus preoperative values.*

patients (11.9%), and marked in one (2.4%). At 24 months follow-up, 10 of 22 (45.5%) patients were found to have some endothelial hyperplasia, minor in 6 (60.0%), moderate in 3 (30.0%), and marked in 1 (10.0%). Urethral obstruction secondary to endothelial hyperplasia did not occur in this series. Neither voiding cysto-urethrography, cysto-urethroscopy, nor urodynamic evaluation demonstrated stenosis of the urethral lumen.

Urinary tract colonization

At the 3, 6, 12 and 24-month follow-up evaluations, 44.5, 47.0, 50.5 and 30.4%, respectively, of the patients' urine cultures revealed bacterial growth, although no prosthesis had to be removed because of infection.

Hydronephrosis

Postoperatively, all but one patient demonstrated improvement or stabilization of hydronephrosis that had been present prior to stent placement (see below). Hydronephrosis actually resolved in 22 of the 28 patients (78.6%) after stent placement. In the remaining patients, stable renal function was observed.

Autonomic dysreflexia

Subjective autonomic dysreflexia symptoms were reported by 110 of the 153 patients (71.9%) preoperatively. These symptoms were effectively reduced by sphincter stent placement. At 3, 6, 12 and 24 months, only 29/96 (30.2%), 24/90 (26.7%), 27/74 (36.5%) and 8/20 patients (40.0%), respectively reported symptoms of autonomic dysreflexia. No patient reported an increase in subjective severity of autonomic dysreflexia after stent insertion.

Complications seen during the trial

Ten patients (6.5%) underwent device explantation during the follow-up period, but seven of the ten were re-implanted with another stent prosthesis. No difference was noted in the stent removal rate between patients with previous sphincterotomy (4/44, 9.1%) and those without (7/109, 6.4%) (p = 0.19). Seven explantations were required because of stent migration, three of which occurred at the time of initial insertion procedure. One explantation was performed because of pain and urethral oedema. Another stent was removed because of incomplete epithelialization, secondary bladder neck contracture and worsening hydronephrosis after 1 year. The remaining explantation was undertaken 1 year after insertion because the patient experienced persistent difficulty in maintaining condom catheter application.[12]

Mild haematuria, without the need for blood transfusion, urethral catheterization or bladder irrigation, occurred in ten patients (6.5%). Oedema of the penis occurred in two patients. One patient noted a superficial penile ulcer caused by excessive wrapping force applied to his condom catheter, while a second patient actually developed a urethrocutaneous fistula due to excessive condom catheter pressure at the base of the penis after 6 months. This small fistula healed spontaneously with suprapubic tube cystostomy drainage.

Two patients experienced epididymo-orchitis which resolved with oral antibiotics. One patient with pre-existing vesico-ureteral reflux demonstrated persistent low-pressure reflux and developed pyelonephritis postoperatively, despite proper prosthesis location documented with low voiding pressure. Subsequently, bilateral ureteral reimplantations were performed, and the patient has not shown any evidence of further upper tract infection. Two patients were hospitalized 1 week after stent insertion because of febrile urinary tract infection with *Pseudomonas*.

Thirteen patients (8.5%) have been reported to suffer from bladder neck obstruction since placement of the device. These patients were managed effectively with either bladder neck incision (seven patients), medical therapy (alpha-1-adrenergic blockade in four patients), or intermittent catheterization (two patients).

Neither perioperative nor postoperative haemorrhage requiring transfusion, nor soft tissue erosion, nor stone formation occurred in any patient as a result of sphincter stent prosthesis placement. Although two patients were noted to have encrustation of the stent at 3 months and one patient at 12 months, none required treatment and all were not obstructed, by urodynamic criteria. Subjective erectile function was not adversely altered in any patient (Table 67.1).

Table 67.1. *Complications of multicentre North American trial (153 patients)*

Complication	No. of patients
Device explant	10
• migration	(7)
• pain	(1)
• incomplete epithelialization and bladder neck contracture	(1)
• difficulty maintaining condom	(1)
Haematuria, mild, resolved spontaneously	10
Penile oedema	2
Urethrocutaneous fistula due to tight condom	1
Epididymo-orchitis	2
Vesico-ureteral reflux (low pressure) requiring reimplantation	1
Hospitalization for febrile UTI	2
Secondary bladder neck contracture	12*
• transurethral incision	(7)
• oral alpha-1-antagonist: terazosin	(4)
• clean intermittent catheterization	(2)

*One patient used both terazosin and catheterization.

Stent removal and sphincter function

Four patients (three quadriplegic and one paraplegic) underwent permanent sphincter stent explantation 6 months or longer after insertion without either stent replacement or surgical sphincteric ablation. Three patients required stent removal because of device migration, while one patient required explantation because of difficulty maintaining condom catheter urinary collection.[13]

Each patient was evaluated with cystoscopy and renal ultrasound prior to sphincter stent insertion, immediately prior to sphincter stent removal, and 1 year after stent removal. The patients' mean voiding pressure of 62.5 ± 39.4 cmH$_2$O prior to stent implantation decreased to 20.7 ± 6.5 cmH$_2$O after stent insertion. One year after stent explantation, the mean voiding pressure had increased to 58.5 ± 21.5 cmH$_2$O.

All stents were completely removed cystoscopically, using a combination technique of neo-epithelial resection and forceps extraction, without perioperative complications. Neither stress urinary incontinence nor urethral stricture has developed in any patient, with over 1 year of follow-up since stent removal. Urethral catheterization and cysto-urethroscopy can be performed in each patient without difficulty. Furthermore, no changes in symptoms of autonomic dysreflexia, renal function, or erectile function have developed in these patients.

One patient subsequently underwent a cutaneous ileocystostomy 6 months later. Urodynamic and cysto-urethroscopy demonstrated no permanent injury to the membranous urethra. The urethral mucosa appeared normal without stricture, while the voiding pressure was quantified at 65 cmH$_2$O 6 months after explantation versus 75 cmH$_2$O prior to initial stent insertion. The patient did not leak urine per urethram after his urinary ileostomy procedure.

Pearls and hints at preventing complications

Proper patient selection is most important to achieving high clinical success rate with sphincter stent implantation. The sphincter stent, even if perfectly placed, will serve as an effective management strategy only if the patient can reliably wear a condom catheter. Patients must be fully counselled and able to demonstrate the effective application and maintenance of an external catheter prior to considering a sphincter-defeating procedure.

Preoperative urodynamic testing is an absolute necessity. Only patients with DH and DESD should be considered candidates for sphincter stent prosthesis placement. This procedure is contraindicated in patients with detrusor areflexia, significantly diminished compliance or a residual volume in excess of 100 ml[14–16] (Table 67.2).

Need for a longer stent for the sphincter

It should be remembered that, because of the elastic recoil of the superalloy mesh of the stent, the diameter of the device increases as the functional length decreases after release from the insertion tool. This consideration is especially important when introducing the device. Care must be taken to initiate implantation with the proximal margin of the device overlying the mid verumontanum. The distant margin of the stent should extend at least 5 mm beyond the end of the membranous urethra into the bulbous urethra. Urethral curvature in the area of the membranous and bulbous urethra mandate that a stent length of at least 3 cm be

Table 67.2. *Contraindications for sphincter stent*

1. **Patient unable to maintain condom catheter placement**

   Any type of sphincter ablation procedure, including sphincter stent placement, is contraindicated in men who cannot consistently apply and maintain condom catheter drainage systems. The surgical placement of a semi-rigid penile prosthesis is an option that may enhance the durability of a condom catheter application; however, the surgeon and patient must both be prepared for the 20–30% erosion and infection rate associated with these devices in SCI patients.

2. **Detrusor areflexia or significantly impaired detrusor contractility with high residual urine volume**

   Patients with lumbosacral injury and no evidence of reflex detrusor contraction during urodynamic evaluation are very poor candidates for any type of sphincter ablation procedure. It is incorrect to assume that defeating external sphincteric function, by any means, will improve urinary drainage in those with absent detrusor activity. The competent bladder neck, prostate and intrinsic urethral coaptation yield enough resistance to bring about large residual urine volumes and poor clinical outcome in these patients.

3. **Possible obstruction of the ejaculatory ducts**

   Men who wish to father children and are candidates for electro-ejaculation should not be recommended for sphincter stent placement because of the risk of decreasing semen quality. However, the recent increasing popularity and success of newer sperm-aspiration and intracytoplasmic sperm-injection techniques may alleviate some concern over the effect of the sphincter stent on semen parameters.

used to cover the external sphincter adequately and prevent stent migration. As can be seen from the multicentre North American trial, over 25% of patients will require a second partially overlapping stent, in addition to an initial 3 cm stent, to expand the external sphincter completely.

Stent migration

One complication that may be increased in patients with stents placed for sphincteric dyssynergia is that of proximal or distal stent migration during the first few weeks postoperatively. This situation, which may require a secondary stent procedure, may be best avoided by placing a 3 cm stent initially, and possibly adding a second stent to overlap the first partially, to ensure complete bridging of the sphincteric mechanism, even allowing for some degree of stent diameter expansion and length shortening. Fortunately, early migration of the stent is usually easily correctable, as the non-epithelialized device can be removed easily with cystoscopic forceps.

Stent release

Complete deployment of the stent from the insertion tool requires the depression of the second of two release catches on the insertion tool. If the second catch is accidently released, the stent may deploy prematurely.[17] It is essential that the stent is in its proper position prior to the release of the second catch. After its release, visual confirmation must ensure separation of the stent from the deployment tool prior to removal of the tool from the urethra. At times, gentle rotation of the tool will be needed for the release mechanism to disengage the stent completely. The zero-degree lens may be extracted to the level of the distal margin and a gentle rocking motion used to ensure that the stent has been released prior to attempts at removing the insertion tool.

It must be remembered that the stent may be completely withdrawn back into the insertion tool as long as the second release catch has not been deployed. This is achieved by sliding the outer sheath forward while pulling back the thumb. Once the stent is withdrawn back into the insertion tool, the device may be repositioned until satisfactorily located for release.

Infertility concerns

Most men with an SCI experience neurogenic ejaculatory failure. The technique of electro-ejaculation is most commonly used to produce a semen specimen, which is then processed to maximize the potential for conception and used for artificial insemination. It is theoretically possible to obstruct the ejaculatory ducts by the proximal edge of the stent. Therefore, great care in proper candidate selection and surgical technique is essential in cases where fertility is an important issue. In general, the sphincter stent is not recommended to men who are considering electro-ejaculation, or in younger men who have not thoroughly considered their fertility potential. However, the recent increasing popularity and success of newer sperm-aspiration and intracytoplasmic sperm-injection techniques may alleviate some concern over the effect of the sphincter stent on semen parameters.

Discussion

The long-term urological needs and costs of spinal cord injury are high. Many SCI patients are eternally hopeful that a cure for SCI will be developed, enabling complete restoration of neurological function, including ambulation. With this belief, some patients refuse or defer irreversible treatments, even if the treatment is medically necessary. Patients prefer sphincter stent prosthesis placement to external sphincterotomy in the authors' clinical trials because the stent is potentially reversible. Although the sphincter prosthesis is designed as a permanent implant for the treatment of DESD, this study has demonstrated that the device may be removed without sequelae, if deemed necessary. Removal of the epithelized UroLume™ stent is a successful but

demanding procedure. Milroy previously reported the removal of three stents, that were completely epithelized over 1 year after insertion, using the technique described above.[13,18–20]

The stents in this series were removed after 6 months without difficulty. Furthermore, follow-up cystoscopy and urodynamic evaluation of these patients revealed no urethral stricture formation after stent insertion and removal. No complications were associated with stent removal or during 1-year of follow-up. Voiding pressure in these patients returned to pre-insertion values, confirming the absence of a permanent effect of the sphincter stent on urethral sphincter function. Indeed, these results question the permanent efficacy of a bioresorbable stent currently under investigation.[21] The authors have *not* encountered a stent that has not been amenable to endoscopic extraction despite its location or duration, the presence of an indwelling catheter, severity of stricture, or hyperplasia[22] (Table 67.3).

Table 67.3. *Conditions that do not contraindicate sphincter stent placement*

Condition	Comment
Age	Older men with possible concurrent bladder neck and prostate obstruction are not contraindicated
Previous external sphincterotomy	In the multicentre study, SCI men with previous sphincterotomy had a success rate similar to that of those without prior sphincterotomy
Previous incision or resection of bladder neck and prostate	
Autonomic dysreflexia	Stent placement at the level of the membranous urethral sphincter does *not* aggravate autonomic dysreflexia
Vesico-ureteral reflux	Effective treatment of outlet obstruction will improve or cure vesico-ureteral reflux
Hydronephrosis	Lowering the voiding pressure and residual urine volume will improve and allow the resolution of hydronephrosis
Small-capacity bladder	Sphincter treatment is independent of bladder capacity
Bladder management	Previously employed urological management, including indwelling catheterization, condom catheter drainage and intermittent self-catheterization have no effect on the success of the sphincter stent
Suprapubic tube cystostomy	Patients with chronically indwelling suprapubic drainage can be treated effectively with the sphincter stent. The cystostomy tube can be removed and the epithelialized tract surgically closed, if necessary

Conclusions

Sphincter stent prosthesis placement effectively decreases detrusor pressure in patients afflicted with DESD. On the basis of experience with Urolume™ stent placement at various levels of the urethra (including the bladder neck, prostate, and bulbous urethra), for various reasons, patients undergoing sphincter stent placement have the least complaints postoperatively. These patients are neurologically impaired and most have ejaculatory dysfunction; therefore few report pain, urinary dribbling, irritation, or haematospermia. In addition, the risk of encrustation, stone formation, and incomplete epithelization is minimal in patients with sphincter stent placement compared with patients with bladder neck or prostate stent placement.

The complications discussed in this chapter are largely associated with the 'learning curve' of utilizing a new device. With greater experience, most could be avoided. The device can be removed completely, even after an extended time period and complete epithelization, without causing damage to the external sphincter function.

The Urolume™ stent prosthesis is an effective device for the treatment of DESD. When compared with conventional sphincterotomy, the reversibility of the device dramatically enhances patient acceptability. The decreased cost and complication rate certainly should enhance its utilization by urologists caring for those afflicted with DH and DESD.

References

1. Hacken H J, Ott R. Late results of bilateral endoscopic sphincterotomy in patients with upper motor neurone lesions. Paraplegia 1976; 13: 268
2. Crane D B, Hackler R H. External sphincterotomy: its effect on erections. J Urol 1976; 116: 316
3. Dollfus P, Jurascheck F, Adli G, Chapuis A. Impairment of erection after external sphincter resection. Paraplegia 1976; 13: 290
4. Kiviat M D. Transurethral sphincterotomy: relationship of site of incision to postoperative potency and delayed hemorrhage. J Urol 1975; 114: 399
5. Lockhart J L, Vorstman B, Weinstein D, Politano V A. Sphincterotomy failure in neurogenic bladder disease. J Urol 1986; 135: 86
6. Perkash I. Modified approach to sphincterotomy in spinal cord injury patients: indications, technique, and results in 32 patients. Paraplegia 1976; 13: 247
7. Schellhammer P F, Hackler R H, Bunts R C. External sphincterotomy: an evaluation of 150 patients with neurogenic bladder. J Urol 1973; 110: 199
8. Whitmore W F, Fam B A, Yalla S V. Experience with anteromedian (12 o'clock) external urethral sphincterotomy in 100 male subjects with neuropathic bladders. J Urol 1978; 50: 99
9. Chancellor M B, Rivas D A, Abdill C K et al. Prospective comparison of external sphincter balloon dilatation and prosthesis placement with external sphincter in spinal cord injured men. Arch Phys Med Rehabil 1994; 75: 297–305
10. Rivas D A, Chancellor M B, Bagley D. Prospective comparison of external sphincter prosthesis placement and external sphincterotomy in men with spinal cord injury. J Endourol 1994; 8: 89–93
11. Chancellor M B, Rivas D A, Ackman D et al. Multicenter trials of Urolume™ endourethral Wallstent[R] prosthesis for the urinary sphincterotomy in spinal cord injured men. J Urol 1994; 152: 924–930
12. Chancellor M B, Karasick S, Erhard M J et al. Placement of a wire mesh prosthesis in the external sphincter of men with spinal cord injuries. Radiology 1993; 187: 551
13. Chancellor M B, Rivas D A, Watanabe T et al. Reversible clinical outcome after sphincter stent removal. J Urol 1996; 155: 1992–1994
14. McInerney P D, Vanner T F, Harris S A B, Stephenson T P. Permanent urethral stents for detrusor sphincter dyssynergia. Br J Urol 1991; 67: 291
15. Sauerwein D, Gross A J, Kutzenberger J, Ringert R H. Wallstents in patients with detrusor–sphincter dyssynergia. J Urol 1995; 154: 495–497
16. Shaw P J R, Milroy E J G, Timoney A G et al. Permanent external striated sphincter stents in patients with spinal injuries. Br J Urol 1990; 66: 297
17. Parikh A M, Milroy E J G. Precautions and complications in the use of the Urolume Wallstent. Eur Urol 1995; 27: 1–7
18. De Vivo M J, Rutt R D, Black K J et al. Trends in spinal cord injury demographics and treatment outcome between 1973 and 1986. Arch Phys Med Rehabil 1992; 73: 424
19. Dewire D M, Owens R S, Anderson G A et al. A comparison of the urological complications associated with long-term management of quadriplegics with and without chronic indwelling urinary catheters. J Urol 1992; 147: 1069–1071
20. Kaplan S A, Chancellor M B, Blaivas J G. Bladder and sphincter behavior in patients with spinal cord lesions. J Urol 1991; 146: 113
21. Kemppainen E, Talja M, Riihela M et al. A bioresorbable stent: an experimental study. Urol Res 1993; 21: 235–238
22. Parikh A M, Milroy E J G. A new technique for removal of the Urolume prostate stent. Br J Urol 1993; 71: 620–621

Vascular stents

XI

68

Metal stents for the treatment of atherosclerotic renovascular disease

G. A. Barbalias, E. N. Liatsikos and D. Siablis

Introduction

Renal artery stenosis is a common disorder and is an established cause of hypertension and renal insufficiency. Renal ischemia resulting from stenosis of the renal artery may lead to systemic arterial hypertension, often difficult to control, with an increased risk of stroke and myocardial infarction, and/or renal atrophy and loss of renal function, finally progressing to end-stage renal disease. Renovascular hypertension is caused either by atherosclerotic plaques, usually located at the origin of the renal artery and occluding the ostium or the proximal portion of the vessel, or by various fibrous and fibrovascular dysplasias, usually located in the middle or distal third of the renal artery and sometimes involving the segmental arterial branches. Approximately two thirds of the cases are of atherosclerotic nature.[1–9]

The main therapeutic goals of renovascular revascularization are improved blood pressure control and renal function, and in the long term, the preservation of renal tissue. Atherosclerotic stenosis located in the truncus of the renal artery can be successfully treated by standard percutaneous transluminal angioplasty (PTA) in most patients. Ostial stenosis is less easy to treat, and the rates of acute failure and late restenosis vary between 9–76% and 25–45%, respectively.[1–9]

Initial experience with renal angioplasty and the 'charm' of percutaneous compared with surgical revascularization, has paved the way to renal artery stent placement. Vascular endoluminal stents were first introduced for coronary and peripheral circulation. Since then they are an alternative, clinically valuable modality that can relieve renal artery obstruction and restore renal blood flow. They provide a mechanical scaffolding, prevent elastic recoil and repair arterial dissection while maintaining vessel patency.[1–13]

Our experience

We report our experience with the use of metal stents for the treatment of ostial atherosclerotic renovascular disease. Since 1996, 62 patients (mean age 67 years) with ostial atherosclerotic renal artery stenosis were treated successfully by placement of metal stents. We used the Palmaz balloon-expandable endoprosthesis (Johnson and Johnson Interventional Systems, Waren, NJ). The Palmaz is a stainless steel mesh mounted on to a percutaneous transluminal coronary angioplasty balloon catheter. The stents were 1–2 cm long and when fully expanded reached a diameter of 5–6 mm.[14,15]

The diagnosis of renal artery stenosis was based on Duplex sonography and intraarterial angiography. Ostial lesions were defined as stenoses of more than 50% of the diameter of the renal artery. In addition, the leading edge of the stenosis was within 5 mm of the opacified aortic lumen. There is a controversy in the literature regarding the degree of renal arterial narrowing that justifies an attempt at revascularization. Angiographic diameter stenosis of less than 50% are generally not considered to be hemodynamically important. Thus, a >50% diameter stenosis usually justifies an attempt at revascularization.[9,16]

All patients had a history of sustained hypertension resistant to intensive antihypertensive treatment. All patients presented with renovascular hypertension and eight had additionally impaired renal function. All the patients gave written informed consent. Prophylactic renal revascularization in patients without clinical manifestations of disease (i.e. hypertension, renal insufficiency, cardiac disturbance) is not well documented in the literature.

The technique of stent insertion has been previously described.[10,11,13–15] Patients were pretreated with oral aspirin (325 mg) and ticlopidine (Ticlid, 500 mg). Angiography, percutaneous transluminal angioplasty (PTA), and stenting were performed transfemorally. Heparin was administered (5000 U). Atheroembolization was minimized by careful and conservative catheter manipulation. Guide catheters were advanced over wires with constant flushing, and care was taken to intubate and manipulate the ostia gently. Initial dilatation was performed with 4–6 mm balloon angioplasty catheters over 0.018 inch wires. Palmaz stents were mounted on appropriately sized balloon catheters (5–8 mm) and deployed at 8–12 atm. For treatment of ostial stenoses, the stent was positioned so that 1–2 mm protruded into the aortic lumen, ensuring complete coverage of the aortic plaque. The balloon was then removed, and an angiography was performed to verify acute patency (Figs 68.1–5). After stenting was performed, aspirin (325 mg daily) and ticlopidine (250 mg twice daily) were continued for 2 weeks.

In 12 patients, stents were placed bilaterally. In 54 patients, the introduction of stents was performed as the primary mode of treatment and in the remaining 8 patients the positioning of the endoprosthesis was deemed necessary due to recurrence of the previously performed renal PTA. The latter patients presented with impaired renal function (i.e. serum creatinine level higher than 2.0 mg per deciliter).

The patients were followed for a mean period of 18 months (range 9–48 months). Blood pressure, drug therapy, and serum creatinine were measured before discharge, at 3, 6 and 12 months, and every year thereafter. Duplex sonography was also performed on a yearly basis. In addition, angiographic evaluation was performed when clinical evidence of restenosis was present.

Positioning of the endoprosthesis was successful in all cases. All patients complained of flank and/or abdominal pain during balloon inflation which disappeared on deflation. No major complications were reported. Patients were given heparin during the procedure and for the first 24 hours. In addition, a combination of aspirin and ticlopidine were given before the procedure and continued for one month; aspirin continued alone for another 6 months.

We did not observe any stent migration. All stents were dilated at the end of the procedure so as to obtain a good expansion and a good anchorage to the arterial wall.

The 18 month patency rate was 77.4% (48 patients). Stenosis of the prostheses was seen in the remaining 14

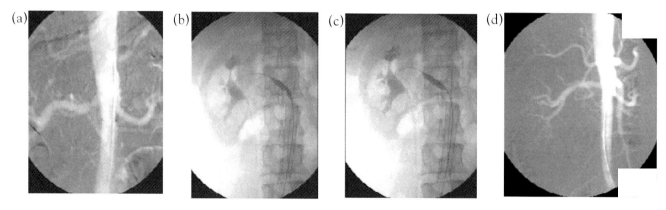

Figure 68.1. *(a) Intraarterial angiography depicting right renal artery stenosis at the level of the ostium. (b) The stenosis is evident during the dilation process with an angioplasty balloon catheter. (c) The stenosis has been dilated and the balloon catheter is fully expanded. (d) After the balloon dilation ended the arterial lumen remained patent.*

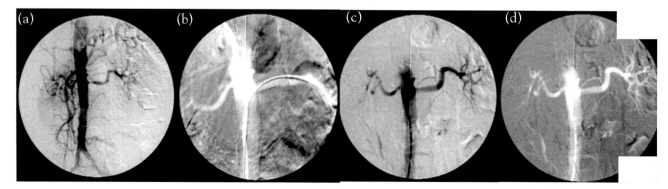

Figure 68.2. *(a) Intraarterial angiography depicting left artery stenosis at the level of the ostium. (b) The guidewire is positioned through the stenosis within the renal artery. (c,d) The stent is finally positioned bypassing the arterial stricture.*

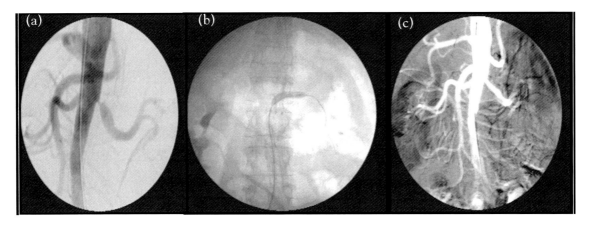

Figure 68.3. (a) Ostial stenosis of the left renal artery. (b) Dilation of the stenosis with a balloon catheter. (c) The metal stent is positioned, incorporated into the arterial wall.

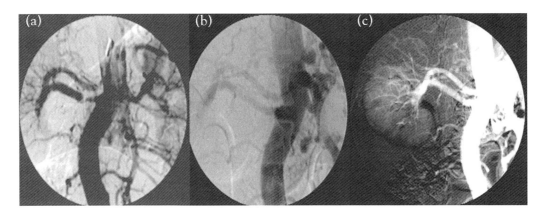

Figure 68.4. (a) Intraarterial angiography depicting two right renal arteries. Both arteries present with ostial stenosis. (b,c) The recanalization of both arteries is achieved with the metal stent.

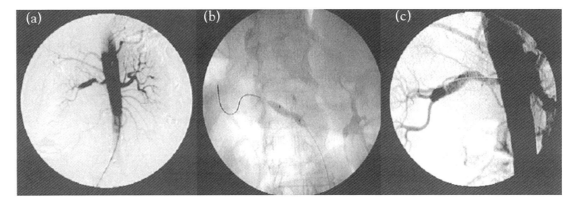

Figure 68.5. (a) Right renal artery stenosis at the level of the ostium. (b) The dilation depicts the stenotic segment of the arterial lumen. (c) The stenosis has been dilated and the stent positioned providing arterial patency.

patients. Restenosis after stent implantation is usually caused by myointimal hyperplasia or by the presence of an organized thrombus. Eight patients were successfully retreated with balloon dilation of the stent lumen. In four cases an additional concentric stent was inserted, and the remaining two cases underwent surgical intervention.

The clinical success of the therapeutic manipulation was evaluated during the hospitalization period and at the first follow-up examination according to the criteria of the Cooperative Study of Renovascular Hypertension. Resolution of hypertension was defined when the diastolic pressure was 90 mmHg or less and there was no need for drug treatment. A trend to improvement was defined as a decrease of at least 10–15% of diastolic pressure, and withdrawal of at least one drug from the treatment regimen.[17]

Hypertension resolved in 39 patients and showed a trend to improve in 15 patients. Renal function was measured by serum creatinine levels and was stable in all patients without significant fluctuations during the follow up evaluation period. Furthermore, we observed no improvement of renal function in the 8 patients who had impaired renal function prior to the procedure.

Discussion

During the past decades, endovascular techniques for atherosclerotic renovascular disease underwent a dramatic development offering a less invasive treatment option to many patients traditionally considered as surgical candidates. Numerous studies have reported excellent technical success, low complication rates, and low rates of restenosis after percutaneous transluminal angioplasty (PTA) and stenting of atherosclerotic renal arteries.[1–9]

Van Jaarsveld et al. presented a prospective randomized study evaluating the effect of percutaneous transluminal renal angioplasty and/or drug therapy in atherosclerotic renal artery stenosis. They showed that in the treatment of patients with hypertension and renal artery stenosis, angioplasty has little advantage over antihypertensive drug therapy.[18]

Baumgartner et al. suggested that renal arterial stent placement considerably improved patency in ostial stenoses, but compared with the technically successful PTA, it does not significantly improve primary patency in proximal and isolated truncal renal arterial stenoses.[5] In addition, Nicita et al. advocated the use of endoluminal stents after percutaneous transluminal angioplasty for the treatment of post-transplant renal artery stenosis with promising results.[19]

Nevertheless, the treatment of an ostial stenosis is technically more demanding, and the rate of late restenosis varies between 25% and 45%. Angioplasty and metal stent placement has been shown to be more

successful, with an acute failure rate of only 0–4% and secondary restenosis rate of 3–39%.[1–13,20]

Leertouwer et al. performed a meta-analysis comparing renal arterial stent placement with renal PTA in patients with renal arterial stenosis. They showed that stent placement had a higher technical success rate and a lower restenosis rate than did renal PTA (98% vs 77% and 17% vs 26%, respectively). The cure rate for hypertension was higher and the improvement rate for renal function was lower after stent placement than after renal PTA (20% vs 10% and 30% vs 38%, respectively). They concluded that renal arterial stent placement is technically superior and clinically comparable to renal PTA alone.[4,14]

Burket et al., in an attempt to determine which factors are predictive of improved blood pressure and renal function when patients with renal artery stenosis are treated with renal artery angioplasty and stent placement, concluded that management of renal artery stenosis with renal artery angioplasty and stent placement is most likely to result in significant improvement in systolic blood pressure among patients with the highest baseline systolic blood pressure.[6]

There are numerous reports in the literature praising PTA and stenting for renal artery stenosis. Nevertheless, revascularization has not yet proved its efficacy improving renal function. Although most authors describe a decrease in systolic and diastolic blood pressure after stent placement, there is lack of standardization of definitions for cure and improvement of hypertension. Thus, the comparison between different studies is often impossible and clinical results vary among different investigators.[21–23]

The lack of straightforward methods to assess individual kidney function creates a major obstacle in the evaluation of the effect of revascularization on the treated organ. In cases of unilateral renal artery stenosis, an abnormal serum creatinine level indicates loss of more than half the nephrons of both kidneys. Thus, the dysfunction of the contralateral kidney masquerades the effect of treatment of unilateral disease on the measurements of overall renal function.[9,16,21–23]

Dorros et al. presented their experience with the use of Palmaz-Schatz stent revascularization of renal artery stenosis on 163 consecutive patients for poorly controlled hypertension and/or preservation of renal function. Renal artery stent revascularization in the presence of normal or mildly impaired renal function had a beneficial effect on blood pressure control and a nondeleterious effect on renal function. Survival was adversely affected by renal dysfunction despite adequate revascularization. They suggested that early diagnosis and adequate revascularization before the onset of renal dysfunction could beneficially affect blood pressure control, preserve or prevent deterioration of renal function, and improve patient survival.[15]

Watson et al. showed that in patients with chronic renal insufficiency and global obstructive atherosclerotic renovascular disease (bilateral renal artery stenosis or unilateral stenosis in the presence of a solitary or single functional kidney), renal artery stenting improved or stabilized renal function and preserved kidney size.[23]

Our results with stenting ostial renal artery stenoses are concurrent with the existing experience of the literature, and are noteworthy since we have a large experience with the use of metal stents in different sites of the urinary system (i.e. renal artery, ureter, urethra).[24–27] In our institution, the initial success rate was 100% and the 18 month patency rate was 77.4% (48 patients). In addition, hypertension resolved in 39 patients and showed a trend to improve in 15 patients. We observed no improvement of renal function in the 8 patients who had impaired renal function prior to the procedure.[27]

The mean incidence of complications reported in the literature after endovascular renal revascularization is 14%. Most of these are not life-threatening and do not result in renal functional loss. Renal artery branch occlusions occur in less than 2% of cases. Cholesterol embolization resulting in decreased renal function, visceral symptoms, or peripheral symptoms is found to be less than 3%. A case of late aortic dislocation of a stent following stent angioplasty for ostial renal artery stenosis has been reported by Zeller et al.[28]

Restenosis after stent implantation is one of the long-term complications, usually caused by myointimal hyperplasia. The normal healing process in patients with vascular stents triggers the formation of an initial thrombotic layer covering the stent mesh and progressively its replacement initially by fibromuscular tissue and later by collagen. Tso et al. tested the in vivo effect of Matrigel on intimal hyperplasia formation using a sheep vascular stent model. They suggested that dedifferentiation of vascular smooth muscle cells with subsequent migration and proliferation was a key event in intimal hyperplasia formation. Matrigel (basement membrane protein) was shown to inhibit dedifferentiation of vascular smooth muscle cells in vitro. They concluded that the sheep renal artery vascular stent model is feasible for the study of stent biology, and that intimal hyperplasia was reduced by Matrigel-coated stents.[29]

A small number of prospective randomized controlled trials exist comparing revascularization techniques with each other or with medical treatment. Van de Ven et al. performed a randomized prospective study comparing PTA with angioplasty with stent placement (PTAS) in patients with ostial atherosclerotic renal artery stenosis. Primary success rate of PTA was 57% compared with 88% for PTAS. Complications were similar. At 6 months, the primary patency rate was 29% for PTA, and 75% for PTAS. Restenosis after a successful primary procedure occurred in 48% of patients for PTA and 14% for PTAS.[20]

Conclusions

Implantation of metal stents is a safe and effective method for the treatment of atherosclerotic renal artery stenosis and certainly presents an important alternative to renal percutaneous transluminal angioplasty. Treatment of ostial renal artery stenoses with vascular endoprostheses is a procedure that requires considerable angiographic skill and judgement and should only be performed by experienced physicians who have familiarized themselves with the technical aspects of angioplasty.

Renal artery stenting is becoming the method of choice to bypass ostial renal artery stenosis. Nevertheless, it is still obscure in the literature whether it is superior to medical therapy, reduces cardiovascular mortality, provides prolonged improvements in blood pressure control, and/or preserves renal size and function. Thus, several questions need to be addressed by further meticulously designed clinical trials.

References

1. Kaatee R, Beek F J A, Verschuyl E J et al. Atherosclerotic renal artery stenosis: ostial or truncal? Radiology 1996; 199: 637–640

2. Strandness D E Jr. Natural history of renal artery stenosis. Am J Kidney Dis 1994; 24: 630–635

3. Blum U, Krumme B, Flugel P, Gabelmann A, Lehnert T, Buitrago-Tellez C, Schollmeyer P, Langer M. Treatment of ostial renal-artery stenoses with vascular endoprostheses after unsuccessful balloon angioplasty. N Engl J Med 1997; 336: 459–465

4. Leertouwer T C, Gussenhoven E J, Bosch J L, van Jaarsveld B C, van Dijk L C, Deinum J, Man In 't Veld AJ. Stent placement for renal arterial stenosis: where do we stand? A meta-analysis. Radiology 2000; 216: 78–85

5. Baumgartner I, von Aesch K, Do D D, Triller J, Birrer M, Mahler F. Stent placement in ostial and nonostial atherosclerotic renal arterial stenoses: a prospective follow-up study. Radiology 2000; 216: 498–505

6. Burket M W, Cooper C J, Kennedy D J, Brewster P S, Ansel G M et al. Renal artery angioplasty and stent placement: predictors of a favorable outcome. Am Heart J 2000; 139: 64–71

7. Eldrup-Jorgensen J, Harvey H R, Sampson L N, Amberson S M, Bredenberg C E. Should percutaneous transluminal renal artery angioplasty be applied to ostial artery atherosclerosis? J Vasc Surg 1995; 21: 909–915

8. Plouin P-F, Darne B, Chatellier G et al. Restenosis after a first percutaneous transluminal renal angioplasty. Hypertension 1993; 21: 89–96

9. Rundback J H, Sacks D, Craig K, Cooper C, Jones D et al, for the AHA Councils on Cardiovascular Radiology, High Blood Pressure Research, Kidney in Cardiovascular Disease, Cardio-Thoracic and Vascular Surgery, and Clinical Cardiology, and the Society of Interventional Radiology FDA Device Forum Committee Guidelines for the Reporting of Renal Artery Revascularization in Clinical Trials. Circulation 2002; 106: 1572

10. Dorros G, Jaff M, Jain A, Dufek C, Mathiak L. Follow-up of primary Palmaz-Schatz stent placement for atherosclerotic renal artery stenosis. Am J Cardiol 1995; 75: 1051–1055

11. MacLeod M, Taylor A D, Baxter G, et al. Renal artery stenosis managed by Palmaz stent insertion: technical and clinical outcome. J Hypertens 1995; 13: 1791–1795

12. van de Ven P J G, Beutler J J, Kaatee R et al. Transluminal vascular stent for ostial atherosclerotic renal artery stenosis. Lancet 1995; 346: 672–674

13. Henry M, Amor M, Henry I et al. Stent placement in the renal artery: three-year experience with the Palmaz stent. J Vasc Interv Radiol 1996; 7: 343–350

14. Leertouwer T C, Gussenhoven E J, van Lankeren W, van Overhagen H. Response of renal and femoropopliteal arteries to Palmaz stent implantation assessed with intravascular ultrasound. J Endovasc Surg 1999; 6: 359–364

15. Dorros G, Jaff M, Mathiak L, Dorros I I, Lowe A, Murphy K, He T. Four-year follow-up of Palmaz-Schatz stent revascularization as treatment for atherosclerotic renal artery stenosis. Circulation 1998; 98: 642–647

16. Martin L G, Rundback J H, Sacks D, Cardella J F, Rees C R et al. for the SIR Standards of Practice Committee. Quality Improvement Guidelines for Angiography, Angioplasty, and Stent Placement in the Diagnosis and Treatment of Renal Artery Stenosis in Adults. J Vasc Interv Radiol 2002; 13: 1069–1083

17. Standards of Practice Committee of the Society of Cardiovascular and Interventional Radiology. Guidelines for percutaneous transluminal angioplasty. Radiology 1990; 177: 619–626

18. van Jaarsveld B C, Krijnen P, Pieterman H, Derkx F H, Deinum J et al. The effect of balloon angioplasty on hypertension in atherosclerotic renal-artery stenosis. Dutch Renal Artery Stenosis Intervention Cooperative Study Group. N Engl J Med 2000; 6; 342: 1007–1014

19. Nicita G, Villari D, Marzocco M, Li Marzi V, Trippitelli A, Santoro G. Endoluminal stent placement after percutaneous transluminal angioplasty in the treatment of post-transplant renal artery stenosis. J Urol 1998; 159: 34–37

20. van de Ven P J G, Kaatee R, Beutler J J, Beek F J A, Woittiez A J et al. Arterial stenting and balloon angioplasty in ostial atherosclerotic renovascular disease: a randomised trial. Lancet 1999; 353: 282–286

21. Gill-Leertouwer T C, Gussenhoven E J, Bosch J L, Deinum J, van Overhagen H, Derkx F H, Pattynama P M. Predictors for clinical success at one year following renal artery stent placement. J Endovasc Ther 2002; 9: 495–502

22. Caps M T, Perissinotto C, Zierler R E, Polissar N L, Bergelin R O et al. Prospective study of atherosclerotic disease progression in the renal artery. Circulation 1998; 98: 2866–2872

23. Watson P S, Hadjipetrou P, Cox S V, Piemonte T C, Eisenhauer A C. Effect of renal artery stenting on renal function and size in patients with atherosclerotic renovascular disease. Circulation 2000; 102: 1671

24. Barbalias G A, Siablis D, Liatsikos E N, Karnabatidis D, Yarmenitis S, Bouropoulos K, Dimopoulos J. Metal stents: a new treatment of malignant ureteral obstruction. J Urol 1997; 158: 54–58

25. Barbalias G A, Liatsikos E N, Kalogeropoulou C, Karnabatidis D, Siablis D. Metallic stents in gynecologic cancer: an approach to treat extrinsic ureteral obstruction. Eur Urol 2000; 38: 35–40

26. Barbalias G A, Liatsikos E N, Karnabatidis D, Yarmenitis S, Siablis D. Ureteroileal anastomotic strictures: an innovative approach with metallic stents. J Urol 1998; 160: 1270–1273

27. Siablis D, Liatsikos E N, Kalogeropoulou C, Karnabatidis D, Tsota I, Perimenis P, Passakos C, Barbalias G A. Metal stents for the management of atherosclerotic renovascular disease. J Endourol 2001; 15: 993–996

28. Zeller T, Buttner H J, Lorenz H M, Frank U, Muller C, Burgelin K, Roskamm H. Late aortic dislocation of a stent following stent angioplasty for ostial renal artery stenosis. Catheter Cardiovasc Interv 2002; 56: 416–420

29. Tso C, Skinner M P, Hawthorne W J, Fletcher J P. Matrigel-coated stents reduce intimal thickening in a large animal vascular stent model. Int Angiol 2002; 21: 244–249

Indications for stent placement in haemodialysis fistulas and grafts

L. Turmel-Rodrigues

69

Introduction

Since the initial descriptions of the technique in 1980, the results of percutaneous transluminal angioplasty (PTA) in haemodialysis access have been much less successful than in the arterial system. Primary patency rates at 1 year range from 17 to 40% for poly tetrafluoroethylene (PTFE) grafts,[1–5] from 16 to 60% for Brescia–Cimino fistulas,[2,5] and from 12 to 30% for central veins.[4,6] These unsatisfactory results gave rise to great hopes for stents when they became available in 1986.

All the articles concerning stent placement in dialysis access published to date describe small series.[4,7–16] In fact, they provide only partial answers with regard to the effectiveness of stents according to type (e.g. Wallstent, Palmaz, Gianturco, Craggstent), the nature of the vessel in which they are placed (native vein, PTFE graft), location (forearm, upper arm, thigh, central vein), graft configuration (straight or loop), and indications for placement (residual stenosis, complication of dilatation, restenosis). However, those papers that reported results according to the life-table method yielded similar results in terms of primary and secondary patency (Tables 69.1 and 69.2). They should however be interpreted with extreme caution as these series are so disparate.

The use of Wallstents in haemodialysis access was first reported by Zollikofer and colleagues[7] in 1988. They reported a gain in patency of some months over simple dilatation in the treatment of a long stenosis of the basilic vein in the outflow of a PTFE graft. In 1989 Rousseau et al.[8] reported a secondary patency of 64% at 1 year after systematic placement of Wallstents in stenoses. In 1989 Günther et al.[9] also reported six cases of Wallstent insertion. They described some early thromboses and development of intimal hyperplasia in three patients with more than 3 months' follow-up (however, three of six lesions were more than 5 cm long). After placement of Wallstents, mainly in early recurring stenoses, Zollikofer et al.[10] reported in 1992

Table 69.1. *Stent placement in dialysis access: primary patency rates reported according to the life-table method*

Reference*	Stent	1-year primary patency (%)
1	Gianturco	19
4	Gianturco	11
17	Wallstent	20
14	Wallstent	31
18	Wallstent + Craggstent	15–27

*Numbered according to reference list.

Table 69.2. *Stent placement in dialysis access: secondary patency rates reported according to the life-table method*

Reference*	Stent	1-year secondary patency (%)	2-year secondary patency (%)
17	Wallstent	33	–
4	Gianturco	78–100	–
14	Wallstent	86	77
18	Wallstent + Craggstent	81–88	80

*Numbered according to reference list.

the presence of intimal hyperplasia in all cases before 10 months in five peripheral lesions, necessitating redilatation but yielding a secondary patency of 29 months in one patient. They determined that stents could double or triple restenosis intervals, but concluded, however, that stents should be reserved for failures of dilatation and for stenoses recurring within 2 months. They described new stenoses developing outside the stent, and cases in which restenosis intervals decreased after initial lengthening.

Beathard[11] in 1991 reported results after placement of 30 Gianturco stents in 28 patients. He demonstrated in this randomized study that Gianturco stents with a unique 15 mm diameter did not delay restenosis at the venous anastomosis of grafts, in comparison with regular dilatation leaving no residual stenosis. Beathard also reported further entanglement of Gianturco stents with Fogarty catheters in cases where secondary thrombectomy was necessary. Quinn et al.[4] confirmed the lack of value of systematic placement of Gianturco stents, even after having matched stent and PTFE graft diameters and having included stents placed for residual stenoses after regular dilatation. They were unable to determine whether what was true for peripheral grafts was also true for central veins. Quinn et al.[12] also reported the death of a patient from septicaemia 48 hours after stent placement. Such a complication suggests the necessity for systematic antibiotic coverage of any haemodialysed patient in whom such a 'foreign body' is placed. Quinn also reported a transient neurological deficit, probably due to the mechanical compression of the stent on an adjacent nerve. On the basis of Quinn and Beathard's studies, it is advisable to avoid placing Gianturco stents for dialysis access.

By 1994, Shoenfeld et al.[13] had placed 17 Wallstents and 8 Palmaz stents in central veins of 19 patients. These authors concluded that primary patency rates at 1 year were clearly greater after stent placement than after regular dilatation; however, the series was small. They reported that stents placed in the subclavian vein are prone to deformity due to the powerful two-point musculoskeletal compression forces causing persistent extrinsic compression of both vein and stent.

The largest series to date was published in 1995 by Vorwerk et al.,[14] who placed 92 Wallstents in 65 patients. They reported patency rates in central veins that were clearly greater than those currently reported for regular dilatation and they concluded that Wallstents decreased the likelihood of restenosis in this location. In contrast, for peripheral sites they reported restenosis intervals after stent placement that were similar to those after regular dilatation. These authors therefore advised restricting stents to cases in which the patency of the shunt was definitively compromised after balloon dilatation, either by considerable residual stenosis or by dissection. Including all indications, Vorwerk et al.[14] reported a mean period of patency of 6.7 ± 7.2 months between two episodes of shunt reobstruction after stent placement. However, they reported a fairly high (10%) thrombosis rate within a week of stent placement, even though most of these thromboses were not due to any underlying stenosis or

restenosis. They reported a short experience with atherectomy catheters to remove secondary intimal hyperplasia occurring in stents, but did not draw any conclusions regarding the superiority of this expensive device over simple redilation. Vorwerk et al. also reported one death shortly after stent placement: this was due to cardiac tamponade, probably linked to unintentional perforation of the right atrium with the guidewire used for balloon dilatation and stent delivery.

Despite a small panel of 10 patients, Kovalik et al.[15] confirmed the usefulness of Wallstents for residual stenoses after dilatation of central veins. However, in cases of early recurring stenoses, they concluded that stents were less effective than simple redilatation leaving no residual stenosis.

After having experienced pulmonary migration of two Palmaz stents in 1994, Gray et al.[16] reported their experience with Wallstents of a flat diameter of 10 mm in 56 lesions in 52 patients.[17] They reported downstream migration due to the underestimation of the true diameter of central veins. They also reported unintentional pulmonary emoblization of two subclavian stents after further attempts at central line placements by nephrologists who were not aware of the presence of the subclavian stents. These stents were easily removed percutaneously using snares. Like Quinn et al.[12] Gray et al.[16] reported a septic complication: a PTFE graft had to be removed because of local infection within 2 weeks of stent placement. This emphasizes the extreme vulnerability of these haemodialysed patients with regard to risk of infection. Gray et al.[16] reported the occurrence of a pseudoaneurysm on contact with the stent 10 months after its placement. In cases of placement in the subclavian vein, these authors emphasized that it was important not to overlap the ostium of the internal jugular vein, in order to keep the way free for central catheter placement or for the outflow of an axillary–jugular graft. Gray and colleagues' primary patency rate after stent placement was 20%, similar to those of other series; their low secondary patency rate of 33% was due to the absence of radiological declotting of thrombosed accesses.

In the present author's recent study in Tours,[18] 48 Wallstents and 14 Craggstents were placed in 47 patients to prevent stenosis recoil after dilatation and to delay the early recurrence of stenoses. The author and colleagues demonstrated that stents doubled restenosis intervals at the venous anastomosis of grafts, as well as in native fistulas. This positive effect was less (and not statistically significant) in central veins. Like previous authors, the present author found that stents were more clearly effective for the treatment of recoiling stenoses than of recurring stenoses.

The relative disenchantment regarding the effectiveness of bare stents gave rise to new hopes for covered stents. The only vascular covered stent to become available since 1993 is a Craggstent covered with Dacron. Unfortunately, in addition to initial transient inflammatory reactions, this first type of Dacron-coated stent has not shown any evidence of superiority over bare stents in hindering restenosis.[19] The only superiority of this covered stent is to ensure the absolute control of rare major vessel rupture induced by dilatation balloons. The coverage of the breach by watertight Dacron stops leakage in all cases, even when prolonged balloon tamponade, manual compression and bare stents have failed, which is rare. Craggstents and Wallstents are compatible and a covered Craggstent can be placed through a Wallstent when the Wallstent does not allow rupture control.

Indications for stenting

From the published data and from personal experience, some general rules can be proposed and some reasonable indications for stent placement in 1997 can be outlined.

Choice of stent

In contrast to the arterial system, vein diameter increases with flow. There is, therefore, a risk of detachment and downstream (pulmonary) migration of any endoprosthesis that was not large enough, or not wall adherent. These anatomical and mechanical constraints mean that self-expandable stents (e.g. Wallstent, Craggstent, Memotherm, Gianturco) are preferable to balloon-expandable stents (Palmaz, Strecker). The stent diameter must be 1–2 mm greater than the diameter of the vessel in order to cling to the intima. Greater oversizing of stents must be avoided because excessive radial force could stimulate reactional intimal hyperplasia.

Dialysis access stenoses are often located in joint spaces (e.g. elbow or shoulder), leading to a preference for highly flexible stents (Wallstent, Craggstent) over the more rigid Gianturco stent.

Even when stents are self-expandable and can increase in diameter after placement, it is important not to accept any residual stenosis in stents. Complementary dilatation immediately after placement is almost the rule, and the use of high-pressure balloons such as the Blue-Max™ (Boston Scientific, Natick, MA, USA), inflatable to 25 atmospheres ($\approx$ 2.53 MPa) may be necessary.

When a stent must be placed in a cannulation area (which is a rare indication), puncturable stents must be used and the author currently recommends the Craggstent.

Because of the disappointing results to date for covered stents, they are recommended only for rupture control when bare stents have failed. Their usefulness and reliability in cases of early restenosis within a bare stent has still to be determined.

Think of the future

The superiority of percutaneous dilatation over conventional surgery lies in the treatment of stenoses 'in situ' and preservation of the patient's 'venous real estate'. It is important to keep this in mind when placing a stent. Stents must not obviate further surgery and must protect the ease of making new anastomoses, especially for the outflow of a new graft. Stents must protrude as little as possible beyond the treated stenosis and must never overlap an adjacent venous confluence. There are three locations where the latter problem is frequently relevant, as follows:

1. A stent placed in the final arch of the cephalic vein must not protrude into the subclavian vein, where it could induce stenosis that would preclude future use of the basilic vein for creation of a direct fistula or for drainage of an upper arm graft.
2. A stent placed in the subclavian vein must not overlap the ostium of the internal jugular vein. This vein is essential for placing a future central catheter or for drainage of a graft running from the axillary vein.
3. A stent placed in the right or left brachiocephalic ('innominate') vein must not protrude into the superior vena cava, in order to respect the flow coming from the contralateral trunk. For stenoses

limited to the right brachiocephalic vein, it is also important to try not to overlap either the subclavian ostium or the internal jugular ostium, i.e. to place the stent in the brachiocephalic trunk only, which is not easy when the trunk is very short (see Fig. 69.4).

Indications

Acute PTA-induced rupture

In these circumstances, a stent can save the vascular access. Slight local extravasations are very common immediately after dilatation: they are simply the evidence of local trauma induced, of necessity, by mechanical enlargement. In contrast, the definition of acute rupture is major extravasation pushed by flow into a rapidly growing haematoma (Figs. 69.1 and 69.2). Diagnosis is first clinical before being imaged: the patient complains of intense pain immediately upon balloon deflation, whereas this manoeuvre should decrease the local pain induced by balloon inflation. Fluoroscopic testing confirms the rupture and it is essential to have left a guidewire through the dilated area because the vast majority of these ruptures are controlled by prolonged (10 minutes) low-pressure (2 atmospheres) balloon tamponade. When the balloon is re-inflated, it is necessary to check by injection through the side-port of the introducer sheath that the balloon is effectively stopping flow and leakage from the fistula. During these (possibly repeated) 10 minutes without flow, the perivascular haematoma starts to coagulate on contact with the ruptured area and it may also be useful to compress the haematoma manually when it is clinically accessible. In rare cases, the breach is too large or the patients' clotting mechanism is impaired, and leakage persists in spite of several 10–minute balloon tamponades; this is the indication for stent placement. Bare stents are effective in the majority of cases because they reopen the vessel at the level of the rupture and there is less resistance in the outflow vein than in the perivascular haematoma. To stop the flow during stent placement, it may be necessary to inflate a balloon at the origin of the fistula, which necessitates an additional retrograde puncture and catheterization. Sometimes, prolonged ballooning and external compression are sufficient to control leakage, but it is necessary to place a stent because of residual stenosis due to the extrinsic compression by the perivascular haematoma (Figs. 69.2 and 69.3). Systematic stent placement in cases of

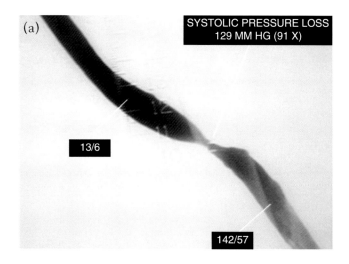

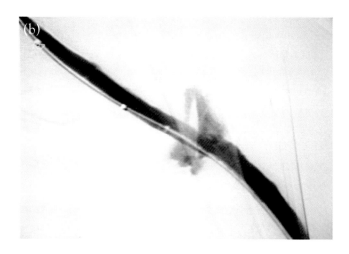

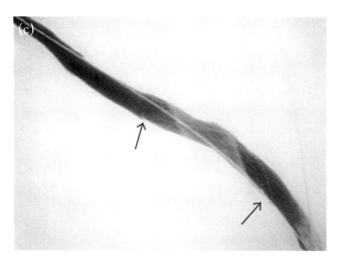

Figure 69.1. (a) Severe stenosis of the axillary outflow of an externalized basilic vein. (b) Major rupture induced by dilatation, not controlled by repeated low-pressure balloon tamponades. (c) Control (immediate) of rupture after placement of a Craggstent (arrows).

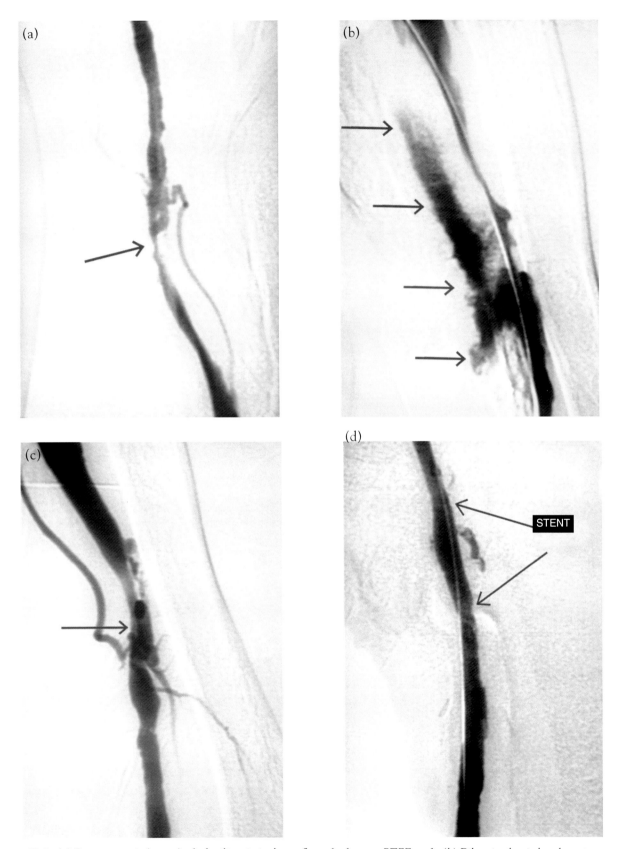

Figure 69.2. (a) Severe stenosis (arrow) of a basilic vein in the outflow of a forearm PTFE graft. (b) Dilatation has induced a rupture, with major extravasation of contrast media (arrows). (c) Leakage has been controlled by a 10-minute low-pressure balloon tamponade, but there is significant residual stenosis (arrow). (d) Absence of residual stenosis after placement of a Wallstent.

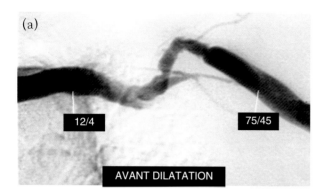

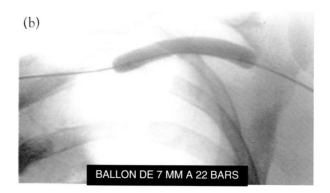

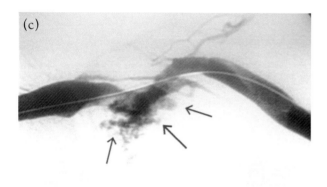

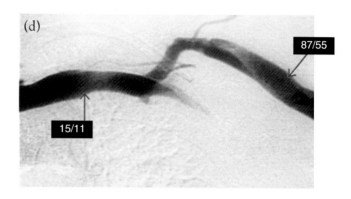

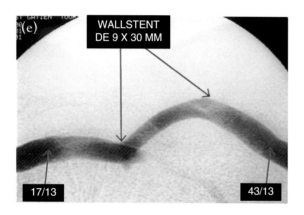

Figure 69.3. *(a) Severe stenosis of the final arch of a cephalic vein with an 84% loss of systolic pressure. (b) Virtual absence of any residual waist after dilatation to 7 mm at 22 atmospheres. (c) Rupture induced by dilatation (arrows). (d) Leakage controlled by prolonged balloon tamponade but with unchanged stenosis and an 83% loss of systolic pressure. (e) Distinct (but not complete) improvement obtained after placement of a Wallstent, giving a 60% residual loss of systolic pressure.*

rupture may also be advocated to prevent formation of secondary pseudoaneurysms from the breach, which remains an area of weakness of the vessel wall.

Some rarer cases have been reported concerning persistent leakage after Wallstent or Craggstent placement. Ruptures were ultimately stopped by placement of covered Craggstents through just previously implanted bare stents, with good results at 5 months' follow-up.[19]

In the author's experience, stenoses located in the final arch of the cephalic vein and in the axillary outflow externalized basilic veins are prone to dilatation-induced rupture.

Soft post-PTA recoiling stenosis

Soft post-PTA recoiling stenosis is the greatest indication for stent placement, unanimously advised by all authors, and it leads to a clear improvement in the management of central veins (Fig. 69.4). However, it is necessary to have a clear definition of a soft recoiling stenosis. A recoiling stenosis is a stenosis that induces no residual 'waist' on the inflated dilatation balloon but in which the vessel wall collapses more or less as soon as the balloon is removed, inducing residual narrowing. Such a recoiling lesion needs a stent when the residual stenosis is greater than 30% in diameter or induces systolic loss greater than 30% at pullback pressure

(a)

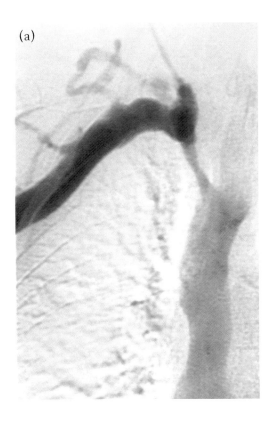

(b)

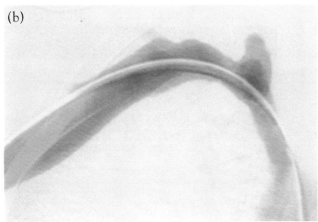

(c)

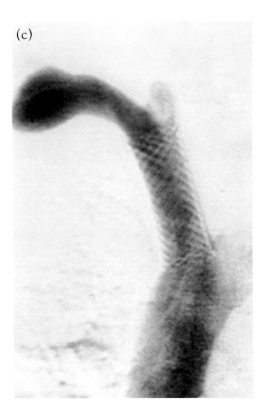

Figure 69.4. (a) Stenosis of the right brachiocephalic trunk, causing arm oedema. (b) Stenosis recoil after dilatation to 12 mm (the diameter of the brachiocephalic trunk is inferior to the diameter of the subclavian vein). (c) Lack of residual stenosis after placement of a Wallstent (14 x 30 mm). Note that the stent does not protrude into the superior vena cava and does not overlap either the subclavian ostium or the internal jugular ostium.

measurement. Before placing the stent, it is important to have achieved sufficient dilatation, i.e. to have a slightly oversized balloon diameter 1–2 mm greater than the diameter of the immediately upstream or downstream normal vein. Because stent placement cannot be recommended lightly, a residual stenosis can be tolerated when it is the first dilatation procedure on the dialysis access but any further residual stenosis must be stented if clinical abnormalities lead to reintervention within 6 months.

These recoiling stenoses are very frequent in central veins (brachiocephalic trunks, superior vena cava) and less common in peripheral veins and grafts, in which slight overdilatation and high-pressure balloons must be used before affirming the presence of a residual stenosis.

The subclavian vein is a situation apart. Definition of a residual stenosis is angiographically difficult because of the presence of final anatomical narrowing. Persistence of collaterals and a pressure gradient greater than 10 mmHg are objective signs of a residual stenosis.

Stent placement must be particularly clearly indicated, as long-term results are frequently disappointing in this location.

Residual stenosis in the axillary vein after dilatation may be due to, or increased by, extrinsic compression of the breast, not only in obese patients but even when the arm is in abduction. The author has placed one stent in such a case with an excellent outcome, the underlying PTFE graft that had thrombosed three times in 2 months before stenting remained patent through 5 months' follow-up.

There are some stenoses that are not abolished despite the highest pressure (25 atmospheres) currently applicable in the strongest balloons. Subsequent residual stenoses are 'hard' stenoses and not soft recoiling stenoses. In the author's opinion, stents are not indicated in these cases and recourse to a direct, mechanically more aggressive, tool (i.e. an atherectomy device or a cutting balloon) is advised.

Pseudoaneurysms

Pseudoaneurysms may become thrombosed after placement of a stent across their neck or base. The mechanism can be easily understood if a covered stent is placed, as for aortic aneurysms, but some thromboses have also occurred after placement of bare stents (Fig. 69.5). The indication seems valuable for pseudoaneurysms originating from PTA-induced ruptures and systematic placement can even be discussed. The indication is far more open to criticism for aneurysms originating from cannulation areas, since surgical repair is a simple procedure that does not consume healthy veins.

Restenosis

The current area for discussion regarding the use of stents is their value in delaying restenosis. Although the author has encountered some cases in which no benefit was gained, there is evidence of a statistically significant increase in mean patency after stent placement. Wallstents and Craggstents can lengthen restenosis intervals in PTFE grafts as well as in native fistulas.

Early recurring stenoses can, of course, be managed by regular repeat dilatation, with good secondary

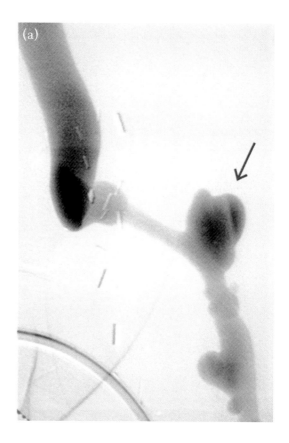

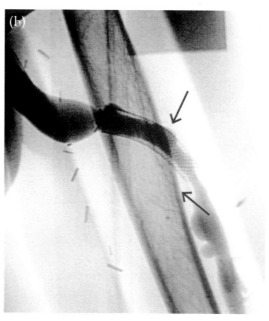

Figure 69.5. (a) Pseudoaneurysm caused by rupture induced by a dilatation performed 2 weeks earlier (arrow). (b) Angiography 6 months after stent placement shows thrombosis of the pseudoaneurysm (arrow) and a new stenosis immediately upstream from the Wallstent (arrows).

patency of 82% at 1 year and 65% at 2 years for PTFE grafts, as reported by Safa et al.[5] However, those authors did not report how many redilatations or declottings per year were necessary to maintain patency. In the overall management of dialysis access stenoses, the present author considers it acceptable to reintervene at intervals of more than 6 months. In contrast, because of patient irradiation, cost and comparison with the efficacy of surgery, it is not considered acceptable to redilate (or to declot) a vascular access every 3 months, except when it is the last possible access before placement of a permanent central catheter. In the author's institutions before the stent era, early recurring stenoses constituted surgical indications. In doubling intervals of free function, stents have yielded acceptable 6-month reintervention periods in these patients and are cost-effective from month 6 after placement, since their price in France is equivalent to the cost of a redilatation procedure. Stenting also means fewer reinterventions for these patients who have undergone multiple operations. In addition, doubling reintervention intervals underestimates the effect of stents on initial stenosis, since further reinterventions are not linked to a restenosis in the area of the stent.

Stents can, however, induce two mid-term problems — inefficacy of redilatation and development of new downstream stenoses. When intimal hyperplasia increases with time and repeated dilatations, it may behave like a slowly recoiling stenosis, the immediate post-PTA result appearing to be adequate but angiography some minutes later revealing recoil. Trials of removal by atherectomy catheters have not been conclusive; placing a new bare stent through the previous stent was ineffective and placement of a covered stent through the bare stent was reported to be helpful in only one in four cases.[19] The development of excessive intimal hyperplasia after stent placement is a phenomenon that appears to be uncommon for stenoses treated only by repeated dilatation. It might be an argument for avoiding placing a stent in a stenosis occurring in the last available vascular access of a patient before placement of a permanent central catheter. The second mid-term problem is the development of a new stenosis immediately downstream

from the stent (Fig. 69.6). This evolution at the venous anastomosis of PTFE grafts occurred in 15% (2/13) of the author's cases 1 year after stent placement and in 56% (5/9) of cases at 2 years, whereas the initial stenosis had not recurred within the stent. In native fistulas, it occurred in 14% (1/7) of cases at 1 year and in 33% (2/6) of cases at 2 years. Such stenoses, diagnosed between 4 and 53 months after stent implantation, were probably due to turbulence created by the difference in compliance between the stent and the native vein that already existed between the graft and the anastomosed vein. Such a development means that, in contrast to simple dilatation and redilatation, stent placement can impair a few centimetres of healthy downstream veins, just as surgical prolongation of the graft to bypass the stenosis would have done. The difference is, however, that, of necessity, surgery immediately takes a few centimetres of healthy vein, whereas only half of the stents placed create a similar situation at 2 years. In addition, patients prefer percutaneous stent placement to open surgery. Before the stent era, patients with rapidly recurring stenoses underwent surgery; nowadays, they undergo surgery only if restenosis recurs every 3 months or less despite stent placement. The author has noted such rapidly recurring restenoses in stents in 7% (1/14) and 25% (2/8) of grafts at 1 year and 2 years respectively, in 22% (2/9) of native fistulas at 1 year and in 1/4 subclavian veins (3 weeks after stent placement).

The author's personal series is too small to confirm the same value of stents in early restenoses of central veins. Vorwerk et al.[14] and Shoenfeld et al.[13] considered stents to be valuable for this indication. In contrast, Kovalik et al.[15] reported restenosis intervals in central veins that were shorter after stent placement than after simple dilatation leaving no residual stenosis. However, this study included only ten patients.

A stenosis that is located less than 10 cm from the wrist in a Brescia–Cimino fistula is the one situation in which, in the author's opinion, stenoses and restenoses must be treated surgically and not by stent. In this specific case, the surgical construction of a new arteriovenous anastomosis immediately downstream from a stenosis is a simple intervention, performed

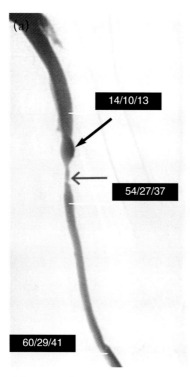

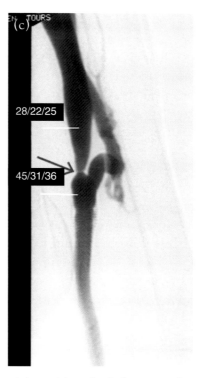

Figure 69.6. (a) Stenosis (arrows) of the venous anastomosis of an upper arm PTFE graft that has recurred twice in 6 months.

(c) New stenosis (arrow) immediately downstream from the Wallstent 8 months after its placement.

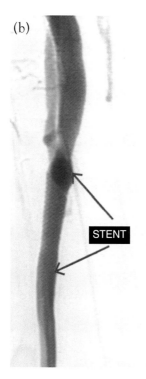

(b) Lack of residual stenosis after stent placement and normalization of outflow vein.

under local anaesthesia, that leaves enough vein for cannulation and yields better primary patency rates than radiological treatments. It is a much easier surgical procedure than the creation of a new fistula, since the forearm vein is already mature. For reasons of cost-effectiveness and low morbidity, such lesions are not good indications for stent placement[20] or even for simple dilatation.

Periprocedural management

The septic complications described in the literature suggest the use of routine antistaphylococcal antibiotic coverage of any haemodialysis patient during stent placement. For the same reason it is not advisable to place a stent during declotting procedures. These are longer interventions which necessitate several percutaneous approaches; fresh thrombi are immediately under the skin and it is better to avoid placing a permanent foreign body in such circumstances and to insert a stent some weeks later, when possible.

There is no need for anticoagulants or antiplatelet drugs before, during or after stenting, as long as excellent flow is restored in the haemodialysis access.

Introducer-sheaths used for placement of larger stents can have a gauge as great as 10 Fr. Problems of haemostasis can therefore occur at a puncture site after removal, with the risk of subsequent pseudoaneurysm. Many teams recommend the femoral route in these cases, but direct puncture of the fistula is possible if a small subcutaneous tunnel is created between the skin entry point and the fistula entry point; this facilitates final compression and stimulates subcutaneous activators of coagulation.

Early thrombosis after stent placement can be due to inappropriate positioning or to secondary migration of the prosthesis. However, no anatomical abnormality is found in many cases after radiological or surgical declotting, and the general condition of patients with subsequent hypercoagulability or chronical hypotension could be questioned.

No lasting mechanical impairment has been reported after the insertion of Wallstents or Craggstents, even after placement in the bend of the elbow. In contrast, transient inflammatory reactions for 1 or 2 weeks are frequent after a covered stent, probably related to the Dacron.

Follow-up

Underlying stenosis is at high risk of recurrence after stenting, even though it may be delayed. Nephrologists must detect clinical and paraclinical signs of restenosis before acute thrombosis occurs. Systematic angiography 1 year after stent placement can be contemplated.

Conclusions

Even if their effectiveness is irregular and limited over time, Wallstents and Craggstents are valuable in selective indications of PTA failures or limitations, such as recoiling stenoses, ruptures and early restenoses. They can sometimes rescue a procedure, and dilatation should not be attempted without the availability of stents. For the controversial problem of rapidly recurring stenoses, it is emphasized that stents are effective if the stenosis

has previously been sufficiently dilated in diameter and pressure and if residual stenoses are not accepted after stent placement. For teams such as that of the author, who worked only with dilatation balloons before 1988, the availability and the selective use of stents has been a major improvement in the treatment of these patients, as valuable as the availability of high-pressure balloons and hydrophilic guidewires.

Acknowledgement

The author thanks Doreen Raine for editing the English.

References

1. Beathard G. Percutaneous transvenous angioplasty in the treatment of vascular access stenosis. Kidney Int 1992; 42: 1390–1397
2. Turmel-Rodrigues L, Pengloan J, Blanchier D et al. Insufficient dialysis shunts: improved long-term patency rates with close hemodynamic monitoring, repeated percutaneous balloon angioplasty, and stent placement. Radiology 1993; 187: 273–278
3. Kanterman R, Vesely T, Pilgram T et al. Dialysis access grafts: anatomic location of venous stenosis and results of angioplasty. Radiology 1995; 195: 135–139
4. Quinn S, Schumann E, Demlow T et al. Percutaneous transluminal angioplasty versus endovascular stent placement in the treatment of venous stenoses in patients undergoing hemodialysis: intermediate results. JVIR 1995; 6: 851–855
5. Safa A, Valji K, Roberts A et al. Detection and treatment of dysfunctional hemodialysis access grafts: effect of a surveillance program on graft patency and the incidence of thrombosis. Radiology 1996; 199: 653–657
6. Glanz S, Gordon D, Lipkowitz G et al. Axillary and subclavian vein stenosis: percutaneous angioplasty. Radiology 1988; 168: 371–373
7. Zollikofer C, Largiader I, Bruhlmann N et al. Endovascular stenting of veins and grafts: preliminary clinical experience. Radiology 1988; 167: 707–712
8. Rousseau H, Morfaux V, Joffre F et al. Treatment of haemodialysis arterio-venous fistula stenosis by percutaneous implantation of new intravascular stent. J Intervent Radiol 1989; 4: 161–167
9. Gunther R, Vorwerk D, Bohndorf K et al. Venous stenoses in dialysis shunts: treatment with self-expanding metallic stents. Radiology 1989; 170: 401–405
10. Zollikofer C, Antonnucci F, Stuckmann G et al. Use of the Wallstent in the venous system including hemodialysis related stenoses. Cardiovasc Intervent Radiol 1992; 15: 334–341
11. Beathard G. The use of the Gianturco intra-vascular stent in stenotic hemodialysis fistulas. Trans Am Soc Artif Intern Organs 1991; 37: M 234–235
12. Quinn S, Schumann E, Hall L et al. Venous stenoses in patients who undergo hemodialysis: treatment with self-expandable endovascular stents. Radiology 1992; 183: 499–504
13. Shoenfeld R, Hermans H, Novick A et al. Stenting of proximal venous obstructions to maintain hemodialysis access. J Vasc Surg 1994; 19: 532–539

14. Vorwerk D, Guenther R, Mann H et al. Venous stenosis and occlusion in hemodialysis shunts: follow-up results of stent placement in 65 patients. Radiology 1995; 195: 140–146

15. Kovalik E, Newman G, Suhocki P et al. Correction of central venous stenoses: use of angioplasty and vascular Wallstents. Kidney Int 1994; 45: 1177–1181

16. Gray R, Dolmatch B, Horton K et al. Migration of Palmaz stents following deployment for venous stenoses related to hemodialysis access. JVIR 1994; 5: 117–120

17. Gray R, Horton K, Dolmatch B. Use of Wallstents for hemodialysis access-related venous stenoses and occlusions untreatable with balloon angioplasty. Radiology 1995; 195: 479–844

18. Turmel-Rodrigues L, Blanchard D, Pengloan J et al. Wallstents and craggstents in hemodialysis grafts and fistulas: results for selective indications. JVIR 1997; 8: 975–982

19. Sapoval M, Turmel-Rodrigues L, Raynaud A et al. Cragg covered stents in hemodialysis access: initial and mid-term results. JVIR 1996; 7: 335–342

20. Bosnjakovic P, Ivkovic T, Ilic M, Arackis S. Strecker stent in stenotic hemodialysis Brescia-Cimino arterio-venous fistulas. Cardiovasc Intervent Radiol 1992; 15: 217–220

Stent-grafts in endovascular management of iliofemoral venous occlusions caused by urologic pelvic malignancies

D. Yachia, G. Faragi, A. Gremitsky and G. Bartal

70

Introduction

Cancer remains the second leading cause of death in the industrial world and worldwide. As life expectancy worldwide continues to increase, so will cases of cancer. Bladder cancer is the sixth most common cancer found in adults, and its incidence has been increasing over the past 30 years. The highest incidence rates of bladder cancer are found in industrial countries, such as the United States, Canada, France, Denmark, Italy and Spain. Bladder cancer is the fourth leading cause of cancer death in people over 75 years old.[1] By the end of the 20th Century 60 000 new cases of bladder cancer were reported annually in the United States and 75 000 in Europe. In the United States its incidence increased by about 10% between 1973 and 1991.[1] Currently patients with non-metastatic invasive primary bladder tumors are treated by endoscopic resection for grading and staging of the tumor. The endourological procedure may be followed by radical cystectomy and a bladder replacement surgery, during which are removed the prostate and the seminal vesicles in males, and the uterus, ovaries and a part of the vagina with the urethra are removed in females. Ninety-four per cent of urologists treat the bladder cancer surgically only when the tumor is superficial, without evidence of local or distant spread. Patients who refuse surgery or are not fit for surgery are referred to radiation oncologists for external beam therapy, or those with distant metastases are referred to oncologists for chemotherapy.

Extrinsic or intrinsic iliofemoral vein occlusion causing venous circulatory disturbance is frequently seen in invasive pelvic malignancies (Fig. 70.1). Patients with such malignancies may develop swelling and pain of the lower extremities as a result of compression and/or occlusions of the tumor on the pelvic veins and lymphatic vessels (Fig. 70.2). Some of the inoperable patients suffer more from the venous occlusion that significantly affects their quality of life than from their primary disease. Generally, compared with the underlying disease, the vascular drainage of the lower extremities is regarded as less important, and is managed conservatively, hoping that the drainage will be obtained by the venous collaterals.

Conventional management

Like the other pelvic malignancies, patients with pelvic urologic invasive malignancies may develop swelling and pain of the lower extremities, as a result of compression and/or occlusions by the tumor the pelvic veins and lymphatic vessels. Treatment of such venous disease is a challenge. Conventional treatment options are limited to: physiotherapy using lymphatic massage, long-term anticoagulation, surgical venous bypass, or no treatment at all. Even without treatment, in some patients some improvement of symptoms can occur over the time that can be explained by the development of collateral circulation. When the swelling is not associated with metastatic tumor, lower extremity elevation, compression stocking and the use of pneumatic boot are the basis of the conservative management.

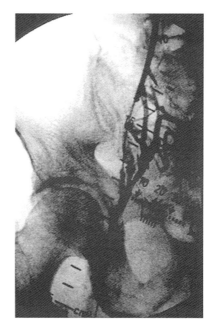

Figure 70.1. *Venography showing iliofemoral vein occlusion and collaterals.*

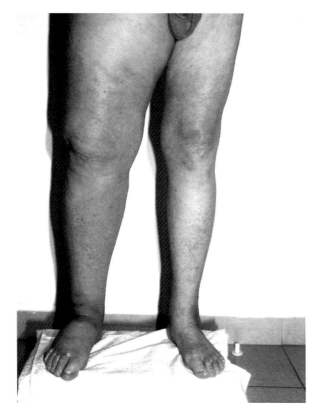

Figure 70.2. *Typical right lower extremity swelling in a bladder cancer patient with pelvic recurrence.*

Conventional treatment for iliofemoral vein thrombosis comprises heparinization followed by oral sodium warfarin (Coumadine). In such treatment, regimen recanalization of the occluded veins depends mainly on the effectiveness of the patient's fibrinolytic system. Several studies on such conventional treatments reported disappointing results with systemic thrombolysis for iliofemoral venous thombosis.[2,3] Only 6% of patients with acute deep vein thrombosis (DVT) may show complete thrombus lysis within 10 days.[4] In the case of venous stenosis or occlusion associated with pelvic malignancy, the chances of success for systemic thrombolysis are almost nil, while major surgery, such as surgical bypass, is very aggressive and associated with its own long-term morbidity.[5,6] Although feasible, iliofemoral vein replacement or bypass is a controversial, often risky procedure. If the pelvic tumor is resectable, the tumor mass can be removed together with the affected vein and the gap can be substituted with a vascular graft. However, the procedure is often ineffective

even without recurrent tumor progression. During the past few years, some innovative approaches are being developed for ameliorating the quality of life of the patients with advanced malignant disease.

Minimally invasive approach

Using interventional radiological techniques for recanalization of occluded venous drainage is a modern approach. Percutaneous transluminal angioplasty (PTA) of an occluded vessel has been successfully used in the arterial system, especially in the treatment of atherosclerotic lesions. The use of such an approach for the venous system is a very logical application of this technology. However, in the treatment of various venous stenoses PTA alone yielded unsatisfactory long-term patency rates of 35–50% after 1 year and only 10–32% after 2 years.[7–9] Venous stenoses have relatively high recurrence rates after PTA or may be completely resistant to PTA even if high pressure balloons are used. The failure rates are higher in malignant disease, even without tumor progression, because the external malignant compression causing venous stenoses often preclude a primary effective dilatation.[10,11]

Since the advent of endovascular metal endoprostheses (stents), a new option has become available for patients with venous stenosis or occlusion by pelvic tumor compression. In patients with invasive urological pelvic tumors causing an iliofemoral venous stenosis and an edematous lower extremity, percutaneous endovascular stent placement is a minimally invasive non-surgical alternative for re-establishing venous flow and sustained relief of pain and edema in the lower extremities. The highest success rates have been achieved when local chemical or mechanical thrombolysis, percutaneous transluminal angioplasty (PTA) and stenting were combined. In 1994, Semba and Drake reported very high patency rates at 3 months (92%) after aggressive multi-modal treatment comprising of thrombolysis, PTA and stenting.[12] Recently, additional excellent results have been reported with similar multi-modal treatments.[13] Vascular stenting has also been found to be successful for treating fibrotic stenoses developing after radiotherapy of the pelvic veins.[11] Although the life expectancy of urological patients with pelvic locally invasive malignancies is not long, reports of 1–4 years patency rates for stents placed in pelvic veins in benign disease are encouraging.[14] Such very reasonable patency rates not only allow the patients to continue living with a reasonable quality of life, it also gives hope to some patients who may benefit from additional applications of chemotherapy. Despite these reports, using vascular stents for venous obstruction as a palliation for severe lower extremity edema in experienced hands, is an underused interventional radiological procedure that can ameliorate or ease the suffering of these urologic patients. Such procedures have been described in the literature especially for invasive gynecological tumors but reports on the use of vascular stents in urologic pelvic malignancies are quite rare. We think that patients with urological pelvic malignancy causing iliofemoral venous circulatory difficulties can benefit enormously from this relatively simple procedure.

In the following, we review the use of endovascular stenting of the iliofemoral vein for relieving the obstruction caused by pelvic malignancies, and we emphasize the benefit of this approach in urological pelvic malignancies or scarring developing after pelvic irradiation for urological tumors.

Diagnosis

Radical cystectomy is considered as the most effective local therapy for patients with invasive bladder tumor. Pelvic recurrence of transitional cell carcinoma following radical cystectomy is relatively uncommon (4–18%), but once it occurs, the prognosis is poor. Symptomatic tumoral pelvic venous obstructions despite chemotherapy and/or radiotherapy or because of radiotherapy, can be successfully palliated with endoluminal stenting. Before approaching such a treatment, conducting a proper and systematic diagnostic workup is mandatory.

Pelvic masses are usually symptomatic and detected during evaluation of clinical symptoms. Lower abdominal, pelvic and rectal pain are the most common presenting complaints. These complaints may be associated with genital and lower extremity edema, priapism, constipation, bowel obstruction, and urethral or vaginal bleeding. Venous and lymphatic occlusion due to compression by a pelvic mass results in ipsilateral lower extremity pain, swelling and occasional venous ulceration. An edematous lower extremity in pelvic

urologic tumors is always evaluated for deep vein thrombosis (DVT). Usually, in the absence of DVT, the symptoms may be attributed to lymphedema, and appropriate conservative treatment is initiated without any further evaluation. In such cases, the edema in the lower extremity may not improve with conservative treatment if a proper diagnostic workup is not performed. It is important to consider that urological pelvic tumors, postoperative radiotherapy, and recurrent cancer increase the risk for an underlying venous occlusion in these patients.

Based on the criteria described by Killewich et al. a diagnosis of venous occlusion should be confirmed initially by venous Duplex Ultrasound.[15] Duplex Ultrasound may detect thrombus and identify the patient who may have proximal venous stenosis. It also can detect decreased or absent phasicity of compressed veins. Phasicity is known to be a normal variant in venous blood flow associated with respiration that is consistent with patent proximal vessels.[15,16] The loss of phasicity in the pelvic or proximal lower extremity veins identifies the patient who may have proximal venous occlusion, such patients should undergo further imaging studies. Direct ascending or descending iliofemoral venography is accepted as a 'gold standard' imaging method, but is invasive and better reserved for patients who require intervention. Noninvasive imaging methods, such as computed tomography (CT) venography or magnetic resonance (MR) venography can provide an accurate diagnosis.

Recent implementation of ultrafast multi-detector spiral CT scanners allows non-invasive quick and accurate diagnosis of vascular pathology. An added value of such cross-sectional imaging methods is that of visualization of surrounding tissues and organs, as well as an accurate evaluation of size of the vessel and the extent of vascular pathology. Multi-planar and three-dimensional reconstructions allow accurate sizing of the altered vessel and pre-procedural planning of the stent size required for the proper and successful treatment. MR venography is an evolving technique that can provide useful information as to the extent of venous pathology.

The absence of collateral vessels on venography does not exclude the existence of significant obstruction, and their presence may indicate an obstruction not visualized.[17]

Types of stents

The aim of intravascular stenting is to obtain and maintain lumen patency providing mechanical support to the endoluminal surface of the stenotic or an occluded vein. Two types of vascular stents are available: balloon-expandable and self-expandable. Any vascular stent, balloon- or self-expandable can be used for this purpose. Recently, new generations of covered stents (stent-grafts) have been developed and became available on the market. A special polyester (PET) material covers the same stent and preserves its basic properties. This stent-graft is similar to the surgical graft, but with its own radial force and lumen 'memory'. Recently, a stent-graft (Wallgraft by Boston Scientific) became available on the market (Fig. 70.3). Covered self-expandable stent-grafts are inserted percutaneously. They function as a surgical graft, have substantial radial force to maintain the lumen diameter and can avoid vessel collapse as well as tumor ingrowth. Balloon-expandable stents or stent-grafts have a high radial force during placement, but growing external pressure by the tumor or any accidental extrinsic mechanical pressure can collapse the stent. Once collapsed, such a balloon-expandable stent will never regain its lumen and this will lead to acute occlusion. Self-expandable stents exposed to external pressure or mechanical force regain their shape and lumen instantaneously. Bare stents are subject to tumor ingrowth through the openings between the struts, which will lead to instant reocclusion. When the indication for stent insertion is a malignancy, preference should be given to covered stents (stent-grafts), in order to prevent tumor ingrowth seen with non-covered stents.

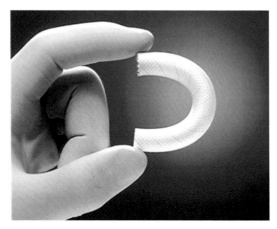

Figure 70.3. *The kink-resistant self-expanding Wallgraft endoprosthesis composed of a 'superalloy' stent body with a polyester (PET) cover material.*

Currently, the Wallgraft is the only self-expandable stent-graft available on the market.

Stent insertion

This is similar to arterial percutaneous transluminal angioplasty (PTA), except that during this procedure the patient is also administered 5000 iu of heparin intravenously.

Ultrasound-guided right internal jugular vein access is used to reach the affected iliofemoral vein segment. If the occluded segment can be passed with a guidewire, the chances for its recanalization by PTA and stenting are good. The obstructed segment is dilated with a PTA balloon catheter before stent insertion, in order to ease the opening of the stent during self-expansion or balloon expansion. If a thrombus is present, a local thrombolysis is initiated using urokinase infusion directly into the thrombus. An alternative procedure is to perform a mechanical thrombectomy using various available percutaneous mechanical thrombectomy systems, such as a Trerotola Percutaneous Thrombectomy Device (PTD Arrow), or a similar one when the thrombus is longstanding. The use of an Inferior Vena Cava (IVC) filter before thrombectomy is not clear-cut. Especially when a thrombolysis is performed there are interventional radiologists who do not deploy a filter and others that do. Our practice is to insert and IVC filter at the end of the procedure.

Stents are placed above the inguinal ligament. In long stenoses more than one stent needs to be inserted to cover the entire length of the compression. In such cases, the stents are placed in-tandem overlapping each other. When stenting iliocaval junction lesions, stents should be inserted well into the inferior vena cava.[17] Occasionally, even self-expanding stents have to be balloon expanded if the stenosis is tight, or there is a rebound after balloon dilatation preventing satisfactory self-expansion. Stent patency and localization is verified at the end of the procedure by venography. Iliofemoral vein stenting gives better results in patients with poorly developed collateral circulation.

Oral warfarin is started the day of the procedure but intravenous heparinization is continued for 2–4 days (800–1000 iu/h). Following stent placement, patients are put on an indefinite warfarin regimen (international normalized ratio; INR 2–3).

Figures 70.4 and 70.5 depict the steps of the entire procedure of thrombectomy, balloon dilatation and stent placement into the iliofemoral vein. In this case, a vana cava filter was deployed before mechanical thrombectomy.

(a)

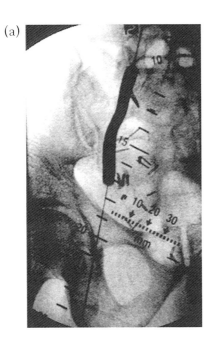

(b)

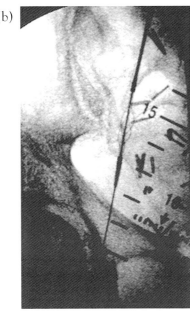

(c)

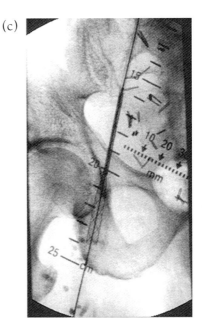

(d)

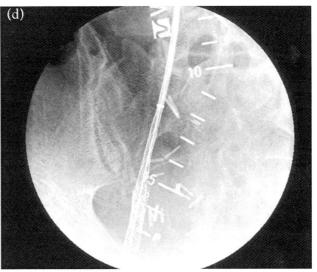

(e)

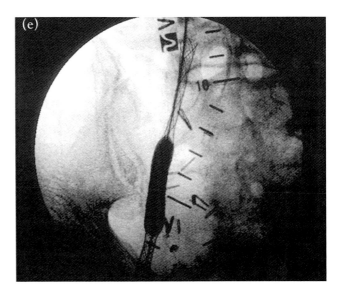

Figure 70.4. *Steps for inserting the stent. (a) balloon dilatation of occlusion; (b) mechanical thrombectomy with Trerotola device; (c) deployment of partially opened stent; (d) deployment of an additional stent in-tandem; (e) balloon dilatation of in-tandem stents.*

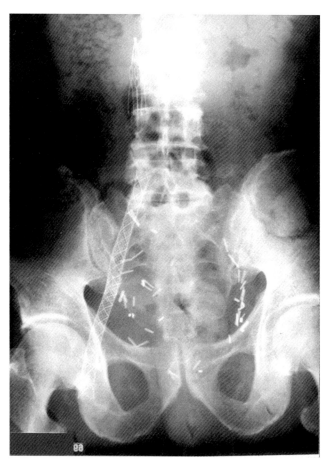

Figure 70.5. *Abdominal X-ray showing the vena cava filter and the iliofemoral in-tandem stents.*

Complications

Most of the periprocedural complications of this procedure are minor and require no additional therapy, but in some cases, the complications may vary from large hematoma formation necessitating blood transfusion, bleeding due to anticoagulant therapy, migration of the stent either proximal or distal to the area of the stenosis or into the inferior vena cava, stent fracture, pulmonary embolism, cardiovascular accident to sepsis and death. Stent migration, after its full expansion, if not caused accidentally by the operator during the procedure is a very rare complication in venous stenting procedures.

Follow-up

Patients are clinically followed monthly for 6 months and then once every 3 months. The follow-up includes measurement of leg and calf circumference and color

duplex flow studies. Stent patency is evaluated with doppler ultrasound at 1 week, then it is reassessed at 1, 3 and 6 months and then at 6 month intervals. In case of reocclusion of the stented segment, a recanalization by thrombus aspiration, thrombolysis (in early occlusions) and thrombectomy is performed. An additional stent may be inserted as a stent-in-stent. In the reported series, patients with a history of malignant disease had more stent occlusions than those with benign disease.[14] These secondary, late reocclusions could be due to the tumor ingrowth into the lumen through the interstices of the stent. Use of stent-grafts can prevent such tumor ingrowth but cannot prevent in-stent clot formation.

Discussion

Patients with urological malignancies may develop stenosis and occlusion of the large pelvic veins. The stenosis and occlusion of the pelvic veins may be due to: metastatic tumor, surgical vascular trauma, fibrosis caused by radiation treatment, or a combination of these factors. The stenosed vessels may cause lower extremity edema, that clinically appears similar to lymphedema. Without any treatment or with a conservative approach, due to the development of collateral circulation, in some patients some improvement in symptoms can occur over time. However, these approaches are time-consuming and add severe mobility limitations to the patient.

Percutaneus insertion of the metallic vascular stent-graft is a novel interventional radiological technique that should be taken into consideration in the management of extrinsically compressed major pelvic veins by urological pelvic tumors. Endovascular stent placement is a non-surgical alternative for re-establishing venous flow and sustained relief of pain and edema of the lower extremities in patients with locally invasive urological pelvic tumors. The stent or stent-graft provides rigidity to the venous wall to counteract the extrinsic compression, regardless of the etiology. The published experience with gynecological and surgical pelvic tumors indicates that satisfactory palliation of iliac vein compression related to local malignancy and scarring related to surgery or radiation therapy can be achieved using endovascular stents. Compared to the conservative management of such a swelling of the lower extremities, the relatively rapid resolution of pain and swelling after stent placement indicates the dramatic effect of restoration of vein patency on symptoms. For patients with malignant disease, the rapid improvement of symptoms after stent placement is necessary in order to experience any palliative effect of the procedure.[14] As well as the subjective well-being reported by the patients, we have observed such a rapid improvement in our invasive bladder cancer patients in whom objective resolution of the edematous extremity could be documented.

Conclusions

The use of vascular stents or stent-grafts is a viable option for urological malignancies involving the iliofemoral veins. Endovascular recanalization of iliac vein occlusion related to local malignancy and/or radiation therapy can be achieved using vascular stents

or stent-grafts. This method is minimally invasive and safe, restores venous return, abolishes the venous engorgement causing severe lower extremity swelling and gives good early results (Fig. 70.6).

Iliac vein stenting is and should be seen as a palliative procedure for tumor compression. It should not preclude a possible definitive approach, such as surgical removal of post-radiotherapy compressing scar tissues, when the patients' life expectancy is long enough.

Despite the initial relatively high cost of this approach, when compared to the total cost of the continuous treatments these patients need (such as physiotherapy, special stockings, medication, frequent hospitalization, loss of working days, etc.) stent-grafts are cost-effective, and provide almost immediate benefit to the patients.

This underused, relatively simple and viable palliative option for reducing the misery of these patients may be used in almost any hospital that has an available trained interventional radiology service.

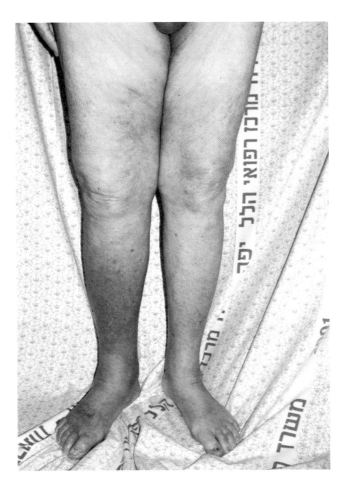

Figure 70.6. *The same patient (see Fig. 70.2) 2 weeks after iliofemoral stenting. Note the reduction of the lower extremity swelling.*

References

1. Ries L A G, Eisner M P, Kosary C L, Hankey B F, Miller B A, Clegg L, Edwards B K (eds). SEER Cancer Statistics Review, 1973–1999. Bethesda, MD: National Cancer Institute, 2002: http://seer.cancer.gov/csr/1973–1999/
2. Hill S L, Martin D, Evans P. Massive vein thrombosis of the extremities. Am J Surg 1989; 158: 131–136
3. Camerota A J. A strategy of aggressive regional therapy for acute iliofemoral venous thrombosis with contemporary venous thrombectomy or catheter-directed thrombolysis. J Vasc Surg 1994; 20: 244–254
4. Sherry S. Thrombolytic therapy for deep vein thrombosis. Semin Intervent Radiol 1985; 4: 331–337
5. Raju S. Experience in venous reconstruction in patients with chronic venous insufficiency. In: Bergan J J, Yao J S T (eds) Venous disorders. Philadelphia: W B Saunders, 1991: 296–305
6. Gloviczski P, Pairolero P C, Toomey B J et al. Reconstruction of large veins for nonmalignant venous occlusive disease. J Vasc Surg 1992; 16: 750–761
7. Hunter D W, Castaneda-Zuniga W R, Coleman C C et al. Failing arteriovenous dialysis fistulas: Evaluation and treatment. Radiology 1984; 152: 631–635
8. Wilms G, Baert A L, Nevelsteen et al. Balloon angioplasty of venous strictures. Journal Belge de Radiologie 1989; 72: 273–277
9. Glanz S. Dialysis fistula stenosis. Treatment by angioplasty. In Kadir S (ed) Current practice of interventional radiology. Philadelphia: Decker, 1991: 280–287
10. Marache P, Asserman P, Jabinet J L et al. Percutaneous transluminal venous angioplasty in occlusive iliac venous thrombosis resistant to thrombolysis. Am Heart J 1993; 125: 362–366
11. Zollikofer C L, Antonucci F, Stuckman G et al. Use of the Wallstent in the venous system including hemodialysis-related stenoses. Cardiovasc Intervent Radiol 1992; 15: 334–341

12. Semba C P, Dake M D. Iliofemoral deep venous thrombosis: aggressive therapy with catheter-directed thrombolysis. Radiology 1994; 191: 487–494

13. AbuRahma A F, Perkins S E, Wulu J T, Ng H K. Iliofemoral deep vein thrombosis: Conventional therapy versus lysis and percutaneous transluminal angioplasty and stenting. Ann Surg 2001; 233: 752–760

14. Nazarian G K, Bjarnason M D, Dietz C A Jr. et al. Iliofemoral venous stenoses: Effectiveness of treatment with metallic endovascular stents. Radiology 1996; 200: 193–199

15. Killewich L A, Bedford R G, Beach K W, Strandness D E. Diagnosis of deep vein thrombosis: A prospective study comparing duplex scanning to contrast venography. Circulation 1989; 79: 810–814

16. Burbidge S J, Finlay D E, Letourneau J G, Longley D G. Effects of central venous catheter placement on upper extremity duplex findings. J Vasc Intervent Radiol 1993; 4: 399–404

17. Neglen P, Raju S. Balloon dilatation and stenting of chronic iliac vein obstruction: technical aspects and early clinical outcome. J Endovasc Ther 2000; 7: 79–91

The future

XI

71

Extra-anatomical urinary diversion
P. J. Paterson

Introduction

It is not uncommon for patients with advanced or recurrent intra-abdominal malignancy to develop obstructive renal failure. The decision to treat or not to treat is sometimes difficult, and quality-of-life assessment is paramount; the wishes of the patient and relatives are of prime importance. However, in the case of previously untreated disease or slowly progressive recurrence, where the patient has not had the opportunity of receiving all available therapeutic modalities, the decision is easy: the majority of urologists would treat the renal failure by some form of drainage.

After initial decompression by nephrostomy it is usually possible to pass a ureteric stent in either an antegrade or retrograde fashion. 'Usually' is not 'always' and in a small minority of patients the ureter is either completely occluded or so deformed that the intraluminal passage of a stent is impossible. In this situation the standard management has historically been long-term nephrostomy. This is not without its problems: tubes become infected or dislodged and the patient has to bear an external appliance. Although some patients are content with this treatment, others feel that their quality of life would be better if they were able to void naturally. It is to meet this need that the concept of extra-anatomical stenting to channel the urine from the kidney to the bladder has developed.

The problem was first addressed by Ahmadzadeh[1] in a group of eight patients with prostatic cancer. He devised a system whereby a fine-bore tube was placed percutaneously in the kidney, tunnelled subcutaneously via the iliac fossa and inserted into the bladder in the manner of a suprapubic catheter. Initial results were encouraging and, significantly, no patient suffered as a result of urine leak into the subcutaneous tissues. Indeed, significant complications were notable by their absence. The Glasgow group[2] modified his technique to make stent insertion and replacement easier, leading to the production of the 'Paterson–Forrester' stent by Cook Urological Inc., Spencer, IN, USA (Figs. 71.1–71.2).

The same problem was considered by Desgrandchamps[3] of Le Duc's unit in Paris. He used a modified vascular graft that took the same route in 13 patients, again with excellent results.

There would seem to be advantages and disadvantages to these two methods, the fine bore and the large bore (see Table 71.1). It must be emphasized that this comparison is purely speculative, as the author's experience is restricted to the fine-bore stent.

The wide-bore tube should not, and to date has not, need to be changed. However, in the event of the (as yet unreported) event of occlusion it cannot be changed — it has the advantages and disadvantages of a 'once and for all' procedure. The converse is true of the fine-bore tube.

Table 71.1. *Advantages and disadvantages of fine-bore and wide-bore stents for extra-anatomical urinary diversion*

Type	Advantage	Disadvantage
Fine bore (Ahmadzadeh Lingham)	Easy to insert	Needs to be changed at intervals of about 6 months
	Easy to change	
Wide bore (Desgrandchamps)	Does not need to be changed	More difficult to insert
	Can be converted to 'anterior cutaneous nephrostomy'	

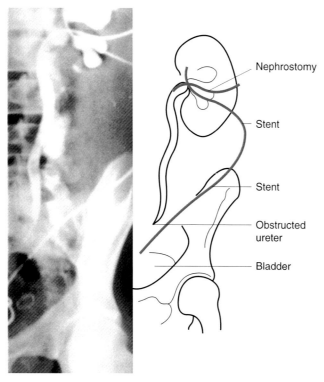

Figure 71.1. *Subcutaneous stent bypassing a completely obstructed ureter.*

Whatever the advantages and disadvantages of the two different methods may be, both offer the potential of a significant improvement of lifestyle when compared with long-term nephrostomy.

Operative technique

The author's experience is entirely with the fine-bore Paterson–Forrester stent. The principle, if not the details, of insertion of the wide-bore stent are similar.

Stent insertion (Figs. 71.1 and 71.2)
This technique is not suitable for emergency decompression of the uraemic patient — initial management should be with one or two nephrostomies, depending on the ultrasonic appearance of the kidneys.

Prior to surgery the patient is given a therapeutic dose of antibiotic as determined by culture. Antibiotic cover is continued for 24 hours.

Although the operation is minimally invasive the operative area is large, extending from the loin to the urethra; the author therefore prefers to use general anaesthesia. Muscle relaxation is not required.

Initially, the patient is placed in a prone position. The kidney is visualized radiologically using contrast instilled via the existing nephrostomy. A new puncture is made into the lower calyx with the skin entry site more infrolateral than usual. Following guidewire insertion the track is dilated until it is possible to introduce a modified vascular dilator and sheath — in effect a 'mini-Amplatz' — into the pelvis. The specially designed drainage tube is passed over the guidewire via the sheath, its position checked and the sheath and guidewire withdrawn. The tube is secured to the skin by a temporary suture to prevent accidental displacement.

A small incision is made above the iliac crest as far anteriorly as possible (the patient is still face down). The dilator and sheath are now tunnelled from the nephrostomy site to this new incision, using a combination of the dilator itself, scissors and blunt finger dissection. The stent is now passed down the sheath so that it also emerges at the new incision. The temporary suture is cut and the nephrostomy site sutured. A second holding suture is used to provide stent stability.

The patient is turned supine and placed in the lithotomy position. A third small incision is made near

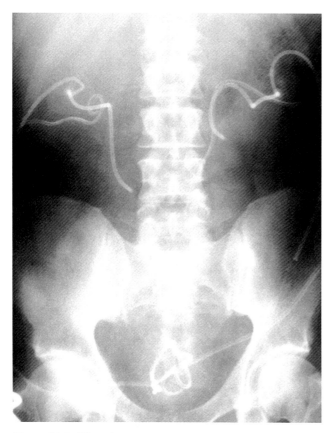

Figure 71.2. *Bilateral stents.*

the anterior superior spine and the stent brought to this, using the same method; finally, the stent is made to emerge from a small midline suprapubic incision. The route taken by the stent may have to be varied if the patient has a stoma, but this in no way contraindicates the procedure. If a bilateral procedure is used, both stents come together at this single wound.

The patient is subjected to cystoscopy and the bladder distended. A trochar with a peel-away sheath is passed from the suprapubic incision into the bladder using both manual and endoscopic guidance. The precise site of entry into the bladder does not seem important. The tube is passed down the sheath and into the bladder, the peel-away sheath is peeled away, and all the remaining skin incisions are sutured.

A urethral catheter is inserted and left on free drainage for at least 24 hours.

Stent replacement

Initially, the author electively changed the stent every 3 months, but later experience suggests that these stents remain patent for at least 6 months.

The author's routine is to perform stent exchange with the patient under general anaesthesia. Positioning of the patient is dependent on whether one or two stents require to be replaced and on the sex of the patient. Unilateral stents in males can be changed with the patient in a lateral position as this provides good access to the loin and also allows introduction of a flexible cystoscope. If the stents are bilateral, or the patient female, s/he is first placed prone and later rotated into lithotomy position. In all cases, appropriate antibiotic cover is used.

A small incision is made in the loin, over the stent, which can be easily palpated. The incision is deepened using diathermy until about 2 cm of the stent are exposed. It is interesting to note that the stent is usually surrounded by a pseudo-capsule.

The stent is cross-clamped with two small haemostats, to prevent spillage of potentially infected urine, and divided. The two ends are secured with fine sutures to prevent retraction into the tissues.

Attention is first directed to the upper segment. A guidewire is passed into the kidney under radiological screening. It is not usually necessary to opacify the kidney. The upper part of the old stent is extracted. Small dilators are used to widen the track and to allow insertion of the modified vascular dilator and sheath. The upper end of the new stent is passed over the guidewire into the renal pelvis, and the sheath is withdrawn. The stent is temporarily secured to the skin with a suture.

A second guidewire is passed down the lower portion of the old stent into the bladder, from whence it is retrieved with the cystoscope and withdrawn from the external meatus. The old stent is removed via the loin incision. While the guidewire is held under moderate tension, a dilator is passed over it and so comes to lie with its tapered end in the loin wound and the other end external to the urethra. Provided that the wire is not allowed to kink, this manoeuvre is surprisingly easy.

The lower end of the new stent is fed over the wire and locked to the dilator. Initially this was achieved by simply forcing the end of the dilator into the stent — the Cook stent provides a customized locking device. The dilator is eased out of the urethra and simultaneously the stent is fed from above into the pseudo-capsule that has formed around the old stent. It is important to ensure that the renal end of the stent is not dislodged at this stage.

When the stent–dilator connection emerges at the meatus the stent is freed, the dilator discarded and the guidewire withdrawn. The bladder end of the stent is placed in the bladder under cystoscopic control.

The incision is closed using an absorbable suture.

Patients and results

This technique is in its infancy and the published data refer to a total of 27 patients treated in three centres (see Table 71.2). All had terminal disease and, clearly, long-term survival is not to be expected; however, good medium-term palliation can be achieved. One of Ahamadzadeh's patients was reported as surviving 30 months (it is unclear whether he was still alive at the time that the seminal paper was published); one of the author's small group lived 24 months after initiation of treatment, and Desgrandchamps reported survival figures ranging from 2 to 16 months.

Complications are surprisingly few and are restricted to short-term urine leakage from the suprapubic incision in one of the Glasgow patients.

Urine leak into the subcutaneous tissues with subsequent cellulitis has not been recorded to date. The

Table 71.2. *Data from published series (three centres) relating to extra-anatomical urinary diversion*

Organ[*]	Desgrandchamps[3]	Series Ahmadzadeh[1]	Lingham[2]
Prostate	4	8	
Colon	2		3
Ovary	2		
Breast	2		
Lymphoma	1		
Body of uterus			1
RPF[†]			1
Cervix	3		

[*]Site of primary malignancy;

[†]RPF = retroperitoneal fibrosis (the patient refused laparotomy).

reason for this must be speculative but the presence of the previously inserted nephrostomy and a urethral catheter, together with the proximity of the stent to skin suture lines, suggests that the line of least resistance for extravasated urine is outwards rather than inwards. Urine will leak onto the dressings rather than force its way through the tissues.

It is interesting to note that work in Israel on experimental dogs, who had neither nephrostomy nor catheter, confirmed that infection of the track is not a problem.[4]

Colostomy is not a contraindication — three of the Glasgow patients and three of the patients treated in Paris had stomata.

The technique is not universally applicable. Desgrandchamps was unable to place a stent satisfactorily in one patient, and the author has declined to operate in the case of a patient with a large incisional hernia involving the projected route of the tube.

Involvement of the bladder in the disease process is a relative contraindication as haematuria leads to clot adherent to the stent and thus occlusion. In this group

of patients the bladder may be initially free from tumour and become involved later in the disease process; this calls for a change of plan.

A small post-radiotherapy bladder is not a contraindication even if the patient requires a urethral catheter. One of the author's patients fell into this group and stated that he found a catheter easier to live with than a nephrostomy as he was able to sleep more comfortably.

Conclusions

Subcutaneous urinary diversion with an extra-anatomical stent provides effective and safe pyelovesical drainage of urine and allows patients with bilateral complete ureteric obstruction to void normally.

Many of these patients have a surprisingly long life expectancy, and quality of life during their terminal illness can be significantly improved by this technique.

The increasing ingenuity of stent manufacturers and inserters allows the majority of patients to be treated with conventional intraluminal stents. Where this is impossible, consideration should be given to subcutaneous diversion rather than leaving the patient with a long-term nephrostomy with its inherent problems.

References

1. Ahmadzadeh M. Clinical experience with subcutaneous urinary diversion: new approach using a double pigtail stent. Br J Urol 1991; 67(6): 596–599
2. Lingham K, Paterson P J, Lingham M K et al. Subcutaneous urinary diversion: an alternative to nephrostomy. J Urol 1994; 152(1): 70–72
3. Desgrandchamps F, Cussenot O, Meria P et al. Subcutaneous urinary diversions for palliative treatment of pelvic malignancies. J Urol 1995; 154(2pt1): 367–370
4. Greenstein A, Koontz W W Jr. Subcutaneous ureteral replacement — a dog model. First International Symposium on Urological Stents. Jerusalem, 27–31 October 1996: abstr O10.6

72

Polymeric endoluminal paving: local endo-urological polymer systems for support, barrier creation and site-specific drug delivery
M. J. Slepian

Introduction

For over two decades stents have been utilized in urology. Early stents were largely temporary implant devices fabricated from rubber or plastic for use in the upper urinary tract. These stents were non-wall-contacting devices, free floating in the lumen, to ensure continued urinary flow and prevent lumen compromise. More recently, metal stents, based on designs originally developed for the vascular system, have been utilized in the urinary tract. These implants have been temporary or permanent, providing direct wall support as well as functioning as moulds to facilitate lumen healing and urinary tract remodelling following endo-urological intervention. As the use of an increasingly wide variety of stents finds clinical application in urology, limitations of current stent designs emerge.

Current urological stents, while effective in generically providing lumen patency for the maintenance of urine flow, have several limitations. Limitations of current stents include incomplete expansion, poor luminal wall apposition, migration, poor wall support, progressive recoil and mechanical collapse, encrustation, infection, obstruction, lumen injury, patient discomfort and progressive epithelial thickening. As such, if stents are to assume an increasing role in the management of a multitude of urologic conditions, improved stents or alternative stenting methods, allowing for more predictable implant deployment, improved wall support, reduced fouling, encrustation and late epithelial thickening are needed.

In 1988, a generic method in which biodegradable structural polymers could be locally deployed on the endoluminal surface of tissue lumens was developed as an alternative to conventional stenting. Using this method solid, gel and liquid polymer systems have been applied to endoluminal surfaces as adherent conformal tubular thin films. This process of tissue resurfacing with polymers was termed 'polymeric endoluminal paving and sealing'. The vision behind this method was that local polymer liner layers might serve as endoluminal supports, barriers and depots for sustained drug delivery.

Since 1988 significant progress has been made in the development of this method, with numerous studies in the vascular tree demonstrating implant success, long-term patency, local barrier creation and long-term sustained drug delivery.

Recently, polymer paving has been examined as a method for endo-urological application. Pilot studies suggest that local mould-in-place polymer systems may be readily deployed providing effective endoluminal structural support in the urethra. In this chapter the potential utility of polymer paving for endo-urological applications is discussed. Four questions are addressed: what are the limitations of conventional stents in the genitourinary (GU) tract; what is polymer paving; in what forms might paving be implemented in the GU tract; and how might paving address specific limitations of endo-urological stenting?

What are the limitations of current endo-urological stents?

Despite the rapid growth in the use of both intraluminal and endoluminal urologic stents, as currently designed they suffer from several significant limitations. These limitations have hampered both the short- and long-term success of endo-urological stenting. Specific limitations of urologic stents, which in the future may be overcome utilizing a paving approach, are outlined below and summarized in Table 72.1.

Incomplete expansion
Incomplete expansion is a problem for endoluminal metal stents. This is particularly a problem with balloon-expandable rather than self-expanding designs. Balloon-expandable stents fabricated out of medical-grade stainless steel require adequate expansile force to achieve complete opening and seating of the stent. Incomplete expansion may result from inadequate inflation pressure, balloon rupture during deployment, presence of an endoluminal non-compliant lesion, such as a stone or fibrous non-compliant lesion, or stent

Table 72.1. *Limitations of endo-urological stents*

Incomplete expansion
Poor luminal wall apposition
Migration
Poor wall support
Progressive recoil and mechanical collapse (stent crush)
Biofouling
Encrustation
Infection
Obstruction
Ureteral injury
Urethral injury
Stent discomfort
Progressive epithelial thickening with lumen compromise

slippage on the balloon catheter resulting in dilatation of only a segment of the stent. Incompletely expanded stents are at increased risk for migration. Further, inadequate expansion may ultimately compromise long-term urinary flow and stent patency.

Poor luminal wall apposition

Inadequate contact of the stent with the endoluminal wall is a limitation of current endoluminal metallic stents. This may occur as a result of inadequate expansion, as outlined above, or as a result of endo-urological anatomic constraints. The three-dimensional endoluminal topography of the GU tract, particularly the trans-prostatic urethra, is complex in shape. Ng, using three-dimensional ultrasonography, demonstrated that the prostatic urethra has a triangular cross-sectional configuration.[2] In addition to a non-circular cross-sectional profile, in the longitudinal axis the urethra is tortuous. The net effect of this architecture is a complex shape to which an endoluminal stent must accommodate. Current permanent metal urologic stents are derived from endovascular designs. As such, they are simple tubular forms that tend to expand and stabilize in a simple cylindrical shape. To date a stent specifically designed for complex endo-urological topographies has not been constructed.

Beyond being geometrically incomplete, poor wall apposition has potential biological consequences. With poor wall contact the possibility of stent migration is increased. Further, point contact with the endoluminal surface rather than uniform conformal contact creates points of increased wall stress and continuous irritation.

This may result in enhanced urothelial hypertrophy and thickening, which may compromise urine flow. In addition, incomplete wall contact creates gaps and voids between the extraluminal surface of the stent and the underlying tissue wall. These gaps prevent the stent wires from becoming effectively covered and passivated by epithelium. As such, these surfaces, as outlined below, may become fouled with biofilm and encrustations leading to infection.

Migration

Stent migration is a problem for both intraluminal and endoluminal stents. Intraluminal internal double-J stents and external endopyelotomy stents have been reported to migrate. Internal endopyelotomy stents have been reported to migrate out through the ureteropelvic junction incision, resulting in gross urinary extravasation into the retroperitoneum.[3] Migration of these stents also leaves the critical ureteral incision site unstented, resulting in subsequent surgical failure. External ureteral stents have been reported to migrate and need repositioning in 14% of cases.[4]

Stent migration has been observed for metallic endoluminal stents as well.[5,6] Stent migration may result in either urinary retention or urinary incontinence, depending upon the position of migration.

Poor wall support

Several of the current stent designs provide only limited wall support. Polymeric and rubber stents, by design, provide only limited wall support. These devices are typically only partially wall contacting and function largely as transluminal bridge devices, facilitating urinary flow in and around their perimeter. The majority of expandable metal designs typically open to a circular cross-sectional profile. As outlined above, the prostatic urethra has been demonstrated to have a non-circular cross-sectional profile. As such, a circular implant device provides only limited points of wall contact and support. Beyond this geometric limitation, several stent designs, such as the Urolume, Ultraflex and Memotherm, are self-expanding, exerting less outward force on the tissue wall for support.

Progressive recoil and mechanical collapse (stent crush)

Progressive narrowing of luminal calibre leading to collapse is a potential problem of several current stent designs. The greatest likelihood for this exists with self-expanding metal stents. These designs have lower hoop strength and crush resistance than balloon-expandable stents, affording a lower level of wall support. In cases of extrinsic compression and fibrosis, these self-expanding stent designs are at greater risk for collapse. Beyond this slow progressive stent collapse, traumatic stent crush may occur with expandable metal stents in the urinary tract in anatomical locations exposed to external mechanical compression. For example, expandable metal stents in the bulbar urethra have been found to crush in cases where patients have been bicycle and horseback riding.

Biofouling

Immediately following stent implantation, stent surfaces become progressively covered with proteinaceous material, cellular and extracellular debris present in the urine flowing over them.[7,8] This film may become progressively complex with time. As such, this film may serve as a soil for bacterial contamination, leading to urinary tract infection and bacteraemia.[9] Conversely, early stent-surface bacterial colonization may lead to further biofouling and biofilm accumulation. Progressive fouling may ultimately lead to lumen compromise, with decreased urinary flow.

Encrustation

Following early biofouling of stent surfaces, elemental deposition from urine may occur. Progressive deposition and crystal formation involving calcium, magnesium and phosphorous salts may lead to eventual crystalline build-up or 'encrustation' of the stent surface.[8,10,11] If this process continues, on chronically implanted devices it may lead to significant thickening with eventual urinary flow reduction. Further, an encrusted implant surface is a supportive surface for bacterial colonization. As outlined above, this may increase morbidity as a result of urinary tract infection and bacteraemia.

Infection

Infection is a complication associated with both intraluminal and endoluminal stents. Biofilm formation and encrustation of a stent surface provides a rich supportive environment for bacterial colonization.[8,9,12,13] Progressive bacterial overgrowth may lead to embolization and infection of the urinary tract and possible spillover bacteraemia. Surface colonization may amplify the propensity for further superinfection. Entrenched colonization of a biofilm layer on an implant is extremely difficult to eradicate with antibiotics or antibacterials.[14] Progression to clinical infection often requires device removal.

Obstruction

In the most extreme form of fouling, endo-urological stents may become obstructed. In the acute setting (e.g. after deployment following endopyelotomy), partial or complete obstruction with accompanying fevers was noted in up to 64% of cases.[15] This type of acute obstruction was commonly due to procedure-related blood clots. More chronically, obstruction may be due to severe calcification and stones. In addition to endoluminal obstruction, stent narrowing may result from progressive wall thickening as a result of urothelial thickening.[16]

Ureteral injury

Expansion of constrained stents in the urinary tract may be associated with urothelial and deeper-layer injury. Care must be taken during deployment to avoid overdilatation and deep injury. In addition to expansion injury, damage related to the anatomical location of stent deployment may occur. Early experimental studies examining metal self-expanding stents in the ureter revealed evidence of interruption of ureteral peristaltic flow. As such, long segments in the ureter should not be bridged with metal wall-contacting stents as they induce hydro-ureter.

Urethral injury

Damage to underlying intact epithelium may occur, particularly with deployment of expandable metal stents. Significant lumen denudation is associated with a higher incidence of bacterial colonization and urinary tract infection. Further, extensive denudation and injury in the peristent zone, associated with stent deployment or removal, may itself lead to stricturing of the urethra.

Stent discomfort

This complication is particular to endo-urological stents. Stents have been noted to cause perineal pain, painful intercourse and continuous 'foreign body' feeling in the genitalia. Ureteral stents have been associated with irritative bladder symptoms.

Progressive epithelial thickening with lumen compromise

Progressive intimal or epithelial thickening is a complication associated with metal endoluminal stents. This complication is a generic one, in that progressive build-up of a pseudointimal or epithelial layer is seen in most lumina in which metallic wall-contacting endoprostheses are placed. In blood vessels this is a particular problem, resulting in pseudointimal thickening known as progressive restenosis.[17,18] For endo-urological devices thickening has been reported, particularly in the urethra, in that placing a stent in contact with skin in the setting of urethral reconstruction results in a very aggressive hypertrophic reaction.[19]

What is polymer paving?

Generic description of the paving process

Polymeric endoluminal paving, in its generic form, is a process in which biocompatible polymers may be applied percutaneously, through a catheter, to the endoluminal surface of hollow tubular organs, organ components or artificially created tissue tracts, forming layers of polymer coating in intimate contact with the underlying tissue surface. This 'tissue re-surfacing' process has been termed 'paving'.[20,21] The initial therapeutic target for paving was the arterial endoluminal surface. Extending beyond vascular applications, endoluminal surfaces of other hollow organ systems (i.e. the GU tract — kidney, ureter, bladder, prostate and urethra) that are amenable to catheter-based polymer application are also potential therapeutic targets for paving.

Generic functional role and advantages of paving

Locally applied polymer coatings, i.e. paving layers, have been developed to provide three broad classes of therapeutic function to the target organ or tissue surface. Paving layers may function as (a) wall or tissue supports, (b) as barriers and/or (c) as local depots for sustained release or retention of therapeutic pharmacological, biochemical or cellular elements.

As a wall support, paving, via local polymer flow into surface irregularities, offers an advantage, relative to stenting, of custom moulding to accommodate irregularities in the underlying surface. Uniformly applied polymer coatings also provide for more symmetrical distribution of wall stress than stents. Different regional polymer thicknesses or compositions provide the ability to vary compliance of the polymer support layer as well. Further, polymers offer surface and interface advantages. These advantages include the ability to provide enhanced surface texture, i.e. smoothness for improved blood flow, or surfaces readily modifiable for improved tissue compatibility to limit surface deposition or thrombosis.

As a barrier, paving offers a unique therapeutic intervention not provided by metal stenting. An applied polymer film can function as a synthetically interposed tissue barrier. This barrier may be utilized to limit underlying tissue exposure to overflowing cellular, microbial or endocrine elements, to prevent tissue ingrowth and to restore natural barrier functions compromised by disease or therapeutic processes. For example, following arterial angioplasty, the de-endothelialized endoluminal surface is highly thrombogenic. Application of thin polymer layers to thrombogenic arterial subintima have been demonstrated to prevent adhesion of platelets to the surface and local thrombosis, mechanically and non-pharmacologically.[22–25]

An additional advantage of paving — and perhaps its most significant — lies in its ability to serve as a local depot for sustained drug or other therapeutic delivery. Drug delivery via adherent endoluminal polymers offers several therapeutic advantages. Local application of a drug via resident polymer affords concentrated delivery of the drug, achieving tissue levels not otherwise attainable. As drug release occurs via diffusion or erosion of the polymer — a time-dependent process — delivery to the target site will be sustained for days to weeks or beyond, depending on the specific characteristics of the polymer utilized. Further, local delivery reduces systemic drug exposure, thereby limiting systemic side effects. Polymer-based systems also allow delivery of agents that might otherwise be difficult or impossible to deliver via oral or intravenous routes owing to problems of solubility or formulation. This method of drug administration also provides the possibility of utilizing agents which might not otherwise be administrable because of dosage range or toxicity limitations encountered with conventional routes of administration. Further, locally applied polymer systems may serve as depots for entrapped or encapsulated biological or cellular elements that may augment or replace diseased organ function.

Three forms of paving

Polymer paving, in its current state of development, may be thought of as a family of therapeutic approaches. Depending upon the choice of polymer system utilized as the substrate for paving, a variety of physical types of endoluminal paving layers may be formed. As such, utilizing materials of differing consistencies raises the possibility of different types of therapeutic effects and duration of polymers at the site of application. Specifically, three forms of polymer paving have been devised and demonstrated to date, including solid paving, gel paving and liquid paving.

Solid paving

'Solid' or 'structural' paving was the initial form of paving to be demonstrated experimentally.[1,19] In this form, thin tubes or sheets of biodegradable polymer are transported intravascularly or intraluminally via catheter, positioned at the desired deployment site and locally remoulded by catheter-based thermoforming. As opposed to stenting, which relies on either the inherent expansile tendency of a constrained stent (i.e. self-expanding stents) or active mechanical deployment or expansion (i.e. balloon-expanding stents), solid paving relies on catheter-based mechanical deformation combined with controlled-phase changes of the polymer material, typically through a local heating and cooling process. Advantage is taken of the thermoplastic nature of several biodegradable, biocompatible polymers, copolymers or blends, in that localized, simultaneous polymer heating and moulding permits the polymer substrate to flow and conform to the irregularities and interstices frequently encountered in many endoluminal surfaces while maintaining a balloon-determined smooth luminal surface. Further, by premodifying the polymer substrate with fenestrations, the flow can be 'directed', to create predetermined forms. The resultant polymer liner may have partially open walls or be a continuous barrier layer of specific permeability. Solid paving, of all the paving forms discussed herein, offers the broadest therapeutic potential, including endoluminal wall support, physical barrier imposition and localized, sustained, intraluminal drug delivery.

To appreciate more fully the process of polymer paving, sequential photographs, taken during an early polymer deployment experiment in a 'mock' urethral lumen, are presented in Figure 72.1. the intraluminal melt–flow thermoforming of the polymer substrate that takes place within a tissue tract can be more clearly appreciated from Figure 72.2, with a pre-deployed polymer paving layer on the left (in this instance with minimal fenestrations) and a post-deployed polymer on the right. Of note, with pressure-directed flow, the bulk polymer is reconfigured with the development of macroporous regions in the polymer surface (Fig. 72.2, right seal). In addition, while the external configuration of the polymer layer on the right appears somewhat irregular, as it has been contoured as a 'relief' of the underlying tissue surface, its internal surface is smooth.

The conformal nature of an endoluminal paving layer may be appreciated from stereomicroscopic and histological cross-sections of a paved bovine coronary artery (Fig. 72.3). In this case, a solid sheet of poly(ϵ-caprolactone) was applied to the endoluminal surface of a bovine coronary artery. The polymer possesses adequate structural stability to maintain the vessel in a overdistended configuration (Fig. 72.3). The applied polymer is seen as a wavy, refractile layer, in intimate contact with the endoluminal surface of the vessel (Fig. 72.4). Of note, the architecture of the vessel wall underlying the paved zone is preserved with an intact media, despite application of the paving layer.

Recently, a new solid paving system has been developed that achieves local polymer melting and flow through a thermoselective approach.[25,26] In this system a photosensitive dye is incorporated within the polymer films to be deployed. The polymer film is then illuminated via a fibre-optic catheter, with light at a specific wavelength chosen to achieve maximum light absorbance by the dye. This intense energy absorbance by the dye results in local conversion of light to heat, resulting in polymer melting (Fig. 72.5). Through selection of a dye-illumination wavelength combination in the near infrared, with absorbance characteristics distinctly different from those of tissue, illumination results in transmission of light through tissue with minimal tissue photothermal heating.[27] Utilizing this system, local, sustained, intraluminal drug delivery has recently been demonstrated.[28]

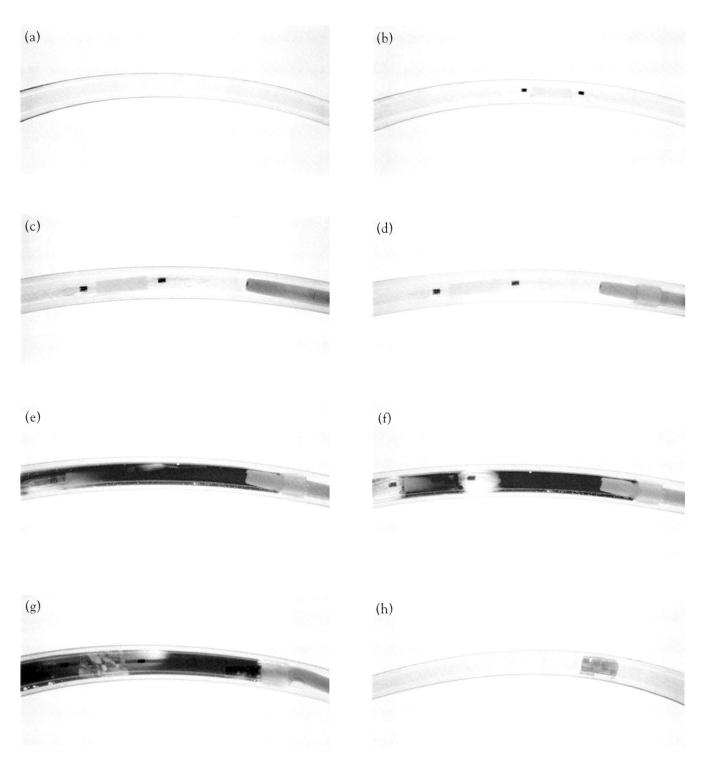

Figure 72.1. *In vitro solid 'structural' paving in a transparent mock urethra. (a) Mock urethra; (b) tubular polymer substrate positioned at desired location within the urethra on a balloon deployment catheter; (c) distal, balloon occlusion catheter placed. Balloon deflated; (d) occlusion catheter with balloon inflated to create a stagnant column of urine around the polymer substrate; (e) heated saline (60°C), in red, is injected via an infusion port to create a column of hot saline surrounding the polymer to facilitate an instant polymer melt; (f) polymer remains in its original form after being surrounded by hot fluid until a mild radial dilating force is exerted by the deployment balloon with resultant progressive expansion; (g) further balloon expanison results in pressure-directed polymer flow forming a lumen encasing 'polymer paving layer', with the external polymer surface geometry being dictated by the shape of the urethral wall, while the new intraluminal surface is smooth; (h) following deflation of the distal flow occlusion balloon, with return of urine flow or operator-directed cool fluid flushing, the polymer paving layer achieves increased mechanical stability. Upon removal of the deployment catheter the applied polymer is left intact with the urethra locally 'paved'.*

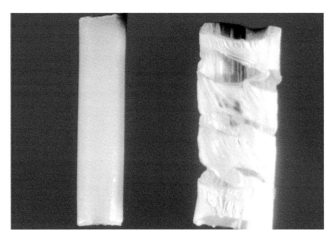

Figure 72.2. *Pre-deployed tube of polymer for structural paving with microscopic fenestrations (left). Expanded, post-deployed tubular polymer paving layer removed from tissue lumen (right). Note development of open regions, engineered to occur in this case.*

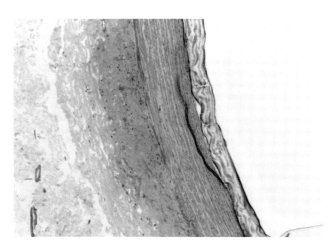

Figure 72.4. *Paved normal bovine coronary artery in cross section (× 100). Paving layer of poly (ε-caprolactone) is visible in intimate contact with the underlying arterial wall. Arterial wall architecture is preserved, with an intact media and adventitia, despite polymer application.*

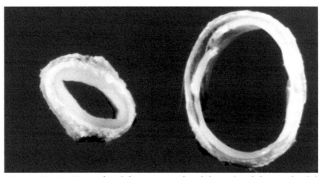

Figure 72.3. *Example of the structural stability of endoluminal solid paving layer. Baseline bovine coronary artery (left). Contiguous segment of identical bovine coronary artery dilated and paved at a balloon: artery ratio of >2:1. Note a thin endoluminal polymer paving layer supports the vessel wall, resisting recoil and collapse, despite the significant over-dilatation.*

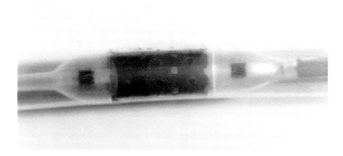

Figure 72.5. *Photothermal solid paving catheter. Note pre-deployed, fenestrated, dye-containing poly (ε-caprolactone) paving thin film on central deployment balloon. Illuminated (red) central fiber optic may be seen.*

Gel paving

Apart from using solid or structural polymers as substrates for paving, the use of polymeric hydrogel or colloidal systems as the applied polymeric material forms the basis for the second form of paving that has been developed — gel paving.[22–24,29,30] Hydrogel polymer systems provide the ability to create in situ short-term, non-structural physical barrier layers that are (a) permeable to fluid, gases and low-molecular-weight solutes, (b) exclusionary of larger-molecular-weight compounds and physically limiting of cell–cell and cell–matrix interactions with the underlying tissue surface. The therapeutic motivation for the development of this form of paving arose in the vascular field from attempts to develop a physical (i.e. non-pharmacological) method of preventing or limiting early interactions between blood and arterial subintima exposed as a result of interventional procedures such as balloon angioplasty. Early blood–tissue interactions, particularly within an injured artery or tissue tract, play an essential role in localized thrombosis and the development of subsequent arterial-wall thickening or tissue-tract narrowing.[31,32] Through the use of polymeric hydrogel or colloidal materials as the substrate for paving, short-term, 'bandage-like', semipermeable endoluminal barriers could be created transiently on a tissue surface — i.e. for days to weeks, more briefly than would be possible with more rigid solid paving systems, which typically take months to be biodegraded. These types of materials also allow the creation of either thin or thick polymer barriers, depending upon the particular indication, chemistry and mode of application of the gel system selected. Gel systems afford an advantage in that, depending upon the particular gel chemistry utilized, they may be either biodegraded by bond cleavage or bioeroded through dissolution or physical thinning. This type of paving may also be utilized as a means of localized drug delivery, although it is typically of shorter duration than that achievable with solid paving. The gel paving process is illustrated in Figure 72.6 in a series of photographs taken during an in vitro gel paving experiment.

Several catheter systems have been designed for localized in situ formation of both thin and thick hydrogel paving layers. The catheter systems vary, depending upon the nature of the flowable material utilized for hydrogel formation as well as the chemical or physical means utilized to convert the pre-gel constituents to a gel locally. Recently, a novel gel-paving catheter system with a contained fibre-optic illuminating element has been developed, allowing for in situ photopolymerization of polyethylene-glycol-lactide thin hydrogel paving layers.[29]

Liquid paving

The third form of paving — 'liquid paving' — involves the use of flowable, polymeric, macromeric or pre-polymeric solutions that have varying levels of avidity for the underlying tissue surface. Interactions may range from non-specific (i.e. weak van der Waals, electrostatic or hydrogen bonding) types to more specific receptor–ligand interactions or potentially to locally formed, covalent interactions. Interactions may also occur due to physical intercalation or trapping. When fluids for liquid paving

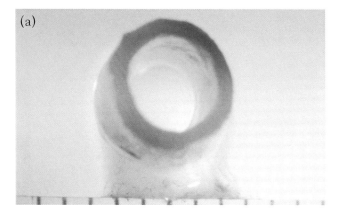
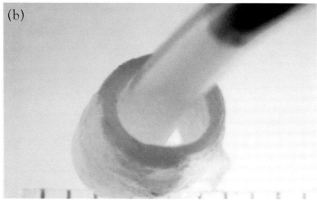
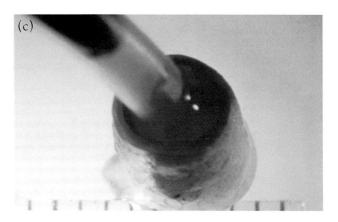
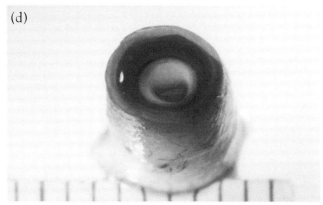

Figure 72.6. *In vitro gel paving with a thermoreversible hydrogel paving system. (a) Bovine coronary artery segment in cross-section; (b) catheter positioned in artery lumen to act as a 'mold-core'; (c) liquid polymer is instilled and fills cavity of 'mold'. The walls of the mold are defined by the central, lumen-obstructing (and preserving) catheter and the arterial endoluminal surface; (d) upon removal of the mold-core catheter a layer of hydrogel, paving the endoluminal surface, remains.*

are applied locally, they interact, coat or adhere to the underlying tissue surface and act as a short-term, thin, chemical interface layer. This type of paving may function as a means of transiently changing the tissue surface charge, porosity, or tissue lubricity, modifying cellular avidity to contacting or overflowing molecules or cells, or as a means of short-term local drug delivery.

In what forms might paving be implemented for endo-urological applications?

It is envisaged that both solid paving and gel paving will have clinical utility in urology. Five broad forms of use are contemplated: (1) solid paving as a stand-alone enhanced stenting method; (2) solid paving combined with metal stenting; (3) gel paving as a stand-alone local barrier and drug-delivery method; (4) gel paving as a second-step therapy applied to metallic stents, and (5) combined solid and gel paving. Each of these envisaged embodiments is outlined below. The advantages of paving for endo-urological applications are outlined in the following section and in Table 72.2.

Solid paving as a stand-alone enhanced stenting method

Solid paving, as described above, may be utilized as a stand-alone stenting method in numerous locations in the urological tract. The prostatic and penile urethra are specific anatomical locations that are particularly amenable to solid paving.

Solid paving: prostatic urethra
Solid paving is well suited to function as an endoluminal support method in the prostatic urethra.

The prostatic urethra, rather than being a simple tubular structure, has a complex three-dimensional luminal configuration. As such, conventional stents, which remain largely tubular, are unable to accommodate to complex urethral three-dimensional geometry. Lack of intimate wall contact with conventional stents is a set-up for migration, encrustation and infection. In contrast, utilizing solid paving in the prostatic urethra will allow formation of a custom-moulded wall support. It is envisaged that polymers will be delivered locally to the prostate, either as a direct therapy for benign prostatic hyperplasia (BPH) or as secondary supports following prostate reduction procedures such as transurethral resection (TURP), transurethral needle ablation or visual laser ablation of the prostate. Solid structural polymers, either in tubular form or as flat rolled sheets, will be delivered via a low–profile transurethral balloon catheter system. Once in place, the polymers will be unfurled and mechanically expanded while simultaneously being heated. Heating may take place by a variety of methods, including intra-balloon heating elements,[1,20,26] or by incorporation in the polymer of an absorbant dye that results in local heating of the polymer.[25,27] The combination of simultaneous heating and mechanical moulding of the polymer, i.e. in situ thermoforming, utilizing an underlying compliant or pre-moulded balloon that facilitates polymer distribution and flow, will result in custom contouring of the polymer to accommodate to the complex geometry of the prostatic urethra. In this system the balloon catheter acts as a mould-core, with the complex prostatic lumen acting as the mould itself. The result of this in situ thermoforming process is the creation of a structurally supportive endoluminal polymer liner that has a large lumen with a similar cross-sectional profile to the underlying native urethral

Table 72.2. *Advantages of paving for endo-urological applications*

Solid paving	Gel paving
Custom contouring of endoluminal support	Custom barrier formation in situ
Conformal to complex 3D anatomy (e.g. prostatic urethra)	Elastomeric
Barrier for hyperplasia or tumour ingrowth	Facilitation of urethral healing
Reduced fouling, encrustation and infection	Reduced risk of epithelial damage
Sustained long-term local drug delivery	Reduced fouling, encrustation and infection
Sustained long-term local radiation delivery	Intermediate-term local drug delivery
Local biological or cell delivery — tissue engineering	Local biological or cell delivery — tissue engineering
Biodegradable or permanent	Biodegradable or bioerodable

shape, although with increased cross-sectional dimension. The external shape of the moulded polymer liner is dictated by the underlying tissue architecture, although in enlarged form, depending upon the degree of balloon dilatation and distension of the lumen at the time of paving. Alternatively, a device that allows polymer to be pumped in, as a viscous fluid that sets in place, could be utilized. This approach would add the advantage of not needing to size the polymer implant specifically, as occurs with metal stenting prior to implantation. The ability to apply a polymer as a continuum would eliminate incomplete tract coverage, which may occur when short specific lengths of polymer tube or sheet are used.

In addition to serving as custom-moulded endoluminal supports, polymer liner layers may provide other therapeutic benefits. Polymer films may serve as local therapeutic barriers to limit exposure of underlying injured tissues. Alternatively, polymer layers, being customizable to provide limited porosity, may serve to limit the excessive epithelial overgrowth that accompanies open-configuration metal stents. In the case of malignancy, polymer films may provide local barriers to prevent tumour ingrowth.

A third function of solid paving layers resides in their drug-delivery potential. Polymer films may also provide a local depot reservoir for targeted sustained delivery of therapeutic agents. It is envisaged that local agents that lead to prostatic tissue involution may be administered for BPH. In the case of malignancy, local chemotherapeutic agents may be administered. Polymer films may also release bioactive compounds that facilitate rapid re-epithelialization of the injured urethral surface.

An additional feature of solid paving is the ability to provide an implant that is biodegradable. Polymer films, depending upon the polymer utilized and physicochemical characteristics of that polymer (i.e. molecular weight, degree of crystallinity, degree of crosslinking, glass-rubber transition), may provide a spectrum of residence times in the lumen. Polymers may be fabricated to biodegrade over a broad spectrum from weeks to months to years following implantation. The degradation time of specific polymer films to be used clinically will be dictated by the specific clinical use scenario. An example of a valuable indication for solid paving is following TURP: a biodegradable endo-urethral support that obviates the need for prolonged catheterization or a second follow-up visit for device removal, as in the case of an implanted metal stent, may be particularly valuable and cost effective.

Solid paving: penile urethra

Solid paving may be utilized in the penile urethra as an endoluminal support, barrier and local drug-delivery device in a manner similar to that described for the prostatic urethra. It is envisaged that polymer may be locally transported to the desired anatomical location and thermoformed in situ as described above. As opposed to the prostatic urethra — where significant rigidity and collapse resistance (i.e. hoop strength) of the deployed polymer is desired — in the penile urethra, ready collapse with rapid recoil and regain of shape are desirable specifications. As such, the polymeric materials utilized in the penile urethra will differ from those used in the prostatic urethra: in general, more elastomeric polymers with less intrinsic crystallinity will be used.

In the penile urethra, polymer films may be utilized for several applications. Polymer films may be used as custom-contoured endoluminal supports and patches. As such, polymer films may serve as local biodegradable 'Band Aids™', providing temporary wall support to facilitate healing of strictured urethra following stricture transection. This may be achieved without the secondary epithelial damage that is associated with the removal of temporary conventional stents. Solid polymer films may also provide local release of bioactive agents and growth factors that may accelerate urethral re-epithelialization.

Solid paving: ureter

In the ureter a modified form of solid paving with clinical utility may be envisaged. Specifically, in the case of extrinsic compression from mass or tumour or from intrinsic narrowing from hyperplastic lesion or tumour, solid paving may be utilized to provide endoluminal support. Short segments of the ureter may be locally paved with several types of material. One embodiment may use structural polymers with some degree of elastomeric character: these polymer films will provide endoluminal support while, at the same time, allowing for bulk urine transport to avoid interruption of peristalsis and creation of an immobile segment with resultant hydro-ureter. Alternatively, utilizing electroconductive elastomeric polymers, short polymer film segments may be made dynamic with expansile and compressive capabilities. These segments would be pulsed via an extrinsic pulse generator akin to a pacemaker and would actively facilitate urine transport to prevent hydro-ureter.

Solid paving combined with metal stenting

Solid paving may be combined with conventional metal stenting to enhance the efficacy of conventional stents. Currently, metal stents are often used as temporary implant devices after endo-urological intervention to provide acute endo-urethral support allowing healing and progressive lumen moulding and remodelling; these stents are then removed. Stent removal is often difficult and frequency results in re-injury of the urethra. Through use of composite implants, composed of metal stents plus overlying solid paving polymer films, metal stents of reduced mass with more open architecture may be utilized; such implants will provide similar (if not greater) endoluminal wall support acutely. As urethral tissues heal and strengthen, polymer films will simultaneously biodegrade. These minimalistic metal stents may then be readily removed, as their open design, with minimal tissue overgrowth, will facilitate simple transluminal recover.

In addition to structural advantages, solid paving may provide surface advantages to metal stents. Application of polymer films utilizing polymers, copolymers or blends possessing hydrophilic surface properties may enhance stent surface characteristics. Polymer films applied over stents may reduce stent biofouling, encrustation and propensity for bacterial colonization and infection. Further, altered surface properties may limit excessive epithelial overgrowth and progressive lumen compromise.

In addition to simple barrier coverage, a solid paving layer applied over a stent provides a local reservoir for sustained local drug delivery. Such polymers may deliver a wide variety of agents for periods up to a year, depending upon the specific clinical use.

Gel paving as a stand-alone endo-urological method

Gel paving may be utilized as a stand-alone procedure independent of conventional stenting. As such, it is envisaged that it will serve as an adjunct method to enhance the acute and chronic efficacy of numerous endo-urological procedures. Gel polymers, locally applied as conformal endoluminal films, may serve as local barriers and means for sustained intermediate-term drug delivery. Such gels may be formed in situ, either as a liquid, which is delivered to the tract site where it then gels in place, or as an in situ photopolymerizable gel, which is 'grown' in place, progressively thickening, from its surface outward toward the lumen.

As barriers, endoluminal gel paving layers may transiently limit underlying injured tissue from exposure to urine, blood, and tissue fluids released as a result of a therapeutic endo-urological procedure. Such local biodegradable tissue barriers will allow underlying tissue to heal while being protected to some degree from luminal exposure. In the arterial tree, gel paving of lesions to limit overflowing blood contact during healing has been demonstrated to result in rapid healing and re-endothelialization of lesions following mechanical disruption. Similarly, in the GU tract, such gel patches may facilitate effective lumen healing of the urethra following cold cutting of a stricture. Local hydrogel barriers may result in reduced recurrence of strictures as a result of more effective healing followed by successful re-epithelialization. Similarly, gel paving may be utilized as an adjunct to endoscopic urethral surgery or balloon dilatation to provide local post-trauma lumen coverage to facilitate re-epithelialization.

In addition to its transient barrier function, gel paving may effectively provide intermediate-term (i.e. days–weeks) delivery of growth factors or other active pharmacological compounds to facilitate rapid and controlled regional lumen re-epithelialization. In the lower GU tract, gel containing pharmacological agents favouring re-epithelialization may be utilized following TURP or stricture lysis. Alternatively, hydrogels may be utilized in a tissue-engineering approach to engraft locally epithelial cells in more radical procedures requiring extensive local plastic reconstruction. In the upper GU tract, hydrogels may be utilized following stone removal, providing local delivery of anti-inflammatory agents to limit post-procedural oedema. A discussion of other advantages of gel paving in the GU tract, as an adjunct to stenting, is provided below.

Gel paving as a second-step therapy applied to metallic GU stents

Gel paving may be utilized as an adjunct method to enhance the efficacy of conventional urological metal stents. Immediately following metal stenting, a thin layer of polymeric hydrogel could be applied over the stent, as well as to the surrounding upstream and downstream urethral segments. Gel would also be applied to adjacent regions of the urethra that may have been subjected to instrumentation or injured during stent deployment. It is envisaged that gel would be applied, as described above, either as preformed flowable polymers that form polymeric hydrogels in situ, or as a precursor system that is photopolymerizable in place. The applied gel would serve as a hydrophilic non-stick surface. This surface has been demonstrated in other systems to limit cell, protein and bacterial adherence; such a non-fouling surface would serve to limit stent encrustation and infection. In addition, this surface would allow healing and re-epithelialization underneath to proceed unimpeded in a protected environment. With time, as the hydrogel bioerodes and degrades, the underlying re-epithelialized surface would slowly be exposed again to direct urinary flow.

In addition to simple barrier coverage, a hydrogel paving layer applied over a stent can provide local delivery of bioactive agents. These agents might facilitate more rapid re-epithelialization of the stent. In addition, agents may be incorporated to retard bacterial colonization and to limit further salt deposition and encrustation, thereby enhancing the already favourable properties of the polymeric biomaterial itself.

Combination solid and gel paving for endo-urological applications

In a further iteration it is readily conceivable that solid and gel paving may be utilized jointly. Solid polymer films may be applied, as outlined above, as conformal custom-moulded endoluminal supports. Gel paving hydrogel polymers may then be applied on a solid paving zone, much like application of gels over stents as described in the section above on second-step therapy.

The use of solid structural polymers as well as hydrogel polymer systems affords the potential for synergy providing the best of both worlds: structural polymers applied via solid paving afford excellent local support; gel polymers provide enhanced tissue compatibility, minimal fouling and maximum long-term patency.

A dual solid and gel paving system also offers advantages as far as local drug delivery is concerned. Use of both solid and gel polymers together affords a wide spectrum of drug-delivery times: solid polymers typically provide weeks to months of drug delivery via polymer erosion and progressive drug diffusion; in contrast, gel systems provide focused local drug delivery at very high concentrations, typically for days to weeks, with drug delivery via diffusion as well as elution retardation. If both of these systems are used together, combination systems that provide high-dose initial delivery of one agent (i.e. via the hydrogel), followed by sustained long-term release from the solid paving matrix polymer, may be possible.

How might paving address specific limitations of current endo-urological stents?

Paving provides superior endoluminal support via conformal moulding and intimate wall apposition, ensuring complete tract expansion

The custom mouldability in situ of solid paving may be particularly valuable for endo-urological applications. The ability to mould a polymeric conduit liner on an individual basis, to adapt to local underlying tissue irregularities, while at the same time guaranteeing a large round or oval luminal cross-sectional profile, would be particularly advantageous. Utilizing structural polymers, with intrinsic strength and good crush resistance, a conformal endoluminal polymer liner within the urethra would provide excellent luminal support. Beyond adequate mechanical support, the ability to limit regions of non-support and stent non-contact (i.e. such as that occurring with conventional metal tubular stents in complex urethral anatomy), is advantageous. Reducing these regions will limit the creation of flow dividers, which may be sites for encrustation and infection due to urine pooling and stagnation. In addition, these unsupported zones are sites allowing for more epithelial ingrowth and overgrowth.

Paving has reduced the propensity for migration

The invagination of the polymer during local application into underlying luminal tissues could further provide an element of tongue-in-groove physical adhesion to the underlying tissue surface; this microcontouring capability is not afforded by current metal stenting. This feature would be particularly valuable as a means of limiting migration and embolization of the implant.

Paving as an adjunct to stenting effectively reduces metal stent surface biofouling and cellular deposition

Paving may be valuable as an approach to limit biofouling due to protein, crystal and microbial deposition on metal endo-urological stents. Recently, several studies have examined the efficacy of gel paving in situ, applied over implanted metal stents, as a means of limiting cell (platelet) and protein deposition on metal stents implanted in the arterial tree. Balloon-expandable stents (Palmaz, 1 cm length) were implanted in bilateral femoral arteries in pigs pretreated with aspirin. Pigs were heparinized during stent implantation only. Polyethylene glycol-lactide hydrogel layers (100 μm) were then photopolymerized in situ in one stented femoral artery per pig, covering a 3.5 cm segment, immediately following stent placement. Contralateral unpaved arteries served as controls. Pigs were allowed to recover and were maintained on aspirin (325 mg daily) during follow-up. Gross thrombosis and platelet deposition were assessed 1 hour and 3 days after stenting. In this study, stented gel-paved arteries uniformly had reduced overt thrombosis, reduced microscopic platelet deposition and enhanced patency compared with unpaved controls (Fig. 72.7).[33] In endo-urological applications, hydrogels photopolymerized in situ may similarly block extrinsic protein, cell and bacterial deposition on implanted stents by virtue of the hydrophilic non-stick properties of these hydrogel materials. Alternatively, a combination of solid paving polymers plus hydrogels may be utilized with metal stents, as outlined above, to achieve the desired non-fouling properties.

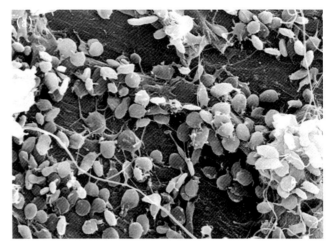
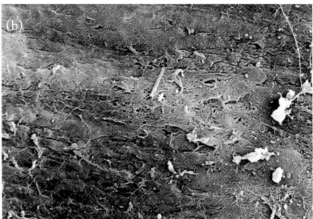

Figure 72.7. *Thrombo-protection of injured arterial surfaces via gel paving. (a) Scanning electron micrograph (× 3000) of abraded rat carotid artery. Note that the damaged intimal surface is coated with activated platelets and fibrin. Identical injured surface 'pre-coated' with endoluminal gel paving layer subsequently exposed to overflowing blood. (b) Note significant reduction in platelet deposition on injured surface, the gel having acted as a thrombo-resistant physical barrier layer.*

Paving as a stand-alone system provides a biodegradable implant with limited potential for surface biofouling, encrustation and infection

The enhanced surface properties of polymers, such as those described above, extend to stand-alone paving systems as well. Stand-alone biodegradable solid paving applied for example, post-TURP or as a stand-alone support for urethral strictures or tumour obstruction, may be fashioned so that the implant polymer selected has the appropriate surface properties (i.e. hydrophilicity, contact angle, surface texture), for minimal biofouling. Further, solid structural polymers may also incorporate — either covalently or as blends — hydrophilic polymer systems, similar to those utilized in gel paving, that have excellent surface properties with minimal surface-fouling potential.

In addition to limitation of fouling and encrustation, via the intrinsic properties of the polymers, incorporation of materials and therapeutic agents to limit organic and inorganic deposits may further enhance the performance of endoluminal polymers. Agents that change the surface charge of polymers, limiting urine 'salting-out', may be utilized to enhance performance. Antimicrobial agents may also be incorporated in the polymers; these may remain active on the surface or be released slowly, limiting local microbial colonization.

Paving offers reduced potential for tissue-tract injury

A further advantage of paving resides in the ability of polymers to be fabricated with material properties that allow for compliance matching of the polymer to the underlying tissue, because creation of an endoluminal implant with compliance similar to the tissue is less likely to create chronic mechanical tissue injury. This phenomenon has been demonstrated in the vascular tree. In urology, implanting a rigid metal stent has increased the risk for trauma to lumen structures over time, from device external impact and crush, device migration and device manipulation from subsequent endo-urological procedures. Further, device removal entails a significant risk for epithelial layer disruption and underlying tissue tract trauma. These limitations are obviated by the use of paving. Through the use of stand-alone biodegradable conformal implants, with intrinsic elasticity, the risk of tissue injury is reduced while the device is in place. Further injury from device-removal procedure is ruled out, as the implant will biodegrade without endo-urological manipulation.

Paving offers the potential for reduced implant discomfort

Endoluminal polymers, which are supportive yet moderately elastic, are less likely to create discomfort for the patient. Further, as the tissue surrounding the polymer liner heals post-procedure (e.g. in the case of TURP), the polymer will, at the same time, start to biodegrade. With late biodegradation, polymers will further soften, thereby reducing the discomfort due to chronic luminal distention or local irritation. The drug-delivery potential of paving offers a means for locally releasing a local anaesthetic, a modification that may be utilized in the early days after implantation, to reduce discomfort from initial placement.

Paving effectively functions as a barrier to physical ingrowth

Polymer-paving layers, particularly if formed from structural polymeric materials, may provide a custom-moulded, physical, barrier layer. The porosity and permeability of this barrier layer may be tailored over a wide spectrum of permeability, ranging from limited permeability to completely non-permeable, as seen with a dense polymer layer. The author has examined the ability of such a non-porous polymer layer, applied to an arterial endoluminal surface following arterial stretch injury, to limit subsequent neointimal ingrowth. In this pilot study, a distinct limitation of tissue ingrowth was observed in regions of solid polymer application, with preserved ingrowth in gapped macroporous regions. Although preliminary, these studies suggest that polymer layers may be fashioned to act as physical barriers in vivo, limiting tissue ingrowth, while still maintaining the viability of underlying tissue parenchyma. Similar applications may be envisaged for endo-urological application to limit epithelial ingrowth in post-traumatic urethral applications. Further, in cases of malignancies, polymer barriers may provide a physical means to limit lumen encroachment.

Paving effectively provides sustained local drug delivery

In addition to acting as a physical, non-pharmacological barrier, paving may further limit biofouling, encrustation, infection and epithelial overgrowth by virtue of local drug delivery. Utilizing a solid paving system in a canine arterial model in vivo, the author has demonstrated that an endoluminal polymer film of poly(ε-caprolactone) could effectively deliver sustained levels of heparin locally to the applied tissue site.[28] Similarly, it has been demonstrated by the author that gel paving layers may effectively deliver a drug to an applied tissue surface, achieving more sustained delivery than is achieved with instillation of a drug by a catheter. For endo-urological applications, a solid, gel or combination paving system, with interspersed antimicrobial or antiproliferative agents, may further enhance lumen patency and function.

Conclusions

Polymer paving is a generic, endoluminal, therapeutic method that holds great potential for endo-urological applications. In the short term, reduced stent fouling, reduced encrustation and colonization, control of epithelial hyperplasia and enhanced stent patency are achievable goals of GU paving. In the future, endo-urological paving may be utilized as a technique for the local delivery of drugs, or of biological or cellular therapeutic agents that target pathological disruption of the GU tract. Methods such as paving may be viewed as a first step toward endoluminal 'tissue engineering' of the GU tract. Continued advances in the fields of biomaterials, cell biology, pharmacology, and genetic engineering may in the future enhance the full potential of paving.

References

1. Slepian M J, Schindler A. Polymeric endoluminal paving/sealing: A biodegradable alternative to intracoronary stenting. Circulation 1988; 78: II–408
2. Ng K J, Gardener J E, Rickards D et al. Three-dimensional imaging of the prostatic urethra—an exciting new tool. Br J Urol 1994; 74: 604–608
3. Hernandex-Graulau J M. Indications for percutaneous nephroscopy in noncalculous disease. In: Sosa R E, Albala D M, Jenkins A D, Perlmutter A P (eds) Textbook of Endourology. Philadelphia: Saunders, 1997: 165
4. Motola J A, Badlani G H, Smith A D. Results of 212 consecutive endopyelotomies: an 8 year follow-up. J Urol 1993; 149: 453
5. Yachia D, Aridogan I A. Comparison between first generation (fixed caliber) and second generation (self-expanding, large caliber) temporary prostatic stents. Urol Int 1996; 57: 165–169
6. Thomas P J, Britton J P, Harrison N W. The prostakath stent: 4 years experience. Br J Urol 1993; 71: 430
7. Reid G. Microbial adhesion to biomaterials and infections of the urogenital tract. Colloid Surfaces B: Biointerfaces 1994; 2: 377–385
8. Hukins D W L, Hickey D S, Kennedy A P. Catheter encrustation by struvite. Br J Urol 1983; 55: 304–305
9. Costerton J W, Cheng K J, Geesey G G. Bacterial biofilms in nature and disease. Annu Rev Microbiol 1987; 41: 435–464
10. Elves A W S, Fenely R C L. Long-term urethral catheterization and the urine biomaterial interface. Br J Urol 1997; 80: 1–5
11. Schulz K A, Wettlauffer J N, Oldani G. Encrustation and stone formation: complication of indwelling urethral stent. Urology 1985; 25: 616–619
12. Cormio L, LaForgia P, Siitonen A, Ruutu M. Is it possible to prevent bacterial adhesion onto ureteric stents? Urol Res 1997; 25: 213–216
13. Morris N S, Stickler D J, Winter C. Which indwelling urethral catheters resist encrustation by Proteus mirabis biofilms? Br J Urol 1997; 80: 58–63
14. Hoyle B D, Costerton J W. Bacterial resistance to antibiotics: the role of biofilms. Prog Drug Res 1991; 15: 91–105
15. Kunkel M, Korth K. Endopyelotomy: long-term follow-up of 143 patients. J Endourol 1990; 4: 109
16. Tillem S M, Press S M, Badlani G H et al. The Urolume endourethral prosthesis for the treatment of recurrent bulbar urethral strictures: results of the North American Urolume Trial. J Urol 1995; 153: 580A
17. Forrester J S, Fishbein M, Helfant R, Fagin J. A paradigm for restenosis based on cell biology: clues for the development of new perspective therapies. J Ma Coll Cardiol 1991; 17: 758–769
18. Califf R M, Fortin D F, Frid D J et al. Restenosis after coronary angioplasty: an overview. J Am Coll Cardiol 1991; 17: 2B–13B
19. Boccon-Gibod L, Barthelemy Y. Late (1–4 years) results of the Wallstent endourethral prosthesis in strictures of the male urethra. J Urol 1995; 153: 579B
20. Slepian M J. Polymeric endoluminal paving and sealing: therapeutics at the crossroad of biomechanics and pharmacology. In: Topol E J (ed) Textbook of Interventional Cardiology. Philadelphia: Saunders, 1989: 647–670
21. Slepian M J. Polymeric endoluminal paving: a family of evolving methods for extending endoluminal therapeutics beyond stenting. Cardiol Clin 1994; 12: 715–737
22. Hill-West J L, Chowdhury S M, Slepian M J, Hubbell J A. Inhibition of thrombosis and intimal thickening by in situ photopolymerization of thin hydrogel barriers. Proc Nat Acad Sci 1994; 91: 5967–5971
23. Slepian M J, Hossainy S F A, Pathak C P, Hubbell J A. Bioerodible endovascular gel paving: a new approach for reducing the thrombogenicity of injured arterial surfaces. Trans Soc Biomater 1993; 16: 235
24. Slepian M J, Hossainy S F A, Pathak C P et al. Thermoreversible polyether hydrogels reduce the thrombogenicity of injured arterial intimal surfaces. Circulation 1993; 88(4 Pt 2): I–319
25. Slepian M J, Berrigan K M, Roth L, Campbell P K. Polymeric endoluminal photo-thermal paving: initial experience in normal and dissected canine carotid arteries in vitro (abstr). J Vasc Intervent Radiol 1994; 5: 10
26. Slepian M J, Berrigan K M, Roth L, Campbell P K. Endovascular photothermal paving: a new paving form – acute in vivo efficacy and patency. Trans Soc Biomater 1994; 17: 17
27. Campbell P K, Berrigan K M, Roth L, Slepian M J. Photothermal intravascular delivery of biodegradable materials: in vitro temperature measurements. Trans Soc Biomater 1994; 17: 16
28. Slepian M J, Campbell P K, Berrigan K et al. Biodegradable endoluminal polymer layers provide sustained transmural heparin delivery to the arterial wall in vivo. Circulation 1994; 90(4 Pt 2): I–20
29. Slepian M J, Massia S P, Sawhney A et al. Endoluminal gel paving using in situ biodegradable photopolymerized hydrogels: acute efficacy in the rabbit. Circulation 1993; 88(4 Pt 2): I–660
30. Slepian M J, Hubbell J A. Polymeric endoluminal gel paving: hydrogel systems for local barrier creation and site-specific drug delivery. Adv Drug Deliv Rev 1997; 24: 11–30
31. Fingerle J, Johnson R, Clowes A et al. Role of platelets in smooth muscle cell proliferation and migration after vascular injury in the rat carotid artery. Proc Nat Acad Sci USA 1989; 86: 8412–8416
32. Steele P M, Cheseboro J H, Holmes D R et al. Balloon angioplasty in pigs: histologic wall injury as a determinant of platelet deposition and thrombus formation. Circ Res 1985; 57: 105–112
33. Slepian M J, Khosravi F, Massia S P et al. Gel paving of intraarterial stents in vivo reduces stent and adjacent arterial wall thrombogenicity (abstr). J Vasc Intervent Radiol 1995; 6: 50

A site-specific dynamic stent for the lower urinary tract

D. Yachia and R. Levy

73

Introduction

In general terms, stenting is the use of a device to create an artificial pathway, support structure or opening for hollow organs that are closed or obstructed due to benign or malignant obstructive diseases. However, by simply looking at the different organs where stenting can be used, we can easily see the differences in their anatomical structure and function. Since Charles Dotter, in 1969, experimented with the polymer stents in canine peripheral arteries, no matter from which material they were manufactured or how they were constructed (solid, helical – in single or double helix formats, knitted or braided – covered or uncovered) all the stents had a cylindrical shape.

In the lower urinary tract, since the first prostatic stent developed by Fabian in the early 1980s, all the stents, either temporary or permanent, were not only cylindrical but also static. All cylindrical stents developed for organs that have a cylindrical lumen, fit the shape and the caliber of the tubular organ it was intended for. Even though the caliber of the arteries reduce toward the periphery and veins enlarge toward the heart, this change is very gradual and the cylindrical vascular stents which have the same caliber at both ends fit perfectly between the walls of the blood vessel. This is not the case in urology. Mono-caliber stents hardly fit the tubular parts of the urinary tract. Although a tubular organ, each segment of the urethra has a different cross-section shape and caliber, and also has an active voluntary sphincter, making this organ entirely different than other tubular organs. Despite these differences, lower urinary tract stents were designed as mono-caliber cylindrical devices, having a bell-shaped sphincter-side end for anchoring purposes. Even the ureters have variable calibers all along their length. These varying calibers make it difficult to stent the urinary tract in the way that blood vessels are stented. In contrast to blood vessels, where the stents used are permanently implanted, in the urinary tract, most stents used are temporary requiring removal after a period of time.

Accumulating experience has shown that adopting and then adapting stents developed for the vascular tree to the prostatic and bulbar urethra does not always fulfill our needs. In many cases, significant lessons have been learned through trial and error which has led to a greater understanding of the abilities or limitations of the available stents.

Before describing the concept of the 'new stent' we provide some basic information on the available stents.

Permanent stents

Permanent stents are devices implanted into tubular organs and remain permanently in the body. If we look at all the permanent stents that were introduced for use in the urinary tract we see that they were adapted for prostatic and urethral or even for ureteral use by changing the caliber and/or the length of the basic vascular design. From the vast vascular stent designs the only ones that were tried in the urinary tract were the balloon-expandable Palmaz stent which was marketed as the Titan; the self-expanding Wallstent and the Strecker stent. Despite encouraging early results with the use of the balloon-expandable permanent Palmaz stent for opening prostatic obstructions, its use was abandoned after a short period. This was due to the longitudinal rigidity of the stent, the unacceptably high early migration rates and the impossibility of expansion to cover the entire surface of the irregular prostatic urethra and then become completely covered by urethral lining.

The era of the self-expanding stent began with the introduction of the braided Wallstent developed by Wallstén for vascular use (see Chapter 5). This stent became the most widely recognized device used in many medical disciplines, including urology. The design of this stent was based on the well-known 'Chinese finger trap' in which one can insert a finger which is trapped when the finger is retracted. This is a widely used wire braiding principle used industrially in the manufacture of coaxial cables and some catheter braids. The

Wallstent was first tried in recurrent bulbar strictures and then as an alternative to benign prostatic hyperplasia (BPH) surgery.

Both the Wallstent and the knitted Strecker stent introduced for use in the urinary tract were self-expanding and highly flexible permanent stents. Like the Wallstent, the Strecker stent (Memotherm) was also used in BPH. Both devices had round cross-sections that did not fit to the prostatic urethra; a segment of the urethra which rarely has a round cross-section.[1] An additional problem with the self-expanding permanent stents was that their anchoring depended on the radial force they exerted on the urethral wall. Especially when short stents (2–3 cm) were used they could migrate almost immediately after their release from their insertion device. Secure anchoring of these stents could begin only after a few days when the urethral lining started to proliferate toward the lumen.

Temporary stents

The temporary stents are devices for insertion into the urethra and then removed after a certain period of time. These stents, such as the fixed-caliber Prostakath and the self-expanding ProstaCoil, were based on the 'Partial Catheter' design developed by Fabian in the early 1980s. Like the original stent, all had a prostatic segment and a bulbar-anchoring segment connected by a trans-sphincteric wire. The Partial Catheter and the Prostakath, which was almost a gold-plated copy of it, because of their design geometry, did not allow passage to any catheter larger than 5–6 Fr through their lumen, but the ProstaCoil with a much larger lumen and a different design in its 'trans-sphincteric segment' allowed passage to catheters and endoscopes up to 17 Fr. The Partial Catheter and the Prostakath had 30% and the ProstaCoil, 5% migration rates. The first two could be left indwelling up to 1 year and the third up to 3 years. There are no published data on migration rates of the partially self-expanding Memokath and the recent Horizon stents, both of which have a bell-like distal end near the sphincter for anchoring and no bulbar segment; or the latest Spanner stent, which looks like a short Foley and has a bulbar anchoring segment. The polyurethane intraurethral catheters (IUC) designed by Nissenkorn and Barnes allowed immediate relief of obstruction but because of their small caliber they occluded after a short while. Their indwelling time was

3–6 months and had high migration rates. Despite its bulbar-anchoring segment the Trestle (which looks like a short, two-part Nelaton catheter) migrated, mainly toward the bladder.

In 1993, the consensus report on prostatic stents prepared for the 2nd International Consultation on Benign Prostatic Hyperplasia (BPH) stated the following:

> If the prostate was spherical externally with a cylindrical urethra of unvarying dimension running through it in a straight line like a drainpipe, with no middle lobe, and with no sensation in the urethra, the problem (of using a prostatic stent) would be quite simple. Unfortunately, this is not so and one must contend with all the known anatomical problems as one positions the stent after careful assessment of the urethra . . . .[2]

The uneven shape of the prostatic urethra was demonstrated by Ng et al. using three-dimensional sonographic imaging.[1]

With further accumulating experience, the stent experts added the following to their next report prepared for the 3rd International Consultation on Benign Prostatic Hyperplasia (BPH) held in 1995, when they tried to define the 'ideal stent':

> When a stent is to be used, it should be [malleable] so that it can conform to the shape of the prostatic urethra and [easy to insert] with an [internal diameter adequate to allow cystoscopy] with a rigid or flexible instrument. In addition the [ideal stent] should [remain in position] for a prolonged period of time without migration, should be [easily removed] and [replaced], and should be [inexpensive]. Though some of the easily removable stents come close to this ideal specification, none as yet, fulfill it completely. [They also added that] Careful positioning of the stent is vital . . . to provide adequate relief of symptoms.[3]

Although the early vision for prostatic stenting for the management of prostatic obstructions is moving closer to reality, unfortunately most companies producing stents are focused on the more lucrative vascular stenting and are investing less on non-vascular, especially on the design of stents for lower urinary tract applications. This can be seen in a more recent statement in the last edition of Campbell's *Urology*: 'It is hard to predict whether further design changes (in temporary stents) will take place. . . . further developments in this type of stent are unlikely'.[4] There is no doubt that design and material improvements should and can be done to prevent the unwanted complications associated with stent use.

Deficiencies in current temporary urethral stents

Most of the existing stent design and technologies only partly address the needs and requirements of urologists who treat patients with prostatic or anterior urethral obstructions. We think that the existing gap between what is available today and what is desired in the field of lower urinary urinary tract stenting can be bridged by new designs based on the specific needs of the site – the urethra.

Shape and conformability
Permanent urethral stents
Stents used in the vascular system are permanent. An ideal vascular stent is about 1.2 times the vessel diameter to ensure appropriate anchoring, without causing unnecessary pressure to the wall of the vessel. After its release, the entire stent is in contact with the vessel wall. As stents expand and press against the entire vessel wall, some traumatic damage to the endothelium occurs. This damage induces a chain tissue reaction until the stent becomes covered with endothelium.

Exactly the same mechanism should occur in the prostatic urethra in that a permanent stent becomes completely covered by urethral epithelium. Although complete coverage occurs when a stent is used in the bulbar urethra, unfortunately this does not always

happen in the prostatic urethra. This is due to the irregular, usually non-cylindrical shape of the prostatic urethra. When we look at the prostatic urethra what we see are different prostatic urethral lumen shapes that can be endoscopically classified as an A-, an I- or an O-shaped lumen (Fig. 73.1). All urologists are very familiar with these shapes. The first two conform poorly to a simple cylindrical stent even if it has a caliber of over 40 Fr. Cylindrical permanent prostatic stents can fit only to an O-shaped prostatic urethra because all the walls of the stent will be in contact with the urethral walls. Using a cylindrical permanent stent in A- and I-shaped prostatic urethras has a risk of partial stent embedding and, as a consequence, development of infection and stone formation on the bare wires. Although, based on their findings, Ng and Milroy recommended new permanent stent shapes, no changes have occurred since the work of Ng et al. was published in 1994.[1]

Temporary prostatic stents
These stents, because they are intended to remain temporarily in the urethral lumen, can be cylindrical, provided that they have a large lumen caliber and good anchoring. However stents with a large caliber may cause more irritative symptoms than those of smaller caliber.

Stent-shortening at deployment/accurate positioning
A problem with the self-expanding metallic permanent and temporary stents is their shortening on release. The

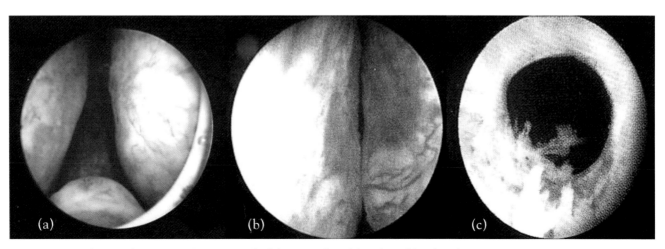

Figure 73.1. *Endoscopic classification of prostatic urethral shapes: A-shape (a), I-shape (b) and O-shape (c) prostatic urethra.*

degree of shortening depends on the caliber the stent is reduced to before insertion, and on the expanded caliber. Careful consideration should be given to the effects of stent-shortening when using self-expandable stents. The deployed Wallstent is about 30% shorter than its constricted length. The ProstaCoil and UroCoil shortens by ~40–50% on deployment. The previous design of the Horizon stent shortens by ~50–60%, and the new design of Horizon and the Memokath by ~10%. In less experienced hands this shortening causes deployment inaccuracies.

Patient discomfort

Urinary urgency after permanent and temporary urethral stent insertion is caused by foreign body irritation. 'Being a foreign body, inevitably all prostatic or bulbar urethral stent is associated with some discomfort'.[3] A frequently encountered early complaint of patients, having a stent inserted into their prostatic or bulbar urethra, is urgency of urination. This can be a distressing irritative symptom which can last from a couple of days to weeks. It is usually manageable by anti-inflammatory or anticholinergic drugs.

In large caliber temporary stents, although they are longitudinally flexible, their downstream end as well as their entire structure are radially stiff. These large caliber, cylindrical, non-lumen-conforming temporary stents may cause more irritative symptoms than lumen-conforming stents. The very hard, large caliber cylindrical stents, by forcing themselves to the lumen of the host organ, cause these symptoms. Sitting on a hard surface, the patient can feel the stiffness of the stent.

Theoretically, a stent tailored to the irregularly shaped prostatic urethra may reduce these irritative symptoms. There was a hope that an in situ formed semi-rigid stent, based on the 'solid paving' principle would be the answer to this problem, but such a stent has not yet been developed (see Chapter 72).

Incontinence

A quite frequently encountered complaint of patients, having a permanent or a temporary urethral stent in their prostatic or bulbar urethra, is incontinence. Incontinence after stent insertion can be from urge incontinence to dribbling during stress or total incontinence. This is usually caused either because of foreign body irritation to the prostatic urethra or

mechanical interference to the sphincter. The reason for urge incontinence, which is seen especially during the first days after insertion of the stent, is the mechanical irritation caused by the foreign body. These irritative symptoms can be managed by anti-inflammatory or anticholinergic drugs and disappear after a few days. In patients who do not complain of irritative symptoms but have some degree of incontinence, the reason is mechanical interference caused by the stent to the contraction ability of the sphincter. In mechanical terms, a sphincter in any part of the body is a formation of muscular tissue encircling a body lumen. Although different sphincters differ in their anatomic shape and composition, the contraction of any sphincter occludes the lumen of the organ it is encircling in order to prevent passage of urine, feces, bile or stomach contents from one side of the sphincter to the other. The mechanics of a sphincter are entirely different from that of a valve (i.e. venous valves), which prevents the back-flow of venous blood. Contraction of a sphincter covers a certain space, narrowing the lumen it encircles in a gradual manner. The diameter of the lumen of the urethra passing through the voluntary sphincteric mechanism changes dynamically for passing or stopping the passage of the urine. In particular, the voluntary urinary sphincter (the external sphincter), during its contraction, gives a fusiform shape to the urethral lumen. This phenomenon is a standard finding seen during ascending urethrographies (Fig. 73.2a). Placing a cylindrical stent with a ring-shaped sphincteric end, in a body lumen adjacent to a sphincter often interferes with the proper functioning of the sphincter. One of the problems encountered with the current permanent or temporary urethral stents (either prostatic or bulbar) is partial or total incontinence, especially when one end of the stent has to be positioned near the external sphincter (Fig. 73.2b and Fig.73.3a–e). The radially outward forces exerted on the inner wall of the lumen near the sphincter by the stent may prevent the sphincteric segment of the lumen from becoming completely occluded by the sphincter.

Temporary stents, although flexible, their ends as well as their entire body are radially stiff. When positioned at the vicinity of the sphincter they disturb the sphincter to fully contract it into normal fusiform shape. Reported incontinence rates after temporary stent insertion are 10–20%. [2]

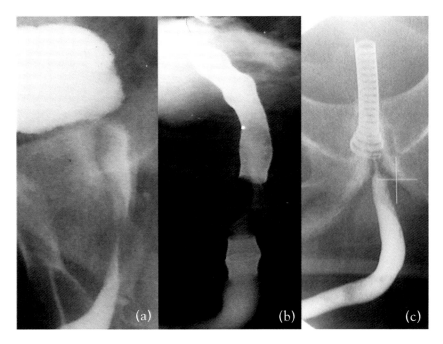

Figure 73.2. *(a) Normal, fusiform shaped external sphincter as seen in an ascending urethrogram. (b) ProstaCoil stent with both its sphincteric ends (of the main body and bulbar segment) in the near vicinity of the external sphincter. (c) The bell-shaped anchoring segment of the new Horizon stent in the near vicinity of the external sphincter.*

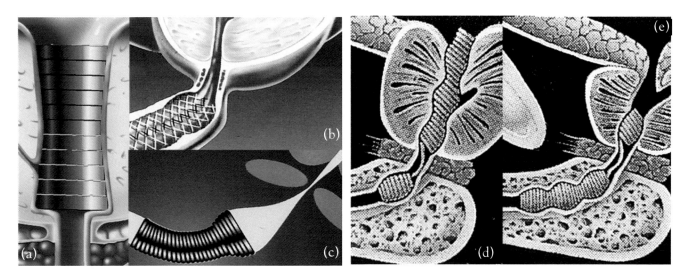

Figure 73.3. *Stent localization near the sphincter as designed by their manufacturers. (a) The Horizon (old design) in the prostatic urethra. (b) The Urolume in the bulbar urethra. (c) The Memokath in the bulbar urethra. (d) The ProstaCoil in the prostatic urethra. (e) The UroCoil-S in the bulbar urethra.*

The large caliber (>40 Fr) permanent stents (including their ends) are radially flexible all along their body but have an equal radial force in all their length. Although these stents are more flexible and despite their radially flexible ends, when they are positioned very near to the sphincter they also interfere with its contraction.

Lumen vs urine flow

In contrast to the function of the lumen of indwelling catheters, where the urine flow is passive, the size of the lumen of the stents is important because the patient actively urinates through the stent. It is obvious that the smaller the lumen of the stent the lower will be the urinary flow. The 16 Fr external caliber intraurethral catheters (IUCs) have an 8–10 Fr lumen caliber. The Spanner, with its reinforced body has a 20 Fr and 22 Fr external caliber but a 12–14 Fr lumen caliber allowing a Q_{max} of 11.6 ml/s, which is still an almost obstructed flow. A larger caliber lumen allows a better flow as can be seen from the flow through the ProstaCoil which has a 22 Fr lumen caliber and a mean Q_{max} of 21.3 ml/s (range 15–36 ml/s).

Transurethral instrumentation through the stent

Only the large caliber urethral stents allow instrumentation through their lumen. In the past, the use of first-generation temporary urethral stents for long-term use was a contraindication in bladder cancer patients who needed endoscopic follow-up. However, with the second-generation, self-expandable large caliber stents, such as the ProstaCoil and UroCoil, the Memokath and the Horizon, this became a relative contraindication. These stents allow passage to flexible cystoscopes and small caliber rigid cystoscopes (15.5–19 Fr), all inserted under vision. With the increase of upper urinary tract endoscopic procedures, the large caliber stents can also be used to perform ureteroscopy with instruments inserted through their large lumen.

Tissue proliferation

Another problem encountered with the current temporary urethral coil stents is tissue ingrowth between the loops of the coils or reactive tissue proliferation at the sphincteric end of the stent. Tissue ingrowth can be prevented if there is no distance between the loops of the coils or the stent is 'covered'. Currently, there is no 'covered stent' in use in the lower urinary tract for preventing such tissue ingrowth. The ProstaCoil, UroCoil and Memokath stents are manufactured in such a way that the loops of the coils tightly touch each other and do not allow tissue ingrowth into the lumen. However, this is not the case with the Horizon Nitinol stent or the self-expanding Biofix biodegradable coil stent (after its expansion) which allows tissue ingrowth between the separated loops of the coils (Fig. 73.4). However, with all the temporary stents, when left indwelling a few months, a reactive proliferative tissue starts to develop at the sphincteric end of the device in some patients. This tissue may cause partial or complete obliteration of the stent. The reason for this reactive

tissue proliferation is the radial stiffness of the sphincteric end of the stent causing repeated friction to the urethral wall during opening and closing of the sphincter. A similar phenomenon occurs in vascular stents, where reactive tissue develops at both ends of the stent. This is called the 'candy wrap effect'.

The new stent design

The concept of a new stent design was born after analysing all the deficiencies of the current urological stents, including the UroCoil and ProstaCoil stents developed by Yachia more than a decade ago. The plan was to develop stents:

1. to have a geometry conforming to the variations of caliber and lumen shapes of the urinary tract;
2. to be more comfortable to the patient;
3. to prevent incontinence and tissue proliferation by designing it as dynamic and 'sphincter-friendly';
4. would not shorten or elongate during deployment;
5. have a large lumen to allow very good urinary flow; and
6. to allow instrumentation through its lumen.

To reach these goals a methodology was developed to answer the deficiencies of the current stents. The resulting technological platform can be adapted for designing permanent urological stents as well as temporary and permanent stents for use in different organs.

Such urological stents based on this technological platform have been designed, prototyped and tested in

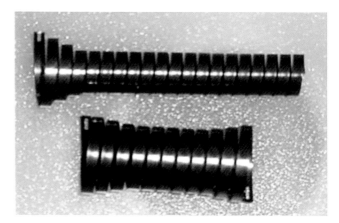

Figure 73.4. *The distances between the loops of the coils cause intraluminal tissue proliferation.*

laboratory conditions, and recently in a small group of patients (patents pending). The new stents will be inserted by endoscopy (Fig. 73.5).

Stent material

The new stent is the first 'covered stent' specially designed for use temporarily in the lower urinary tract. The self-expanding components of the stent are made of nickel-titanium alloy (Nitinol or NiTi), which is an alloy having a super-elasticity and also a thermally activated shape memory. The entire stent, including the distances between the metal parts, are covered with a biocompatible polymer to make it an impermeable tube preventing tissue ingrowth into the lumen. Despite its large caliber, the new stents are designed to allow easy endoscopic removal.

Shape and conformability

For prostatic use, the new stent has a main body, a bulbar-anchoring segment and a trans-sphincteric segment to connect both parts (Fig. 73.6a,b). The main body of the stent can have different cross-sectional

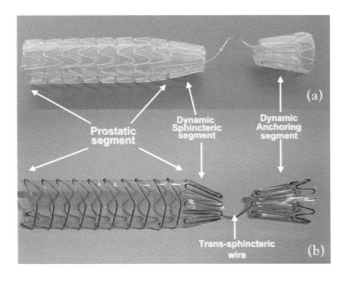

Figure 73.5. *The endoscopic delivery tool of the new stent.*

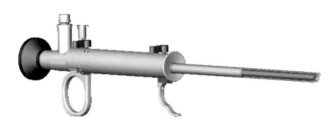

shapes. For bulbar urethral use the stent is designed as a single part: a conical segment near the sphincter and a cylindrical body of 45 Fr to tutor the bulbar urethra (Fig. 73.6c). Its large caliber will prevent the new stent from migrating downstream.

Currently, the new prostatic stents are designed as two different cross-sectional shapes:

A *triangular cross-section design* for the A- or I-shaped prostatic urethral lumen (Fig. 73.7a). This design allows the pushing aside of the two lateral lobes by the side walls of the main body, reinforced by the base of the triangle which expands laterally. The shape of the cross-section changes at its sphincteric end to a round cross-section to fit the shape of the pre-sphincteric urethra. The bulbar-anchoring segment is also designed so that it contracts and relaxes in concert with the sphincter.

A *round-cross section design* for the O-shaped prostatic urethral lumen (Fig. 73.7b). This design also has a similar sphincteric segment to that above.

Both new stents are very flexible longitudinally as well as radially, but are strong enough to keep the urethra open (Fig. 73.8).

In contrast to the available temporary stents which force themselves to the lumen they have inserted, the new stent will be able to negotiate with the tissues surrounding it. This is important, especially when a stent is inserted after one of the various thermotherapies for benign prostatic hyperplasia (BPH) and brachytherapy, or cryotherapy for prostate cancer,

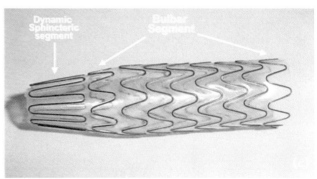

Figure 73.6. *The new stent designs. The segments of the new round (a) and triangular (b) prostatic stents, and the round bulbar urethral stent (c).*

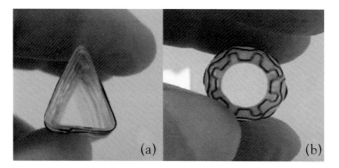

Figure 73.7. *(a) Triangular cross-section of the prostatic stent. (b) Round cross-section of the prostatic and bulbar stent.*

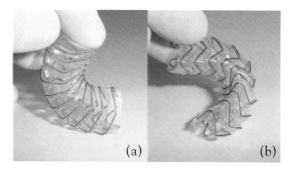

Figure 73.8. *The highly flexible main body of the triangular prostatic stent. (a) Anterior flexibility. (b) Lateral flexibility.*

during the stage of tissue edema developing following treatment. During the edematous stage the two designs of the new stent will temporarily reduce in caliber, but will never become occluded by external compression (this has been checked and proved under laboratory conditions). With the gradual resolution of edema the stent will regain its original shape (Fig. 73.9).

Ease of removal

In removing this very large caliber new stent from the urethra without trauma, a new and simple concept emerged to bridge the existing gap between what is available today and what is needed in the field of lower urinary tract stenting. The easily removable new large caliber stent will further the possibility of stent use in the treatment and/or management of many benign and malignant prostate and urethral diseases.

Non-shortening stent at deployment for accurate positioning

The new stent does not shorten during its deployment. The stent is reduced in caliber by crimping it into 24 Fr

overtube for straightforward endoscopic insertion. This caliber reduction technique does not cause any changes to the length of the crimped stent, and thus allows for very accurate positioning. After its release, the stent self-expands.

The use of a stent having a 'sphincter-friendly' segment of low resistance in a lumen adjacent to a sphincter also has a major advantage. It allows the stent to be more accurately positioned in the lumen with the sphincteric end touching the sphincter.

Reduced patient discomfort

Blood vessels do not have sensation and the presence of a stent in a blood vessel does not cause any discomfort to the patient. The urethra, especially the prostatic urethra, has high levels of sensation. Inserting a softer and tissue-negotiating stent may significantly reduce the discomfort felt by patients.

Sphincter conforming for incontinence prevention

The new stent design has a main body of high resistance in both the triangular and round cross-sectional

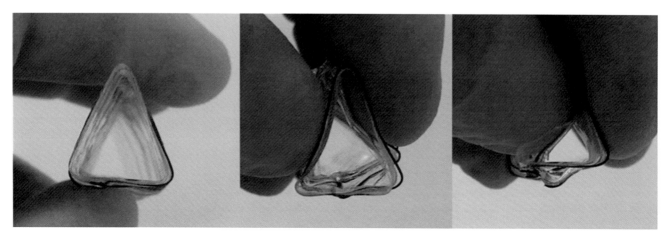

Figure 73.9. *Different stages of external compression of the triangular stent. Note the permanency of the lumen.*

versions. There is also a segment near the sphincter with a resistance lower than the main body in order to prevent mechanical interference to sphincteric function. Such a stent fits itself dynamically to the diameter and shape changes of the sphincter. The sphincteric end of such a stent has a lower resistance and a good caliber and shape conformation. The diameter of the low resistance segment dynamically fluctuates with the diameter of the lumen so as to remain in contact with the lumen wall at all times. When the sphincter closes and the diameter of the lumen adjacent to the sphincter decreases, the diameter of the end segment of the stent also decreases in a conical shape almost to zero, while remaining in contact with the lumen wall. When the sphincter opens for voiding, and the diameter of lumen adjacent to the sphincter increases, the diameter of the end segment also increases, but always remains in contact with the lumen wall allowing unobstructed urination (Fig. 73.10). Thus, the end segment of the stent dynamically conforms to the lumen shape adjacent to the sphincter during opening and urination (cylindrical) and closing of the sphincter (conical).

Large lumen for unobstructed urine flow

Although urine flow not only depends on the bladder outlet caliber but also on the detrusor, past experience with the large caliber ProstaCoil showed that mean Q_{max} values of 21.3 ml/s (range 15–36 ml/s) can easily be reached after large caliber stent insertion. The surface of the round cross-section of the ProstaCoil was 80 mm^2. The surface of the cross-section of the triangular new stent is ~110 mm^2, and the round one ~175 mm^2, which will allow an excellent urinary flow.

Transurethral instrumentation through the stent

Experience with the large caliber UroCoil and ProstaCoil stents has shown that it is possible to pass endoscopes through their lumen for diagnostic and therapeutic goals in bladder disease. The very large lumen of the new stent will allow the passage of endoscopes up to 17 Fr through the bladder, and will also allow ureteroscopic procedures, without removing the stent.

Tissue proliferation

In contrast to the current temporary stents in which there is a sudden drop of caliber tutored by the radially rigid stent and the dynamic part of the urethra (sphincter) the new stent is designed to adapt itself to the function of the sphincter without interfering with its contraction ability, and soft enough to prevent induction of development of reactive tissue proliferation. Use of a stent having an end segment of low resistance eliminates the sharp pressure gradient that otherwise exists on the lumen wall around the sphincteric end of the stent, reducing the possibility of friction and the resulting reactive tissue growth. The presence of the low resistance covered sphincteric segment of low resistance near the sphincter also provides some support to the pre-sphincteric lumen wall without interfering with its functioning.

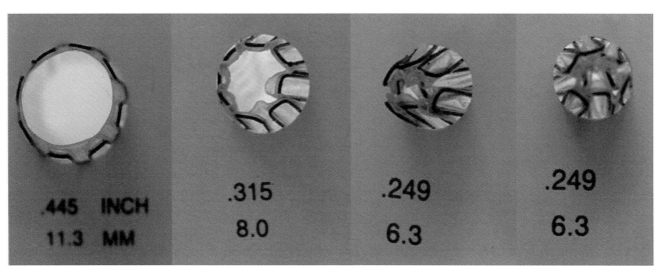

Figure 73.10. *A demonstration of lumen conformability of the dynamic sphincteric segment.*

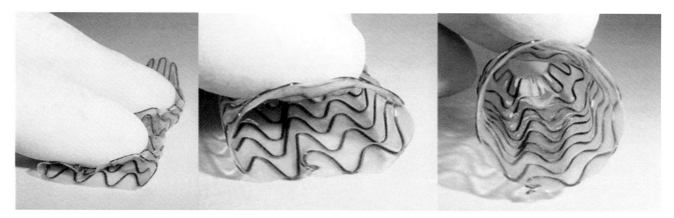

Figure 73.11. *Crush-proof new stent. Even after being compressed for long periods, the stent returns to its original shape with reduction of compression.*

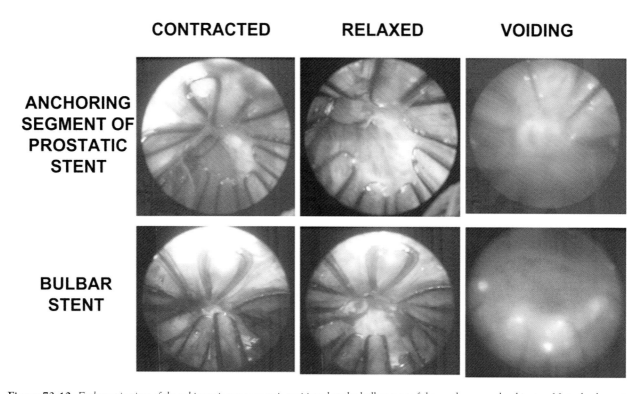

Figure 73.12. *Endoscopic view of the sphincteric segment as is positioned at the bulbar part of the urethra near the shincter. Note the dynamic changes in the shape of the stent during contraction and relaxation of the sphincter, as well as during voiding.*

Shape-regaining ability

In the currently available self-expanding temporary stents, once expanded they cannot go back to a smaller caliber. The new stent, after its deployment, continues to expand with gentle radial pressure until it reaches its maximal expansion. Even after this stage, the stent can be compressed to a reduced caliber (i.e. when sitting on a hard surface with a stent in the bulbar urethra, or during the edematous phase after thermotherapy or brachytherapy). The stent will return to its original shape and caliber when the compressing force no longer exists (Fig. 73.11). Under laboratory conditions, the new stent was found to have the ability of fitting itself dynamically to diameter changes in the urethra.

Initial clinical experience

The new stent designs were used satisfactorily in a small group of patients (4 BPH and 4 recurrent bulbar urethral stricture). This study proved the dynamic ability of the sphincteric segment of the stents. Figure 73.12 shows the dynamic adaptability of the new stents to the dynamics of the external sphincter, during its contraction and relaxation.

It is hoped that the new stent designs will answer, if not all most of the deficiencies of the current stents, but their efficacy will have to be proven.

References

1. Ng K J, Gardener J E, Rickards G et al. 3-Dimensional imaging of the prostatic urethra – an exciting new tool. Br J Urol 1994; 74: 604–608

2. Nordling J, Conort P, Milroy E, Williams G, Yachia D. B. Stents. The 2nd International Consultation on Benign Prostatic Hyperplasia (BPH) 1993. Jersey, Channel Islands: Scientific Communication International Ltd, 1993: 468–481

3. Yachia D, Nordling J, Milroy E, Williams G. II Stents. The 3rd International Consultation on Benign Prostatic Hyperplasia (BPH) 1995. Jersey, Channel Islands: Scientific Communication International Ltd, 1996: 577–583

4. Fitzpatrick J M, Mebust W K. Minimally invasive and endoscopic management of benign prostatic hyperplasia. In: Campbell's urology, 8th edn. Philadelpha: W B Saunders, 2002: 1379–1422

Index

Note: Page numbers in **bold** text refer to figures in the text; those in *italics* to tables or boxes